U0294706

The Chinese Medicine Study Guide Series

Fundamentals

Diagnostics

Acupuncture and Moxibustion

Materia Medica

Formulae

Chinese Medicine Study Guide

Materia Medica

Project Editors: **Li Rui, Zhou Ling & Liu Shui**

Copy Editor: **Liu Yang**

Book Designer:**Yin Yan**

Cover Designer: **Yin Yan**

Typesetter: **Wei Hong-bo**

Chinese Medicine Study Guide

Materia Medica

Zhong Gan-sheng
Prof. of Chinese Pharmacology

Translated by

Liu En-zhao, M.S. TCM & Zhou Ling, M.S. TCM

Edited by

Katrina Beth Nott Blalack, M.S.O.M., Dipl. O.M., L.Ac.
Andrea Kurtz, L.Ac., Dipl.O.M.
Lara Deasy, B.Sc. TCM

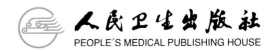

人民卫生出版社
PEOPLE'S MEDICAL PUBLISHING HOUSE

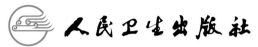

PMPH   PEOPLE'S MEDICAL PUBLISHING HOUSE

Website: http://www.pmph.com

Book Title: Chinese Medicine Study Guide: Materia Medica
中药学图表解

Copyright © 2007 by People's Medical Publishing House. All rights reserved. No part of this publication may be reproduced, stored in a database or retrieval system, or transmitted in any form or by any electronic, mechanical, photocopy, or other recording means, without the prior written permission of the publisher.

Contact address: Bldg 3, 3 Qu, Fang Qun Yuan, Fang Zhuang, Beijing 100078, P. R. China, phone/fax: 86 10 6761 7315, E-mail: pmph@pmph.com

Disclaimer

This book is for educational and reference purposes only. In view of the possibility of human error or changes in medical science, neither the author, editor nor the publisher nor any other party who has been involved in the preparation or publication of this work guarantees that the information contained herein is in every respect accurate or complete. The medicinal therapy and treatment techniques presented in this book are provided for the purpose of reference only. If readers wish to attempt any of the techniques or utilize any of the medicinal therapies contained in this book, the publisher assumes no responsibility for any such actions.

It is the responsibility of the readers to understand and adhere to local laws and regulations concerning the practice of these techniques and methods. The authors, editors and publishers disclaim all responsibility for any liability, loss, injury, or damage incurred as a consequence, directly or indirectly, of the use and application of any of the contents of this book.

First published: 2009
ISBN: 978-7-117-10640-5/R · 10641

Cataloguing in Publication Data:
A catalog record for this book is available from the CIP-Database China.

Printed in The People's Republic of China

ISBN 978-7-117-10640-5

9 787117 106405 >

About the Author

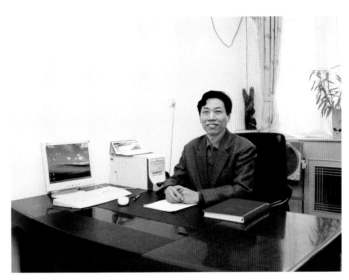

钟赣生　教授

Prof. **Zhong Gan-sheng**, is the dean of the Department of Chinese Pharmacology, in the School of Preclinical Medicine, Beijing University of Chinese Medicine, he is the director of the "Project of Quality Curriculum—Chinese Pharmacology" managed by the Ministry of Education, a tutor of doctoral students, the vice chairman and secretary-general of the China Association of Chinese Medicine Branch of Basic Chinese Pharmacology, a member of the Evaluation Committee of SFDA and the CMA expert for the database for malpractice.

Studying under Prof. Yan Zhenghua, a famous expert on Chinese medicine, Professor Zhong graduated from the Beijing College of Chinese Medicine (now Beijing University of Chinese Medicine) with a master's degree in Chinese Pharmacology in July 1987. After graduation, Prof. Zhong worked at the University (Department of Chinese Pharmacology), teaching and engaged in scientific research on Chinese Pharmacology till now. He was the Deputy Editor-in-Chief of such teaching materials as standardized *"Chinese Pharmacology"* by the "New Century Project" for students at Chinese medicine colleges all over the country; *"Clinical Chinese Pharmacology"* by the "New Century Project" for students on the 7-year academic system (long term academic structure) at colleges of Chinese medicine, and *"Chinese Pharmacology"* by the state's 11th five-year plan and the state's Chinese medicine colleges' foreign education plan.

Prof. Zhong has, as the first author or independently, published 62 articles, edited 19 academic books and teaching materials; he has been in charge of ten, and has participated in nine research projects. The main research work focuses on alcoholic poisoning, the nature of incompatibility of nineteen medicinal herbs, comparisons between Chinese and foreign pharmacy histories, and, research and development of the teaching materials for Chinese Pharmacology. One piece of course material in particular, developed by Prof. Zhong, has received many awards. "The Shennong Chinese Medicine Teaching Assistant System" by Prof. Zhong won "The First Prize of Excellent Teaching Material of the State Administration of Traditional Chinese Medicine" from 1990 to 1994.

Preface

Chinese materia medica is a subject specializing in the study of the basic theories of Chinese medicinals and their origin, production area, methods of collection and processing, the property, flavor, function and the practical principles, which are significant components in Chinese medicine. It is also set as a requisite course in universities and colleges of Chinese medicine (CM) in China. Chinese materia medica is one of the test subjects in the graduation examination, postgraduate entrance examination for Chinese medicine and the Chinese pharmacy major, the certified physician and pharmacist examination, and the overseas graduation examination of Chinese medicine in China. However, due to its wide coverage and dull memory process, it is considered to be one of the most difficult subjects in universities and colleges of Chinese medicine. Therefore, in this book, various figures and tables are presented to show the relations among different medicinals, so as to attract students' interest and strengthen their understanding and recall.

During the compiling process, we consulted the fifth and sixth edition of _Chinese Materia Medica_ by Professor Gao Xue-min. According to the requirements of the course syllabus of Chinese Materia Medica, different charts and tables were designed to explain important and difficult points in each chapter. The book serves as a reference for students learning Chinese materia medica, for teachers, and for those preparing for examinations of Chinese medicine. Meanwhile, it is also helpful for researchers in clinical practice and basic research work.

In this book, each medicinal is marked with "★★★", "★★" or "★" in figures and tables separately, which indicates the different learning requirements in course syllabi. Medicinals marked with "★★★" are for mastering; medicinals marked with "★★" are for getting familiar with; medicinals marked with "★" are just for getting to know. Medicinals with no mark are just for reference.

The book is a summary of my years' experience in teaching and research of Chinese materia medica, and is an attempt to explain the main contents of Chinese pharmacy in the forms of figures and tables. To continually increase the quality of this manual, I sincerely welcome and greatly appreciate the opinions and corrections from readers and experts of the field.

Zhong Gan-sheng
Beijing University of Chinese Medicine
January, 2004

Table of Contents

001   **Introduction**

Part 1   General Discussion

005   **Chapter 1   The Origins and Development of the Chinese Materia Medica**

011   **Chapter 2   Producing Areas and Collection of Chinese Medicinals**

011   Section 1   Producing Area

013   Section 2   Collection

014   **Chapter 3   Processing and Preparation**

014   Section 1   Purposes of Processing and Preparation

014   Section 2   Methods of Processing and Preparation

017   **Chapter 4   Characters and Functions of Chinese Medicinals**

018   Section 1   Property

019   Section 2   Flavor

024   Section 3   Ascending, Descending, Floating and Sinking

026   Section 4   Channel Entering

029   Section 5   Toxicity

032   **Chapter 5   Compatibility**

035   **Chapter 6   Contraindications**

041   **Chapter 7   Dosage and Administration**

041   Section 1   Dosage

043   Section 2   Administration

Part 2   Systematic Discussions

051   **Chapter 8   Medicinals that Release the Exterior**

052   Section 1   Medicinals that Disperse Wind Cold

052   Má huáng (Herba Ephedrae)

053   Guì zhī (Ramulus Cinnamomi)

054   Zǐ sū yè (Folium Perillae)

054   Zǐ sū gěng (Caulis Perillae)

054   Shēng jiāng (Rhizoma Zingiberis Recens)

054   Shēng jiāng pí (Exodermis Zingiberis Recens)

054   Shēng jiāng zhī (Succus Rhizomatis Zingiberis)

055   Xiāng rú (Herba Moslae)

056	Jīng jiè (Herba Schizonepetae)	060	Cāng ěr zǐ (Fructus Xanthii)
057	Fáng fēng (Radix Saposhnikoviae)	061	Xīn yí (Flos Magnoliae)
058	Qiāng huó (Rhizoma et Radix Notopterygii)	061	Cōng bái (Bulbus Allii Fistulosi)
058	Bái zhǐ (Radix Angelicae Dahuricae)	062	É bù shí cǎo (Herba Centipedae)
059	Xì xīn (Radix et Rhizoma Asari)	062	Hú suī (Herba Coriandri Sativi)
059	Gǎo běn (Rhizoma Ligustici)	062	Chéng liǔ (Cacumen Tamaricis)

063   Section 2   Medicinals that Disperse Wind Heat

063	Bò he (Herba Menthae)	068	Shēng má (Rhizoma Cimicifugae)
064	Niú bàng zǐ (Fructus Arctii)	068	Gé gēn (Radix Puerariae Lobatae)
064	Chán tuì (Periostracum Cicadae)	068	Gé huā (Flos Puerariae Lobatae)
065	Sāng yè (Folium Mori)	069	Dàn dòu chǐ (Semen Sojae Praeparatum)
066	Jú huā (Flos Chrysanthemi)	070	Fú píng (Herba Spirodelae)
067	Màn jīng zǐ (Fructus Viticis)	071	Mù zéi (Herba Equiseti Hiemalis)
067	Chái hú (Radix Bupleuri)		

079   **Chapter 9   Medicinals that Clear Heat**

080   Section 1   Medicinals that Clear Heat and Purge Fire

080	Shí gāo (Gypsum Fibrosum)	085	Yā zhí cǎo (Herba Commelinae)
081	Zhī mǔ (Rhizoma Anemarrhenae)	085	Zhī zǐ (Fructus Gardeniae)
082	Hán shuǐ shí (Glauberitum)	086	Xià kū cǎo (Spica Prunellae)
082	Lú gēn (Rhizoma Phragmitis)	087	Jué míng zǐ (Semen Cassiae)
083	Tiān huā fěn (Radix Trichosanthis)	087	Gǔ jīng cǎo (Flos Eriocauli)
084	Zhú yè (Folium Phyllostachydis Henonis)	088	Mì méng huā (Flos Buddlejae)
084	Dàn zhú yè (Herba Lophatheri)	088	Qīng xiāng zǐ (Semen Celosiae)

089   Section 2   Medicinals that Clear Heat and Dry Damp

090	Huáng qín (Radix Scutellariae)	095	Kǔ shēn (Radix Sophorae Flavescentis)
091	Huáng lián (Rhizoma Coptidis)	095	Bái xiān pí (Cortex Dictamni)
092	Huáng bǎi (Cortex Phellodendri Chinensis)	096	Kǔ dòu zǐ (Sophora Alopecuroides)
093	Lóng dǎn cǎo (Radix et Rhizoma Gentianae)	096	Sān kē zhēn (Radix Berberidis)
094	Qín pí (Cortex Fraxini)	097	Mǎ wěi lián (Radix et Rhizoma Thalictri Baicalensis)

097   Section 3   Medicinals that Clear Heat and Detoxify

097	Jīn yín huā (Flos Lonicerae Japonicae)	103	Zǐ huā dì dīng (Herba Violae)
097	Rěn dōng téng (Caulis Lonicerae Japonicae)	103	Yě jú huā (Flos Chrysanthemi Indici)
098	Lián qiào (Fructus Forsythiae)	104	Chóng lóu (Rhizoma Paridis)
099	Chuān xīn lián (Herba Andrographis)	104	Quán shēn (Rhizoma Bistortae)
100	Dà qīng yè (Folium Isatidis)	105	Lòu lú (Radix Rhapontici)
100	Bǎn lán gēn (Radix Isatidis)	106	Tǔ fú líng (Rhizoma Smilacis Glabrae)
101	Qīng dài (Indigo Naturalis)	106	Yú xīng cǎo (Herba Houttuyniae)
102	Guàn zhòng (Rhizoma Cyrtomii)	107	Jīn qiáo mài (Rhizoma Fagopyri Dibotryis)
102	Pú gōng yīng (Herba Taraxaci)	107	Dà xuè téng (Caulis Sargentodoxae)

107   Bài jiàng cǎo (Herba Patriniae)

108   Shè gān (Rhizoma Belamcandae)

109   Shān dòu gēn (Radix et Rhizoma Sophorae
Tonkinensis)

109   Běi dòu gēn (Rhizoma Menispermi)

109   Mǎ bó (Lasiosphaera seu Calvatia)

110   Qīng guǒ (Fructus Canarii)

110   Jǐn dēng lóng (Calyx seu Fructus Physalis)

111   Jīn guǒ lǎn (Radix Tinosporae)

111   Mù hú dié (Semen Oroxyli)

112   Bái tóu wēng (Radix Pulsatillae)

112   Mǎ chǐ xiàn (Herba Portulacae)

119   Section 4   Medicinals that Clear Heat and Cool Blood

119   Shēng dì huáng (Radix Rehmanniae)

120   Xuán shēn (Radix Scrophulariae)

121   Mǔ dān pí (Cortex Moutan)

124   Section 5   Medicinals that Clear Deficient Heat

124   Qīng hāo (Herba Artemisiae Annuae)

125   Bái wēi (Radix et Rhizoma Cynanchi Atrati)

125   Dì gǔ pí (Cortex Lycii)

113   Yā dǎn zǐ (Fructus Bruceae)

114   Dì jǐn cǎo (Herba Euphorbiae Humifusae)

114   Wěi líng cài (Herba Potentillae Chinensis)

115   Fān bái cǎo (Herba Potentillae Discoloris)

115   Bàn biān lián (Herba Lobeliae Chinensis)

115   Bái huā shé shé cǎo (Herba Hedyotis Diffusae)

116   Shān cí gū (Pseudobulbus Cremastrae seu Pleiones)

117   Xióng dǎn (Ursi Fel)

117   Qiān lǐ guāng (Herba Senecionis Scandentis)

118   Bái liǎn (Radix Ampelopsis)

118   Sì jì qīng (Folium Illics Purpureae)

119   Lǜ dòu (Semen Phaseoli Radiati)

122   Chì sháo (Radix Paeoniae Rubra)

123   Zǐ cǎo (Radix Arnebiae)

123   Shuǐ niú jiǎo (Cornu Bubali)

126   Yín chái hú (Radix Stellariae)

127   Hú huáng lián (Rhizoma Picrorhizae)

143   **Chapter 10   Medicinals that Drain Downwards**

144   Section 1   Medicinals that Promote Defecation by Purgation

144   Dà huáng (Radix et Rhizoma Rhei)

145   Máng xiāo (Natrii Sulfas)

146   Fān xiè yè (Folium Sennae)

146   Lú huì (Aloe)

147   Section 2   Medicinals that Promote Defecation by Moistening Intestines

147   Huǒ má rén (Fructus Cannabis)

147   Yù lǐ rén (Semen Pruni)

148   Sōng zǐ rén (Semen Pini Koraiensis)

149   Section 3   Medicinals that Drastically Promote Defecation and Purge Fluids

149   Gān suì (Radix Kansui)

149   Jīng dà jǐ (Radix Euphorbiae Pekinensis)

149   Hóng dà jǐ (Radix Knoxiae)

150   Yuán huā (Flos Genkwa)

151   Shāng lù (Radix Phytolaccae)

151   Qiān niú zǐ (Semen Pharbitidis)

152   Bā dòu (Semen Crotonis)

152   Qiān jīn zǐ (Semen Euphorbiae)

157   **Chapter 11   Medicinals that Expel Wind and Damp**

158   Section 1   Medicinals that Expel Wind, Cold and Damp

158   Dú huó (Radix Angelicae Pubescentis)

159   Wēi líng xiān (Radix et Rhizoma Clematidis)

159   Xú cháng qīng (Radix et Rhizoma Cynanchi
Paniculati)

160   Chuān wū (Radix Aconiti)

160   Cǎo wū (Radix Aconiti Kusnezoffii)

161   Qí shé (Agkistrodon)

161   Wū shāo shé (Zaocys)

162   Mù guā (Fructus Chaenomelis)

162   Cán shā (Faeces Bombycis)

163   Shēn jīn cǎo (Herba Lycopodii)

163   Xún gǔ fēng (Herba Aristolochiae Mollissimae)

163   Sōng jié (Lignum Pini Nodi)

164   Hǎi fēng téng (Caulis Piperis Kadsurae)

164   Qīng fēng téng (Caulis Sinomenii)

165   Dīng gōng téng (Caulis Erycibes)

165   Kūn míng shān hǎi táng (Radix Tripterygium Hypoglaucum)

166   Xuě shàng yī zhī hāo (Radix Aconiti Brachypodi)

166   Lù lù tōng (Fructus Liquidambaris)

167   Section 2   Medicinals that Expel Wind, Heat and Damp

167   Qín jiāo (Radix Gentianae Macrophyllae)

167   Fáng jǐ (Radix Stephaniae Tetrandrae)

168   Sāng zhī (Ramulus Mori)

169   Xī xiān cǎo (Herba Siegesbeckiae)

169   Chòu wú tóng (Folium Clerodendri Trichotomi)

170   Hǎi tóng pí (Cortex Erythrinae)

170   Luò shí téng (Caulis Trachelospermi)

171   Léi gōng téng (Radix Tripterygii Wilfordii)

171   Lǎo guàn cǎo (Herba Erodii)

172   Chuān shān lóng (Rhizoma Dioscoreae Nipponicae)

172   Sī guā luò (Fructus Retinervus Luffae)

172   Section 3   Medicinals that Expel Wind, Cold and Damp, and Strengthen Bones and Muscles

173   Wǔ jiā pí (Cortex Acanthopanacis)

173   Sāng jì shēng (Herba Taxilli)

173   Gǒu jǐ (Rhizoma Cibotii)

174   Qiān nián jiàn (Rhizoma Homalomenae)

175   Xuě lián huā (Herba Saussureae Lanicepsis)

175   Lù xián cǎo (Herba Pyrolae)

176   Shí nán yè (Folium Photiniae)

182   **Chapter 12   Aromatic Medicinals that Transform Damp**

183   Huò xiāng (Herba Agastachis)

183   Pèi lán (Herba Eupatorii)

184   Cāng zhú (Rhizoma Atractylodis)

184   Hòu pò (Cortex Magnoliae Officinalis)

186   Shā rén (Fructus Amomi)

186   Bái dòu kòu (Fructus Amomi Kravanh)

187   Cǎo dòu kòu (Semen Alpiniae Katsumadai)

187   Cǎo guǒ (Fructus Tsaoko)

190   **Chapter 13   Medicinals that Promote Water Flow and Drain Damp**

191   Section 1   Medicinals that Promote Water Flow to Reduce Edema

191   Fú líng (Poria)

191   Fú líng pí (Cutis Poriae)

192   Fú shén (Sclerotium Poriae Paradicis)

192   Yì yǐ rén (Semen Coicis)

192   Zhū líng (Polyporus)

193   Zé xiè (Rhizoma Alismatis)

194   Dōng guā pí (Exocarpium Benincasae)

194   Dōng guā zǐ (Semen Benincasae)

194   Yù mǐ xū (Stigma Maydis)

195   Hú lu (Fructus Lagenariae)

195   Xiāng jiā pí (Cortex Periplocae)

195   Zhǐ jù zǐ (Semen Hoveniae)

196   Zé qī (Herba Euphoribiae Helioscopiae)

197   Lóu gū (Gryllotalpa)

197   Jì cài (Herba Capsellae)

197   Section 2   Medicinals that Induce Diuresis to Relieve Stranguria

198   Chē qián zǐ (Semen Plantaginis)

198   Huá shí (Talcum)

199   Guān mù tōng (Caulis Aristolochiae Manshuriensis)

199   Chuān mù tōng (Caulis Clematidis Armandii)

199   Tōng cǎo (Medulla Tetrapanacis)

200   Qú mài (Herba Dianthi)

200   Biǎn xù (Herba Polygoni Avicularis)

201   Dì fū zǐ (Fructus Kochiae)

201   Hǎi jīn shā (Spora Lygodii)

201   Shí wéi (Folium Pyrrosiae)

202   Dōng kuí zǐ (Fructus Malvae)

203   Dēng xīn cǎo (Medulla Junci)

203 Bì xiè (Rhizoma Dioscoreae Hypoglaucae)

203 Section 3 Medicinals that Drain Damp to Relieve Jaundice

204 Yīn chén (Herba Artemisiae Scopariae)

205 Chuí pén cǎo (Herba Sedi)

204 Jīn qián cǎo (Herba Lysimachiae)

206 Jī gǔ cǎo (Herba Abri)

204 Hǔ zhàng (Rhizoma Polygoni Cuspidati)

207 Zhēn zhū cǎo (Herba Phyllanthi Urinariae)

205 Dì ěr cǎo (Herba Hyperici Japonici)

213 **Chapter 14　Medicinals that Warm the Interior**

214 Fù zǐ (Radix Aconiti Lateralis Praeparata)

220 Gāo liáng jiāng (Rhizoma Alpiniae Officinarum)

215 Gān jiāng (Rhizoma Zingiberis)

221 Hú jiāo (Fructus Piperis)

216 Ròu guì (Cortex Cinnamomi)

221 Huā jiāo (Pericarpium Zanthoxyli)

218 Wú zhū yú (Fructus Evodiae)

222 Bì bá (Fructus Piperis Longi)

218 Xiǎo huí xiāng (Fructus Foeniculi)

222 Bì chéng qié (Fructus Litseae)

219 Dīng xiāng (Flos Caryophylli)

226 **Chapter 15　Medicinals that Regulate Qi**

227 Chén pí (Pericarpium Citri Reticulatae)

233 Lì zhī hé (Semen Litchi)

227 Jú hé (Semen Citri Reticulatae)

234 Xiāng fù (Rhizoma Cyperi)

227 Jú luò (Vascular Aurantii)

235 Fó shǒu (Fructus Citri Sarcodactylis)

227 Jú yè (Folium Citri Reticulatae)

235 Xiāng yuán (Fructus Citri)

227 Huà jú hóng (Exocarpium Citri Grandis)

236 Méi gui huā (Flos Rosae Rugosae)

227 Qīng pí (Pericarpium Citri Reticulatae Viride)

236 Lǜ è méi (Flos Mume)

229 Zhǐ shí (Fructus Aurantii Immaturus)

237 Suō luó zǐ (Semen Aesculi)

229 Zhǐ qiào (Fructus Aurantii)

237 Xiè bái (Bulbus Allii Macrostemi)

230 Mù xiāng (Radix Aucklandiae)

238 Tiān xiān téng (Herba Aristolochiae)

231 Chén xiāng (Lignum Aquilariae Resinatum)

238 Dà fù pí (Pericarpium Arecae)

231 Tán xiāng (Lignum Santali Albi)

239 Gān sōng (Radix et Rhizoma Nardostachyos)

232 Chuān liàn zǐ (Fructus Toosendan)

239 Jiǔ xiāng chóng (Aspongopus)

232 Wū yào (Radix Linderae)

239 Dāo dòu (Semen Canavaliae)

233 Qīng mù xiāng (Radix Aristolochiae)

240 Shì dì (Calyx Kaki)

245 **Chapter 16　Medicinals that Eliminate Food Retention**

246 Shān zhā (Fructus Crataegi)

248 Lái fú zǐ (Semen Raphani)

246 Shén qū (Massa Medicata Fermentata)

248 Jī nèi jīn (Endothelium Corneum Gigeriae Galli)

247 Mài yá (Fructus Hordei Germinatus)

250 Jī shǐ téng (Herba Paederiae)

247 Gǔ yá (Fructus Setariae Germinatus)

250 Gé shān xiāo (Radix Cynanchi Wilfordii)

247 Dào yá (Fructus Oryzae Germinatus)

251 Ā wèi (Resina Ferulae)

254 **Chapter 17　Medicinals that Expel Worms**

255 Shǐ jūn zǐ (Fructus Quisqualis)

257 Hè cǎo yá (Herba et Gemma Agrimoniae)

255 Kǔ liàn pí (Cortex Meliae)

257 Léi wán (Omphalia)

256 Bīng láng (Semen Arecae)

258 Hè shī (Fructus Carpesii)

256 Nán guā zǐ (Semen Cucurbitae)

259 Fěi zǐ (Semen Torreyae)

259   Wú yí (Fructus Ulmi Macrocarpae Praeparata)

262   **Chapter 18   Medicinals that Stop Bleeding**

263   Section 1   Medicinals that Cool Blood and Stop Bleeding

263   Xiǎo jì (Herba Cirsii)   266   Cè bǎi yè (Cacumen Platycladi)

263   Dà jì (Herba seu Radix Cirsii Japonici)   266   Bái máo gēn (Rhizoma Imperatae)

264   Dì yú (Radix Sanguisorbae)   267   Zhù má gēn (Radix Boehmeriae)

265   Huái huā (Flos Sophorae)   267   Yáng tí (Radix Rumicis Japonici)

265   Huái jiǎo (Fructus Sophorae)

268   Section 2   Medicinals that Transform Stasis to Stop Bleeding

268   Sān qī (Radix et Rhizoma Notoginseng)   270   Huā ruǐ shí (Ophicalcitum)

269   Qiàn cǎo (Radix et Rhizoma Rubiae)   270   Jiàng xiāng (Lignum Dalbergiae Odoriferae)

270   Pú huáng (Pollen Typhae)

271   Section 3   Medicinals that Astringe to Stop Bleeding

272   Bái jí (Rhizoma Bletillae)   274   Xuè yú tàn (Crinis Carbonisatus)

272   Xiān hè cǎo (Herba Agrimoniae)   274   Ǒu jié (Nodus Nelumbinis Rhizomatis)

273   Zǐ zhū (Folium Callicarpae Formosanae)   275   Jì mù (Flos Loropetali Chinensis)

273   Zōng lǘ tàn (Petiolus Trachycarpi)

275   Section 4   Medicinals that Warm Channels to Stop Bleeding

275   Ài yè (Folium Artemisiae Argyi)   277   Zào xīn tǔ (Terra Flava Usta)

276   Páo jiāng (Rhizoma Zingiberis Praeparatum)

283   **Chapter 19   Medicinals that Invigorate Blood and Transform Stasis**

284   Section 1   Medicinals that Invigorate Blood to Relieve Pain

284   Chuān xiōng (Rhizoma Chuanxiong)   287   Mò yào (Myrrha)

285   Yán hú suǒ (Rhizoma Corydalis)   287   Wǔ líng zhī (Faeces Trogopterori)

285   Yù jīn (Radix Curcumae)   288   Xià tiān wú (Rhizoma Corydalis Decumbentis)

285   Jiāng huáng (Rhizoma Curcumae Longae)   288   Fēng xiāng zhī (Resina Liquidambaris)

286   Rǔ xiāng (Olibanum)

289   Section 2   Medicinals that Invigorate Blood to Regulate Menstruation

289   Dān shēn (Radix et Rhizoma Salviae Miltiorrhizae)   293   Niú xī (Radix Achyranthis Bidentatae)

290   Hóng huā (Flos Carthami)   294   Jī xuè téng (Caulis Spatholobi)

291   Táo rén (Semen Persicae)   294   Wáng bù liú xíng (Semen Vaccariae)

292   Yì mǔ cǎo (Herba Leonuri)   295   Yuè jì huā (Flos Rosae Chinensis)

292   Zé lán (Herba Lycopi)   295   Líng xiāo huā (Flos Campsis)

296   Section 3   Medicinals that Invigorate Blood to Treat Trauma

296   Tǔ biē chóng (Eupolyphaga seu Steleophaga)   297   Gǔ suì bǔ (Rhizoma Drynariae)

296   Mǎ qián zǐ (Semen Strychni)   298   Xuè jié (Sanguis Draconis)

297   Zì rán tóng (Pyritum)   299   Ér chá (Catechu)

297   Sū mù (Lignum Sappan)   299   Liú jì nú (Herba Artemisiae Anomalae)

300   Section 4   Medicinals that Invigorate Blood to Remove Blood Stasis

300   É zhú (Rhizoma Curcumae)   301   Sān léng (Rhizoma Sparganii)

301   Shuǐ zhì (Hirudo)

301   Méng chóng (Tabanus)

302   Bān máo (Mylabris)

303   Chuān shān jiǎ (Squama Manitis)

311   **Chapter 20   Medicinals that Stop Cough, Calm Panting and Transform Phlegm**

312   Section 1   Medicinals that Warm and Transform Cold Phlegm

312   Bàn xià (Rhizoma Pinelliae)

313   Tiān nán xīng (Rhizoma Arisaematis)

313   Dǎn nán xīng (Arisaema cum Bile)

314   Yǔ bái fù (Rhizoma Typhonii)

314   Guān bái fù (Radix Aconiti Coreani)

315   Bái jiè zǐ (Semen Sinapis)

316   Zào jiá (Fructus Gleditsiae)

316   Xuán fù huā (Flos Inulae)

317   Bái qián (Rhizoma et Radix Cynanchi Stauntonii)

317   Māo zhuǎ cǎo (Radix Ranunculi Ternati)

318   Section 2   Medicinals that Clear Heat and Transform Phlegm

318   Chuān bèi mǔ (Bulbus Fritillariae Cirrhosae)

318   Zhè bèi mǔ (Bulbus Fritillariae Thunbergii)

319   Guā lóu (Fructus Trichosanthis)

320   Zhú rú (Caulis Bambusae in Taenia)

320   Zhú lì (Succus Bambusae)

321   Tiān zhú huáng (Concretio Silicea Bambusae)

321   Qián hú (Radix Peucedani)

322   Jié gěng (Radix Platycodonis)

323   Pàng dà hǎi (Semen Sterculiae Lychnophorae)

323   Hǎi zǎo (Sargassum)

324   Kūn bù (Thallus Laminariae)

324   Huáng yào zǐ (Rhizoma Dioscoreae Bulbiferae)

325   Hǎi gé qiào (Concha Meretricis seu Cyclinae)

325   Hǎi fú shí (Pumex)

325   Wǎ léng zǐ (Concha Arcae)

326   Méng shí (Chlorite-schist)

327   Section 3   Medicinals that Stop Cough and Calm Panting

327   Kǔ xìng rén (Semen Armeniacae Amarum)

327   Tián xìng rén (Semen Armeniacae Dulce)

328   Zǐ sū zǐ (Fructus Perillae)

329   Bǎi bù (Radix Stemonae)

329   Zǐ wǎn (Radix et Rhizoma Asteris)

329   Kuǎn dōng huā (Flos Farfarae)

330   Mǎ dōu líng (Fructus Aristolochiae)

330   Pí pá yè (Folium Eriobotryae)

331   Sāng bái pí (Cortex Mori)

331   Tíng lì zǐ (Semen Lepidii)

332   Bái guǒ (Semen Ginkgo)

332   Yín xìng yè (Folium Ginkgo)

333   Ǎi dì chá (Herba Ardisiae Japonicae)

333   Yáng jīn huā (Flos Daturae)

334   Huà shān shēn (Radix Physochlainae)

334   Luó hàn guǒ (Fructus Momordicae)

335   Mǎn shān hóng (Folium Rhododendri Daurici)

335   Hú tuí zǐ yè (Folium Elaegni Pungentis)

343   **Chapter 21   Medicinals that Calm the Mind**

344   Section 1   Heavy Medicinals that Calm the Mind

344   Zhū shā (Cinnabaris)

345   Cí shí (Magnetitum)

345   Lóng gǔ (Os Draconis)

346   Lóng chǐ (Dens Draconis)

346   Hǔ pò (Succinum)

347   Section 2   Medicinals that Nourish the Heart to Calm the Mind

347   Suān zǎo rén (Semen Ziziphi Spinosae)

348   Bǎi zǐ rén (Semen Platycladi)

348   Líng zhī (Ganoderma)

349   Xié cǎo (Rhizoma et Radix Valerianae Pseudoofficinalis)

349   Shǒu wū téng (Caulis Polygoni Multiflori)

350   Hé huān pí (Cortex Albiziae)

350   Yuǎn zhì (Radix Polygalae)

354   **Chapter 22   Medicinals that Calm the Liver and Extinguish Wind**

355   Section 1   Medicinals that Suppress the Liver Yang

355   Shí jué míng (Concha Haliotidis)

356   Zhēn zhū mǔ (Concha Margaritiferae Usta)

356   Mǔ lì (Concha Ostreae)

357   Zǐ bèi chǐ (Concha Cypraeae Violacae)

358   Dài zhě shí (Haematitum)

359   Cì jí lí (Fructus Tribuli)

360   Luó bù má (Folium Apocyni Veneti)

360   Shēng tiě luò (Frusta Ferri)

361   Section 2   Medicinals that Extinguish Wind to Relieve Convulsions

361   Líng yáng jiǎo (Cornu Saigae Tataricae)

362   Niú huáng (Calculus Bovis)

363   Zhēn zhū (Margarita)

363   Gōu téng (Ramulus Uncariae Cum Uncis)

364   Tiān má (Rhizoma Gastrodiae)

365   Dì lóng (Pheretima)

365   Quán xiē (Scorpio)

366   Wú gōng (Scolopendra)

366   Jiāng cán (Bombyx Batryticatus)

371   **Chapter 23   Medicinals that Open the Orifices**

372   Shè xiāng (Moschus)

373   Bīng piàn (Borneolum Syntheticum)

373   Sū hé xiāng (Styrax)

373   Shí chāng pú (Rhizoma Acori Tatarinowii)

377   **Chapter 24   Medicinals that Tonify Deficiency**

378   Section 1   Medicinals that Replenish Qi

379   Rén shēn (Radix et Rhizoma Ginseng)

380   Xī yáng shēn (Radix Panacis Quinquefolii)

381   Dǎng shēn (Radix Codonopsis)

381   Tài zǐ shēn (Radix Pseudostellariae)

383   Huáng qí (Radix Astragali)

384   Bái zhú (Rhizoma Atractylodis Macrocephalae)

385   Shān yào (Radix Discoreae)

386   Bái biǎn dòu (Semen Lablab Album)

387   Gān cǎo (Radix et Rhizoma Glycyrrhizae)

387   Dà zǎo (Fructus Jujubae)

388   Cì wǔ jiā (Radix et Rhizoma seu Caulis Acantho-panacis Senticosi)

388   Jiǎo gǔ lán (Rhizoma seu Herba Gynostemmatis Pentaphylli)

388   Hóng jǐng tiān (Radix et Rhizoma Rhodiolae Crenulatae)

389   Shā jí (Fructus Hippophae)

389   Yí táng (Saccharum Granorum)

390   Fēng mì (Mel)

391   Section 2   Medicinals that Supplement Yang

391   Lù róng (Cornu Cervi Pantotrichum)

391   Lù jiǎo (Cornu Cervi)

391   Lù jiǎo jiāo (Colla Cornus Cervi)

391   Lù jiǎo shuāng (Cornu Cervi Degelatinatum)

392   Zǐ hé chē (Placenta Hominis)

393   Yín yáng huò (Herba Epimedii)

393   Bā jǐ tiān (Radix Morindae Officinalis)

394   Xiān máo (Rhizoma Curculiginis)

395   Dù zhòng (Cortex Eucommiae)

395   Xù duàn (Radix Dipsaci)

396   Ròu cōng róng (Herba Cistanches)

396   Suǒ yáng (Herba Cynomorii)

397   Bǔ gǔ zhī (Fructus Psoraleae)

397   Yì zhì rén (Fructus Alpiniae Oxyphyllae)

398   Tù sī zǐ (Semen Cuscutae)

398   Shā yuàn zǐ (Semen Astragali Complanati)

399   Gé jiè (Gecko)

400   Hé táo rén (Semen Juglandis)

400   Dōng chóng xià cǎo (Cordyceps)

401   Hú lú bā (Semen Trigonellae Callorhimi)

401   Jiǔ cài zǐ (Semen Allii Tuberosi)

402   Yáng qǐ shí (Actinolitum)

402   Zǐ shí yīng (Fluoritum)

402   Hǎi gǒu shèn (Testis et Penis Callorhini)

403   Hǎi mǎ (Hippocampus)

403   Há ma yóu (Oviductus Ranae)

404   Section 3   Medicinals that Enrich Blood

404   Dāng guī (Radix Angelicae Sinensis)

405   Shú dì huáng (Radix Rehmanniae Praeparata)

406   Bái sháo (Radix Paeoniae Alba)

408   Ē jiāo (Colla Corii Asini)

411   Section 4   Medicinals that Nourish Yin

411   Běi shā shēn (Radix Glehniae)

411   Nán shā shēn (Radix Adenophorae)

412   Bǎi hé (Bulbus Lilii)

413   Mài dōng (Radix Ophiopogonis)

413   Tiān dōng (Radix Asparagi)

414   Shí hú (Caulis Dendrobii)

415   Yù zhú (Rhizoma Polygonati Odorati)

415   Huáng jīng (Rhizoma Polygonati)

404   Yáng hóng shān (Radix Seu Herba Pimpinelae)

409   Hé shǒu wū (Radix Polygoni Multiflori)

410   Lóng yǎn ròu (Arillus Longan)

410   Chǔ shí zǐ (Fructus Broussonetiae)

417   Míng dǎng shēn (Radix Changii)

417   Gǒu qǐ (Fructus Lycii)

418   Mò hàn lián (Herba Ecliptae)

418   Nǔ zhēn zǐ (Fructus Ligustri Lucidi)

419   Sāng shèn (Fructus Mori)

419   Hēi zhī ma (Semen Sesami Nigrum)

420   Guī jiǎ (Carapax et Plastrum Testudinis)

420   Biē jiǎ (Carapax Trionycis)

435   **Chapter 25   Astringent Medicinals**

436   Section 1   Medicinals that Consolidate the Exterior to Arrest Sweats

436   Má huáng gēn (Radix et Rhizoma Ephedrae)

437   Fú xiǎo mài (Fructus Tritici Levis)

437   Nuò dào gēn xū (Radix Oryzae Glutinosae)

438   Section 2   Medicinals that Astringe the Lung and Large Intestine

438   Wǔ wèi zǐ (Fructus Schisandrae Chinensis)

439   Wū méi (Fructus Mume)

440   Wǔ bèi zǐ (Galla Chinensis)

440   Yīng sù qiào (Pericarpium Papaveris)

441   Hē zǐ (Fructus Chebulae)

442   Shí liú pí (Pericarpium Granati)

442   Ròu dòu kòu (Semen Myristicae)

443   Chì shí zhī (Halloysitum Rubrum)

443   Yǔ yú liáng (Limonitum)

444   Section 3   Medicinals that Consolidate the Kidney Essence, Reduce Urination and Arrest Leukorrhea

444   Shān zhū yú (Fructus Corni)

445   Fù pén zǐ (Fructus Rubi)

446   Sāng piāo xiāo (Ootheca Mantidis)

446   Jīn yīng zǐ (Fructus Rosae Laevigatae)

447   Hǎi piāo xiāo (Endoconcha Sepiae)

447   Lián zǐ (Semen Nelumbinis)

447   Lián xū (Stamen Nelumbinis)

447   Lián fáng (Receptaculum Nelumbinis)

447   Lián zǐ xīn (Plumula Nelumbinis)

448   Hé yè (Folium Nelumbinis)

448   Hé gěng (Petiolus Nelmbinis)

448   Qiàn shí (Semen Euryales)

449   Cì wei pí (Corium Erinacei)

449   Chūn pí (Cortex Ailanthi)

450   Jī guān huā (Flos Celosiae Cristatae)

456   **Chapter 26   Emetics**

457   Cháng shān (Radix Dichroae)

457   Guā dì (Pedicellus Melo)

457   Dǎn fán (Chalcanthitum)

460   **Chapter 27   Medicinals that Attack Toxins, Kill Parasites and Stop Itching**

461   Xióng huáng (Realgar)

461   Liú huáng (Sulphur)

462   Bái fán (Alumen)

464   Mù biē zǐ (Semen Momordicae)

462   Shé chuáng zǐ (Fructus Cnidii)

465   Tǔ jīng pí (Cortex Pseudolaricis)

463   Chán sū (Venenum Bufonis)

465   Fēng fáng (Nidus Vespae)

463   Zhāng nǎo (Camphora)

465   Dà suàn (Bulbus Allii)

469   **Chapter 28   Medicinals that Draw out Toxins, Expel Pus and Rejuvenate Flesh**

470   Shēng yào (Hydrargyrum Oxydatum Crudum)

472   Qiān dān (Minium)

470   Qīng fěn (Calomelas)

472   Lú gān shí (Calamina)

471   Pí shí (Arsenicum)

472   Péng shā (Borax)

475   Index by Disease Names and Symptoms
485   Index by Chinese Medicinals — Pin Yin Names
490   Index by Chinese Medicinals — Pharmaceutical Names

Introduction

Chinese Medicinals

"Chinese medicinals" is a general name for the traditional medicines used in China. They are characterized by the following aspects:

1. Most Chinese medicinals originate in China.

2. The recognition and use of Chinese medicinals are based on the theories of Chinese medicine (CM), which have unique theoretical and practical application systems.

3. The use of Chinese medicinals reflects certain characteristics of the history, culture and natural resources in China.

In brief, Chinese medicinals are used in the prevention, treatment and diagnosis of diseases under the guidance of the theories of Chinese medicine. They play an important role in protecting people's health in China. More than 3,000 medicinals are recorded in ancient herbal texts. At present, over 12,800 medicinals have been collected and identified.

Herbal Materia Medica

Chinese medicinals come from natural medicines and their processed products. Sources include plants, animals, minerals and some chemicals and biomedicines. As plant materials (accounting for over 80% of medicinals) are most widely used in Chinese medicine, it is said that medicinal herbs are the foundation of Chinese medicinals. Therefore, Chinese medicinals have been known as "herbs" and have been passed down from ancient times.

Herbal Medicine

Herbal medicine is widely used among the people, but not often used in hospitals of Chinese medicine. Herbal medicine is frequently used by civil physicians and most of them lack processing standards.

Chinese Herbal Medicine

Chinese herbal medicine is a mix of Chinese medicine and herbal medicine. Thus it can be seen that herbal medicine and Chinese medicine are similar in nature. The concepts of herbal medicine, Chinese medicine and Chinese herbal medicine should be integrated and unified as Chinese medicine.

Indigenous Medicine

Indigenous medicine means herbs commonly used in the autonomous (ethnic minority) regions of China. The origins of these herbs are essentially the same as Chinese medicinals. As with the theories and experience of both Chinese medicine and Western medicine, these indigenous medicines have gradually developed characteristic herbal medicines with distinct regional features, such as Tibetan medicine, Mongolian medicine, Uighur medicine, *Dai* medicine, *Miao* medicine and *Yi* medicine. Indigenous medicine and Chinese materia medica are both important components in Chinese medicine.

Chinese Patent Medicines

Chinese patent medicines are produced from raw Chinese medicinals under the guidance of Chinese medical theory. They are made in specified dosages and forms according to standard formulas and preparation technologies. Physicians and patients can choose patent medicines according to the actions, indications, dosage and administration instructions noted on them. Essentially, Chinese patent medicines are prepared forms of herbal prescriptions or single Chinese medicinals. Patent medicines are also an important component of Chinese medicine.

Clinical Chinese Materia Medica (Pharmacology)

Since ancient times, Chinese medicinals have been called herbs, and written records describing the Chinese materia medica have formed the classic texts of the study of Chinese herbal medicine up to modern times. With the development of modern science, the study of Chinese herbal medicine has expanded into a number of branches, including the clinical use, pharmacology, cultivation, the botanical study, chemistry, processing, pharmaceutical preparation, and identification of Chinese medicinals, and Chinese patent medicines.

The clinical study of Chinese medicinals refers to specific research on fundamental theory, origins, and areas of production, collection, processing, properties, effects and rules of the clinical use of Chinese medicinals. The clinical study of Chinese medicinals forms the backbone of study in Chinese medicine colleges and universities, and is an important component in the treasure chest of traditional Chinese medical science.

PART 1

General Discussion

Chapter 1
The Origins and Development of the Chinese Materia Medica

I. THE ORIGINS OF MEDICINE IN PRIMITIVE SOCIETY (FROM ANCIENT TIMES TO THE 21ST CENTURY B.C.)

While searching for food, our ancestors inevitably ate some poisonous plants which caused adverse reactions such as vomiting, diarrhea, coma or even death. They sometimes came across other plants and found that these could alleviate or eliminate the above symptoms. After countless tests, tasting and feeling, they accumulated valuable experience in distinguishing food and medicinals, and gradually acquired an understanding of herbal medicine. This describes the early discovery of herbal medicine. Upon the development of clan society, with the invention and use of bows and arrows, human society began a stage of hunting and fishing, and they therefore came to understand animal medicine as well. With the development of farming and animal husbandry in the later periods of clan society, more medicinals were discovered and early drug therapy was developed. Therefore, the Chinese materia medica has originated over a long course of human history and medical practice.

With the evolution of the economy, culture and medical science, there were increasing demands for medicine. Accordingly, medicinals were collected from wild areas and also cultivated and domesticated. Natural minerals and processed medicine were included as well. Moreover, written records have been developed in order to record knowledge and clinical experience of medicinals.

II. THE *XIA*, *SHANG* AND *ZHOU* DYNASTIES (FROM 21ST CENTURY B.C. TO 221 B.C.)

Wine is the earliest discovered stimulant (when used in a small dose) and anesthetic (when used in a large dose). It was found to activate the blood and improve the efficacy of other drugs and to work as a fine solvent. Therefore, wine is honored as "the first of all medicinals." Wine is also used as an adjuvant for processing other medicinals. After people developed an understanding of medicinals, wine came to gradually be used for making medicinal wines. The invention and use of medicinal wines are helpful to enhance a curative effect, which brings a significant influence in propelling Chinese medicine.

The method of decocting medicinals was invented by Yi Yin of the *Shang* Dynasty, who was reknown for cooking and Chinese medicine, which indicates that the invention of the decoction was closely related to the advance in food processing techniques. The decoction was found to be convenient as well as enhancing the curative effect of medicinals, while reducing their side effects. Meanwhile, it propels the development of compound prescriptions. Therefore, the decoction is one of the most common preparation forms of Chinese medicinals and its use is constantly expanding.

Pharmaceutical science developed early in China. Formal written records on Chinese pharmaceutical sciences date back to the *Western Zhou* Dynasty (1066 B.C. to 771 B.C.). For example, *The Book of History–Elaboration on Fate* (*Shàng Shū–Shuō Mìng Piān*, 尚书·说命篇) says: *"To treat stubborn and chronic diseases, if medicine does not cause dizziness or other reactions, it will not take effect at all"* (药不瞑眩，厥疾弗瘳). The *Rites of the Zhou – Officials under the Lead of Tianguanzhongzai* (*Zhōu Lǐ – Tiān Guān Zhǒng Zǎi Xià*, 周礼·天官冢宰下) says: *"Physicians are in charge of medical services. They collect medicinals to treat diseases"* (医师掌医之政令，聚毒药以供医事).

The Book of Songs (*Shī Jīng*, 诗经) is a literary work from the *Western Zhou* Dynasty. It is the first document specifically on Chinese medicinals that exists in China. It includes over 100 kinds of medicinal animals and plants.

The Book of Mountains and Seas (*Shān Hǎi Jīng*, 山海经) from the early *Qin* Dynasty documented famous mountains and rivers in China. Though it is not a monograph on medicinals, it recorded as many as 126 medicinals, describing their production area, character and function, further deepening people's knowledge of medicinals.

The Yellow Emperor's Inner Classic (*Huáng Dì Nèi Jīng*, 黄帝内经) laid the foundation of Chinese medicine and greatly influenced the development of the Chinese materia medica, including theories on the four properties, five flavors, channel entering, and actions of ascending, descending, floating and sinking. (Contemporary to, or possibly much earlier this, *Fifty-two Formulae* (*Wǔ Shí Èr Bìng Fāng*, 五十二病方) contained over 240 medicinals and 280 formulas. It included internal medicine, surgery, gynecology, otorhinolaryngology, etc. It is the first medicinal monograph describing the processing and preparations of medicinals.)

III. THE *QIN* AND *HAN* DYNASTIES (FROM 221 B.C TO 220 A.D.)

Representative herbal works from the *Qin* and *Han* dynasties are included in Table 1-1 (see p.10).

IV. THE *SOUTHERN* AND *NORTHERN* DYNASTIES (FROM 265 A.D. TO 581 A.D.)

① Representative Herbal Works

Representative herbal works from the *Southern* and *Northern* Dynasties are included in Table 1-1 (see p.10).

② Other Famous Herbal Works in the *Southern* and *Northern* Dynasties

Herbal works

Lei Xiao's Discussion of Herbal Preparations (*Léi Gōng Páo Zhì Lùn*, 雷公炮炙论) by Lei Xiao of the Southern *Song* Dynasty. The first processing and preparation monograph of medicinals in China: A symbol for the emergence of a new branch of the Chinese materia medica.

Wu Pu's Materia Medica (*Wú Pǔ Běn Cǎo*, 吴普本草).
Li Dang-zhi's Medicinal Record (*Lǐ Dāng Zhì Yào Lù*, 李当之药录)
Miscellaneous Records of the Materia Medica (*Míng Yī Bié Lù*, 名医别录).
Xu Zhi-cai's Medicinal Combining (*Xú Zhī Cái Yào Duì*, 徐之才药对).

V. THE *SUI* AND *TANG* DYNASTIES (FROM 581 A.D. TO 907 A.D.)

① Representative Herbal Texts from the *Sui* and *Tang* Dynasties

Representative herbal texts from the *Sui* and *Tang* Dynasties are included in Table 1-1 (see p.10).

② Other Famous Herbal Works

```
                  ┌─ Omissions from the Classic of Materia Medica (Běn Cǎo Shí Yí, 本草拾遗), written by Chen Zang-qi.
                  │  The "Ten Prescriptions" introduced in this book are considered the origin of the classification of the
                  │  Chinese materia medica according to clinical efficacy.
                  │
                  ├─ Materia Medica of Diet Therapy (Shí Liáo Běn Cǎo, 食疗本草), initially written by Meng Shen, and
                  │  revised and supplemented by Zhang Ding. This is the most representative monograph on dietary
                  │  therapy from this period.
                  │
 Herbal Works ───┼─ Materia Medica from the Southern Seaboard Area (Hǎi Yào Běn Cǎo, 海药本草) written by Li Xun. This
                  │  book documents medicinals coming from abroad and from the south of China.
                  │
                  ├─ Discussion of Medicinal Properties (Yào Xìng Lùn, 药性论), also known as the Properties of the Materia
                  │  Medica (Yào Xìng Běn Cǎo, 药性本草), was written by Zhen Quan. This book elaborated on the basic
                  │  theories of the Chinese materia medica.
                  │
                  └─ Materia Medica of Sichuan (Shǔ Běn Cǎo, 蜀本草), written by Han Bao-shen, et al.
```

VI. THE *SONG*, *JIN* AND *YUAN* DYNASTIES (FROM 960 A.D. TO 1368 A.D.)

① Authorized Herbal Works in the *Song* Dynasty

Herbal books in the *Song* Dynasty were compiled by the government as in the *Tang* Dynasty. Authorized herbal works include:

② Representative Herbal Works

Representative herbal works of the *Song* Dynasty are included in Table 1-1 (see p.10).

```
                              ┌─ Materia Medica of the Kaibao Era (Kāi Bǎo Xīn Xiáng Dìng Běn Cǎo, 开宝新祥定本草): The
                              │  first authorized herbal work of the Song Dynasty, compiled by Liu Han, Ma Zhi, et al.
                              │
                              ├─ Revised Materia Medica of the Kaibao Era (Kāi Bǎo Chóng Dìng Běn Cǎo, 开宝重定本草) by
                              │  Li Fang, Zhi Zhi-hao, et al.
                              │
                              ├─ Materia Medica of the Jiayou Era (Jiā Yòu Bǔ Zhù Shén Nóng Běn Cǎo, 嘉佑补注神农本草)
                              │  by Zhang Yu-xi, Lin Yi, Su Song, et al.
                              │
 Authorized Herbal Works ─────┼─ Illustrated Classic of the Materia Medica (Tú Jīng Běn Cǎo, 图经本草) by Su Song. This book
   of the Song Dynasty         │  includes the earliest carving figures of the Chinese materia medica.
                              │
                              ├─ Materia Medica Arranged According to Pattern (Jīng Shǐ Zhèng Lèi Dà Guān Běn Cǎo, 经史证
                              │  类大观本草) often shortened to Dà Guān Běn Cǎo (大观本草).
                              │
                              ├─ Materia Medica of the Zhenghe Era (Zhèng Hé Xīn Xiū Zhèng Lèi Bèi Yòng Běn Cǎo, 政和新修
                              │  证类备用本草) often shortened to Zhèng Lèi Běn Cǎo (证类本草).
                              │
                              └─ Materia Medica of Shaoxing (Shào Xīng Jiào Dìng Jīng Shǐ Zhèng Lèi Bèi Jí Běn Cǎo, 绍兴校
                                 定经史证类备急本草) often shortened to Shào Xīng Běn Cǎo (绍兴本草).
```

③ *Jin* and *Yuan* Periods

During the *Jin* and *Yuan* periods, herbal works were usually written by single physicians. These books were characterized by concise contents and distinct features of clinical Chinese medicinals. Representative works are Liu Wan-su's *Notes on Medicinals in Plain Questions* (*Sù Wèn Yào Zhù*, 素问药注), *Discussion on the Materia Medica* (*Běn Cǎo Lùn*, 本草论), Zhang Yuan-su's *Origins of Medicine* (*Yī Xué Qǐ Yuán*, 医学启源), *Pouch of Pearls* (*Zhēn Zhū Náng*, 珍珠囊) and *Medication based on Differentiation of Zang-fu Theory* (*Zàng Fǔ Biāo Běn Yào Shì*, 脏腑标本药式), Li Dong-yuan's *Systematic Summary of the Theories of Chinese Medicine* (*Yào Lèi Fǎ Xiàng*, 药类法象) and *Key Principles in Medicine* (*Yòng Yào Xīn Fǎ*, 用药心法), Wang Hao-gu's *Materia Medica for Decoctions* (*Tāng Yè Běn Cǎo*, 汤液本草), Zhu Dan-xi's *Supplement to the Extension of the Materia Medica* (*Běn Cǎo Yǎn Yì Bǔ Yí*, 本草衍义补遗), etc.

The herbal works of the *Jin* and *Yuan* periods have two major features:

1. Development and systematization of the basic theories of the Chinese materia medica, including differentiation of the actions of ascending, descending, floating and sinking and channel entering.

2. The establishment by physicians, of this period, of a complete set of pharmacological principles corresponding with different *zang* and *fu* organs, based on the shape, color and taste of Chinese medicinals and the theory of qi transformation, movement of qi, yin-yang and five element theories.

However, this simple and mechanical reasoning style resulted in some negative consequences.

Hu Si-hui of the *Yuan* Dynasty wrote the *Proper and Essential Things for the Emperor's Food and Drink* (*Yǐn Shàn Zhèng Yào*, 饮膳正要), a treatise on dietary therapy. This book recorded dietary prescriptions of the *Hui* and Mongolian ethnic groups and food characteristics and cooking methods of the Mongolian royal family.

During this time, the establishment of the *Huihui* Institute of Medicine promoted medical communication between Chinese and Arabic cultures.

VII. THE *MING* DYNASTY (FROM 1368 A.D. TO 1644 A.D)

① Representative Herbal Works of the *Ming* Dynasty

Representative herbal works of the *Ming* Dynasty are included in Table 1-1 (see p.10).

② Authorized Herbal Works

Essentials of Materia Medica Distinctions (*Běn Cǎo Pǐn Huì Jīng Yào*, 本草品汇精要) by Liu Wen-tai includes 1815 herbs. This book contains 1385 exquisite colorful charts of herbs and examples of herbal preparation technology, and is considered a treasure of ancient paintings. It is the last large-scale authorized herbal work from Chinese feudal society.

③ Topical Herbal Works

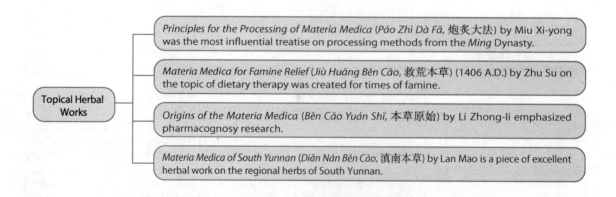

Topical Herbal Works

Principles for the Processing of Materia Medica (*Páo Zhì Dà Fǎ*, 炮炙大法) by Miu Xi-yong was the most influential treatise on processing methods from the *Ming* Dynasty.

Materia Medica for Famine Relief (*Jiù Huāng Běn Cǎo*, 救荒本草) (1406 A.D.) by Zhu Su on the topic of dietary therapy was created for times of famine.

Origins of the Materia Medica (*Běn Cǎo Yuán Shǐ*, 本草原始) by Li Zhong-li emphasized pharmacognosy research.

Materia Medica of South Yunnan (*Diān Nán Běn Cǎo*, 滇南本草) by Lan Mao is a piece of excellent herbal work on the regional herbs of South Yunnan.

VIII. *QING* DYNASTY (FROM 1644 A.D. TO 1911 A.D.)

① Characteristics of Herbal Research of the *Qing* Dynasty

② Representative Herbal Works in the *Qing* Dynasty

Representative herbal works are included in Table 1-1 (see p.10).

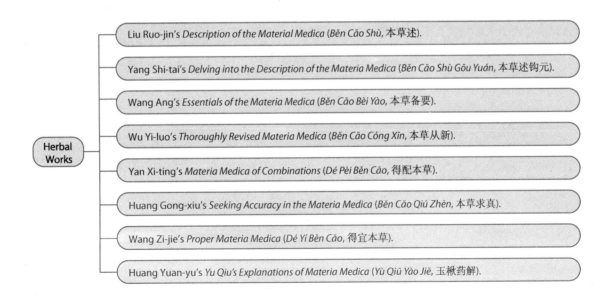

Characteristics of Research of the *Qing* Herbal Works
- It was necessary to further supplement and revise the *Grand Materia Medica* (*Běn Cǎo Gāng Mù*, 本草纲目), with the development of medical science.
- Following the principles of practical use, herbal works were compiled in the form of chapters and absorb the essence from the *Grand Materia Medica*.
- Influenced by the trend of textual research, Shen *Nong's Herbal Classic* (*Shén Nóng Běn Cǎo Jīng*, 神农本草经) was recompiled from ancient documents.
- A large number of herbal works from the *Qing* Dynasty provided new content for the compilation of comprehensive herbal works.
- There were a number of excellent herbal works on specific topics produced in the *Qing* Dynasty.

③ Practical Herbal Works Based on the *Grand Materia Medica*

Herbal Works
- Liu Ruo-jin's *Description of the Material Medica* (*Běn Cǎo Shù*, 本草述).
- Yang Shi-tai's *Delving into the Description of the Materia Medica* (*Běn Cǎo Shù Gōu Yuán*, 本草述钩元).
- Wang Ang's *Essentials of the Materia Medica* (*Běn Cǎo Bèi Yào*, 本草备要).
- Wu Yi-luo's *Thoroughly Revised Materia Medica* (*Běn Cǎo Cóng Xīn*, 本草从新).
- Yan Xi-ting's *Materia Medica of Combinations* (*Dé Pèi Běn Cǎo*, 得配本草).
- Huang Gong-xiu's *Seeking Accuracy in the Materia Medica* (*Běn Cǎo Qiú Zhēn*, 本草求真).
- Wang Zi-jie's *Proper Materia Medica* (*Dé Yí Běn Cǎo*, 得宜本草).
- Huang Yuan-yu's *Yu Qiu's Explanations of Materia Medica* (*Yù Qiū Yào Jiě*, 玉楸药解).

IX. REPRESENTATIVE CONTEMPORARY HERBAL WORKS

Representative contemporary and ancient herbal works are included in Table 1-1.

Table 1-1: Representative Works in Ancient times

Dynasty	Name of Work	Author	Date of Completion	Number of Medicinals Recorded	Remarks
Han Dynasty	*Shen Nong's Herbal Classic*	Anonymous	From the end of the Western *Han* to the early Eastern *Han*	365	The first medicinal monograph in China.
The Southern and Northern Dynasties	*Collection of Commentaries on the Classic of the Materia Medica*	Tao Hong-jing	Around 500 A.D.	730	First established a method of differentiating medicinals based on their natural attributes.
Sui and *Tang* Dynasties	*Newly Revised Materia Medica*	Su Jing, et al	659 A.D.	844-850	The first authorized pharmacopoeia in the world.
Song, Jin and *Yuan* Dynasties	*Revised Zhenghe Materia Medica for Emergencies from the Classics and Historical Documents*	Tang Shen-wei	1082 A.D.	1558	Preserved a large number of classic and historical documents from before the *Song* Dynasty.
Ming Dynasty	*Grand Materia Medica*	Li Shi-zhen	1578 A.D.	1892	The most famous herbal work from the *Ming* Dynasty.
Qing Dynasty	*Omissions from the Grand Materia Medica*	Zhao Xue-min	1765 A.D.	921	An updated herbal work including newly added medicinals.
Contemporary	*Chinese Herbal Medicine*	Editorial Committee of *Chinese Herbal Medicine*	1999 A.D.	8980	A comprehensive herbal work reflecting the development of the Chinese materia medica in the 20th century in China.

Chapter 2
Producing Areas and Collection of Chinese Medicinals

Chinese medicinals mainly come from plants, animals, minerals and processed products. The production area, collection and storage directly influence the quality and curative effect of Chinese herbal medicinals. As recorded in *Shen Nong's Herbal Classic*: "*There are particular notes for each herb, such as the specific processing methods (dried in the shade or in the sun), collecting season, production area, quality, and storage period*" (阴干曝干、采造时月生熟，土地所出，真伪存新，并各有法。).

Section 1　Producing Area

I. AUTHENTIC CHINESE MEDICINALS

Authentic Chinese medicinals refers to medicinals with excellent quality and reliable therapeutic effects. Such medicinals have a long history of use as medication, and of having a proper production area, good quality, abundant production, fine processing and preparation, and remarkable curative effects.

II. PRODUCTION OF AUTHENTIC CHINESE MEDICINALS

1. The distribution and production of

Chinese medicinals calls for a certain natural environment.

2. China is located in East Asia and covers an extensive territory. Most of China is located in a northern temperate zone, with some colder areas in the north of Daxing'anling, subtropical areas in the south part of Qinling and the Huai River, and tropical areas in southern China. Oceans, rivers, lakes, mountains and plains contribute to China's sophisticated geological environment, which allows for the production of various plants. Consequently, each medicinal is naturally confined to a certain production area. This is why physicians of Chinese medicine put so much emphasis on authentic Chinese medicinals.

3. Through years of use, observation and comparison, physicians in ancient times came to understand that although some medicinals have a wide distribution, due to different natural conditions, the quality of herbs grown in different regions varies a great deal. Therefore, the concept of authentic Chinese medicinals is proposed.

The confirmation of authentic Chinese medicinals is related to numerous factors, such as production area, variety and quality. The decisive factor is the clinical curative effect. Famous authentic Chinese medicinals are highly prized. Examples are *huáng lián* (黄连, Rhizoma Coptidis, Coptis Root), *chuān xiōng* (川芎, Rhizoma Chuanxiong, Chuanxiong Root) and *fù zǐ* (附子, Radix Aconiti Lateralis Praeparata, Aconite Root) from Sichuan, *bò he* (薄荷, Herba Menthae, Peppermint) and *cāng zhú* (苍术, Rhizoma Atractylodis, Atractylodes Rhizome) from Jiangsu, *shā rén* (砂仁, Fructus Amomi, Villous Amomum Fruit) from Guangdong, *rén shēn* (人参, Radix et Rhizoma Ginseng, Ginseng), *xì xīn* (细辛, Radix et Rhizoma Asari, Manchurian Wildginger) and *wǔ wèi zǐ* (五味子, Fructus Schisandrae Chinensis, Chinese Magnolivine Fruit) from northeast China, *fú líng* (茯苓, Poria, Indian Bread) from Yunnan, *dì huáng* (地黄, Radix Rehmanniae, Rehmannia Root) from Henan, and *ē jiāo* (阿胶, Colla Corii Asini, Donkey-hide Glue) from Shandong.

III. ATTITUDE TOWARD AUTHENTIC CHINESE MEDICINALS

1. Long term clinical practice has proven that the quality of medicinals is closely related to their curative effects. The *Extension of the Materia Medica* (*Běn Cǎo Yǎn Yì*, 本草衍义) says: "*For medicinals, the selection of the production area is important. High quality medicinals are able to guarantee their curative effect, so physicians then know whether medicinals, in a particular dosage, work well or not.*" (凡用药必择土地所宜者，则药力具，用之有据。) The climate, soil and water are all important in the production, taste and curative effects of medicinals. As early as *Shen Nong's Herbal Classic, Part Record of Famous Physicians* (*Míng Yī Bié Lù*, 名医别录) many herbal documents had records of the varieties and production areas of precious medicinals, such as *dāng guī* (当归, Radix Angelicae Sinensis, Chinese Angelica Root) from Gansu, *gǒu qǐ* (枸杞, Fructus Lycii, Barbary Wolfberry Fruit) from Ningxia, *dà huáng* (大黄, Radix et Rhizoma Rhei, Rhubarb Root and Rhizome) from Qinghai, *huáng qí* (黄芪, Radix Astragali, Astragalus Root) from Neimenggu, *rén shēn* (Radix et Rhizoma Ginseng), *xì xīn* (Radix et Rhizoma Asari) and *wǔ wèi zǐ* (Fructus Schisandrae Chinensis) from northeast China, *dǎng shēn* (党参, Radix Codonopsis, Tangshen Root) from Shanxi, *dì*

huáng (Radix Rehmanniae), *niú xī* (牛膝, Radix Achyranthis Bidentatae, Twotoothed Achyranthes Root), *shān yào* (山药, Rhizoma Dioscoreae, Common Yam Rhizome) and *jú huā* (菊花, Flos Chrysanthemi, Chrysanthemum Flower) from Henan, *sān qī* (三七, Radix et Rhizoma Notoginseng, Notoginseng) and *fú líng* (Poria) from Yunnan, *huáng lián* (Rhizoma Coptidis), *chuān xiōng* (Rhizoma Chuanxiong), *chuān bèi mǔ* (川贝母, Bulbus Fritillariae Cirrhosae, Sichuan Fritillaria Bulb) and *chuān wū* (川乌, Radix Aconiti, Common Monkshood Mother Root) from Sichuan, *ē jiāo* (Colla Corii Asini) of Shandong, *zhè bèi mǔ* (浙贝母, Bulbus Fritillariae Thunbergii, Thunberg Fritillary Bulb) from Zhejiang, *bò he* (Herba Menthae) from Jiangsu and *chén pí* (陈皮, Pericarpium Citri Reticulatae, Aged Tangerine Peel) and *shā rén* (Fructus Amomi) from Guangdong. Since ancient times, these have been considered authentic Chinese medicinals.

2. The yield of authentic Chinese medicinals is limited, and so in fact, some medicinals from other producing areas are used, as long as the curative effects are not influenced. However, it is still necessary to research the ecosystems and cultivation techniques of authentic Chinese medicinals, which is helpful for developing high-quality medicinals and exploring new sources of medicine.

3. At present, a large number of studies on authentic Chinese medicinals are investigating the relationship between geographical distribution, ecosystem and ecological type, growing conditions (including sunlight, temperature, humidity, soil), and chemical composition, and there are also pharmacological studies and ecological studies on wild variants. At the same time, domesticated animal products are being developed to meet the demand for medicinals that are in short supply. To further improve the production of authentic Chinese medicinals, new GAP (Good Agricultural Practice of Medicinal Plants and Animals) production bases have been established to promote the development of authentic Chinese materials. Of course, it must be made certain that the introduced or domesticated types maintain the properties, functions and curative effect of the original ones.

4. Authentic Chinese medicinals have developed over long periods of study and practice of medicine, and continue to evolve. *Rén shēn* (Radix et Rhizoma Ginseng) produced in the Shangdang area of Shanxi became extinct due to environmental changes, so people began to use *rén shēn* (Radix et Rhizoma Ginseng) produced in the northeast China. *Chuān xiōng* (Rhizoma Chuanxiong) did not become an authentic medicinal until the *Song* Dynasty. *Sān qī* (Radix et Rhizoma Notoginseng) was initially produced in Guangxi, and was called *guǎng sān qī* (Radix et Rhizoma Notoginseng) or *tián qī* (Radix et Rhizoma Notoginseng). The *sān qī* (Radix et Rhizoma Notoginseng) produced in Yunnan was later discovered and called *diān sān qī* (Radix et Rhizoma Notoginseng) and is considered better in quality. As a result, Yunnan became a new producing area for *sān qī* (Radix et Rhizoma Notoginseng).

Section 2   Collection

I. THE RELATIONSHIP BETWEEN COLLECTION AND CURATIVE EFFECT

The quality of medicinals is closely related to their collection season and method of collection. During different growing periods, active and poisonous components contained in the medicinal parts of plants and animals vary greatly. Therefore, medicinals must be collected at the proper time.

II. COLLECTION TIME

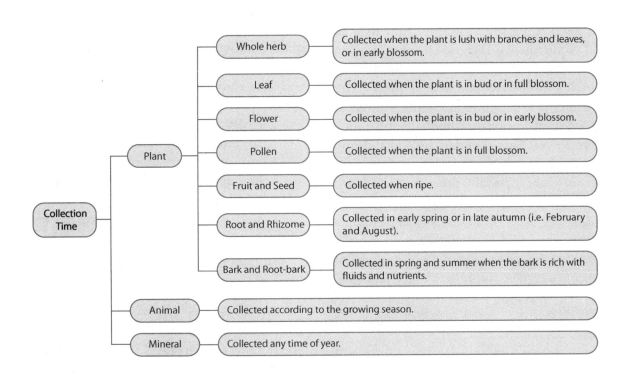

Chapter 3
Processing and Preparation

Processing and preparation, called *Páo Zhì* (炮炙), *Xiū Shì* (修事) or *Xiū Zhì* (修治), refers to the necessary treatment of medicinals before they are used. *Páo Zhì* is a traditional pharmaceutical technology in China.

Most Chinese medicinals are crude substances which need to be processed in order to meet clinical requirements. There are many processing methods which are used according to the different properties of medicinals and requirements of treatment. Poisonous medicinals must be processed to insure safety before administration. Appropriate auxiliary materials are added during processing. Preparations and control of time and temperature are especially noted as recorded in the *Hidden Aspects of the Materia Medica* (*Běn Cǎo Méng Quán*, 本草蒙筌): "*Processing and preparation of medicinals should be properly performed. The curative effect will not be achieved if medicinals are not processed to a certain quality, while over-processing will cause the loss of some properties and tastes*" (凡药制造，贵在适中，不及则功效难求，太过则气味反失).

Section 1　Purposes of Processing and Preparation

There are eight reasons for which medicinals are processed:

1. To purify crude medicinals, guarantee quality and separate crude medicinals into ranks.

2. To cut or shred medicinals into pieces in order to make them convenient for use as medication.

3. To dry medicinals for storage.

4. To eliminate bad tastes and odors and ease oral administration.

5. To reduce toxicity and ensure safety.

6. To enhance curative effects.

7. To change properties and expand the use of medicinals.

8. To guide medicinals to specific channels.

Section 2　Methods of Processing and Preparation

Methods of processing have been gradually developed and enhanced over time. These methods are classified as follows:

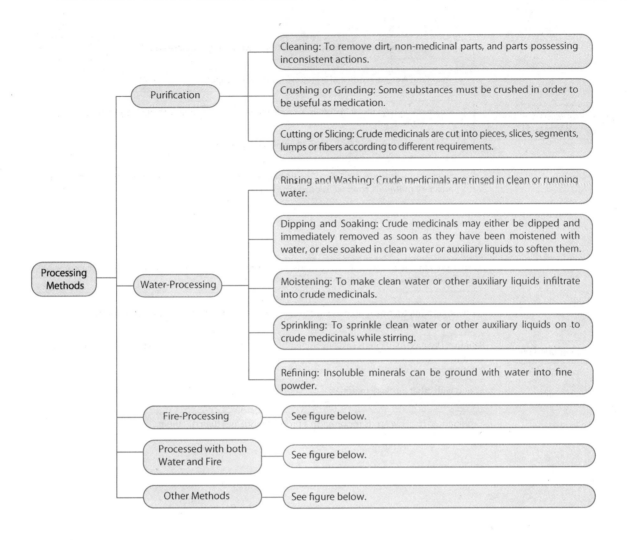

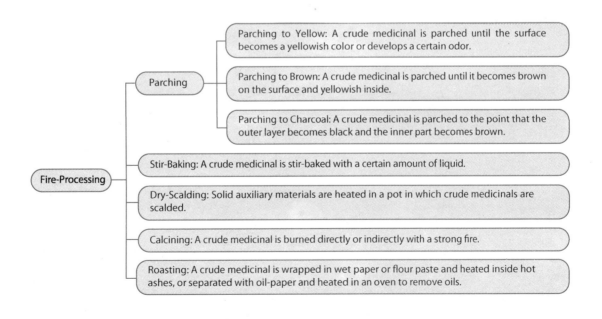

Processed with both Water and Fire

- Boiling: A crude medicinal is boiled in water or with other auxiliary liquids.
- Steaming: A crude medicinal is steamed with water vapor.
- Steaming with Auxiliary Materials: A crude medicinal is steamed with auxiliary materials.
- Scalding: A crude medicinal is quickly dipped into boiling water.
- Quenching: A crude medicinal is calcined red and then quickly put into cold water or other auxiliary materials to make it crisp.

Other Methods

- Frosting: To remove the oils from toxic medicinals, or to put crude medicinals in a well-ventilated place until a frostlike powder emerges on its surface.
- Fermenting: Induce fermenting under a certain condition to change the features of a medicinal.
- Refining: Dissolve medicinals (usually minerals) in water, condense and then leave to sit until crystals emerge.
- Mixing with other auxiliary materials.
- Germinating: To allow seeds to sprout to a proper length and then dry them.

Chapter 4
Characters and Functions of Chinese Medicinals

I. BASIC PRINCIPLES OF TREATING DISEASES WITH CHINESE MEDICINALS

Practitioners of Chinese medicine believe that diseases are caused by an excess or deficiency of qi, blood, yin or yang, or dysfunction of the viscera, channels and collaterals due to pathological factors fighting with healthy qi.

Therefore, the basic functions of Chinese medicinals are to strengthen healthy qi and eliminate pathogenic qi in order to eliminate the causes of disease and to correct imbalances of yin, yang, qi and blood, to restore normal physiological functioning.

Chinese medicinals are therefore used to treat imbalances of yin and yang through their characters and actions.

II. CHARACTER OF CHINESE MEDICINALS

The character of Chinese medicinals refers to their nature and function, and relates to their therapeutic effects. It includes basic fundamentals and actions during therapy.

III. BASIC THEORY OF THE CHARACTER OF CHINESE MEDICINALS

The basic theory of the character of Chinese medicinals is about the principles of applications for the specific character of a Chinese medicinal and the mechanism by which this character is formed, which includes four properties, five flavors, ascending, descending, floating and sinking, channel entering, toxicity, etc. It is based on the theories of yin and yang, viscera, channels and collaterals, and is summed up throughout a long history of clinical practice. It is an important part of Chinese medicine and is the basis for learning, studying and using Chinese medicinals.

IV. THE EFFECT OF CHINESE MEDICINALS

The basic principle in clinical use of medicinals is

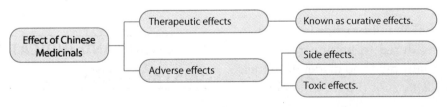

17

to ensure safety and efficacy while using Chinese medicinals.

V. DIFFERENCE BETWEEN CHARACTER AND DESCRIPTION

Character and description are two different concepts. The properties of Chinese medicinals are concluded after administration, which is a summary of the actions and characteristics of Chinese medicinals, and their specific effects on the human body. Description refers to shape, color, odor, taste and texture (light or heavy, loose or dense, hard or soft, moist or dry).

Section 1　Property

I. CONCEPT OF NATURE

The four natures of Chinese medicinals are cold, hot, warm or cool. These natures reflect the actions of medicinals towards yin and yang, cold and hot in the human body, which is a significant component of the basic theory of Chinese medicinals. The nature of the medicinals provides theoretical evidence for medicinal action.

Cold and cool natures belong to yin, while warm and hot natures belong to yang. These are of opposite nature. Cold is different from cool only in degree, as is warm from hot. Some herbal documents may have descriptions of "extremely hot", "extremely cold", "slightly warm," or "slightly cool", which are further distinctions.

II. NEUTRAL MEDICINALS

When a medicinal is neither hot nor cold in nature, it is considered to be neutral. These medicinals are usually mild and moderate in their actions, such as *dǎng shēn* (Radix Codonopsis),

shān yào (Rhizoma Dioscoreae) and *gān cǎo* (甘草, Radix et Rhizoma Glycyrrhizae, Licorice Root). Actually, neutral medicinals tend to be either cool or warm. *Gān cǎo* (Radix et Rhizoma Glycyrrhizae) for example, when unprepared, has a cool nature. While it is stir-baked, it has a slightly warm nature. Therefore, the neutral property is not separate from the four natures of cold, hot, warm or cool.

III. THE APPLICATION OF MEDICINALS WITH DIFFERENT PROPERTIES

Four properties are determined according to different curative effects and reactions of the human body after administration. The determination of properties should be based on reactions to medicinals, as well as the cold or hot nature of a disease. Medicinals with the actions of relieving or eliminating heat syndrome are usually considered cold or cool and vice versa, warm or hot medicinals often alleviate or eliminate cold syndrome.

Symptoms of high fever and thirst, flushing, blood-shot eyes, and a flooding and rapid pulse belong to yang heat syndrome. Medicinals with cold or cool properties such as *shí gāo* (石膏, Gypsum Fibrosum, Gypsum), *zhī mǔ* (知母, Rhizoma Anemarrhenae, Common Anemarrhena Rhizome) and *zhī zǐ* (栀子, Fructus Gardeniae, Cape Jasmine Fruit) can be used to treat such syndromes. If patients have symptoms of yin cold syndrome, such as coldness of the limbs, pale complexion, abdominal cold pain and a faint pulse, hot or warm natured herbs such as *fù zǐ* (Radix Aconiti Lateralis Praeparata), *ròu guì* (肉桂, Cortex Cinnamomi, Cassia Bark) and *gān jiāng* (干姜, Rhizoma Zingiberis, Dried Ginger Rhizome), can be used to eliminate symptoms.

IV. ACTIONS AND INDICATIONS OF THE FOUR PROPERTIES

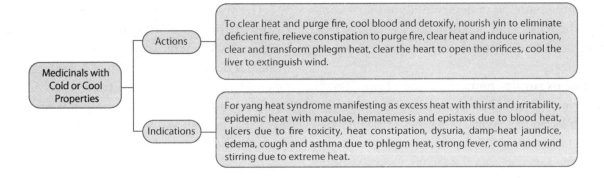

V. SENSE OF FOUR PROPERTIES

1. *Plain Questions – The Most Important Discussion* (*Sù Wèn – Zhì Zhēn Yào Dà Lùn*, 素问·至真要大论): "*Treat cold syndrome with warm medicinals and treat heat syndrome with cold medicinals*" (寒者热之，热者寒之). This statement demonstrates the general principle of the use of the four properties in clinical medications.

2. If cold medicinals are used to treat cold syndrome or hot medicinals to treat heat syndrome, this will aggravate the pathological condition or even cause death. Wang Shu-he said: "*Guì zhī (Ramulus Cinnamomi, Cassia Twig) will cost the patient's life if there is a yang hyperactivity condition. Chéng Qì Tāng (Qi-Coordinating Decoction, 承气汤) may cause death if there is a yin hyperactivity syndrome.*"

3. Note the use of medicinals with different properties. If a medicinal with a cool property is used instead of a cold medicinal, or a warm medicinal is used instead of a hot one, curative effects will not be achieved. If a hot medicinal is used instead of a warm one or cold instead of cool, this will impair yin or yang respectively.

4. As for syndromes of exterior cold and interior heat, heat in the upper and cold in the lower, and a mix of cold and heat, cold and hot medicinals should be used together.

5. "*Avoiding hot medicinals on hot days and cold medicinals on cold days*" (寒无犯寒，热无犯热) proposed in *Plain Questions – Discussion on the Changes and Symbols of the Five Elements's Motion and the Six Kinds of Weather in the Cycle of Sixty Years* (*Sù Wèn – Liù Yuán Zhèng Jì Dà Lùn*, 素问·六元正纪大论) instructs the clinical principle of medication in different seasons according to the four properties. It points out that during the winter, cold medicinals should be avoided if no excess heat syndrome is seen, and in summer, hot medicinals should be avoided to prevent yin consumption.

6. In cases of cold syndrome with the appearance of heat, hot medicinals should be used, assisted by some cold medicinals if necessary. In cases of heat syndrome with the appearance of cold, cold medicinals are chosen, assisted by some hot medicinals if necessary.

Section 2   Flavor

I. CONCEPT OF FLAVOR

Flavor refers to the taste of medicinals, such as sour, bitter, sweet, acrid, and salty. Some medicinals are bland or astringent.

II. FORMING OF FIVE FLAVORS

1. The five flavors are identified by tastes, which reflect the actual tastes of the medicinals.

2. More importantly, the tastes of medicinals have been determined over time through clinical practice and by observing the various reactions on the human body after administration. With the ongoing use of medicinals, there is a

constantly evolving understanding of the actions of medicinals. Some medicinals have tastes that are difficult to distinguish, so they are defined by their effects.

For example, neither *gé gēn* (葛根, Radix Puerariae Lobatae, Kudzuvine Root) nor *zào jiǎo cì* (皂角刺, Spina Gleditsiae, Chinese Honeylocust Spine) have an acrid taste. However, *gě gēn* (Radix Puerariae Lobatae) can release the exterior and is usually applied in exterior syndrome, while *zào jiǎo cì* (Spina Gleditsiae) can eliminate carbuncles and stagnation and is often used in early-stage suppurative infections, or pus without ulceration. The actions of these two medicinals correspond with the effect of the acrid flavor; therefore, they are classified into the category of having an acrid flavor. *Cí shí* (磁石, Magnetitum, Magnetite) does not have a salty taste. However, it enters the kidney channel to suppress floating yang, so it is attributed with a salty flavor.

The five flavors not only reflect the actual tastes of the medicinals but summarize their actions. This is why some medicinals recorded in herbal documents sometimes differ from their original tastes when identifying their flavors. In all, flavor indicates the original taste of a medicinal as well as its actions, which constitute the main theory of "five flavors".

III. THE ACTUAL MEANING OF FIVE FLAVORS

"*Five flavors*" refers to both the real tastes of medicinals as well as their effects.

IV. ACTIONS AND INDICATIONS OF THE "FIVE FLAVORS"

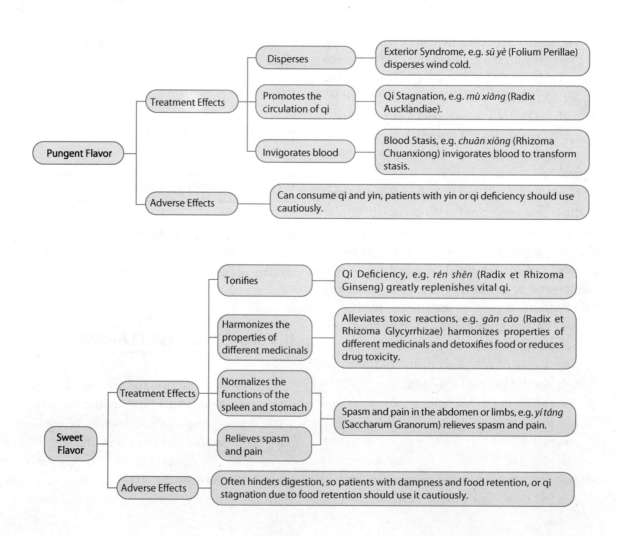

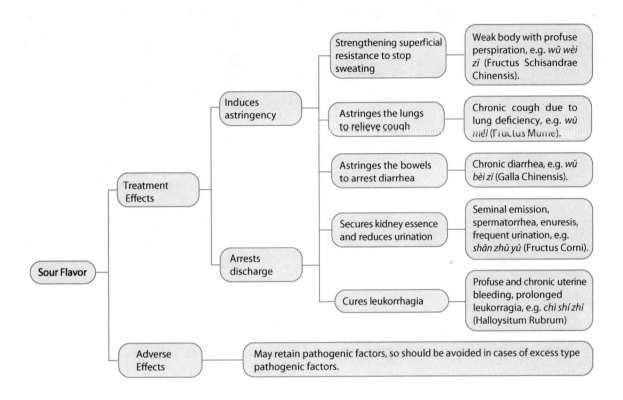

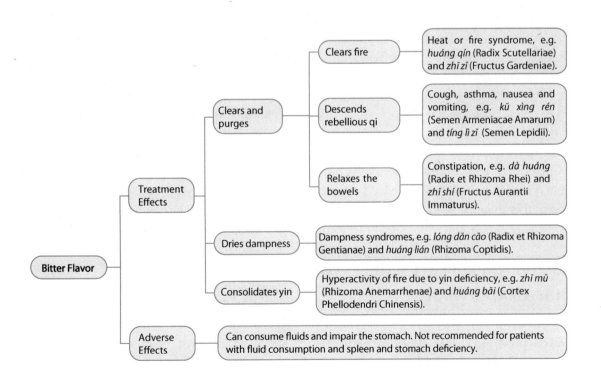

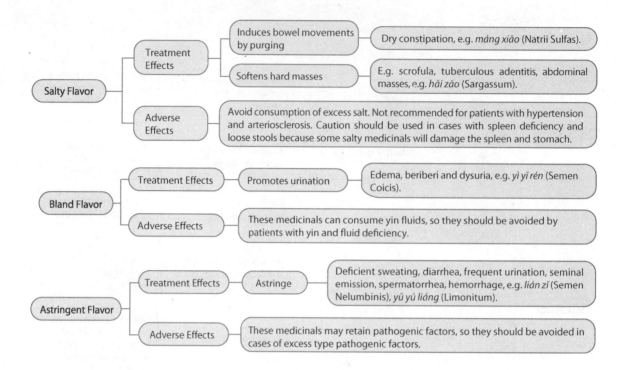

V. RELATIONSHIPS BETWEEN THE FIVE FLAVORS AND FIVE *ZANG*–ORGANS

The five flavors are related to the five elements and five zang-organs. As noted in the *Plain Questions – Treatise Explaining the Five Qi (Sù Wèn – Xuān Míng Wŭ Qì Piān,* 素问·宣明五气篇)*: "The sour flavor enters the liver (wood), bitter flavor enters the heart (fire), sweet flavor enters the spleen (earth), pungent flavor enters the lung (metal) and salty flavor enters the kidney (water)"* (酸入肝（属本）、苦入心（属火）、甘入脾（属土）、辛入肺（属金）、咸入肾（属水）)*. However, in practice, the rules may change. For example, *huáng băi* (Cortex Phellodendri Chinensis) is bitter in flavor and cold in nature, but is used to purge the kidney fire rather than the heart fire.

VI. LOOKING AT PROPERTY AND FLAVOR AS AN INTEGRATED WHOLE

1. Each medicinal has its own property and flavor, and they should be considered as an integrated whole. Miu Xi-yong of the *Qing* Dynasty said: *"Property and flavor are interdependent, determining the character of a medicinal"* (物有味

必有气，有气斯有性)*. That is to say, property and flavor should be considered as a whole in a medicinal to correctly distinguish its action.

2. Generally speaking, medicinals of a certain category always have similar properties and flavors, and therefore similar actions. For example, medicinals with an acrid flavor and warm property usually disperse wind cold, while sweet and warm medicinals often replenish qi and strengthen yang.

3. There are cases of medicinals with the same flavor and property but which differ in actions. For example, *huáng qí* (Radix Astragali) is sweet and warm, but the emphasis is on the sweet flavor, so that it mainly replenishes qi. *Suŏ yáng* (锁阳, Herba Cynomorii, Songaria Cynomorium Herb) is also sweet and warm, with the emphasis on the warmth, so that it mainly strengthens the yang. Medicinals differing in property and flavor will have different actions. *Huáng lián* (Rhizoma Coptidis) is bitter and cold, and acts to clear heat and dry dampness. *Dăng shēn* (Radix Codonopsis) is sweet and warm and acts to replenish qi and supplement the middle *jiao*.

4. Medicinals having the same property but differing in flavor, or having the same flavor but differing in property also have different actions. *Má huáng* (Herba Ephedrae), *xìng rén* (Semen Armeniacae Amarum), *dà zăo* (大枣, Fructus Jujubae, Chinese date), *wū méi* (Fructus Mume)

and *ròu cōng róng* (肉苁蓉, Herba Cistanches, Desert-living Cistanche) are all warm medicinals. However, *má huáng* (Herba Ephedrae) is also acrid in flavor and disperses cold to relieve exterior syndromes; *xìng rén* (Semen Armeniacae Amarum) has a bitter flavor which acts to astringe qi to arrest cough; *dà zǎo* (Fructus Jujubae) is sweet in flavor and nourishes the spleen and replenishes qi; *wū méi* (Fructus Mume) is sour in flavor and astringes both the lung and intestines and *ròu cōng róng* (Herba Cistanche) has a salty flavor and nourishes the kidneys and strengthens yang. *Guì zhī* (Ramulus Cinnamomi), *bò he* (Herba Menthae), *fù zǐ* (Radix Aconiti Lateralis Praeparata) and *shí gāo* (Gypsum Fibrosum) are all acrid in flavor, however, *guì zhī* (Ramulus Cinnamomi) is warm in nature and acts to disperse cold to relieve the exterior syndrome, *bò he* (Herba Menthae) has a cold nature and disperses wind heat, *fù zǐ* (Radix Aconiti Lateralis Praeparata) is hot in nature and supplements the kidney fire and strengthens yang, *shí gāo* (Gypsum Fibrosum) is cold in nature and clears heat and descends fire.

5. A medicinal with several flavors indicates the variety of its functions. *Dāng guī* (Radix Angelicae Sinensis) is pungent, sweet and warm, and it nourishes and invigorates blood, relieves pain, warms the channels and collaterals and disperses cold pathogens. It is used to treat diseases caused by blood deficiency, blood stagnation and blood cold.

6. In clinical practice, medicinals are used in different combinations to treat different diseases. *Shēng má* (升麻, Rhizoma Cimicifugae, Large Trifolious Bugbane Rhizome) is pungent, sweet and slightly cold. When it is used with *huáng qí* (Radix Astragali) to treat collapse of the middle qi, its sweet flavor is emphasized. If it is used in combination with *gé gēn* (Radix Puerariae Lobatae), its acrid flavor is emphasized to release the exterior and to promote the eruption of rashes. When it is used with *shí gāo* (Gypsum Fibrosum) to treat toothache due to stomach fire, its cold property is emphasized to clear heat and descend fire.

7. Property and flavor indicate the character of a medicine, and only reflect the general nature and basic actions. Therefore, they should be considered in combination with the specific function of a certain medicinal to get a complete and exact understanding of the medicinal. Both *sū yè* (Folium Perillae) and *xīn yí* (辛夷, Flos Magnoliae, Blond Magnolia Flower) are pungent and warm, and act to disperse wind cold. However, *sū yè* (Folium Perillae) has a strong action in dispersing, and can promote qi circulation as well. *Xīn yí* (Flos Magnoliae) is less effective than *sū yè* (Folium Perillae) for dispersing wind cold, but is better for opening the nasal passages. Therefore, it is important to give consideration to all aspects of property, flavor and function.

8. As discussed above, the actions expressed by property and flavor and the rules of their combination are rather complex. To direct clinical prescribing, practitioners should master the general principles of property and flavor as well as the therapeutic effects of particular medicinals, and combination principles of property and flavor.

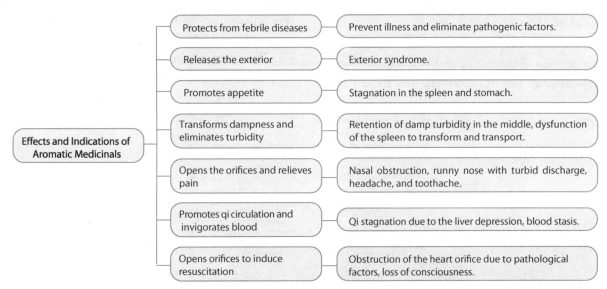

Effects and Indications of Aromatic Medicinals		
	Protects from febrile diseases	Prevent illness and eliminate pathogenic factors.
	Releases the exterior	Exterior syndrome.
	Promotes appetite	Stagnation in the spleen and stomach.
	Transforms dampness and eliminates turbidity	Retention of damp turbidity in the middle, dysfunction of the spleen to transform and transport.
	Opens the orifices and relieves pain	Nasal obstruction, runny nose with turbid discharge, headache, and toothache.
	Promotes qi circulation and invigorates blood	Qi stagnation due to the liver depression, blood stasis.
	Opens orifices to induce resuscitation	Obstruction of the heart orifice due to pathological factors, loss of consciousness.

Section 3   Ascending, Descending, Floating and Sinking

I. CONCEPTS OF ASCENDING, DESCENDING, FLOATING AND SINKING

Actions of ascending, descending, floating and sinking refer to the upward, downward, outward and inward directions in which medicinals tend to act on the body. They are used in correspondence to the location of disease but against the tendency of the disease. Ascending is the opposite of descending, and floating is the opposite of sinking. Ascending and floating are similar in some cases, and so are descending and sinking. They represent the orientation of actions and are the basic theory of medicinal function.

II. ATTRIBUTES OF ASCENDING, DESCENDING, FLOATING AND SINKING

Ascending and floating belong to yang, while descending and sinking belong to yin.

III. TENDENCIES OF MEDICINALS WITH ASCENDING, DESCENDING, FLOATING AND SINKING ACTIONS

As tendencies of diseases are divided into upward (e.g. vomiting, hiccup, asthma), downward (e.g.

anal prolapse, enuresis, irregular uterine bleeding), outward (e.g. spontaneous sweating or night sweating), inward (e.g. internal transmission of exterior syndrome), and locations of disease are different with some in the exterior (e.g. exterior syndrome), in the interior (e.g. constipation), in the upper part of the body (e.g. sore red swollen eyes) and in the lower (e.g. ascites, urinary block), medicinals used to treat such diseases possess corresponding tendencies as well.

IV. FORMATION OF ASCENDING, DESCENDING, FLOATING AND SINKING

The formation of ascending, descending, floating and sinking actions of medicinals have close relationships with their properties, flavors, processing, preparation and compatibility. Moreover, these actions are mainly associated with the therapeutic effects and tendencies on the human body. This is basic theory just like property and flavor.

V. THE INFLUENCING FACTORS FOR ASCENDING, DESCENDING, FLOATING AND SINKING

The influencing factors are: Properties, flavors, textures and weights of medicinals. In addition, the actions can be influenced or even altered by processing and combining.

Therefore, ascending, descending, floating and sinking actions of medicinals can be altered under

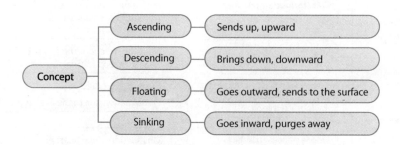

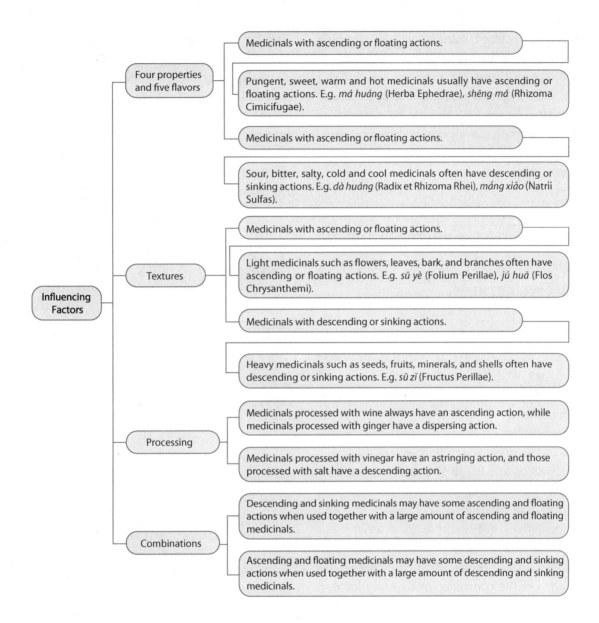

certain conditions (processing, combination). Li Shizhen said: "*Ascending, descending, floating and sinking actions are associated with the character and clinical application of medicinals*" (升降在物，亦在人也).

VI. ACTIONS OF ASCENDING, DESCENDING, FLOATING AND SINKING

1. Generally speaking, ascending and floating medicinals have upward and outward actions and are used for relieving exterior syndrome, venting rashes, detoxifying, eliminating sores, relieving cough by opening restricted lung qi, warming the interior and dispersing cold, warming the liver and removing stasis, warming and activating the channels and collaterals, eliminating painful obstruction, promoting qi circulation and relieving depression, invigorating blood to remove hard masses, opening the orifices and reviving consciousness, raising yang, inducing vomiting, and so forth.

2. Descending and sinking medicinals have downward and inward actions and are usually used for clearing heat and draining fire, purging the bowels, promoting urination, quietening the spirit, calming the liver and subduing yang, extinguishing wind to relieve convulsions, directing

rebellious qi downward, calming asthma, stopping vomiting, relieving hiccup, improving digestion to eliminate stagnant food, securing the exterior and stopping sweating, astringing the lung to relieve cough, astringing the intestines to stop diarrhea, stopping hemorrhage, stopping vaginal discharge, securing the kidney essence, reducing urination, and eliminating dampness, etc.

VII. THE CLINICAL APPLICATIONS OF ASCENDING, DESCENDING, FLOATING AND SINKING ACTIONS

1. Actions of ascending, descending, floating and sinking can regulate qi circulation. They are able to act on different parts of the body and cure diseases when used in accordance with their general tendencies.

2. The principle corresponds with the disease locations but against the tendencies.

For diseases located in the upper or exterior parts of the body, it is appropriate to use ascending and floating medicinals instead of descending and sinking medicinals. For example, for exterior wind heat syndrome, choose *bò he* (Herba Menthae) and *jú huā* (Flos Chrysanthemi) or similar dispersing medicinals. On the contrary, for diseases located in the lower part or the interior of the body, such as constipation, it is proper to use *dà huáng* (Radix et Rhizoma Rhei) and *máng xiāo* (Natrii Sulfas) to unblock the bowels.

For diseases of upward counterflow, medicinals with descending actions should be used. For example, in the treatment of headache and dizziness due to hyperactivity of liver yang, *dài zhě shí* (代赭石, Haematitumm, Haematite) and *shí jué míng* (石决明, Concha Haliotidis, Sea-ear Shell) are used to calm the liver and subdue yang. On the contrary, for diseases which manifest with downward tendencies, medicinals with lifting actions should be used. For example, in the treatment of chronic diarrhea and prolapse due to collapse of qi in the middle *jiao, huáng qí* (Radix Astragali), *shēng má* (Rhizoma Cimicifugae) and

chái hú (柴胡, Radix Bupleuri, Bupleurum) are used to raise the yang and upbear the qi.

3. In conclusion, the most important principle in clinical application is to choose proper medicinals according to disease locations and tendencies.

4. In addition, in order to appropriately treat complex pathological conditions and to regulate visceral functions, medicinals with ascending, descending, floating and sinking actions may be used together. For example, in syndromes of exterior cold and interior heat manifesting as sweating and asthma due to an unresolved exterior syndrome and accumulation of pathogenic heat in the lung, *shí gāo* (Gypsum Fibrosum) and *má huáng* (Herba Ephedrae) are used together. *Shí gāo* (Gypsum Fibrosum) has the action of purging lung fire and descending lung qi, while *má huáng* (Herba Ephedrae) disperses cold to relieve the exterior, opens the lung qi to relieve cough and opens and descends the lung qi. In the treatment of upper heat and lower cold syndrome manifesting as irritability and insomnia, cold low back and loose stools due to an imbalance between the heart yang and the kidney yin, *huáng lián* (Rhizoma Coptidis) and *ròu guì* (Cortex Cinnamomi) are used together. *Huáng lián* (Rhizoma Coptidis) has the action of clearing the heart and descending fire to calm the mind, while *ròu guì* (Cortex Cinnamomi) invigorates the kidney and leads fire to its source in order to restore normal communication between the heart and kidney.

Section 4 Channel Entering

I. THE CONCEPT OF MEDICINALS ENTERING CHANNELS

Channel entry refers to a medicinal's selective therapeutic effects on a certain part of the body. A medicinal exerts obvious or specific therapeutic action on the pathological changes in a certain channel or some viscera, but little effect on the others. The concept of entering channels indicates the direction for application of medicinals in treating diseases, and is one of the basic aspects in the theory of medicinals.

II. FORMATION OF ENTERING CHANNELS

The theory of channel tropism is based on the theory of the viscera, the theory of channels and collaterals, and has been summarized through long term clinical practice. It is closely related to physiological features of viscera, channels and collaterals, accumulation of clinical experiences, constant revision of the system of Chinese differentiation and the characteristics of Chinese medicinals. As channels and collaterals connect the interior and exterior and all parts of the body, a pathological change in the exterior may affect the viscera while disease in the viscera may, in turn, express itself on the exterior of the body. The location of the disease and channels and collaterals it travels are different, therefore, clinical manifestations can vary. For example palpitations and insomnia are usually seen in pathological changes of the heart channel, and chest distress and cough are seen in pathological changes of the lung channel, hypochondriac pain and convulsions are mostly seen in pathological changes of the liver channel. Accordingly, *zhū shā* (朱砂, Cinnabaris, Cinnabar) and *yuǎn zhì* (远志, Radix Polygalae, Thinleaf Milkwort Root) can be used to cure palpitations and insomnia, so they are attributed to the heart channel. *Jié gěng* (桔梗, Radix Platycodonis, Platycodon Root) and *sū zǐ* (Fructus Perillae) are able to cure cough and chest distress, so they are attributed to the lung channel. *Bái sháo* (白芍, Radix Paeoniae Alba, White Peony Root) and *gōu téng* (钩藤, Ramulus Uncariae Cum Uncis, Gambir Plant) are chosen to cure hypochondriac pain and convulsions, so they are attributed to the liver channel. A medicinal may be attributed to several channels at once, which indicates the scope of its use. For example, *má huáng* (Herba Ephedrae) is attributed to the lung and urinary bladder channels, and it acts to induce sweating, promote the flow of lung qi and allay asthma, and is used to treat wind cold syndrome in the exterior. It can also promote urination, and is used to treat edema. The above examples show that the theory of entering channels has developed through clinical practice.

III. METHODS OF ENTERING CHANNELS

Determination of channels entered is based on the nature of medicinals, such as shape, color, odor and taste.

Although there are different ideas of entering channels, channel affinity generally has a close relationship with viscera, channels and collaterals. The theory of viscera and the theory of channels and collaterals are the basis for the theory of entering channels. To discuss the essence of channels entered, one should first grasp the theory of the viscera, channels and collaterals.

Differentiation of channels and collaterals differs from that of the viscera, and was the earlier system of differentiation. Therefore, in history, physicians of Chinese medicine placed emphasis on one or the other in determining the channel

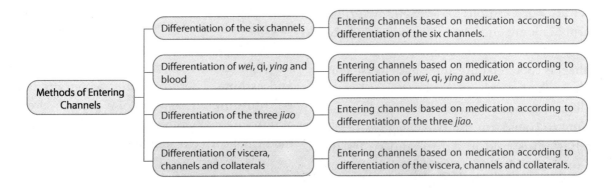

affinity of a medicinal. As a result, there may be different ideas on the entering channels of one medicinal. E.g. *qiāng huó* (羌活, Rhizoma et Radix Notopterygii, Incised Notoptetygium Rhizome and Root) and *zé xiè* (泽泻, Rhizoma Alismatis, Oriental Waterplantain Rhizome) are attributed to the bladder channel. *Qiāng huó* (Rhizoma et Radix Notopterygii) treats headache and general pain and aching of the limbs and joints due to exterior pathogenic cold and dampness. The channel affinity of *qiāng huó* (Rhizoma et Radix Notopterygii) is based on differentiation of channels and collaterals,

because the foot *taiyang* bladder channel dominates the surface and is the first line of defense on the body. *Zé xiè* (Rhizoma Alismatis) has the action of promoting urination and leaching out dampness and is attributed to the viscera of the bladder. Therefore, although the two medicinals enter the same channel, they have different meanings.

IV. SIGNIFICANCE OF CHANNELS ENTERED

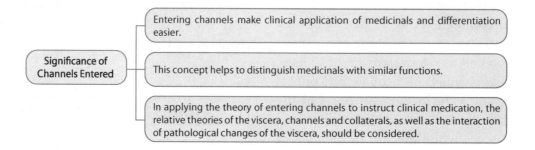

V. THE THEORY OF ENTERING CHANNELS SHOULD BE ASSOCIATED WITH THE FOUR PROPERTIES, FIVE FLAVORS, AND ACTIONS OF ASCENDING, DESCENDING, FLOATING AND SINKING

The channel entering theory should be associated with the theories of the four properties and five flavors, and actions of ascending, descending, floating and sinking of medicinals. Medicinals attributed to the lung channel may have different therapeutic effects due to their differences in properties. For example, *sū yè* (Folium Perillae) is warm in nature and acts to disperse wind cold pathogens from the lung channel. *Bò he* (Herba Menthae) is cool in nature and can disperse wind heat from the lung channel. *Gān jiāng* (Rhizoma Zingiberis) is hot in nature and acts to warm the lung to transform fluids. *Huáng qín* (Radix Scutellariae) is cold in nature and clears fire from the lung. Medicinals attributed to the lung

channel have different therapeutic effects owing to their differences in flavor. For example, *wū méi* (Fructus Mume) is sour in flavor and acts to astringe the lungs to relieve cough. *Má huáng* (Herba Ephedrae) is pungent in flavor and acts to release the exterior and open the lung qi to relieve asthma. *Dǎng shēn* (Radix Codonopsis) is sweet in flavor and replenishes the lung qi. *Chén pí* (Pericarpium Citri Reticulatae) is bitter and can stop cough and transform phlegm. *Gé jiè* (Gecko) is salty in flavor and can invigorate the kidneys and the lungs to relieve asthma. Medicinals which enter the same channels have diverse therapeutic effects due to their different actions of ascending, descending, floating and sinking. For example, *jié gěng* (Radix Platycodonis) and *má huáng* (Herba Ephedrae) have floating actions, so they can open restricted lung qi to relieve cough and asthma. Therefore, only when attention is paid to different aspects of a medicinal can its actions be comprehensively analyzed and the medicinal correctly employed.

Section 5   Toxicity

In documents on herbs, some are marked as "toxic" and "non-toxic". Toxicity is also an important aspect of the characters of medicinals.

I. CONCEPT OF TOXICITY

In ancient times, "*toxicity*" had a broad meaning. All medicinals may generally be considered to be potentially toxic, hyperactive or hypoactive medicinals, or be an indication of side effects. However, in herbal documents of later generations, medicinals were differentiated as "*toxic*", "*extremely toxic*", or "*slightly toxic*" depending on

their adverse effects.

Toxicity generally refers to adverse effects exerted on the human body by medicinals. Toxicity is further divided into acute toxicity, subacute toxicity, subchronic toxicity, chronic toxicity and special toxicity, such as carcinogens, mutagens, affects of abnormal embryo development and addiction. Toxic medicinals are medicinals which may cause impairment, functional disturbance or death due to their chemical or physical actions on the body. Deadly-toxic medicinals are those for which the therapeutic dosage is near the toxic dosage, or is already within the toxic dosage and over dosage may cause a toxic reaction; or it refers to medicinals which may cause irreversible damage to tissues or organs of the human body.

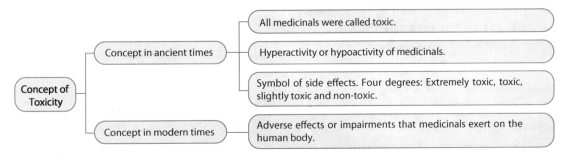

II. DIFFERENCE BETWEEN SIDE EFFECTS AND TOXIC REACTIONS

Side effects of Chinese medicinals refer to any discomfort occurring within the normal dosage, which are unrelated to the therapeutic effects. They are often mild and will vanish once the medicinals are discontinued. Potential side effects of Chinese medicinals are related to various factors, including character, processing, preparation and compatibility of medicinals. Side effects can usually be avoided to a large extent. An allergic reaction is also a potential side effect, which may manifest as itching, skin rash, chest oppression, or rapid breathing. In severe cases, there may be allergic shock. Along with the medicinals, allergic reaction is usually associated with the constitution of the patient. In addition, some medicinals have several functions,

such as *cháng shān* (常山, Radix Dichroae, Dichroa Root). *Cháng shān* can treat malaria as well as induce vomiting. If it is used to treat malaria, the action of inducing vomiting will be the side effect. Therefore, side effects are sometimes relative.

Toxic reactions refer to any damage on the human body resulting from medication, often caused by overdose or long term use. Toxic reactions also are dependant on body constitution.

III. CORRECT ATTITUDE TOWARD TOXICITY

Approaching toxicity of Chinese medicinals correctly is the key to safe administration of medicinals. Several points should be considered, one should:

1. Have a comprehensive evaluation of

toxicity.

2. Be conscientious in the approach to records in herbal documents.

3. Note clinical reports of toxic actions of medicinals.

4. Correctly administer toxic medicinals.

IV. MAIN REASONS FOR TOXIC REACTIONS

The main reasons are:

1. Overdose. For example, medicinals such as *mǎ qián zǐ* (马钱子, Semen Strychni, Nux Vomica) and *fù zǐ* (Radix Aconiti Lateralis Praeparata) can lead to toxic reactions when they are used for a long time or in large doses.

2. Taking incorrect medicinals by mistake. For example, *huà shān shēn* (华山参, Radix Physochlainae, Funnelid Physochlaina Root) or *shāng lù* (商陆, Radix Phytolaccae, Pokeberry Root) are sometimes mistaken for *rén shēn* (Radix et Rhizoma Ginseng), and *dú jiǎo lián* (独角莲, Rhizoma Typhonii, Giant Typhonium Rhizome) is used instead of *tiān má* (Rhizoma Gastrodiae).

3. Improper processing and preparation. For example, *fù zǐ* (Radix Aconiti Lateralis Praeparata) and *chuān wū* (Radix Aconiti) are toxic when unprepared.

4. Improper administration of medicinals. *Fù zǐ* (Radix Aconiti Lateralis Praeparata) and *chuān wū* (Radix Aconiti) are toxic when decocted for only a short period. Many prescriptions will cause toxic reactions when patients catch cold or eat raw or cold food after medication.

5. Incompatibility of medicinals. For example, poisoning caused by simultaneous application of *gān suì* (甘遂, Radix Kansui, Gansui Root) with *gān cǎo* (Radix et Rhizoma Glycyrrhizae), *chuān wū* (Radix Aconiti), *cǎo wū* (草乌, Radix Aconiti Kusnezoffii, Kusnezoff Monkshood Root) or *fù zǐ* (Radix Aconiti Lateralis Praeparata) with *guā lóu* (瓜蒌, Fructus Trichosanthis, Snakegourd Fruit) or *tiān huā fěn* (天花粉, Radix Trichosanthis, Snakegourd Root).

6. Other factors include improper storage, difference in variety, prescription form, medication approach and syndrome patterns, long term application of a certain medicinal, improper medication, self-medication, and medication of nursing mothers and individual differences (constitution, age, etc.).

Therefore, all aspects mentioned above should be well understood to avoid toxic reactions from toxic medicinals.

It should be noted that while toxic medicinals more easily cause toxic reactions, it is not to say that non-toxic medicinals will not induce toxic reactions in any case. There have been reports of toxic reactions from *rén shēn* (Radix et Rhizoma Ginseng), *ài yè* (艾叶, Folium Artemisiae Argyi, Argy Wormwood Leaf) and *zhī mǔ* (Rhizoma Anemarrhenae), which were closely related to overdose or long term use. It is said that:"*Non-toxic medicinals may do harm to the human body if used improperly*" (所谓无毒，亦可伤人) and "*Dà huáng (Radix et Rhizoma Rhei) can be used as a tonic if used according to syndrome differentiation, and tonics like rén shēn (Radix et Rhizoma Ginseng) or lù róng* (鹿茸, *Cornu Cervi Pantotrichum, Deer Velvet*) *can be toxic if used improperly*"(药证相符，大黄也补；药不对证，参茸亦毒).

V. THE MEANING OF MASTERING TOXICITY OF CHINESE MEDICINALS IN CLINICAL PRACTICE

1. When using toxic medicinals, one must properly select medicinals and determine dosages according to the patient's constitution and disease depth. Such medicinals should not be overused and should be discontinued as soon as possible to prevent overdose and cumulative poisoning. At the same time, one must consider incompatibility, and make careful decisions to reduce toxicity. For some toxic medicinals, appropriate preparations are required. In addition, individual differences should be accommodated by increasing or decreasing the dosage of medicine. Self-medication should be avoided. As for the pharmaceutical sector, they must make efforts toward proper identification

and supervision of Chinese medicinals and safeguard toxic medicinals to ensure medication safety and avoid toxic reactions.

2. Some toxic medicinals have remarkable medical effects when chosen properly. Their use is based on the principle of "attacking toxin with toxin," with a prerequisite of safety. For example, *xióng huáng* (雄黄, Realgar, Realgar) is used to treat toxic sores and swellings; *shuǐ yín* (水银, Hydrargyrum, Mercury) is used to treat scabies and syphilis; and *pī shuāng* (砒霜, Arsenicum

Sublimatum, Arsenic Sublimate) is used to treat leukemia.

3. The toxicity of medicinals and clinical manifestations of poisoning should be thoroughly understood so that appropriate and effective treatment will be given in case of toxic reactions. This contributes to the first aid for toxic reactions of Chinese medicinals.

Tables to test your herbal knowledge of the Four Properties and Five Flavors are as follows (Tables 4-1 and 4-2).

Table 4-1: Test your Herbal Knowledge of the Four Properties:

	Cold and Cool Medicinals	**Warm and Hot Medicinals**
Clear heat		
Warm the interior		
Purge fire		
Dispel cold		
Cool blood		
Detoxify		
Supplement fire to strengthen yang		
Warm and activate channels and collaterals		
Rescue devastated yang		

Table 4-2: Test your Herbal Knowledge of the Five Flavors:

Actions \ Flavors	**Pungent**	**Sweet**	**Sour**	**Bitter**	**Salty**	**Astringent**	**Bland**
Promote qi circulation							
Invigorate blood							
Tonify							
Disperse							
Moderate actions of other medicinals							
Purge fire							
Astringe							
Descend rebellious qi							
Harmonize the spleen and stomach							
Promote urination							
Relieve constipation							
Soften hard masses							
Relieve spasms and pain							
Consolidate yin							
Dry dampness							

Chapter 5
Compatibility

I. CONCEPT OF COMPATIBILITY

Compatibility refers to the selective use of two or more medicinals for different diseases according to their character and function.

II. PURPOSE OF COMPATIBILITY

Purpose of Compatibility

To strengthen the therapeutic effects. For example, *má huáng* (Herba Ephedrae) is used in combination with *guì zhī* (Ramulus Cinnamomi) to strengthen its action of dispelling pathogenic factors from the exterior through sweating.

To reduce or eliminate toxicity or side effects. For example, the toxicity of *bàn xià* (Rhizoma Pinelliae) is reduced when used in combination with *shēng jiāng* (Rhizoma Zingiberis Recens).

To adapt to complex pathological conditions in order to treat both the principal and secondary symptoms. For example, applying both tonification and purgation for syndromes with mixed excess and deficiency.

To expand on the indications. For example, *huáng lián* (Rhizoma Coptidis) is used with *wú zhū yú* (Fructus Evodiae) to treat vomiting of sour materials and hypochondriac distending pain caused by fire transformed from liver depression attacking the stomach.

III. CONTENT OF COMPATIBILITY

The Concept of the Seven Relations

In the application of medicinals, sometimes a single medicinal is used alone, and sometimes two or more medicinals are used together. Seven relations refer to the seven types of herbal combinations. These are acting alone, mutual accentuation, mutual enhancement, mutual counteraction, mutual suppression, mutual antagonism and mutual incompatibility.

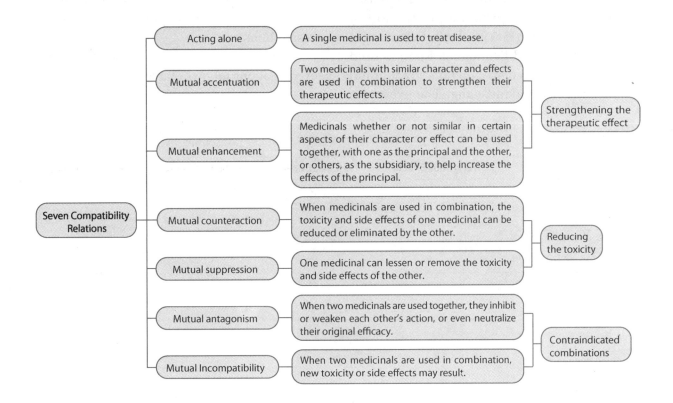

Acting alone	A single medicinal is used to treat disease.	
Mutual accentuation	Two medicinals with similar character and effects are used in combination to strengthen their therapeutic effects.	Strengthening the therapeutic effect
Mutual enhancement	Medicinals whether or not similar in certain aspects of their character or effect can be used together, with one as the principal and the other, or others, as the subsidiary, to help increase the effects of the principal.	
Mutual counteraction	When medicinals are used in combination, the toxicity and side effects of one medicinal can be reduced or eliminated by the other.	Reducing the toxicity
Mutual suppression	One medicinal can lessen or remove the toxicity and side effects of the other.	
Mutual antagonism	When two medicinals are used together, they inhibit or weaken each other's action, or even neutralize their original efficacy.	Contraindicated combinations
Mutual Incompatibility	When two medicinals are used in combination, new toxicity or side effects may result.	

Seven Compatibility Relations

IV. PRINCIPLES IN COMPATIBILITY

1. Mutual accentuation and mutual enhancement can enhance therapeutic effects and are commonly used in clinical practice.

2. Mutual counteraction and mutual suppression can reduce or eliminate side effects and therefore guarantee safety. These combinations are used for medicinals with severe toxicity or side effects, as well as in the processing and preparation of toxic medicinals and as antidotes for poisoning.

3. Mutual antagonism and mutual incompatibility should be avoided in clinical use.

In short, mutual accentuation and mutual enhancement make medicinals work in coordination and enhance therapeutic effects. Mutual counteraction and mutual suppression can reduce or eliminate positive or negative effects, and mutual antagonism and mutual incompatibility should be avoided.

V. COMPATIBILITY OF PAIRED MEDICINALS

Paired medicinals refer to medicinals used in combination in order to strengthen their effects, to reduce or eliminate toxicity and side effects, or to generate new effects. For example, *guì zhī* (Ramulus Cinnamomi) used in combination with *bái sháo* (Radix Paeoniae Alba) acts to regulate the *ying* and *wei,* and relieve exterior syndromes. *Chái hú* (Radix Bupleuri) is used together with *huáng qín* (Radix Scutellariae) to harmonize the *shaoyang* channel to eliminate fever. Together, *zhǐ shí* (Fructus Aurantii Immaturus) and *bái zhú* (Rhizoma Atractylodis Macrocephalae) can both tonify and purge. *Gān jiāng* (Rhizoma Zingiberis) with *wǔ wèi zǐ* (Fructus Schisandrae Chinensis) can descend and diffuse the lung qi. *Huáng lián* (Rhizoma Coptidis) used with *gān jiāng* (Rhizoma Zingiberis) is able to regulate yin and yang. *Ròu guì* (Cortex Cinnamomi) and *huáng lián* (Rhizoma Coptidis) are used to treat heart and kidney miscommunication. *Huáng qí* (Radix Astragali) is used with *dāng guī* (Radix Angelicae Sinensis) to supplement qi to promote production of blood. *Shú dì huáng* (熟地黄, Radix Rehmanniae Praeparata, Prepared Rehmannia Root) is used with *fù zǐ* (Radix Aconiti Lateralis Praeparata) to nourish both yin and yang. The examples mentioned above have all been handed down through clinical experience. Paired medicinals make up of the main part of many herbal prescriptions.

A table to test your herbal knowledge of the seven relations follows (Table 5-1):

Table 5-1: Test your Herbal Knowledge of the Seven Relations:

	Strengthen Effects	Reduce Effects	Increase Toxicity	Reduce Toxicity
Mutual accentuation				
Mutual enhancement				
Mutual counteraction				
Mutual suppression				
Mutual antagonism				
Mutual incompatibility				

Chapter 6
Contraindications

Contraindications in the use of herbs must be taken note of in order to ensure therapeutic effects and medication safety, as well as to prevent toxic reactions and side effects. Four main aspects are addressed: Incompatible combinations in prescriptions, contraindicated patterns, contraindications during pregnancy and dietary contraindications.

I. INCOMPATIBILITY IN PRESCRIPTIONS

① Concept of Incompatibility in Prescriptions

Incompatibility in prescriptions refers to the use of medicinal combinations which can cause toxic reactions or side effects, or reduce their original therapeutic effects. Such combinations should be avoided.

② Main Contents of Incompatibility in Prescriptions

Incompatibilities in prescriptions are summarized by the "eighteen incompatibilities" and "nineteen antagonisms."

(1) Eighteen incompatibilities

Chuān wū (Radix Aconiti), *cǎo wū* (Radix Aconiti Kusnezoffii) and *fù zǐ* (Radix Aconiti Lateralis Praeparata, Monkshood Root) are incompatible with *bàn xià* (Rhizoma Pinelliae), *guā lóu* (Fructus Trichosanthis), *tiān huā fěn* (Radix Trichosanthis, Snakegourd Root), *chuān bèi mǔ* (Bulbus Fritillariae Cirrhosae), *zhè bèi mǔ* (Bulbus Fritillariae Thunbergii), *bái liǎn* (白蔹, Radix Ampelopsis, Ampelopsis) and *bái jí* (白及, Rhizoma Bletillae, Bletilla Rhizome).

Gān cǎo (Radix et Rhizoma Glycyrrhizae) is incompatible with *hǎi zǎo* (Sargassum), *jīng dà jǐ* (京大戟, Radix Euphorbiae Pekinensis, Spurge), *gān suì* (Radix Kansui) and *yuán huā* (芫花, Flos Genkwa, Lilac Daphne Flower Bud).

Lí lú (藜芦, Radix et Rhizoma Veratri Nigri, Eranthis Hyemalis) is compatible with *rén shēn* (Radix et Rhizoma Ginseng), *shā shēn* (沙参, Radix Glehniae, Root of Straight Ladybell), *dān shēn* (Radix et Rhizoma Salviae Miltiorrhizae), *xuán shēn* (玄参, Radix Scrophulariae, Figwort Root), *xì xīn* (Radix et Rhizoma Asari), *bái sháo* (Radix Paeoniae Alba) and *chì sháo* (赤芍, Radix Paeoniae Rubra, Red Peony Root).

(2) Nineteen antagonisms

Liú huáng (硫黄, Sulphur, Sulphur) antagonizes *pò xiāo* (朴硝, Mirabilitum, Mirabilite), *shuǐ yín* (Hydrargyrum) antagonizes *pī shuāng* (Arsenicum Sublimatum); *láng dú* (狼毒, Radix Euphorbiae Fischerianae, Leopard's Bane) antagonizes *mì tuó sēng* (密陀僧, Lithargyrum, Lithargyrum); *bā dòu* (巴豆, Semen Crotonis, Croton Seed) antagonizes *qiān niú zǐ* (牵牛子, Semen Pharbitidis, Pharbitidis Seed); *dīng xiāng* (丁香, Flos Caryophylli, Clove) antagonize *yù jīn* (郁金, Radix Curcumae,

Turmeric Root Tuber); *ròu guì* (Cortex Cinnamomi) antagonizes *chì shí zhī* (Halloysitum Rubrum); *chuān wū* (Radix Aconiti) and *cǎo wū* (Radix Aconiti Kusnezoffii) antagonize *xī jiǎo* (犀角, Cornu Rhinocerotis, Rhinoceros Horn); *yá xiāo* (牙硝, Mirabilitum, Crystallized Mirabilite) antagonizes *sān léng* (三棱, Rhizoma Sparganii, Common Burreed Tuber); and *rén shēn* (Radix et Rhizoma Ginseng) antagonizes *wǔ líng zhī* (五灵脂, Faeces Trogopterori, Excrementum Pteropi).

③ Conscientious Approach to the Eighteen Incompatibilities and Nineteen Antagonisms

(1) There are different opinions as to whether the medicinals named in the eighteen incompatibilities may be used together or not. Some physicians believe that using these medicinals together will cause increased toxicity and damage to the human body. It has been reported that incompatible medicinals such as *chuān wū* (Radix Aconiti) or *cǎo wū* (Radix Aconiti Kusnezoffii) used with *chuān bèi mǔ* (Bulbus Fritillariae Cirrhosae) or *zhè bèi mǔ* (Bulbus Fritillariae Thunbergii), and *bā dòu* (Semen Crotonis) used with *qiān niú zǐ* (Semen Pharbitidis) resulted in toxic reactions. Therefore, it is stipulated in the 1963 edition of the *Pharmacopeia of the People's Republic of China*: "*Medicinals noted as antagonists or as incompatible should not be used together*" (畏、恶、反，系指一般情况下不易同用).

(2) However, there are also documents recording simultaneous use of incompatible medicinals. In these cases, it is believed that the simultaneous use of incompatible medicinals complement each other and cure obstinate and critical diseases. Relative reports range from the treatment of cirrhosis and nephritic edema with the combination of *gān suì* (Radix Kansui) and *gān cǎo* (Radix et Rhizoma Glycyrrhizae), and the treatment of coronary artery disease with *rén shēn* (Radix et Rhizoma Ginseng) and *wǔ líng zhī* (Faeces Trogopterori), to the treatment of tuberculous pleurisy with *yuán huā* (Flos Genkwa), *jīng dà jǐ* (Radix Euphorbiae Pekinensis) and *gān suì* (Radix Kansui) with *gān cǎo* (Radix et Rhizoma Glycyrrhizae). In all the above cases,

good therapeutic effects were achieved, which affirmed this viewpoint.

(3) Thus it can be seen that since there is no conclusive agreement in either document research or clinical and experimental study, further research must be undertaken.

(4) It is prudent to use incompatible medicinals cautiously and under no circumstances should these medicinals be used in combination before sound experimental basis and clinical experience are obtained.

II. CONTRAINDICATED PATTERNS

There are indications for each of the medicinals. Use of medicinals for diseases or syndromes other than those which are indicated are "*contraindicated patterns*".

For instance, *má huáng* (Herba Ephedrae) is pungent and warm and acts to dispel wind cold pathogens from the exterior through sweating, and opens the lung qi to relieve asthma and promote urination. Thus it is usually used for excess type exterior syndrome due to exogenous wind cold manifesting with no sweating and coughs with dyspnea due to impaired dispersion of the lung qi. It is contraindicated for spontaneous sweating due to exterior deficiency, night sweats due to yin deficiency and deficiency type asthma due to failure of the kidney to regulate respiration. *Huáng jīng* (黄精, Rhizoma Polygonati, Solomonseal Rhizome), sweet and neutral, acts to nourish yin and the lung, invigorate the spleen and replenish qi and is used for dry cough due to lung deficiency, and diseases caused by spleen and stomach weakness and kidney essence deficiency. As it may cause stagnation and dampness, it is not suitable for patients with cough and profuse phlegm due to dampness from spleen deficiency, and loose stools due to coldness in the middle *jiao*. Therefore, except for some mild and moderate medicinals, most medicinals have contraindications. Details are found under "*precautions*" of each medicinal.

III. CONTRAINDICATIONS DURING PREGNANCY

① Concept of Contraindications during Pregnancy

Some medicinals can harm the original qi of the fetus and lead to miscarriage; therefore they are contraindicated or given cautiously during pregnancy. Contraindicated medicinals refer to medicinals prohibited during pregnancy other than those used for to assist post-miscarriage.

② Why Contraindicated Medicinals are not Intended to Induce Abortion

(1) From an historical perspective, abortion was against the traditional moral values in ancient China. Records on abortive medicinals were mainly collected to understand contraindications during pregnancy rather than to induce abortion.

(2) It is dangerous and unreliable to use contraindicated medicinals for abortion.

(3) Contraindicated medicinals were initially collected for preventing miscarriage during early pregnancy.

③ Reasons for Contraindications during Pregnancy

(1) Detrimental to pregnant women.
(2) Detrimental to the fetus.
(3) Detrimental to the reproductive process.
(4) Detrimental to infants.

④ Classification for Prohibited and Taboo Medicinals

There are many classifications of contraindicated medicinals, which cause different kinds of damage to the human body, therefore they should be understood and treated individually. In ancient times, mainly prohibited and contraindicated medicinals were mentioned. In modern times, based on clinical practice according to the damage caused to the fetus, medicinals are classified into contraindicated medicinals and medicinals given cautiously during pregnancy.

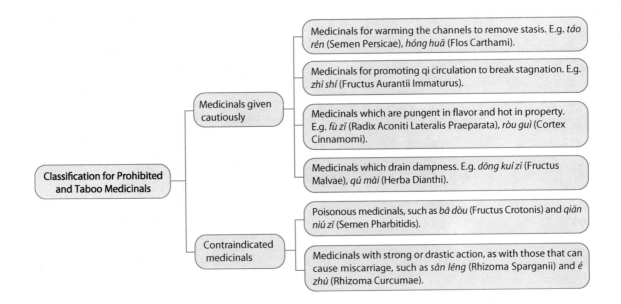

Classification for Prohibited and Taboo Medicinals

Medicinals given cautiously:
- Medicinals for warming the channels to remove stasis. E.g. *táo rén* (Semen Persicae), *hóng huā* (Flos Carthami).
- Medicinals for promoting qi circulation to break stagnation. E.g. *zhǐ shí* (Fructus Aurantii Immaturus).
- Medicinals which are pungent in flavor and hot in property. E.g. *fù zǐ* (Radix Aconiti Lateralis Praeparata), *ròu guì* (Cortex Cinnamomi).
- Medicinals which drain dampness. E.g. *dōng kuí zǐ* (Fructus Malvae), *qú mài* (Herba Dianthi).

Contraindicated medicinals:
- Poisonous medicinals, such as *bā dòu* (Fructus Crotonis) and *qiān niú zǐ* (Semen Pharbitidis).
- Medicinals with strong or drastic action, as with those that can cause miscarriage, such as *sān léng* (Rhizoma Sparganii) and *é zhú* (Rhizoma Curcumae).

⑤ Application Principles in Prohibited and Taboo Medicinals

(1) Contraindicated medicinals should be avoided under any circumstance.

(2) Medicinals to be given cautiously can be used in pathological conditions with attention to proper dosage and therapeutic course and with correct differentiation. Appropriate processing, preparation and combinations are used to reduce as much possibility of damage to the pregnancy as possible. If not absolutely necessary, they should not be used so as to avoid any adverse consequences.

IV. DIETARY RESTRICTIONS

① Concept of dietary restrictions

During the course of treatment with medicinals, certain foods which are inappropriate for the disease or contraindicated for use with a certain medicinal should be avoided or limited.

② Contents of dietary restrictions

Dietary restrictions may include restrictions during diseases and restrictions during administration of medicinals.

Tables to test your herbal knowledge of contraindications follow (Tables 6-1~6-3, p.39 & 40):

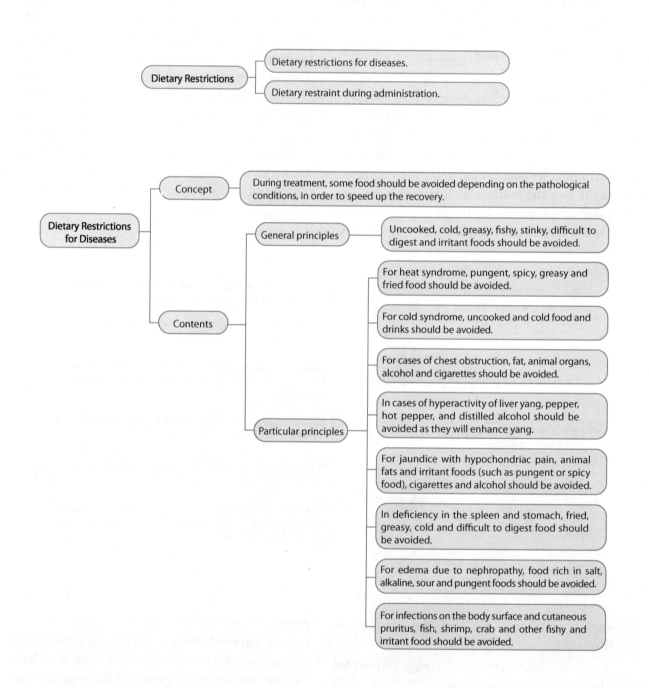

Dietetic Restraint during Administration

Concept — During a course of medication, the intake of some medicinals should be avoided so as not to reduce the therapeutic effects or cause toxic reactions

Records in documents —

Gān cǎo (Radix et Rhizoma Glycyrrhizae), *huáng lián* (Rhizoma Coptidis), *jié gěng* (Radix Platycodonis) and *wū méi* (Fructus Mume) are counteracted by pork.

Biē jiǎ (Carapax Trionycis) is counteracted by edible amaranth.

Cháng shān (Radix Dichroae) is counteracted by raw scallion.

Dì huáng (Radix Rehmanniae) and *hé shǒu wū* (Radix Polygoni Multiflori) are counteracted by raw scallion, garlic and radish.

Dān shēn (Radix et Rhizoma Salviae Miltiorrhizae), *fú líng* (Poria) and *fú shén* (Sclerotium Poriae Pararadicis) are counteracted by vinegar.

Tǔ fú líng (Rhizoma Smilacis Glabrae) and *shǐ jūn zǐ* (Fructus Quisqualis) are counteracted by tea.

Bò he (Herba Menthae) is counteracted by crab.
Honey is antagonistic to raw scallion; and persimmon is antagonistic to crabs.

Table 6-1: Test your Herbal Knowledge on the Eighteen Incompatibilities:

	Chuān wū	Cǎo wū	Fù zǐ	Lí lú	Gān cǎo
Chì sháo					
Bái sháo					
Gān suì					
Chuān bèi mǔ					
Zhè bèi mǔ					
Rén shēn					
Bàn xià					
Dān shēn					
Xuán shēn					
Guā lóu					
Shā shēn					
Bái jí					
Jīng dà jǐ					
Bái sháo					
Bái liǎn					
Xì xīn					
Tiān huā fěn					
Hǎi zǎo					
Chì sháo					
Yuán huā					

Table 6-2: Test your Herbal Knowledge of the Nineteen Antagonisms:

	Liú huáng	Láng dú	Bā dòu	Dīng xiāng	Shuǐ yín	Chuān wū	Cǎo wū	Pò xiāo	Ròu guì	Rén shēn
Wǔ líng zhī										
Sān léng										
Qiān niú zǐ										
Chì shí zhī										
Mì tuó sēng										
Pí shuāng										
Xī jiǎo										
Yù jīn										
Yá xiāo										

Table 6-3: Test your Herbal Knowledge of Classification of Contraindications during Pregnancy:

	Medicinals which dredge the channels to remove stasis	Drastic medicinals	Toxic medicinals	Draining medicinals	Pungent and hot medicinals	Miscarriage inducing medicinals	Medicinals which promote qi circulation and break stasis
Contraindicated medicinals							
Medicinals given cautiously							

Chapter 7
Dosage and Administration

Section 1   Dosage

I. THE CONCEPT OF DOSAGE

Dosage means the amount of medicinals to be used. It mainly refers to the daily amount of each medicinal for an adult (note: the dosage of each medicinal in this book refers to an adult's daily dose of dried medicinal in a decoction if not otherwise noted). Dosage also refers to the relative amount of different medicinals in a formula.

II. MEASUREMENT UNITS FOR CHINESE MEDICINALS

Measurement units are:

1. Weight units. Chinese units are *jin, liang, qian, fen* and *li*. Metric units are kilogram, gram and milligram.

2. Amount units, such as three slices of *shēng jiāng* (Rhizoma Zingiberis Recens), two strips of *wú gōng* (蜈蚣, Scolopendra, Centipede), seven pieces of *dà zǎo* (Fructus Jujubae), a segment of *lú gēn* (芦根, Rhizoma Phragmitis, Reed Rhizome), a leaf of *hé yè* (荷叶, Folium Nelumbinis, Lotus Leaf) or two segments of *cōng bái* (葱白, Bulbus Allii Fistulosi, Scallion).

3. Imperial units, such as foot (*chi*) and inch (*cun*).

4. Volume units such as *dou* (10 liters), *sheng* (liter), *he* (deciliter) and *shao* (centiliter).

In addition, there are other rough measurement methods as "*dao gui*" (special measure for medicinal powder), "*fang cun bi*" (Chinese square inch), "*cuo*" (a pinch) and "*mei*" (a small amount).

With the modern changes in weight and measurement systems, weight is now used to measure solid medicinals.

III. CONVERSION BETWEEN ANCIENT AND MODERN WEIGHT OF CHINESE MEDICINALS

Since the *Ming* and *Qing* Dynasties, imperial units have been extensively used in China, i.e. 1 *jin* = 16 *liang* = 160 *qian*. From the year of 1979, metric units have been used for the measurement of Chinese medicinals, in which 1 kg = 1,000 g = 1,000,000 mg. For convenient calculation, they are converted as the following approximate values: 1 *liang* (hexadecimal system) = 30 g; 1 *qian* = 3 g; 1 *fen* = 0.3 g; 1 *li* = 0.03 g.

IV. FACTORS WHICH INFLUENCE DOSAGE

Since most Chinese medicinals are raw medicinals,

the range of safe dosages are wide and the dosage of medicinals is not as strict as that of chemicals. However, the proper dosage of medicinals directly determines the therapeutic effects. Small doses of medicinals may not take effect and therefore influence pathological conditions. Overdose will lead to side effects or cause waste. In general, the following aspects should be considered when deciding the dosage of a medicinal.

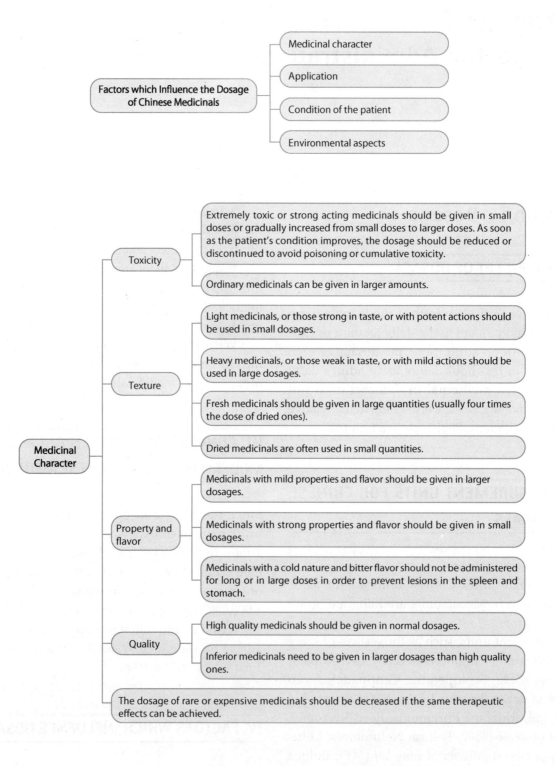

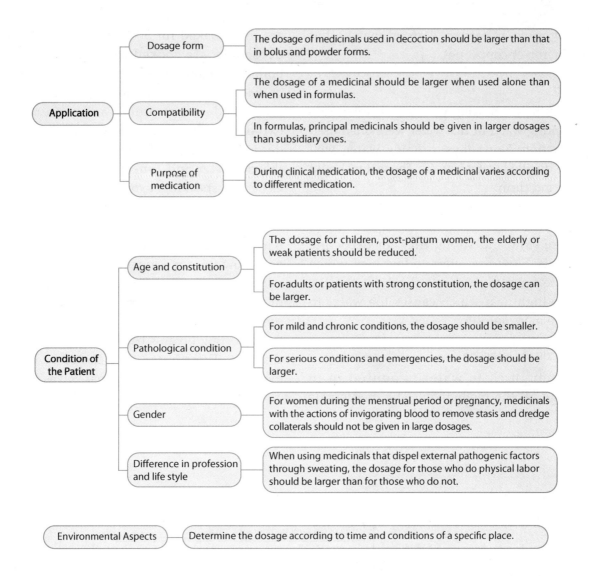

V. DOSAGE CONSIDERATIONS RELATED TO REGION, SEASONAL CHANGES, AND LOCAL ENVIRONMENT

When determining dosage, factors such as season, climate and natural environment should be taken into consideration. In summer, medicinals that dispel external pathogens through sweating, and pungent and warm or extremely hot medicinals are not recommended for use. However, in the winter, they can be used frequently. In summer, bitter and cold medicinals which descend fire can be used in large dosages, while in winter, the dosage should be reduced.

Except for some extremely toxic, harsh, refined or precious medicinals, the oral dosage for plant medicinals or animal gelatins is about 5-10 g. The common dosage for mineral and shell medicinals without toxicity is often 15-30 g. For fresh medicinals, the common dosage is 30-60 g.

Section 2   Administration

I. DECOCTING METHODS

① Container

When preparing a decoction, medicinals are put into a container with a relatively stable chemical property, such as earthenware or enamel, but never an iron or copper pot.

② Water

In ancient times, flowing water, well water, rain water, spring water or rice water were often used for decoction. Nowadays, running water, well water or distilled water is used. The water should be fresh and clean.

③ Fire

There are slow and strong fires for decocting medicinals. Slow fire refers to low heat which allows the water to evaporate slowly. Strong fire refers to high heat which causes the water to evaporate more quickly.

④ Methods of Decocting

First, enough clean water is poured in to submerge all the medicinals. The medicinals are then soaked for 30-60 minutes. In general, decoctions are cooked twice. For the second boiling, the amount of water should be 1/3-1/2 of that in the first decoction. The two decoctions are mixed and strained, and then taken in two doses. The amount of water used and the decocting time should be decided according to the character and function of the medicinals. Generally speaking, exterior-resolving and heat clearing medicinals should be decocted with strong fire for a short period of time, usually 3-5 minutes after boiling. Tonics should be simmered on a slow fire for a longer period, usually 30-60 minutes after boiling. To guarantee the quality of the decoction and increase the therapeutic effects, some medicinals require special treatment during the decocting process because of their particular character. These instructions should be noted on the prescription and are summarized as follows:

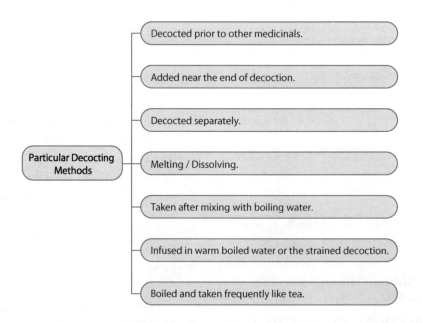

Particular Decocting Methods

- Decocted prior to other medicinals.
- Added near the end of decoction.
- Decocted separately.
- Melting / Dissolving.
- Taken after mixing with boiling water.
- Infused in warm boiled water or the strained decoction.
- Boiled and taken frequently like tea.

Decocted Prior to other Medicinals

As some mineral or shell medicinals are so hard that their active components cannot be easily extracted, they should be boiled before adding other medicinals. Such medicinals include *cí shí* (Magnetitum) and *dài zhě shí* (Haematitum).

Some toxic medicinals such as *fù zǐ* (Radix Aconiti Lateralis Praeparata), *chuān wū* (Radix Aconiti) and *cǎo wū* (Radix Aconiti Kusnezoffii) should also be decocted first to reduce side effects.

Added near the End of Decoction

Some aromatic medicinals, such as *bò he* (Herba Menthae) and *chén xiāng* (Lignum Aquilariae Resinatum) must be added near the end to preserve their aromatic properties.

After decocting for a long period, the active components in some medicinals may be destroyed, such as *gōu téng* (Ramulus Uncariae Cum Uncis) and *dà huáng* (Radix et Rhizoma Rhei).

Decocted Separately

Also known as simmering alone, this method is mainly used for expensive medicinals such as *rén shēn* (Radix Ginseng), *xī yáng shēn* (Radix Panacis Quinquefolii) and *líng yáng jiǎo* (Cornu Saigae Tataricae).

Melting/ Dissolving

Gelatins or other sticky medicinals should be melted or dissolved in boiling water or in the finished decoction for oral administration. E.g. *ē jiāo* (Colla Corii Asini), *lù jiǎo jiāo* (Colla Cornus Cervi).

Taken after Mixing with Boiling Water

The active components in some medicinals are easily extracted with water or they are susceptible to rapid break down by decocting for a long time. E.g. *fān xiè yè* (Folium Sennae).

Infused in Warm Boiled Water or the Strained Decoction

Some precious medicinals such as *shè xiāng* (Moschus) and *niú huáng* (Calculus Bovis).

Medicinals used to improve therapeutic effects, such as *sān qī* (Radix et Rhizoma Notoginseng).

The therapeutic effects of some medicinals will be reduced or the active components are not easily extracted in water. E.g. *léi wán* (Omphalia), *hè cǎo yá* (Gemma Agrimoniae).

Some liquid medicinals, such as *zhú lì* (Succus Bambusae), *jiāng zhī* (Succus Rhizomatis Zingiberis).

Boiled and Taken Frequently like Tea

Some medicinals are difficult for direct oral administration, such as *zào xīn tǔ* (Terra Flava Usta)

Some light medicinals are used in large dosages and will absorb a large amount of water, such as *yù mǐ xū* (Stigma Maydis).

II. METHODS OF ADMINISTRATION

① Time of Administration

Usually one packet of medicinals is given per day in two doses, the interval period being 4-6 hours. In clinical practice, this can be adjusted according to the patient's condition. For example, for acute or febrile disease, two packets may be given per day.

Most medicinals should not be taken immediately before or after meals so as not to influence digestion and therapeutic effects.

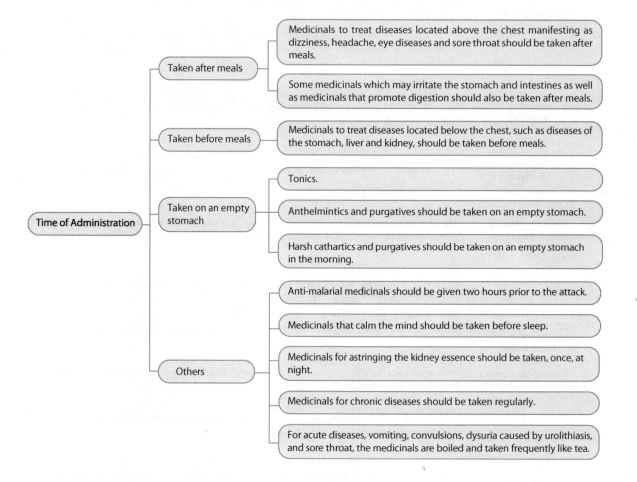

② Methods of Administration

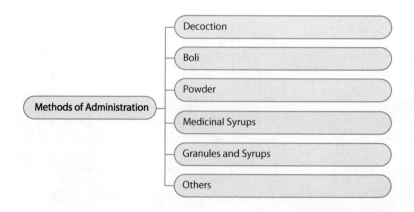

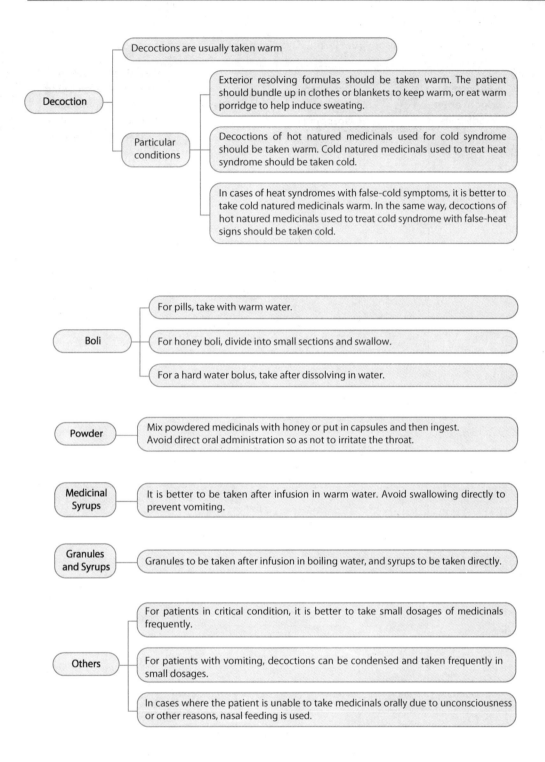

Decoction
- Decoctions are usually taken warm
- Particular conditions
  - Exterior resolving formulas should be taken warm. The patient should bundle up in clothes or blankets to keep warm, or eat warm porridge to help induce sweating.
  - Decoctions of hot natured medicinals used for cold syndrome should be taken warm. Cold natured medicinals used to treat heat syndrome should be taken cold.
  - In cases of heat syndromes with false-cold symptoms, it is better to take cold natured medicinals warm. In the same way, decoctions of hot natured medicinals used to treat cold syndrome with false-heat signs should be taken cold.

Boli
- For pills, take with warm water.
- For honey boli, divide into small sections and swallow.
- For a hard water bolus, take after dissolving in water.

Powder
- Mix powdered medicinals with honey or put in capsules and then ingest. Avoid direct oral administration so as not to irritate the throat.

Medicinal Syrups
- It is better to be taken after infusion in warm water. Avoid swallowing directly to prevent vomiting.

Granules and Syrups
- Granules to be taken after infusion in boiling water, and syrups to be taken directly.

Others
- For patients in critical condition, it is better to take small dosages of medicinals frequently.
- For patients with vomiting, decoctions can be condensed and taken frequently in small dosages.
- In cases where the patient is unable to take medicinals orally due to unconsciousness or other reasons, nasal feeding is used.

A table to test your herbal knowledge of particular decocting methods follows overleaf (Table 7-1):

Table 7-1: Test your Herbal Knowledge of Decocting Methods:

Decocting methods / Medicinals	Decocted prior to other medicinals	Decocted later than other medicinals	Decocted with wrapping	Decocted alone	Dissolved	Taken after mixing with boiling water	Taken after being infused with boiled water	Boiled and taken frequently like tea
Mineral and shell								
Powders								
Expensive medicinals								
Medicinals with active components difficult to extract with water								
Light medicinals used in large amounts, large volumes and absorbing large amounts of water								
Medicinals with toxicity or side effects								
Villous medicinals								
Aromatic medicinals								
Medicinals not suitable for extensive decocting								
Sticky fruits and seeds which are difficult to dissolve								
Gelatins								
Sticky and soluble medicinals								

PART 2

Systematic Discussions

Chapter 8
Medicinals that Release the Exterior

Medicinals whose principal effect is to disperse pathogenic factors from the superficial levels of the body and relieve exterior syndrome are called medicinals that release the exterior.

Character and Actions

Medicinals in this chapter are usually light, pungent and dispersing, and they mainly enter the lung and bladder channels. They often travel in the superficial aspects of the body and promote sweating, thereby dispersing pathogenic factors from the exterior and treating exterior syndrome. *The Yellow Emperor's Inner Classic* states: *"To treat diseases in the superficial aspects of the body, sweating can be used"* (其在皮者，汗而发之). In addition, some of these medicinals promote urination to reduce edema, relieve cough and asthma, vent rashes, arrest pain and heal sores.

Indications

Medicinals that release the exterior are used to treat exterior syndrome manifesting as fever with aversion to cold, headache, general aching, lack of or inadequate sweating, and a floating pulse. Some medicinals are also used for edema, cough and wheezing, measles, urticaria, wind-damp *bi* (痹), and early-stage infections on the surface of the body accompanied by exterior syndromes.

Combinations

Medicinals for dispersing wind-cold or wind-heat should be chosen accordingly. Medicinals with the actions of relieving summer heat, transforming dampness and moistening dryness should be added according to seasonal changes and their respective pathogenic factors. For patients with weak constitutions and excess pathogens, medicinals with the actions of boosting qi, reinforcing yang, supplementing yin and nourishing blood should be used according to the patient's constitution. For early-stage febrile diseases with pathogens in the *wei* level, medicinals with the actions of clearing heat and toxins should be used together with medicinals for dispersing wind heat.

Precautions

The dosage of exterior releasing medicinals must be carefully attended to, and these medicinals should be discontinued as soon as the patient's condition has improved. Otherwise, excessive sweating may lead to consumption of yang qi and damage to the body fluids, and cause depletion of yang or yin. Sweat is also a body fluid, and blood and sweat share the same source. For symptoms of spontaneous sweating, night sweating due to yin deficiency, prolonged sores, urinary strangury, and patients with blood loss, medicinals for releasing the exterior should be used cautiously even when there is an exterior syndrome. Dosages of these medicinals should also be adjusted according to region and season. In spring and summer, people tend to perspire easily, so the dosage should be lighter, while in winter, it should be larger. In the north of China where it is colder, the dosage should be larger, while in the south, it should be lighter. Most of these medicinals are aromatic. Therefore, to prevent any decrease in efficacy, prolonged boiling should be avoided.

Classification

According to their character and function, medicinals that release the exterior are divided into two groups: Medicinals that disperse wind-cold and medicinals that disperse wind-heat. These are also called "warm acrid medicinals for resolving the exterior" and "cool, acrid medicinals for resolving the exterior."

Section 1   Medicinals that Disperse Wind Cold

Medicinals of this kind have strong dispersing actions, chiefly for dispersing wind cold. They are indicated for exterior syndrome due to wind cold, manifesting as fever with aversion to cold, lack of sweating, headache, general body aches, nasal obstruction and discharge, a thin white tongue coating, and a floating and tight pulse. Some of these medicinals can be used to dispel wind to relieve itching, stop pain, relieve cough and asthma, promote urination to reduce edema, eliminate infections on the body surface, as well as urticaria with itching, wind damp *bi*, cough with shortness of breath, edema and early stage skin diseases accompanied by wind cold exterior syndrome.

① *Má huáng* (麻黄, Herba Ephedrae, Ephedra) ★ ★ ★

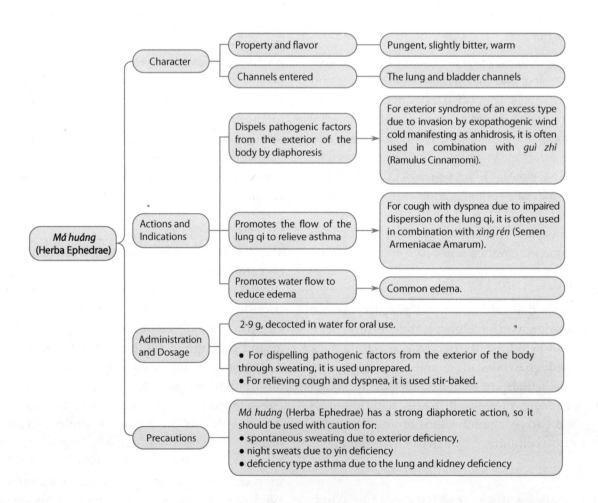

	Character	Property and flavor	Pungent, slightly bitter, warm
		Channels entered	The lung and bladder channels
Má huáng (Herba Ephedrae)	Actions and Indications	Dispels pathogenic factors from the exterior of the body by diaphoresis	For exterior syndrome of an excess type due to invasion by exopathogenic wind cold manifesting as anhidrosis, it is often used in combination with *guì zhī* (Ramulus Cinnamomi).
		Promotes the flow of the lung qi to relieve asthma	For cough with dyspnea due to impaired dispersion of the lung qi, it is often used in combination with *xìng rén* (Semen Armeniacae Amarum).
		Promotes water flow to reduce edema	Common edema.
	Administration and Dosage	2-9 g, decocted in water for oral use.	
		• For dispelling pathogenic factors from the exterior of the body through sweating, it is used unprepared. • For relieving cough and dyspnea, it is used stir-baked.	
	Precautions	*Má huáng* (Herba Ephedrae) has a strong diaphoretic action, so it should be used with caution for: • spontaneous sweating due to exterior deficiency, • night sweats due to yin deficiency • deficiency type asthma due to the lung and kidney deficiency	

② *Guì zhī* (桂枝, Ramulus Cinnamomi, Cassia Twig)
★ ★ ★

Both *má huáng* (Herba Ephedrae) and *guì zhī* (Ramulus Cinnamomi) are pungent in flavor and warm in nature, and enter the lung and bladder channels. They dispel pathogenic factors from the exterior through sweating and can be used for excess type exterior disorders due exogenous wind cold, manifesting as aversion to cold, fever, headache, body aches, absence of sweating, and a floating and tight pulse. The two medicinals are frequently used in combination for mutual accentuation. However, *má huáng* (Herba Ephedrae) has a bitter flavor, promotes the flow of lung qi, opens the interstices and has a stronger diaphoretic action, and is regarded as the most important medicinal for inducing sweating. It is mainly indicated for excess type exterior disorders due to wind cold without sweating. It is also used to diffuse the lung qi to

calm wheezing and promotes urination to reduce edema. It is therefore indicated for cough with shortness of breath due to impaired dispersion of the lung qi or retention of a heat pathogen in the lung, and edema. In addition, it can be used for wind cold *bi*, yin abscesses and phlegm nodules. *Guì zhī* (Ramulus Cinnamomi) is pungent, sweet and warm, and also enters the heart channel. It can warm and activate the defensive yang to release the exterior through sweating, but its diaphoretic action is not as strong as that of *má huáng* (Herba Ephedrae). *Guì zhī* (Ramulus Cinnamomi) therefore can be used for both excess and deficient type exterior disorders. It is also used for warming and activating the channels and vessels, and for reinforcing yang to promote the flow of qi. It is indicated for pain due to cold congealing and blood stasis, such as heart pain caused by devitalization of chest yang and obstruction of heart vessels; vague pain in the

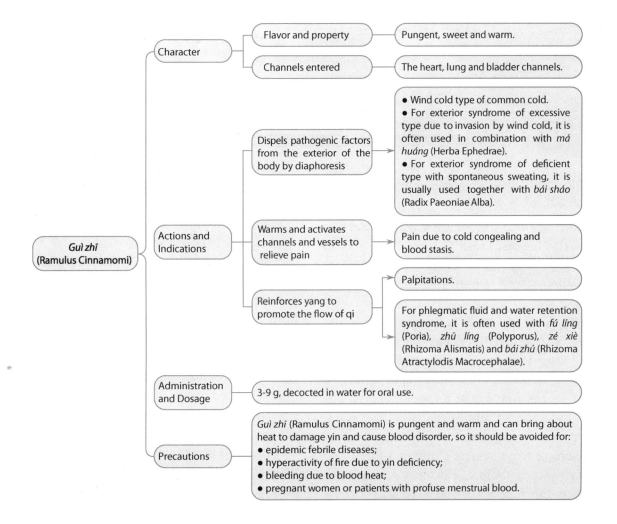

epigastrium and abdomen which is relieved by warmth and pressure due to deficient cold in the middle *jiao*, irregular menstruation, amenorrhea, dysmenorrhea, postpartum abdominal pain caused by blood stasis due to pathogenic cold in the blood, and aching joints of the shoulders and limbs due to wind-cold dampness. It is also used for vertigo, palpitations, cough due to water retention; edema and dysuria due to poor qi transformation in the urinary bladder; palpitations, slow-irregular or slow-weak pulse

with regular intervals caused by failure to activate blood vessels due to hypofunction of chest yang.

③ *Zǐ sū yè* (紫苏叶, Folium Perillae, Perilla Leaf) ★★★
Addition: *Zǐ sū gěng* (紫苏梗, **Caulis Perillae, Perilla Stem**) can soothe the chest and diaphragm, guide qi downwards and prevent miscarriage. It is indicated for qi stagnation and distension in the chest and diaphragm, excessive fetal movement, threatened miscarriage and hypochondriac distending pain.

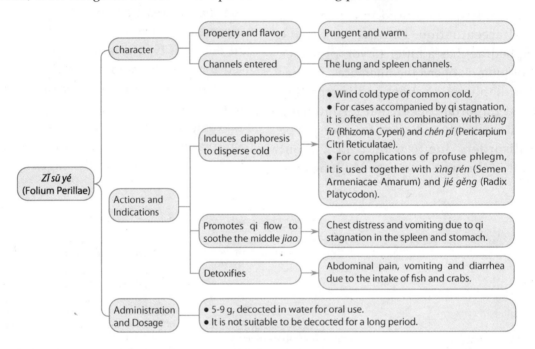

Zǐ sū yé
(Folium Perillae)

- Character
  - Property and flavor —— Pungent and warm.
  - Channels entered —— The lung and spleen channels.
- Actions and Indications
  - Induces diaphoresis to disperse cold
    - Wind cold type of common cold.
    - For cases accompanied by qi stagnation, it is often used in combination with *xiāng fù* (Rhizoma Cyperi) and *chén pí* (Pericarpium Citri Reticulatae).
    - For complications of profuse phlegm, it is used together with *xìng rén* (Semen Armeniacae Amarum) and *jié gěng* (Radix Platycodon).
  - Promotes qi flow to soothe the middle *jiao* —— Chest distress and vomiting due to qi stagnation in the spleen and stomach.
  - Detoxifies —— Abdominal pain, vomiting and diarrhea due to the intake of fish and crabs.
- Administration and Dosage
  - 5-9 g, decocted in water for oral use.
  - It is not suitable to be decocted for a long period.

④ *Shēng jiāng* (生姜, Rhizoma Zingiberis Recens, Fresh Ginger) ★★

Addition: *Shēng jiāng pí* (生姜皮, **Exodermis Zingiberis Recens, Fresh Ginger Peel**) acts to harmonize the spleen to promote urination to reduce edema, and is indicated for edema and dysuria.

Shēng jiāng zhī (生姜汁, **Succus Rhizomatis Zingiberis, Zingiber Juice**) has the same actions as *shēng jiāng* (Rhizoma Zingiberis Recens) and is especially good for relieving vomiting by removing phlegm, and is convenient for emergencies. For symptoms such as numbness, swelling pain, constant vomiting and an inability to eat caused by poisoning from *bàn xià* (Rhizoma Pinelliae) and *tiān nán xīng* (天南星, Rhizoma Arisaematis, Jackinthepulpit Tuber), it can be taken after soaking

in boiling water. It is used in combination with *zhú lì* (竹沥, Succus Bambusae, Bamboo Juice) to treat syncope due to stroke via nasal feeding or ingesting after soaking in boiled water.

Both *zǐ sū yè* (Folium Perillae) and *shēng jiāng* (Rhizoma Zingiberis Recens) are pungent and warm and are attributed to the lung and spleen channels. Both can induce sweating to disperse cold and detoxify. They are indicated for fever with aversion to cold, headache and nasal obstruction due to pathogenic wind cold; and vomiting, diarrhea, abdominal pain due to poisoning from seafood. They have a moderate exterior releasing action, and can be used alone in mild cases. For severe cases, they are used in combination with other medicinals which release the exterior. *Zǐ sū yè* (Folium Perillae) acts to induce sweating to disperse cold in the

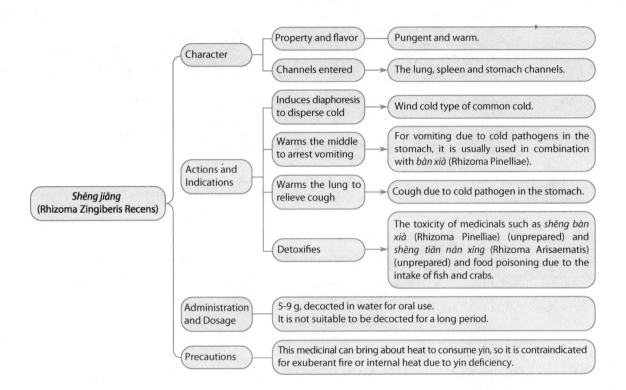

exterior, and promote qi flow to soothe the middle in the interior, as well as transform phlegm to relieve cough. It is indicated for chest and epigastric fullness and distress, nausea, vomiting or cough with profuse phlegm due to wind cold type exterior syndrome accompanied by qi stagnation. *Zǐ sū yè* (Folium Perillae) also can regulate qi circulation to prevent miscarriage, and is used for chest distress and vomiting due to qi stagnation in the spleen and stomach or upward flow of fetal qi, excessive fetal movement due to qi stagnation and plum-pit qi due to phlegm congealing and qi stagnation caused by depression. *Shēng jiāng* (Rhizoma Zingiberis Recens) warms the middle to relieve vomiting, and is regarded the best medicinal to stop vomiting. It can also warm the lung to relieve cough and detoxify, and is usually used for cold syndromes in the spleen and stomach, including cold invading the middle *jiao* and deficient type cold syndrome in the middle, manifesting as gastric cold pain, poor appetite and vomiting. It is effective for relieving vomiting, and is used for various vomiting when combined using herbal compatibility. *Shēng jiāng* (Rhizoma Zingiberis Recens) is a medicinal for warming the stomach; therefore, it is most suitable for vomiting due to cold in the stomach. As for cough due to cold in the lung, it can be used

whether or not there is an exterior syndrome of wind-cold type or phlegm. It can be used to treat poisoning by *bàn xià* (Rhizoma Pinelliae) and *tiān nán xīng* (Rhizoma Arisaematis), and is used for processing *bàn xià* (Rhizoma Pinelliae) and *tiān nán xīng* (Rhizoma Arisaematis) so as to reduce their toxicity.

⑤ *Xiāng rú* (香薷, Herba Moslae, Haichow Elsholtzia Herb) ★ ★

Both *má huáng* (Herba Ephedrae) and *xiāng rú* (Herba Moslae) are pungent and warm. They both can dispel external pathogenic factors through sweating as well as promote urination to reduce edema. Both are indicated for symptoms such as aversion to cold, fever, headache, lack of sweating and edema with an exterior syndrome. *Má huáng* (Herba Ephedrae) has a stronger diaphoretic action but cannot transform dampness and harmonize the middle. It is used for wind cold type exterior syndrome. It can also promote the flow of the lung qi to relieve asthma and promote urination to reduce edema. *Xiāng rú* (Herba Moslae) is inferior to *má huáng* (Herba Ephedrae) in dispersing cold and inducing sweating. It is better at transforming dampness and harmonizing the middle to remove summer-

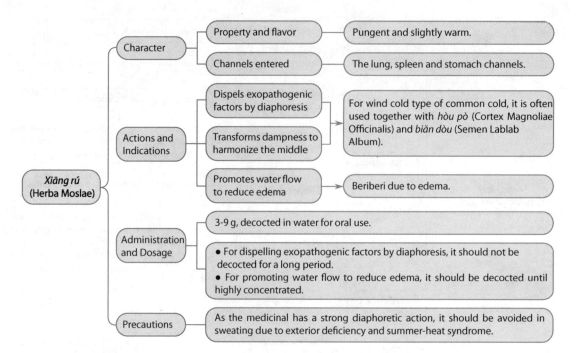

heat. Therefore, it is often used for retention of dampness in the spleen and stomach with wind cold type of common cold, manifesting as aversion to cold, fever, headache, heavy body, absence of sweating, gastric fullness, poor appetite, a greasy tongue coating, or nausea, vomiting and diarrhea (yin type summer heat

syndrome). As the above symptoms are mostly seen in patients who consume cold food and drinks during the summer, *xiāng rú* (Herba Moslae) is known as "summertime *má huáng*."

⑥ *Jīng jiè* (荆芥, Herba Schizonepetae, Fineleaf Schizonepeta Herb) ★ ★ ★

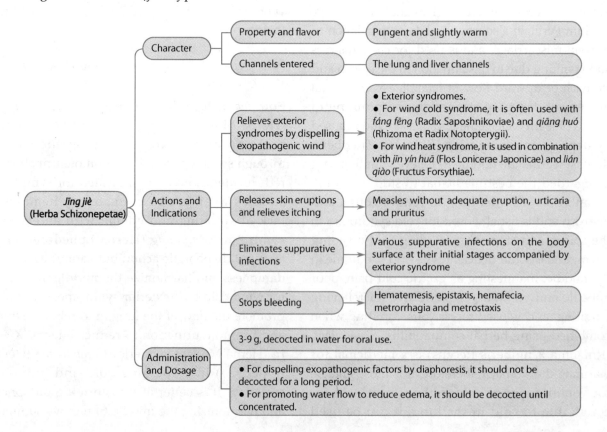

⑦ *Fáng fēng* (防风, Radix Saposhnikoviae, Divaricate Saposhnikovia Root) ★ ★ ★

Both *jīng jiè* (Herba Schizonepetae) and *fáng fēng* (Radix Saposhnikoviae) are pungent and slightly warm; both release the exterior by dispelling wind. Both are indicated for exterior syndromes manifesting as common cold of either wind cold type manifesting with fever, aversion to cold, headache and absence of sweat, or wind heat type manifesting with fever, slight aversion to cold and wind, headache, sore throat, as well as urticaria and pruritus. However, *jīng jiè*'s (Herba Schizonepetae) airy texture has a stronger diaphoretic action than *fáng fēng* (Radix Saposhnikoviae) and is usually chosen for common cold of either wind cold type or wind heat type. It can also vent rashes, eliminate various suppurative infections on the body surface and stop bleeding, so it is used for early stage measles with inadequate eruption, suppurative infections on the body surface in

their initial stages, with exterior syndromes, and various bleeding disorders such as hematemesis, epistaxis, hemafecia, and heavy or chronic uterine bleeding. *Fáng fēng* (Radix Saposhnikoviae) is spongy and moist in texture and is considered a moist medicinal in dispelling wind or a versatile medicinal in dispelling pathogenic wind. It can remove dampness to relieve pain and relieve spasm. It is indicated for headache, heavy body and pain of the four limbs caused by wind cold exterior syndrome, joint pain and spasm of the sinews caused by wind-cold damp *bi*, spasm of muscles, convulsion of the four limbs and opisthotonus due to tetanus. In addition, owing to its ascending nature and ability to dry dampness, it is also used for diarrhea due to the inability of the clear yang to ascend due to spleen deficiency causing damp accumulation, and diarrhea with pain due to disharmony between the liver and spleen.

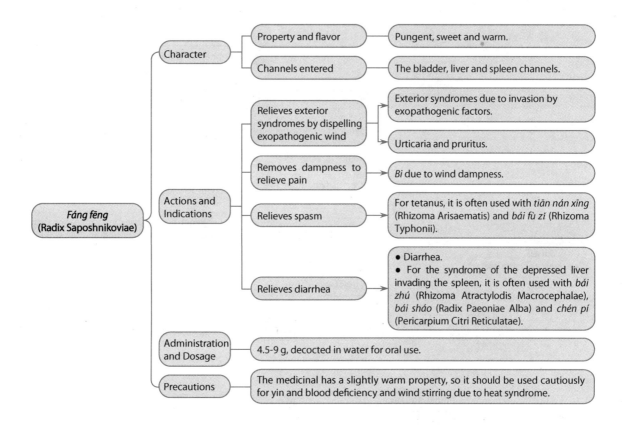

⑧ *Qiāng huó* (羌活, Rhizoma et Radix Notopterygii, Incised Notoptetygium Rhizome and Root) ★ ★ ★

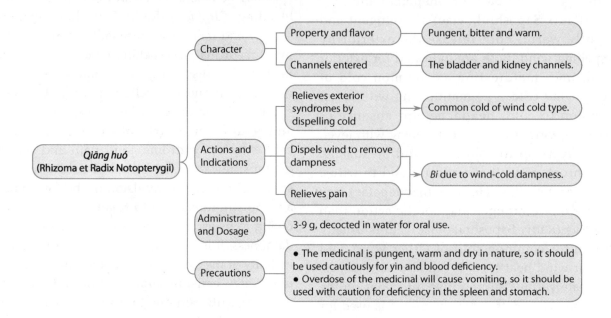

⑨ *Bái zhǐ* (白芷, Radix Angelicae Dahuricae, Dahurian Angelica Root) ★ ★ ★

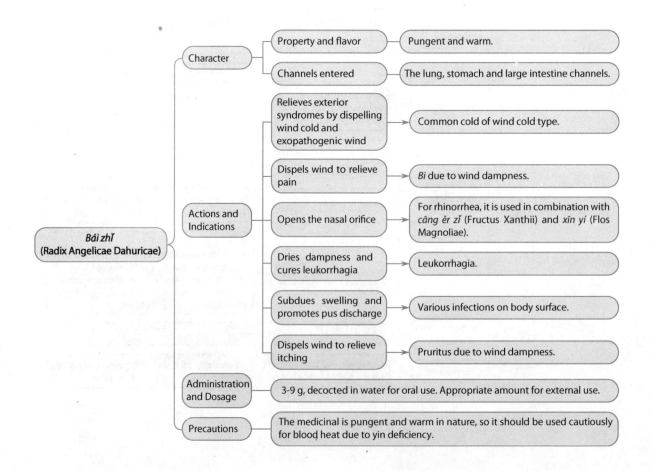

⑩ *Xì xīn* (细辛, Radix et Rhizoma Asari, Manchurian Wildginger) ★★

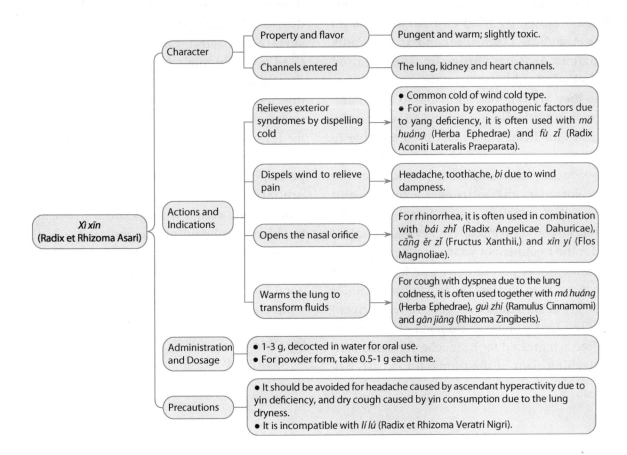

⑪ *Gāo běn* (藁本, Rhizoma Ligustici, Chinese Lovage) ★★

Qiāng huó (Rhizoma et Radix Notopterygii), *bái zhǐ* (Radix Angelicae Dahuricae), *xì xīn* (Radix et Rhizoma Asari) and *gǎo běn* (Rhizoma Ligustici) are all pungent, warm, aromatic and dry in nature. They all release the exterior by dispelling cold, dispel wind to relieve pain, and are effective at relieving pain. *Qiāng huó* (Rhizoma et Radix Notopterygii), *bái zhǐ* (Radix Angelicae Dahuricae) and *gǎo běn* (Rhizoma Ligustici) also can remove dampness. These four medicinals are

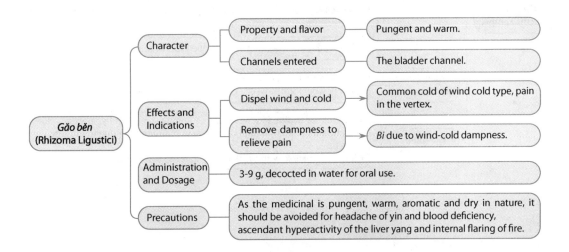

indicated for common cold with severe headache or general body aches due to wind cold or wind cold with dampness, and joint and general body pain caused by wind-cold damp *bi*. *Bái zhǐ* (Radix Angelicae Dahuricae) and *xì xīn* (Radix et Rhizoma Asari) are aromatic, and are used to dispel wind-cold and open the nasal orifices, and so they are especially suitable to treat nasal obstruction with discharge due to wind cold. These two medicinals are often used together to treat runny nose with nasal obstruction, discharge and headache. However, *qiāng huó* (Rhizoma et Radix Notopterygii) is strongly aromatic, and therefore has a strong action in releasing the exterior, dispelling wind and relieving pain. It is used for the treatment of joint, shoulder and back pain in the upper part of body due to wind-cold damp *bi*, because it enters the foot *taiyang* bladder channel. *Bái zhǐ* (Radix Angelicae Dahuricae) enters the foot *yangming* stomach channel and therefore is indicated for headache, forehead pain and swelling pain of the gums. It can also dry

dampness to cure leukorrhagia, reduce swelling and promote pus discharge, dispel wind to relieve itching and is used to treat leukorrhagia due to wind dampness, infections on the body surface and wind damp type pruritus. *Xì xīn* (Radix et Rhizoma Asari) has a strong cold-dispelling action and is used for both exterior and interior cold syndromes. It warms the lungs to transform fluids as well. It is therefore indicated for fever with aversion to cold, lack of sweating and a deep pulse due to contraction of external pathogens due to yang deficiency, headache, orbital pain, and toothache along the *shaoyin* channel, and cough with shortness of breath due to either wind cold or accumulated cold fluids caused by cold in the lung. *Gǎo běn* (Rhizoma Ligustici) ascends to the top of the head, so it is good for treating severe pain in the vertex due to wind-cold.

⑫ *Cāng ěr zǐ* (苍耳子, Fructus Xanthii, Canthium Fruit) ★★

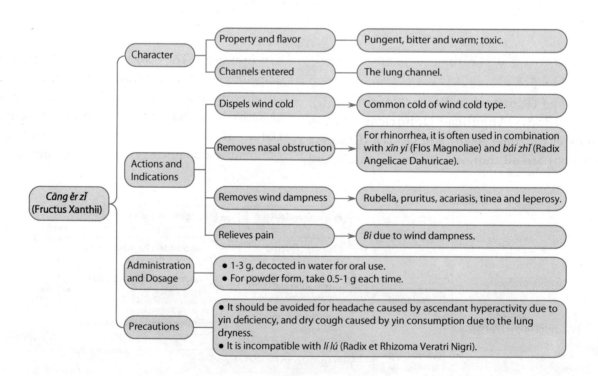

⑬ *Xīn yí* (辛夷, Flos Magnoliae, Blond Magnolia Flower) ★★

Both *cāng ěr zǐ* (Fructus Xanthii) and *xīn yí* (Flos Magnoliae) dispel wind cold and remove nasal obstruction; therefore they are indicated for runny nose with symptoms such as headache, nasal obstruction and discharge. They are also used to treat headache and nasal obstruction caused by wind cold. However, the two should be carefully differentiated. *Cāng ěr zǐ* (Fructus Xanthii) is slightly toxic, and removes wind dampness and relieves pain. It is used for spasm of the limbs due to wind damp *bi*, urticaria, pruritus, scabies, tinea and leprosy. *Xīn yí* (Flos Magnoliae) has an ascending nature, and mainly treats diseases on the face and head, so it is used to open the orifices. It is considered especially effective in treating runny nose with headache, nasal obstruction and discharge.

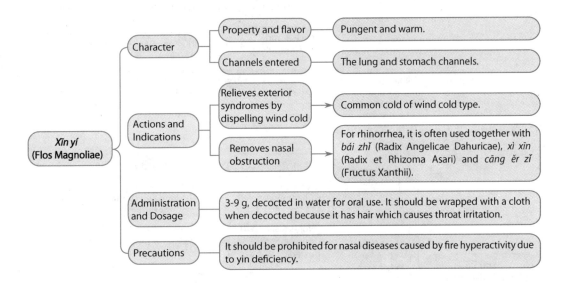

⑭ *Cōng bái* (葱白, Bulbus Allii Fistulosi, Scallion)

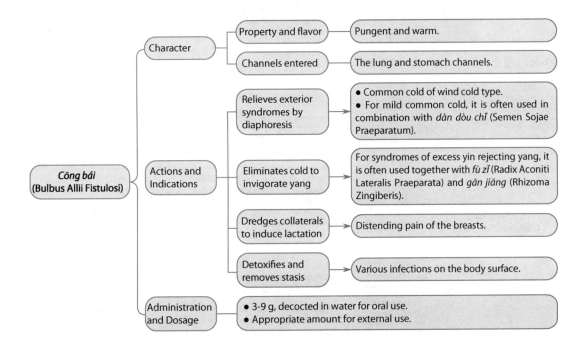

⑮ *É bù shí cǎo* (鹅不食草, Herba Centipedae, Small Centipeda Herb)

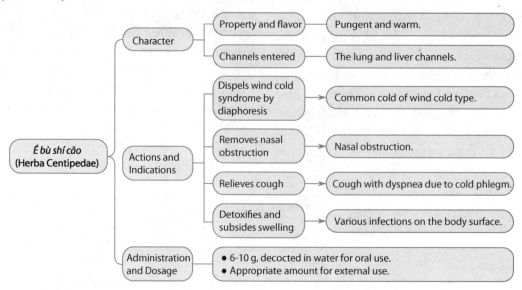

⑯ *Hú suī* (胡荽, Herba Coriandri Sativi, Coriander Herb)

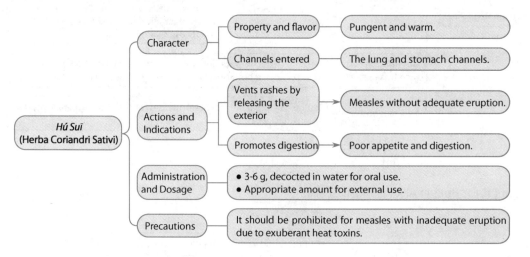

⑰ *Chéng liǔ* (柽柳, Cacumen Tamaricis, Chinese Tamarisk Twig)

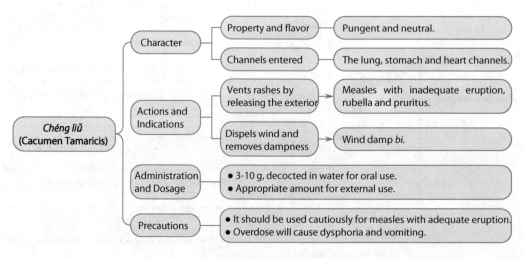

Section 2 Medicinals that Disperse Wind Heat

Medicinals that disperse wind heat usually have a pungent or bitter flavor and cold or cool nature. Their diaphoretic action is comparatively mild and they are mainly used for expelling pathogenic wind heat. These medicinals are indicated for wind heat exterior syndrome, with signs and symptoms such as high fever with slight aversion to cold, thirst, headache, conjunctival congestion, a red tongue tip and a thin yellow coating, and a floating and rapid pulse. Some of these medicinals can be used for clearing the head, improving eyesight, relieving sore throat, venting rashes, relieving itching and cough. They are also indicated for blood-shot eyes, excessive tearing, sore and swollen throat, measles with inadequate eruption, urticaria, pruritus and cough caused by wind heat.

① *Bò he* (薄荷, Herba Menthae, Peppermint) ★ ★ ★

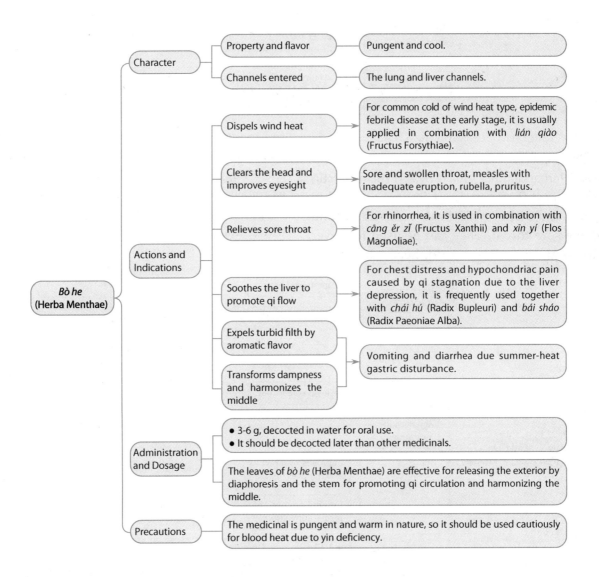

② *Niú bàng zǐ* (牛蒡子, Fructus Arctii, Great Burdock Achene) ★★★

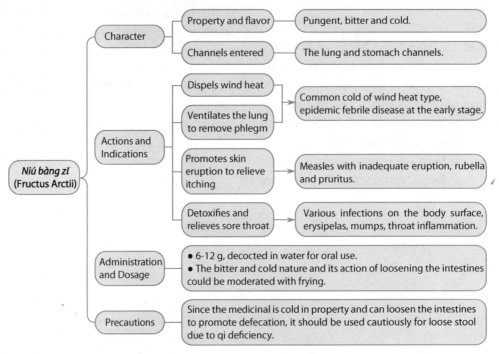

③ *Chán tuì* (蝉蜕, Periostracum Cicadae, Cicada Molting) ★★

Bò he (Herba Menthae), *niú bàng zǐ* (Fructus Arctii) and *chán tuì* (Periostracum Cicadae) are cold in nature and dispel wind heat, vent rashes, and relieve sore throat. They can be used for fever with slight aversion to cold, headache, thirst, red tongue tip, thin yellow tongue coating and a floating and rapid pulse due to wind heat or early stage epidemic febrile disease manifesting as measles in the initial stage with inadequate eruption, urticaria, pruritus, sore and a swollen throat due to flaring-up of wind heat. However, *bò he* (Herba Menthae) is pungent, aromatic

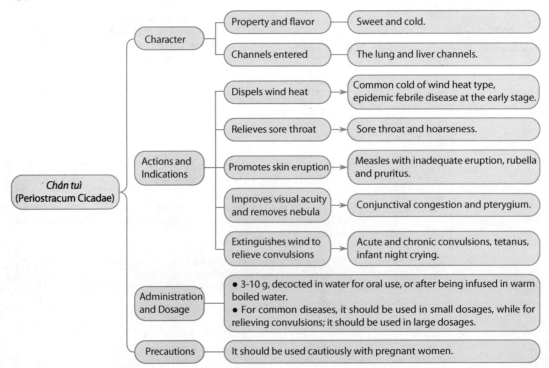

and cool, has a strong diaphoretic action, and so is the first choice for wind heat manifesting as fever without sweating. It can also clear the head, improve eyesight and soothe the liver to promote qi flow. Therefore, it is indicated for headache, conjunctival congestion, excessive tearing due to wind heat flaring upward, chest distress, hypochondriac distending pain, and irregular menstruation with a wiry pulse caused by qi stagnation due to the liver depression. *Niú bàng zǐ* (Fructus Arctii) is pungent, bitter and cold, and can disseminate the lung to eliminate phlegm, so it is most suitable for fever, cough with incomplete expectoration due to wind heat or lung heat. It can dispel wind heat from the exterior, detoxify internal heat toxins, and reduce swelling. It is often used for heat toxin syndrome manifesting as infections on the body surface and erysipelas. It can also moisten the intestines to promote bowel movements;

therefore, it can be used to treat the above symptoms accompanied by constipation. *Chán tuì* (Periostracum Cicadae) is sweet and cold, and has a light texture. Its diaphoretic action is inferior to that of *bò he* (Herba Menthae), and its heat-clearing action is inferior to that of *niú bàng zǐ* (Fructus Arctii). It can dispel wind heat in the lung channel to relieve sore throat and hoarseness, promote skin eruption to relieve itching, as well as dispel wind heat in the liver channel to promote visual acuity and remove nebulae, and cool the liver to extinguish wind to relieve convulsions. It is often indicated for conjunctival congestion and nebulae due to wind heat flaring upward or ascendant hyperactivity of the liver fire, acute or chronic convulsions and tetanus. In addition, *chán tuì* (Periostracum Cicadae) is usually used to treat infant night-crying.

④ *Sāng yè* (桑叶, Folium Mori, Mulberry Leaf) ★ ★ ★

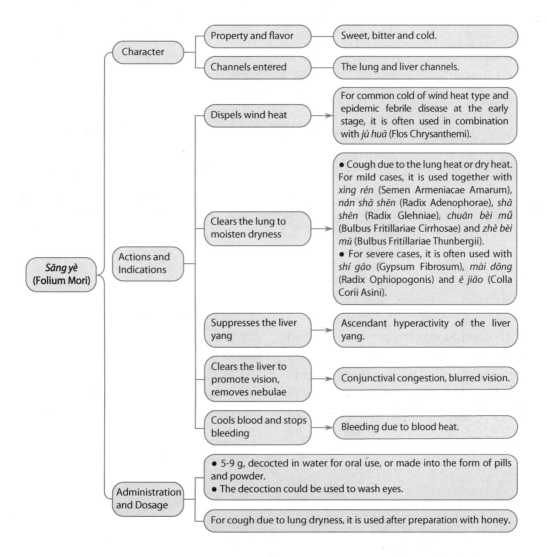

⑤ *Jú huā* (菊花, Flos Chrysanthemi, Chrysanthemun Flower) ★★★

Both *sāng yè* (Folium Mori) and *jú huā* (Flos Chrysanthemi) are sweet and bitter in flavor, cold or cool in property, and dispel wind heat, suppress liver yang, and clear the liver to improve vision. They can be used for fever with slight aversion to cold, headache and cough caused by wind heat or early stage epidemic febrile disease, headache and dizziness due to ascendant hyperactivity of the liver yang, conjunctival congestion due to wind heat flaring upward or liver fire. They are indicated for blurred vision due to kidney and liver deficiency, if combined with medicinals with actions of nourishing the liver and kidney to improve vision.

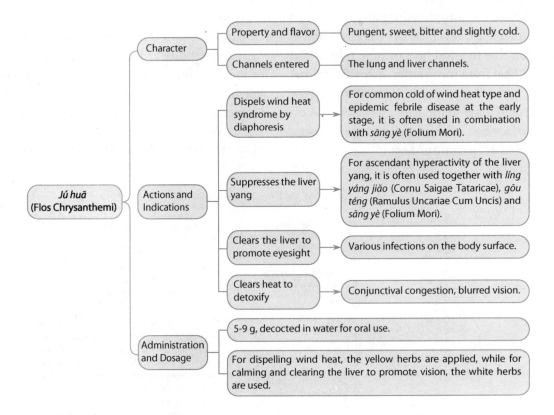

Sāng yè (Folium Mori) strongly dispels wind heat, and is effective for clearing the lung and drying dampness as well as cooling the blood and stopping bleeding. It is indicated for cough with scanty yellow phlegm, dry cough and itchy throat due to lung heat or impairment of the lung by dry heat, hemoptysis, hematemesis and epistaxis due to blood heat.

Jú huā (Flos Chrysanthemi) strongly calms and clears the liver to improve eyesight. It can also clear heat to detoxify, and is used for various infections on the body surface.

⑥ *Màn jīng zǐ* (蔓荆子, Fructus Viticis, Shrub Chastetree Fruit) ★★★

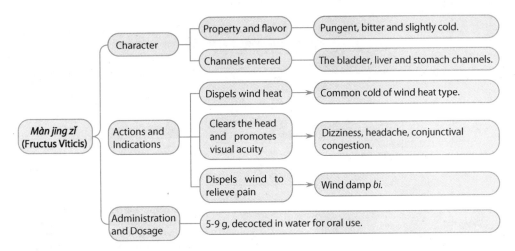

⑦ *Chái hú* (柴胡, Radix Bupleuri, Bupleurum) ★★★

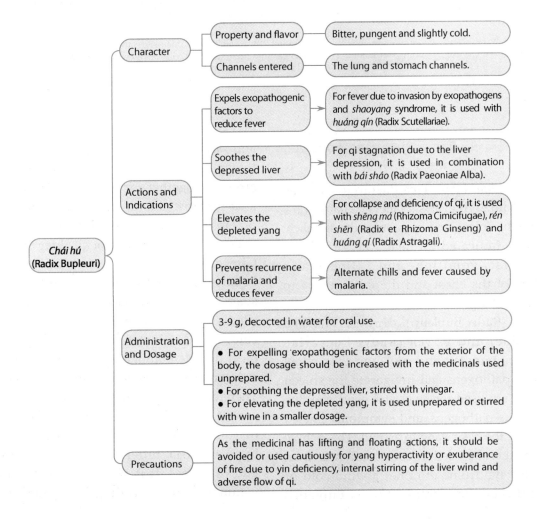

⑧ *Shēng má* (升麻, Rhizoma Cimicifugae, Large Trifoliolious Bugbane Rhizome) ★ ★ ★

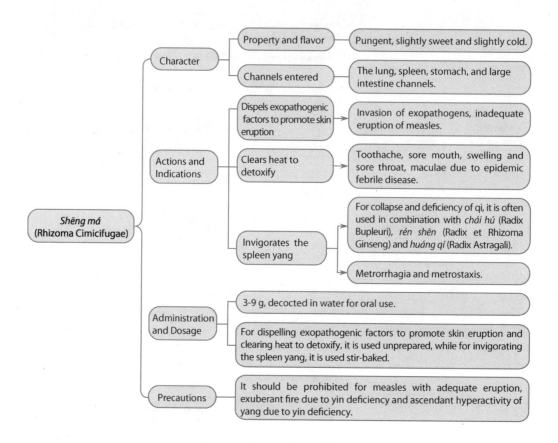

⑨ *Gé gēn* (葛根, Radix Puerariae Lobatae, Kudzuvine Root) ★ ★ ★

Addition: *Gé huā* (葛花, **Flos Puerariae Lobatae, Flower of Kudzuvine**) acts to alleviate hangovers, invigorate the spleen and harmonize the stomach. It is mainly indicated for headache, dizziness, severe thirst, vomiting, and fullness and distension of the chest and diaphragm due to excessive drinking.

Chái hú (Radix Bupleuri), *shēng má* (Rhizoma Cimicifugae) and *gé gēn* (Radix Puerariae Lobatae) are pungent and cool, and they expel exogenous pathogens and invigorate the spleen yang. They are used for fever and headache due to exogenous pathogens, and symptoms caused by failure of the clear yang to ascend. These three medicinals can be used in combination to treat an exterior syndrome of either a wind cold or wind heat type. Both *chái hú* (Radix Bupleuri)

and *shēng má* (Rhizoma Cimicifugae) invigorate the spleen yang to lift prolapsed organs. They are used together for poor appetite, loose stool, anal prolapse due to chronic diarrhea, stomach prolapse, renal prolapse and uterine prolapse due to deficiency and sinking of qi. *Shēng má* (Rhizoma Cimicifugae) and *gé gēn* (Radix Puerariae Lobatae) can vent rashes and are used for early stage measles with inadequate eruption. *Chái hú* (Radix Bupleuri) is pungent, bitter and slightly cold, and dominates the liver and gallbladder qi. It dispels pathogens between the interstitial striae, reduces fever and soothes liver depression. Therefore, it is often used for *shaoyang* syndrome manifesting as alternate chills and fever, feelings of fullness and discomfort in the chest and hypochondria, bitter taste in the mouth, thirst and dizziness. It is also used for fever due to common cold, distending hypochondriac pain,

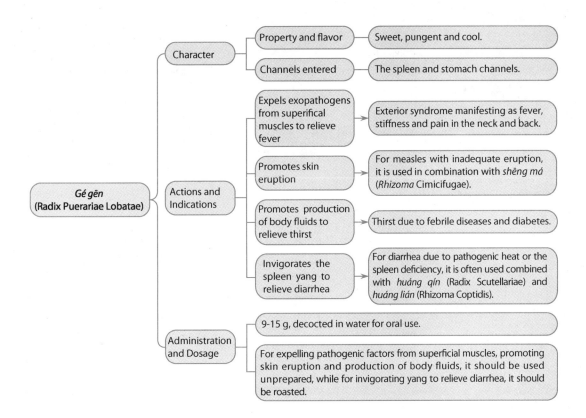

irregular menstruation, dysmenorrhea caused by qi stagnation due to liver depression, and malaria. *Shēng má* (Rhizoma Cimicifugae) mainly lifts the clear yang in the spleen and stomach, and has a stronger lifting action than *chái hú* (Radix Bupleuri). It clears toxic heat and is used for heat toxin syndrome manifesting as toothache, sore mouth, swollen and sore throat, maculae due to febrile diseases and erysipelas. *Gé gēn* (Radix Puerariae Lobatae) is sweet, pungent and cool. It lifts the clear yang in the spleen and stomach and generates fluids to relieve thirst and diarrhea. It is usually used for thirst due to febrile diseases, diabetes due to yin deficiency, heat diarrhea and diarrhea due to spleen deficiency. It also reduces fever by expelling exogenous pathogens and relieves stiffness and pain in the neck and back due to lack of nourishment of the sinews.

⑩ *Dàn dòu chǐ* (淡豆豉, Semen Sojae Praeparatum, Prepared Soybean) ★

Both *dàn dòu chǐ* (Semen Sojae Praeparatum) and *dà dòu huáng juǎn* (大豆黄卷, Semen Sojae Germinatus, Black Soybean Sprout) originate from black soybean, but are processed differently.

Dàn dòu chǐ (Semen Sojae Praeparatum) is pungent and ascending with a light texture, has a moderate diaphoretic action, and can be used for exterior syndromes of both wind cold and wind heat. It also can disperse depressed heat to eliminate irritability, therefore, it can be used for restlessness and insomnia caused by heat accumulation due to pathogenic heat. When fermented with *sāng yè* (Folium Mori) and *qīng hāo* (Herba Artemisiae Annuae), it has a cold property and is often used for irritability due to common cold of the wind heat type, and heat syndrome. When fermented with *má huáng* (Herba Ephedrae) and *sū yè* (Folium Perillae), it is warm in property and is indicated for wind cold.

Dà dòu huáng juǎn (Semen Sojae Germinatus) is able to release the exterior, remove summer heat, clear heat and drain dampness. It is indicated for fever with scanty sweating, aversion to cold, heavy body, chest distress and a greasy tongue coating due to summer damp, damp heat at an early stage, and damp heat accumulation.

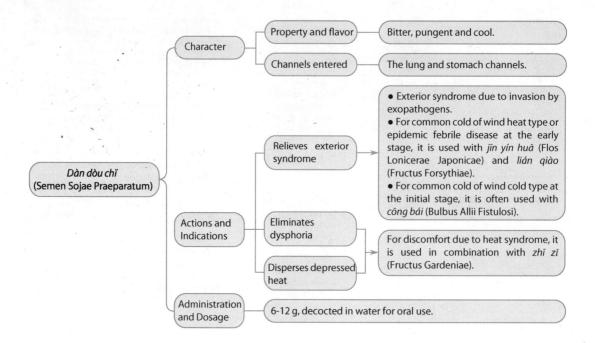

⑪ *Fú píng* (浮萍, Herba Spirodelae, Duckweed)

Both *má huáng* (Herba Ephedrae) and *fú píng* (Herba Spirodelae) disseminate the lungs, open the pores, unblock water channels to release the exterior through sweating, and promote urination to reduce edema. Both can be used for fever with aversion to cold, absence of sweating, edema and dysuria due to external attack.

Má huáng (Herba Ephedrae) is pungent and warm, and is indicated for excess type exterior wind cold syndromes manifesting as aversion to cold without sweating. It is also used for cough with shortness of breath caused by lung qi accumulation.

Fú píng (Herba Spirodelae) is pungent and cold, and is indicated for exterior syndrome due to wind heat manifesting as fever without sweating. It is also used for measles with

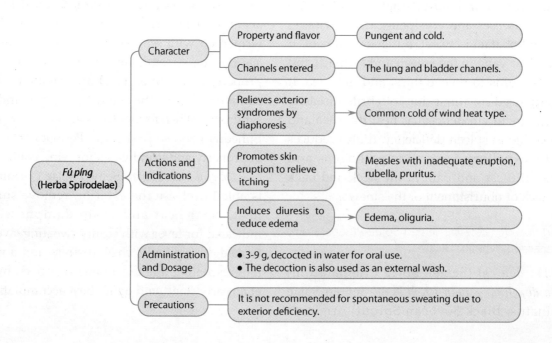

inadequate eruption, urticaria and pruritus by venting rashes to relieve itching.

⑫ *Mù zéi* (木贼, Herba Equiseti Hiemalis, Common Scouring Rush Herb)

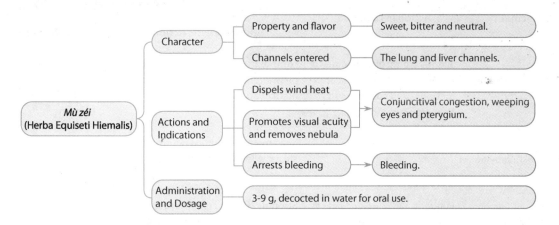

Actions of medicinals that release the exterior are summarized in the following tables (Table 8-1 and 8-2):

Table 8-1: Summary of Medicinals that Release Exterior Wind Cold:

Medicinal	Action in Common	Individual Character	
		Characteristic Actions	**Other Actions**
Má huáng (Herba Ephedrae)	Releases the exterior through sweating	Releases the exterior by disseminating the lung qi, opens the pores, indicated for excess type exterior syndromes without sweating	Disseminates the lung to relieve asthma, promotes urination to reduce edema
Guì zhī (Ramulus Cinnamomi)		Releases the exterior by warming and activating the *wei* yang, indicated for both excess type without sweat and deficiency type with sweat	Warms and activates channels and vessels, reinforces yang to promote qi flow
Sū yè (Folium Perillae)	Releases the exterior through sweating, detoxifies seafood poisoning	Promotes qi circulation and soothes the middle, transforms phlegm to relieve cough, indicated for wind cold type common cold accompanied by qi stagnation or cough with profuse phlegm	Regulates qi circulation to prevent miscarriage
Shēng jiāng (Rhizoma Zingiberis Recens)		Warms the middle to relieve vomiting	Warms the lung to relieve cough, relieves poisoning from *bàn xià* (Rhizoma Pinelliae) and *tiān nán xīng* (Rhizoma Arisaematis).
Xiāng rú (Herba Moslae)	Releases the exterior through sweating, transforms dampness to harmonize the middle, promotes urination to reduce edema, indicated for yin syndrome in summer		

Table 8-1: Summary of Medicinals that Release Exterior Wind Cold:

continued

Medicinal	Action in Common		Individual Character	
			Characteristic Actions	Other Actions
Jīng jiè (Herba Schizonepetae)	Slightly warm, dispels wind to release the exterior, indicated for both wind cold or wind heat type common cold		Light texture and a stronger diaphoretic action than *fáng fēng* (Radix Saposhnikoviae)	Promotes skin eruption, eliminates infections on the body surface, arrests bleeding
Fáng fēng (Radix Saposhnikoviae)			Spongy texture, moist nature, and a strong wind-dispelling action	Removes dampness to relieve pain, relieves convulsions
Xì xīn (Radix et Rhizoma Asari)	Pungent, warm, aromatic and dry, Releases the exterior by dispelling cold, dispels wind to relieve pain	Opens nasal orifice	Strongly dispels cold, warms the lung to transform fluids, indicated for cold syndrome both in the exterior and interior	
Bái zhǐ (Radix Angelicae Dahuricae)			Various types of pain on the face and head along the *yangming* channel	Dries dampness to cure leukorrhagia, subsides swelling and promotes discharge of pus, dispels wind to relieve itching
Qiāng huó (Rhizoma et Radix Notopterygii)		Removes dampness	Strongly releases the exterior by dispelling cold, dispels wind to remove dampness and relieve pain. Indicated for *bi* due to wind cold dampness in the upper part of body	
Gǎo běn (Rhizoma Ligustici)			Severe vertex headache due to wind cold	
Cāng ěr zǐ (Fructus Xanthii)	Dispels wind cold, opens the nasal orifices, indicated for runny nose		Toxic	Dispels wind dampness, relieves pain
Xīn yí (Flos Magnoliae)			A major medicinal for treating runny nose	
É bù shí cǎo (Herba Centipedae)				Relieves cough, detoxifies
Cōng bái (Bulbus Allii Fistulosi)	Releases the exterior through sweating, dispels cold and activates yang, removes stasis and dredges the collaterals to promote the production of milk			
Hú suī (Herba Coriandri Sativi)	Releases the exterior, vents rashes		Promotes digestion	
Chéng liǔ (Cacumen Tamaricis)			Dispels wind to remove dampness	

Table 8-2: Summary of Medicinals that Release Exterior Wind Heat:

Medicinal	Action in common	Individual character	
		Characteristic actions	**Other actions**
Bò he (Herba Menthae)	Dispels wind heat, relieves sore throat, vents rashes	Pungent, cool and aromatic, with a stronger wind-heat dispelling action than other medicinals of the same category	Clears the head and improves eyesight, soothes the liver to promote qi circulation
Niú bàng zǐ (Fructus Arctii)		Pungent, bitter and cold, disseminates the lungs to eliminate phlegm, indicated for cough due to wind heat	Clears heat, detoxifies to relieve swelling, moistens the intestines to promote bowel movements
Chán tuì (Periostracum Cicadae)		Sweet and cold with a light texture. Disperses wind heat in the lung channel to relieve sore throat and hoarseness, vents rashes to relieve itching, as well as disperses wind heat in the liver channel to improve eyesight and remove nebula, cools the liver to extinguish wind to relieve convulsions	
Sāng yè (Folium Mori)	Disperses wind heat, calms the liver yang, clears the liver to improve eyesight	More strongly dispels wind heat than jú huā (Flos Chrysanthemi)	Clears the lung to moisten dryness, cools the blood and arrests bleeding
Jú huā (Flos Chrysanthemi)		Strongly calms and clears the liver to improve eyesight	Clears heat and detoxifes
Màn jīng zǐ (Fructus Viticis)	Disperses wind heat, clears the head and improves eyesight, dispels wind to relieve pain. Indicated for diseases caused by flaring up of wind heat		
Chái hú (Radix Bupleuri)	Raises the yang and releases the exterior	Invigorates the spleen yang	Dominates the liver and gallbladder qi, dispels pathogens in the shaoyang channel	Reduces fever, relieves liver depression
Shēng má (Rhizoma Cimicifugae)			Raises the clear yang in the spleen and stomach	Clears heat and detoxifies
Gé gēn (Radix Puerariae Lobatae)			Raises the clear yang in the spleen and stomach to generate fluids, relieves diarrhea. Indicated for stiffness and pain in the neck and back due to malnutrition of the channels and vessels caused by retention of external pathogens	Vents rashes
Dàn dòu chǐ (Semen Sojae Praeparatum)	Releases the exterior, relieves irritability, disperses depressed heat		
Fú píng (Herba Spirodelae)	Releases the exterior through sweating, vents rashes, promotes urination to reduce edema		
Mù zéi (Herba Equiseti Hiemalis)	Dispels wind heat, improves eyesight, removes nebula and arrests bleeding. Indicated for eye diseases due to wind heat flaring upward.		

Tables to test your herbal knowledge of the actions and indications of medicinals that release the exterior are as follows (Tables 8-3~8-6, see p.74~78):

Table 8-3: Test your Herbal Knowledge of the Actions of Medicinals that Release Exterior Wind Cold:

Medicinal / Effects	Má huáng	Guì zhī	Zǐ sū yè	Shēng jiāng	Xiāng rú	Jīng jiè	Fáng fēng	Qiāng huó	Bái zhǐ	Xì xīn	Gǎo běn	Cāng ěr zǐ	Xīn yí	Cōng bái	É bù shí cǎo	Hú suī	Chéng liǔ
Dispels wind cold																	
Disseminates the lung to relieve asthma																	
Transforms dampness and harmonizes the middle																	
Disperses cold to remove stagnation																	
Warms and activates the channels and vessels																	
Disperses cold and activates the yang																	
Promotes qi circulation and soothes the middle																	
Warms the middle to relieve vomiting																	
Warms the lung to relieve cough																	
Treats seafood poisoning																	
Promotes urination to relieve edema																	

Table 8-3: Test your Herbal Knowledge of the Actions of Medicinals that Release Exterior Wind Cold:

continued

Medicinal / Effects	Má huáng	Guì zhī	Zǐ sū yè	Shēng jiāng	Xiāng rú	Jīng jiè	Fáng fēng	Qiāng huó	Bái zhǐ	Xì xīn	Gǎo běn	Cāng ěr zǐ	Xīn yí	Cōng bái	É bù shí cǎo	Hú suī	Chéng liǔ
Dispels wind to remove dampness																	
Improves appetite and promotes digestion																	
Warms the lung to reduce watery phlegm																	
Relieves edema and promotes the discharge of pus																	
Reinforces the yang to promote the flow of qi																	
Dries dampness to reduce leukorrhagia																	
Opens the nasal orifice																	
Arrests bleeding																	
Eliminates ulcers																	
Relieves convulsions																	
Vents rashes																	
Relieves pain																	
Detoxifies																	

Table 8-4: Test your Herbal Knowledge of the Actions of Medicinals that Release Exterior Wind Heat:

Effects \ Medicinal	Bò he	Niú bàng zǐ	Chán tuì	Sāng yè	Jú huā	Màn jīng zǐ	Chái hú	Shēng má	Gé gēn	Gé huā	Dàn dòu chǐ	Mù zéi
Disperses wind heat												
Clears the head and eyes												
Relieves sore throat												
Vents rashes												
Clears the lungs to moisten dryness												
Detoxifies to reduce swelling												
Relieves itching												
Arrests diarrhea												
Relieves convulsions												
Soothes liver depression												
Calms the liver to improve eyesight												
Cools the blood and stops bleeding												
Expels wind to relieve pain												
Elevates depleted yang to prevent prolapse												
Releases the exterior through sweating												
Generates fluids to relieve thirst												
Improves eyesight and remove nebula												
Alleviates hangover												
Harmonizes the spleen and stomach												
Relieves the superficial muscle layer to reduce fever												
Eliminates irritability												
Promotes urination to reduce edema												

Table 8-5: Test your Herbal Knowledge of the Indications of Medicinals that Release Exterior Wind Cold:

Medicinal / Indications	Má huáng	Guì zhī	Zǐ sū yè	Shēng jiāng	Xiāng rú	Jīng jiè	Fáng fēng	Qiāng huó	Bái zhǐ	Xì xīn	Gǎo běn	Cāng ěr zǐ	Xīn yí	Cōng bái	É bù shí cǎo	Hú suī	Chēng liǔ
Edema, dysuria																	
Summer heat of yin type																	
Forehead pain																	
Measles without adequate eruption																	
Urticaria with itching																	
Suppurative infections on the body surface																	
Hematemesis, epistaxis																	
Tetanus																	
Abdominal pain with diarrhea due to the depressed liver invading the spleen																	
Phlegm fluids																	
Water retention																	
Wind heat type common cold																	
Leukorrhagia																	
Toothache																	
Initial stage ulcer accompanied by exterior syndrome																	
Invasion by exogenous pathogens due to yang deficiency																	
Runny nose																	
Cough with shortness of breath due to cold fluid																	
Yin cold hyperactivity repressing yang																	

Table 8-6: Test your Herbal Knowledge of the Indications of Medicinals that Release Exterior Wind Heat:

Medicinal\ Indications	Bò he	Niú bàng zĭ	Chán tuì	Sāng yè	Jú huā	Màn jīng zĭ	Chái hú	Shēng má	Gé gēn	Dàn dòu chĭ	Fú píng	Mù zéi
Suppurative infections on the body surface												
Early stage epidemic febrile diseases												
Wind cold type common cold												
Infant's convulsions and night crying												
Measles without adequate eruption												
Urticaria with itching												
Headache and blood-shot eyes												
Wind heat type common cold												
Mumps												
Blood-shot eyes and pterygium												
Swollen and painful throat												
Tetanus												
Dry cough due to lung heat												
Chest distress and heat type irritability												
Liver constraint with qi stagnation												
Heat type diarrhea and dysentery												
Alternating chills and fever												
Collapse due to qi deficiency												
Profuse and chronic uterine bleeding												
Thirst due to febrile diseases												
Diabetes due to yin deficiency												
Hematemesis and epistaxis due to blood heat												
Toothache and mouth sores												
Vertigo due to hyperactivity of liver yang												
Common edema												
Hemafecia and bleeding hemorrhoids												

Chapter 9
Medicinals that Clear Heat

Concept

Medicinals whose principal effect is to clear heat in the interior and relieve internal heat syndrome are called medicinals that clear heat.

Character and Actions

Medicinals of this kind are cold or cool and usually have a descending action, which can clear heat, purge fire, cool the blood, detoxify, and clear deficient heat. The treatment principle is mainly one of *"treating heat syndrome with medicinals that are cold or cool"*, as was mentioned in the *Yellow Emperor's Inner Classic* and *Shennong's Herbal Classic* (《内经》: 热者寒之;《神农本草经》: 疗热以寒药).

Indications

Medicinals that clear heat are indicated for heat syndrome in the interior manifesting with vexation and thirst with high fever, diarrhea and dysentery of a damp heat type, suppurating infections on the body surface, and fever due to yin deficiency.

Classification

Internal heat syndromes are divided into heat in the qi level, heat in the *xue* level, heat of an excessive type and heat of a deficient type. This is done in accordance with different types of onset, pathological conditions and body constitutions.

Therefore, medicinals that clear heat are classified into five categories according to their actions and indications: Medicinals that clear heat and purge fire, medicinals that clear heat and dry dampness, medicinals that clear heat and cool the blood, medicinals that clear heat and detoxify and medicinals that clear deficient heat.

Combinations

When using heat-clearing medicinals, a differentiation between excessive heat syndrome and deficient heat syndrome should be made. Excessive heat syndrome involves heat in the qi level, heat in the *ying* level, and heat in the *xue* level. Therefore principles of clearing heat and purging fire, clearing and cooling the *ying* and *xue* levels and a simultaneous clearing of heat in the qi and *xue* levels should be applied accordingly. Deficient heat syndrome includes pathogenic heat impairing the yin, liver and kidney yin deficiency, and interior heat due to yin deficiency. Therefore principles of clearing heat, nourishing yin to expel heat, and nourishing yin and cooling blood to relieve steaming bone fever are applied accordingly. For interior heat syndromes associated with exterior syndromes, medicinals for relieving the exterior syndrome should be used first, or medicinals for relieving the exterior and interior syndrome should be given simultaneously. For interior heat syndromes with food retention, purgatives should be used in combination with heat clearing medicinals.

Precautions

Medicinals that clear heat have cool or cold properties and can easily damage the spleen and stomach; therefore they should be given with caution in cases of poor appetite and loose stools due to deficiency of the spleen and stomach. Medicinals that are bitter and cold can easily transform dryness and damage yin, so they should be used cautiously in cases of yin damage due to heat syndrome or yin deficiency. In cases of excessive yin repelling yang or cold syndrome with false-heat symptoms, heat-clearing medicinals should be avoided.

Section 1　Medicinals that Clear Heat and Purge Fire

Medicinals of this kind are usually bitter and cold or sweet and cold with a relatively strong action in clearing heat. They are indicated for high fever, thirst, sweating, vexation and agitation, or even coma and delirium. There will be a red tongue with a yellow coating, and a strong and rapid pulse due to pathogenic heat invading the qi level. In addition, because the medicinals enter into different channels, they are indicated for different fire heat syndromes in the viscera such as lung heat, stomach heat, heart fire and liver fire.

① *Shí gāo* (石膏, Gypsum Fibrosum, Gypsum) ★ ★ ★

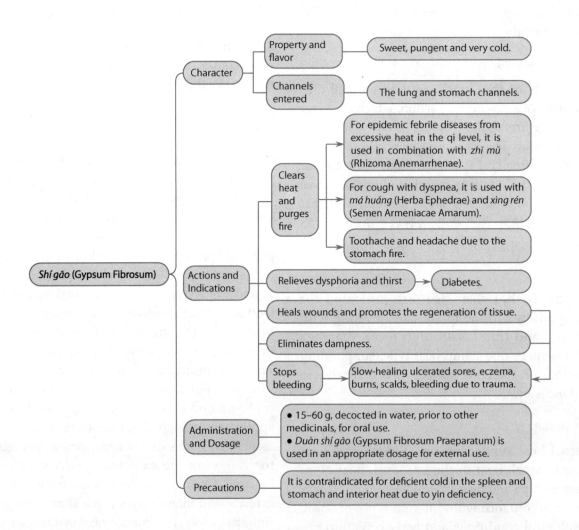

② *Zhī mǔ* (知母, Rhizoma Anemarrhenae, Common Anemarrhena Rhizome) ★ ★ ★

Both *shí gāo* (Gypsum Fibrosum) and *zhī mǔ* (Rhizoma Anemarrhenae) are cold and enter the lung and stomach channels. They can clear heat and purge fire, eliminate vexation and relieve thirst and are indicated for excessive heat syndrome in the lung and stomach manifesting with strong fever, thirst, sweating with a powerful and big pulse. They can also be used for cough due to lung heat. *Shí gāo* (Gypsum Fibrosum) is pungent sweet and cold and has a strong action of clearing heat and purging fire. It emphasizes clearing heat and relieving exterior syndromes from the muscles, and clearing and purging excessive fire in the lung and stomach. Therefore it is used for cough with dyspnea due to lung heat, as well as headache and swelling pain of the gums due to stomach fire flaring upward. Calcined *shí gāo* (Gypsum Fibrosum) can relieve vexation and thirst, heal wounds and promote regeneration of tissue, eliminate dampness and stop bleeding. It is used for slow-healing ulcerated sores, eczema, burns, scalds, bleeding due to trauma, etc. *Zhī mǔ* (Rhizoma Anemarrhenae) is bitter, cold and moist. It is inferior to *shí gāo* (Gypsum Fibrosum) in its actions to clear heat and purge fire. It is effective for nourishing lung and stomach yin to moisten dryness as well as for nourishing the kidney to descend fire. It is often used for dry cough due to yin deficiency, diabetes due to internal heat from yin deficiency, steaming bone fever, night sweating, vexation due to yin deficiency with fire hyperactivity, and constipation due to yin deficiency with dry intestines. *Zhī mǔ* (Rhizoma Anemarrhenae) can clear lung heat and moisten lung dryness in the upper *jiao*, clear the stomach heat and moisten stomach dryness in the middle *jiao*, and nourish kidney yin and descend deficient fire in the lower *jiao*. It can clear heat of either an excessive or deficient type.

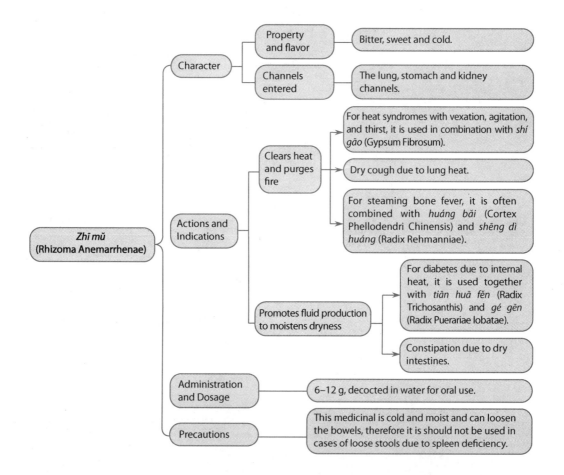

③ *Hán shuǐ shí* (寒水石, Glauberitum, Calcitum)

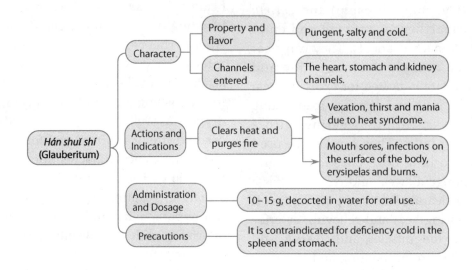

④ *Lú gēn* (芦根, Rhizoma Phragmitis, Reed Rhizome) ★★

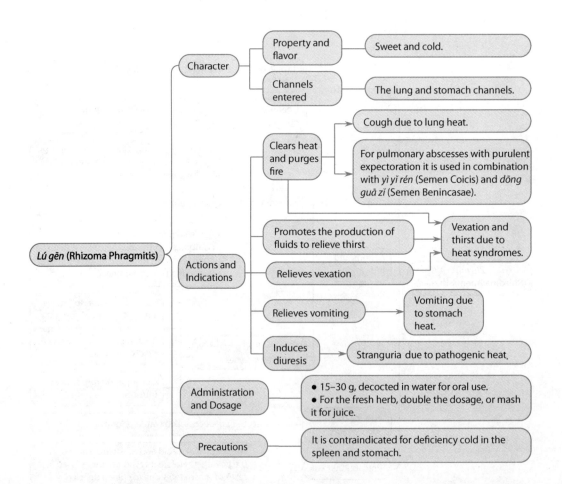

⑤ *Tiān huā fěn* (天花粉, Radix Trichosanthis, Snakegourd Root) ★ ★

Lú gēn (Rhizoma Phragmitis) and *tiān huā fěn* (Radix Trichosanthis) are both sweet and cold and enter the lung and stomach channels. Both medicinals can clear heat, purge fire and promote fluid production to relieve thirst. They are indicated for fluid consumption, vexation, thirst, a dry tongue with scanty fluids, and cough due to lung heat. *Lú gēn* (Rhizoma Phragmitis), is sweet and cold and has stronger actions of clearing heat, purging fire and relieving vexation than *tiān huā fěn* (Radix Trichosanthis). It can clear the lung to eliminate phlegm and promote the discharge of pus, clear the stomach to relieve vomiting, and clear heat to induce diuresis. Therefore it is used for pulmonary abscesses with chest pain, purulent expectoration, vomiting and hiccup due to the stomach heat, stranguria due to pathogenic heat, and reddish scanty urine. *Tiān huā fěn* (Radix Trichosanthis) is effective for promoting the production of fluids to relieve thirst, therefore it is indicated for diabetes with polydipsia due to yin deficiency. At the same time, it can clear the lung to moisten dampness, decrease swellings and promote the discharge of pus. It is indicated for dry cough with scanty phlegm or bloody phlegm caused by lung damage due to dry heat; and skin diseases in the early stages due to exuberant heat toxins. It can eliminate skin infections when there is no pus, while promoting ulceration and pus discharge for infections that are pustulant.

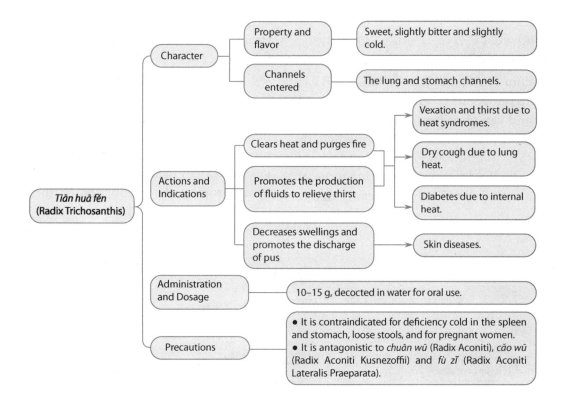

⑥ *Zhú yè* (竹叶, Folium Phyllostachydis Henonis, Henon Bamboo Leaf)

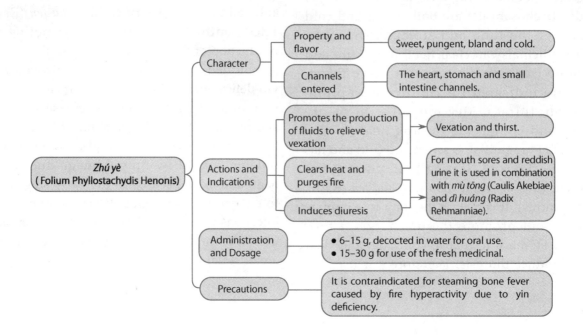

⑦ *Dàn zhú yè* (淡竹叶, Herba Lophatheri, Lophatherum Herb) ★

Zhú yè (Folium Phyllostachydis Henonis) and *dàn zhú yè* (Herba Lophatheri) are both sweet, bland and cold, and can clear heat, purge fire, relieve vexation and induce diuresis. Both medicinals are used for vexation and thirst due to heat consuming the fluids; mouth sores due to heart fire flaring upward; reddish and scanty urine,

stranguria due to heart heat invading the small intestine. There are differences, including that *zhú yè* (Folium Phyllostachydis Henonis) is from the leaf of Phyllostachyl *nigra* (Lodd. Ex Lindl.) Munro var. henonis (Mitf.) Stapf et Rendle, of the family Poaceae, and it has stronger actions for clearing the heart, purging fire and removing vexation than *dàn zhú yè* (Herba Lophatheri). It can promote the production of fluids, so it is

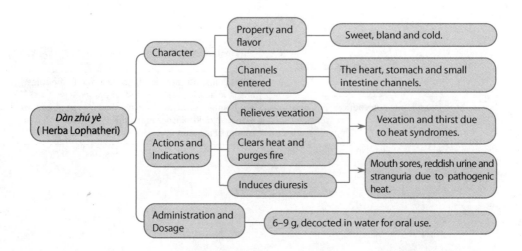

often used for vexation and thirst due to heat syndrome. *Dàn zhú yè* (Herba Lophatheri) is the dried herb of *Lophatherum gracile* Brongn., of the family Poaceae. It is effective for clearing heat and inducing diuresis, hence is used for mouth sores, vexation, scanty and reddish urine, stranguria due to heart fire attacking the small intestine, edema of a damp heat type and reddish urine due to jaundice. In addition, *zhú*

yè juǎn xīn is the immature curved leaf of *zhú yè* (Folium Phyllostachydis Henonis). It is able to clear the heart and purge fire, and is used for heat invading the pericardium due to febrile diseases, with strong fever, coma and delirium.

⑧ *Yā zhí cǎo* (鸭跖草, Herba Commelinae, Common Dayflower Herb)

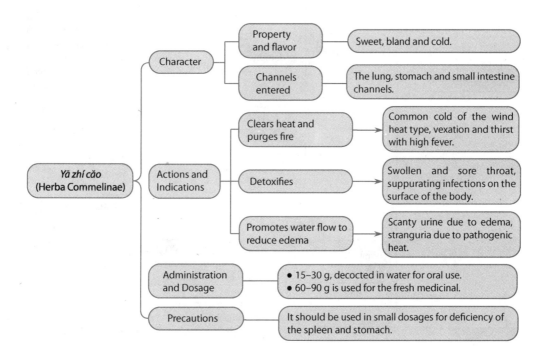

⑨ *Zhī zǐ* (栀子, Fructus Gardeniae, Cape Jasmine Fruit) ★ ★ ★

Zhī zǐ (Fructus Gardeniae) and *yā zhí cǎo* (Herba Commelinae) are both bitter and cold and can clear heat, purge fire, detoxify and drain damp. Both medicinals are used for heat syndrome with vexation, thirst, suppurating infections on the surface of the body, jaundice of a damp heat type, and stranguria of a heat type. *Zhī zǐ* (Fructus Gardeniae) has a descending nature and it is effective for clearing heat, purging fire and detoxifying. It is used for vexation, depression, and strong fever, coma and delirium, by clearing and purging fire in the heart, lung, stomach and

san jiao. In addition, *zhī zǐ* (Fructus Gardeniae) can clear fire in both the qi and *xue* levels, cool blood, stop bleeding, and reduce swelling to relieve pain. Therefore it is used for vomiting, epistaxis, and conjunctival congestion due to blood heat, and used externally it can treat trauma. *Yā zhí cǎo* (Herba Commelinae) has a strong action of promoting the flow of water to reduce edema, as well as an action to dispel exterior pathogens. Therefore it is used for common cold of the wind heat type, epidemic febrile diseases in the initial stage with pathogen retention in the *wei* level, edema, and scanty urine of a damp heat type.

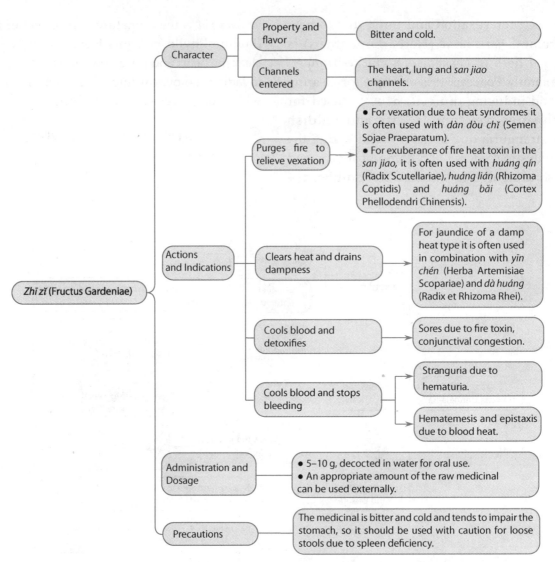

Zhī zǐ (Fructus Gardeniae)

- **Character**
  - **Property and flavor** — Bitter and cold.
  - **Channels entered** — The heart, lung and *san jiao* channels.
- **Actions and Indications**
  - **Purges fire to relieve vexation** —
    - For vexation due to heat syndromes it is often used with *dàn dòu chǐ* (Semen Sojae Praeparatum).
    - For exuberance of fire heat toxin in the *san jiao,* it is often used with *huáng qín* (Radix Scutellariae), *huáng lián* (Rhizoma Coptidis) and *huáng bǎi* (Cortex Phellodendri Chinensis).
  - **Clears heat and drains dampness** — For jaundice of a damp heat type it is often used in combination with *yīn chén* (Herba Artemisiae Scopariae) and *dà huáng* (Radix et Rhizoma Rhei).
  - **Cools blood and detoxifies** — Sores due to fire toxin, conjunctival congestion.
  - **Cools blood and stops bleeding** —
    - Stranguria due to hematuria.
    - Hematemesis and epistaxis due to blood heat.
- **Administration and Dosage** —
  - 5–10 g, decocted in water for oral use.
  - An appropriate amount of the raw medicinal can be used externally.
- **Precautions** — The medicinal is bitter and cold and tends to impair the stomach, so it should be used with caution for loose stools due to spleen deficiency.

⑩ *Xià kū cǎo* (夏枯草, Spica Prunellae, Common Selfheal Fruit-spike) ★ ★ ★

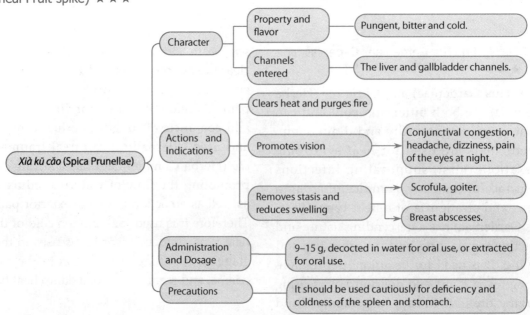

Xià kū cǎo (Spica Prunellae)

- **Character**
  - **Property and flavor** — Pungent, bitter and cold.
  - **Channels entered** — The liver and gallbladder channels.
- **Actions and Indications**
  - **Clears heat and purges fire**
  - **Promotes vision** — Conjunctival congestion, headache, dizziness, pain of the eyes at night.
  - **Removes stasis and reduces swelling** —
    - Scrofula, goiter.
    - Breast abscesses.
- **Administration and Dosage** — 9–15 g, decocted in water for oral use, or extracted for oral use.
- **Precautions** — It should be used cautiously for deficiency and coldness of the spleen and stomach.

⑪ *Jué míng zǐ* (决明子, Semen Cassiae, Cassia Seed) ★★

Xià kū cǎo (Spica Prunellae) and *jué míng zǐ* (Semen Cassiae) are both cold and can clear the liver to promote vision and relieve hypertension. Both medicinals can be used for conjunctival congestion, photophobia and excessive tearing due to liver fire flaring upward. They are medicinals commonly used in ophthalmology. They are also used to treat dizziness and headache from hypertension due to ascendant hyperactivity of liver heat. However, there are many differences between the two medicinals. *Xià kū cǎo* (Spica Prunellae) is pungent, bitter and cold and has a much stronger action of clearing liver fire compared with *jué míng zǐ* (Semen Cassiae). It can also remove depressed stasis. Therefore it is used for scrofula, goiter, and breast abscesses due to a stagnation of phlegm and fire. *Jué míng zǐ* (Semen Cassiae) has a strong action of promoting vision, and is indicated for conjuctival congestion due to wind heat or liver fire flaring upward, and blurred vision due to yin deficiency in the liver and kidney. In addition, it has a moist texture, and therefore is also used for constipation due to dry intestines of an internal heat type.

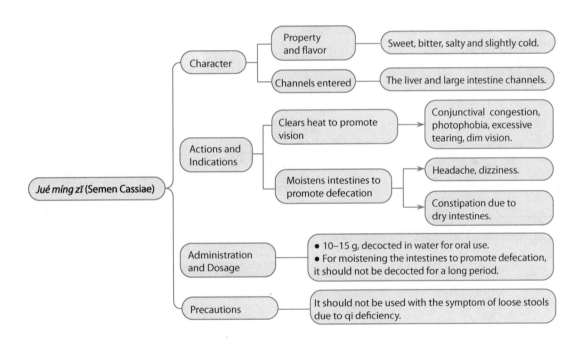

⑫ *Gǔ jīng cǎo* (谷精草, Flos Eriocauli, Pipewort Flower)

Both *mù zéi* (Herba Equiseti Hiemalis) and *gǔ jīng cǎo* (Flos Eriocauli) can dispel wind heat, promote vision and remove nebula, and are indicated for wind heat upwardly invading with conjunctival congestion, nebulae, photophobia and excessive tearing. However, *mù zéi* (Herba Equiseti Hiemalis) has a stronger action of dispelling wind heat but with mild bleeding-arresting ability, so it is often used in combination with other blood regulating medicinals to treat blood in the stools and hemorrhoids of a blood heat type. *Gǔ jīng cǎo* (Flos Eriocauli) is better than *mù zéi* (Herba Equiseti Hiemalis) in clearing heat and purging fire and is used for headache, toothache and sore throat due to wind heat.

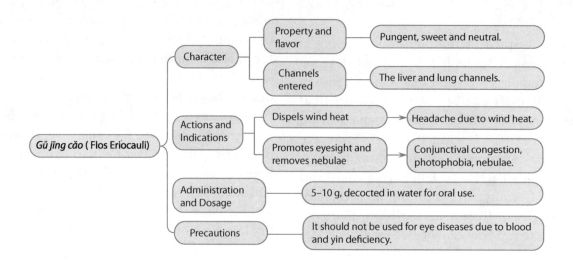

⑬ *Mì méng huā* (密蒙花, Flos Buddlejae, Pale Butterflybush Flower)

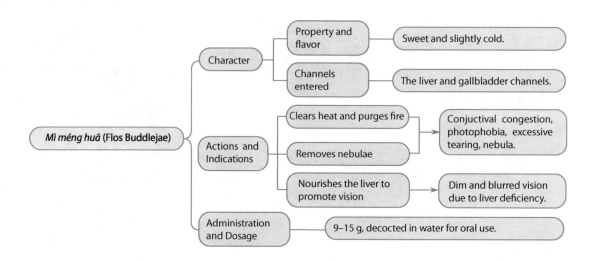

⑭ *Qīng xiāng zǐ* (青葙子, Semen Celosiae, Feather Cockscomb Seed)

Both *qīng xiāng zǐ* (Semen Celosiae) and *mì méng huā* (Flos Buddlejae) can clear the liver, purge fire, promote vision and remove nebula. They are indicated for conjunctival congestion, photophobia, excessive tearing, and nebulae due to liver fire upwardly flaring. *Qīng xiāng zǐ* (Semen Celosiae) has a strong action of clearing and purging liver fire, and is also used for headache, dizziness and insomnia with vexation due to the transformation of liver yang into fire. *Mì méng huā* (Flos Buddlejae) can clear liver heat as well as nourish liver blood. It is used for blurred vision with dry eyes due to liver deficiency with heat. It can also be used for both eye diseases of both excess and deficiency types.

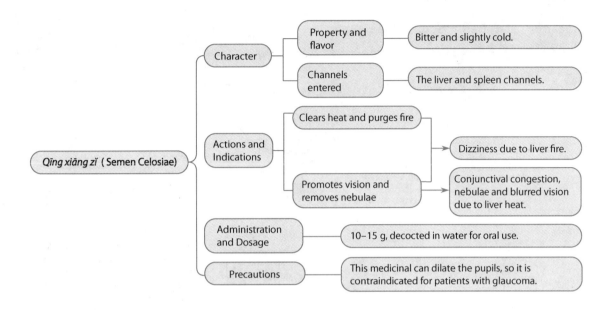

Section 2　Medicinals that Clear Heat and Dry Damp

Medicinals of this kind are usually bitter and cold, and have strong actions of clearing heat and drying damp. Therefore they are mainly used for damp heat syndrome. Since they are bitter and can purge fire, they are often used for fire heat syndrome affecting the *zang* and *fu* organs. Clinical symptoms can vary greatly in accordance with the different locations of damp heat in the body. In cases of damp heat accumulation and unsmooth circulation of qi due to damp warmth or summer-heat damp, there are manifestations such as low fever, chest and epigastric masses and distress, scanty and reddish urine, and a yellow and greasy tongue coating. For damp heat retention in the spleen and stomach leading to dysfunction of ascending and descending, manifestations include epigastric and abdominal distension and fullness, vomiting, diarrhea, and dysentery. If there is a transportation and transformation disturbance due to damp heat stagnating in the intestines, symptoms are diarrhea, dysentery and hemorrhoids. For damp heat accumulation in the liver and gallbladder, the symptoms are jaundice with reddish urine, hypochondriac distending pain, and swelling of the ears with pustular discharge. For damp invasion of the lower *jiao*, there are manifestations that include yellow leukorrhea or stranguria of a heat type. For damp heat invading the joints, manifestations include red, swollen, and painful joints. For damp heat invading the skin and flesh, manifestations include eczema and sores. Medicinals that clear heat and dry damp are used for the diseases mentioned above which are induced by damp heat.

① *Huáng qín* (黄芩,Radix Scutellariae, Baical Skullcap Root) ★★★

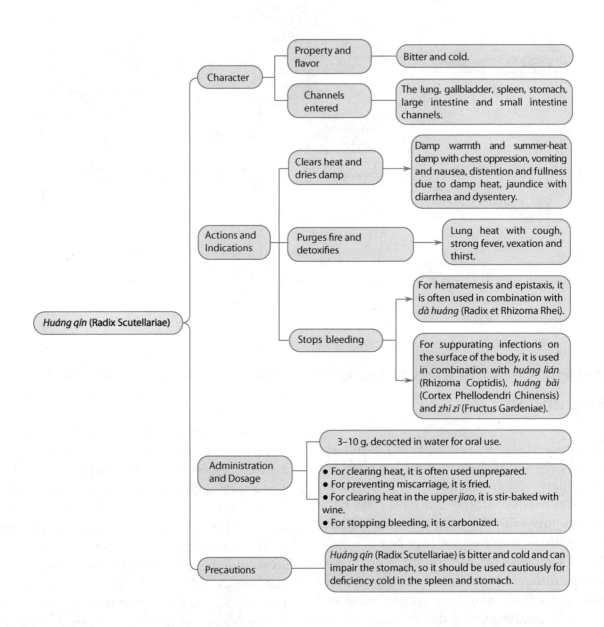

Huáng qín (Radix Scutellariae)

- **Character**
  - **Property and flavor** — Bitter and cold.
  - **Channels entered** — The lung, gallbladder, spleen, stomach, large intestine and small intestine channels.

- **Actions and Indications**
  - **Clears heat and dries damp** → Damp warmth and summer-heat damp with chest oppression, vomiting and nausea, distention and fullness due to damp heat, jaundice with diarrhea and dysentery.
  - **Purges fire and detoxifies** → Lung heat with cough, strong fever, vexation and thirst.
  - **Stops bleeding** →
    - For hematemesis and epistaxis, it is often used in combination with *dà huáng* (Radix et Rhizoma Rhei).
    - For suppurating infections on the surface of the body, it is used in combination with *huáng lián* (Rhizoma Coptidis), *huáng bǎi* (Cortex Phellodendri Chinensis) and *zhī zǐ* (Fructus Gardeniae).

- **Administration and Dosage**
  - 3–10 g, decocted in water for oral use.
  - For clearing heat, it is often used unprepared.
  - For preventing miscarriage, it is fried.
  - For clearing heat in the upper *jiao*, it is stir-baked with wine.
  - For stopping bleeding, it is carbonized.

- **Precautions** — *Huáng qín* (Radix Scutellariae) is bitter and cold and can impair the stomach, so it should be used cautiously for deficiency cold in the spleen and stomach.

② *Huáng lián* (黄连, Rhizoma Coptidis, Coptis) ★ ★ ★

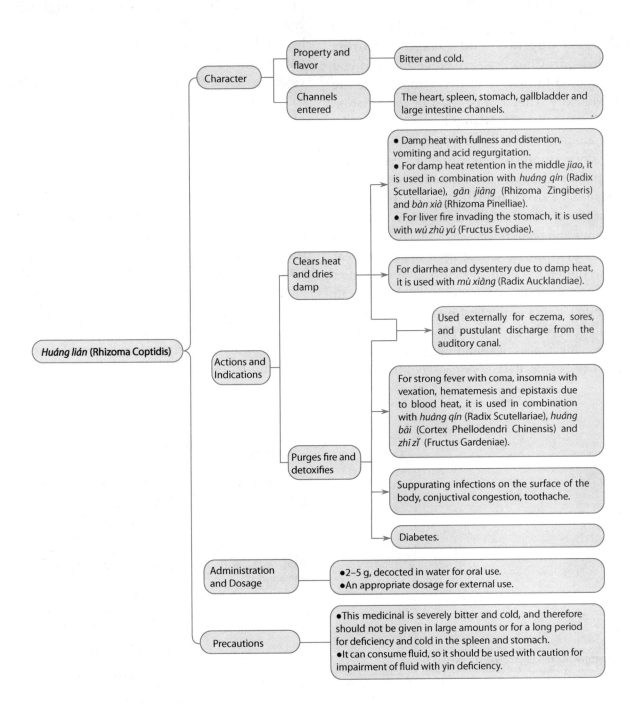

③ *Huáng bǎi* (黄柏, Cortex Phellodendri Chinensis, Phellodendron Bark) ★ ★ ★

Huáng qín (Radix Scutellariae), *huáng lián* (Rhizoma Coptidis) and *huáng bǎi* (Cortex Phellodendri Chinensis) are bitter and cold and can be used to clear heat, dry damp, purge fire and detoxify. They can be used in combination for diseases caused by damp heat and fire toxin. They are indicated for damp heat with diarrhea, dysentery, jaundice, leukorrhagia, eczema and damp sores. They can also be used for exuberance of fire heat toxin manifesting with various infections on the surface of the body, with red swellings and pain. *Huáng qín* (Radix Scutellariae) has a milder flavor, and is used for damp heat in the upper *jiao*, and therefore it is indicated for damp warmth and summer-heat, damp in the initial stages with chest oppression, nausea, vomiting, low fever, and a yellow greasy tongue coating. It can also clear and purge lung fire and excessive heat in the upper *jiao*, cool blood, stop bleeding, remove heat and prevent miscarriage. Therefore it is often used to treat cough with yellow thick phlegm due to lung heat; exuberant heat in the upper and middle *jiao* due to exterior pathogenic heat manifesting as a strong fever, vexation, thirst, flushing, dry lips, reddish urine, constipation, a yellow tongue coating and a rapid pulse; seasonal febrile disease with alternate chills and fever; sore throat due to flaring up of fire toxin; hematemesis, epistaxis, hemafecia, excessive uterine bleeding and menstrual spotting due to blood heat; excessive fetal movement, and vaginal bleeding during pregnancy due to heat accumulation. *Huáng lián* (Rhizoma Coptidis) is severely bitter and cold, and has the strongest action of the three medicinals to clear heat, dry damp, purge fire and detoxify. It is effective for clearing damp heat in the middle *jiao*; therefore it is regarded as the first choice in cases of damp heat with diarrhea, dysentery, fever, abdominal pain and tenesmus. At the same time, it can be

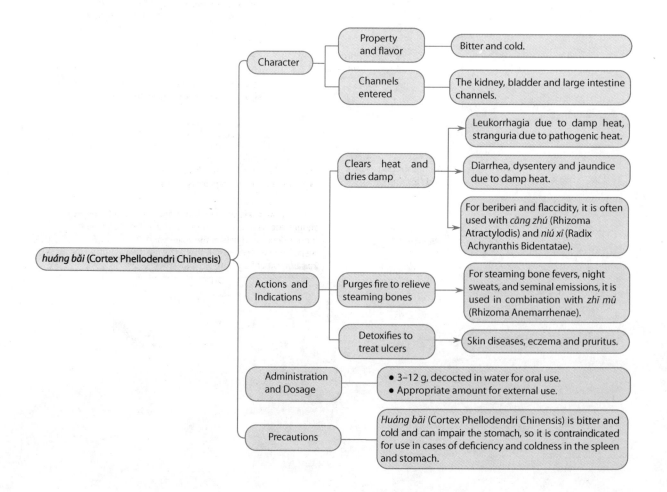

huáng bǎi (Cortex Phellodendri Chinensis)

- Character
  - Property and flavor — Bitter and cold.
  - Channels entered — The kidney, bladder and large intestine channels.
- Actions and Indications
  - Clears heat and dries damp
    - Leukorrhagia due to damp heat, stranguria due to pathogenic heat.
    - Diarrhea, dysentery and jaundice due to damp heat.
    - For beriberi and flaccidity, it is often used with *cāng zhú* (Rhizoma Atractylodis) and *niú xī* (Radix Achyranthis Bidentatae).
  - Purges fire to relieve steaming bones
    - For steaming bone fevers, night sweats, and seminal emissions, it is used in combination with *zhī mǔ* (Rhizoma Anemarrhenae).
  - Detoxifies to treat ulcers — Skin diseases, eczema and pruritus.
- Administration and Dosage
  - 3–12 g, decocted in water for oral use.
  - Appropriate amount for external use.
- Precautions — *Huáng bǎi* (Cortex Phellodendri Chinensis) is bitter and cold and can impair the stomach, so it is contraindicated for use in cases of deficiency and coldness in the spleen and stomach.

used for clearing and purging fire in the heart and stomach so as to relieve vexation and vomiting. It is also chosen for cases of fire heat exuberance in the *san jiao* with strong fever, restlessness, or even coma and delirium; heart fire hyperactivity with insomnia, vexation, mouth sores; hematemesis, epistaxis due to blood heat; disharmony between the liver and stomach with hypochondriac distending pain, vomiting and acid regurgitation; diabetes with excessive appetite due to stomach fire exuberance; swelling and pain in ears and eyes and septicemia induced by boils. *Huáng bǎi* (Cortex Phellodendri Chinensis) is bitter and cold with a descending action, and is able to clear damp heat in the lower *jiao*. It is indicated for

yellow turbid and foul leukorrhagia due to damp heat, swelling and pain in the knees and feet. It is effective for clearing and purging kidney fire in the lower *jiao* so as to reduce deficiency heat. Therefore it is used for fevers, steaming bone fevers, night sweats, and seminal emissions due to yin deficiency.

④ *Lóng dǎn cǎo* (龙胆草, Radix et Rhizoma Gentianae, Chinese Gentian) ★ ★

The differences between the actions of *huáng qín* (Radix Scutellariae), *huáng lián* (Rhizoma Coptidis), *huáng bǎi* (Cortex Phellodendri Chinensis) and *lóng dǎn cǎo* (Radix et Rhizoma Gentianae) are shown in the following table (Table 9-1):

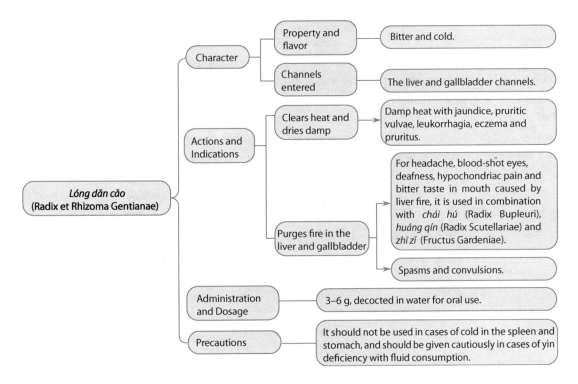

Both *lóng dǎn cǎo* (Radix et Rhizoma Gentianae) and *xià kū cǎo* (Spica Prunellae) are cold and can clear liver fire. They are indicated for headache and blood-shot eyes due to liver fire. The differences between them are that *lóng dǎn cǎo* (Radix et Rhizoma Gentianae) mainly purges excessive fire from the liver and gallbladder, and is usually chosen for fire of an excess type in the liver and gallbladder with hypochondriac pain, bitter taste in the mouth, deafness; and strong fever with convulsions due to wind syndrome induced by

heat exuberance in the liver channels. It has a very bitter and cold nature, and therefore is effective for clearing heat and drying damp especially in the lower *jiao*. Therefore it is used to treat scrotal swelling and pain, yellow thick leukorrhagia, pruritic vulvae, eczema and pruritus due to damp invasion of the lower *jiao*, as well as jaundice, hypochondriac pain, bitter taste in the mouth and reddish urine due to damp heat in the liver and gallbladder. *Xià kū cǎo* (Spica Prunellae) is pungent, bitter and cold, and has a stronger action in

Table 9-1

	Clears Damp Heat	Clears and Purges Fire and Heat
huáng qín (Radix Scutellariae)	upper *jiao*	lung
huáng lián (Rhizoma Coptidis)	middle *jiao*	heart and stomach
huáng bǎi (Cortex Phellodendri Chinensis)	lower *jiao*	kidney
lóng dǎn cǎo (Radix et Rhizoma Gentianae)	lower *jiao*	liver and gallbladder

clearing liver fire to promote vision, and therefore is chosen for blood-shot, swollen and painful eyes with nebula due to liver fire flaring upward. At the same time it is used to clear liver heat, scatter accumulations, decrease swellings, and descend blood pressure. Also it is often used for liver stasis transforming into fire, phlegm fire congealing and accumulations, nodules on the neck like scrofula, phlegm nodes, and breast abscesses. It can also treat high blood pressure from liver yang hyperactivity, headache and dizziness.

⑤ *Qín pí* (秦皮, Cortex Fraxini, Ash Bark) ★

Qín pí (Cortex Fraxini) and *chūn pí* (椿皮, Cortex Ailanthi, Ailanthus Bark) are bitter and cold, can clear heat and dry damp to relieve diarrhea and leukorrhagia, and are indicated for diarrhea with abdominal pain, dysentery due to damp heat accumulation, and leukorrhagia with bloody and purulent discharge due to damp heat invasion of the lower *jiao*. Differentiation: *Qín pí* (Cortex Fraxini) can clear heat, detoxify, and relieve diarrhea and dysentery. It is used for diarrhea and dysentery with bloody and purulent discharge due to heat toxins. It can also clear the liver and purge fire to promote vision and remove nebula, and therefore is indicated for blood-shot, swollen and painful eyes and nebulae due to depressed fire in the liver channel. *Chūn pí* (Cortex Ailanthi) has an astringent flavor and can clear heat, and dry damp to relieve diarrhea and leukorrhagia. It is used for diarrhea, dysentery and leukorrhagia with bloody and purulent discharge due to damp heat. It can also relieve diarrhea and leukorrhagia through its astringency, and is used for chronic diarrhea and dysentery due to loose intestines, as well as chronic leukorrhagia due to spleen and kidney deficiency. Meanwhile, it can clear heat, dry damp, astringe blood and is indicated for excessive uterine bleeding and menstrual spotting, excessive menstrual blood, blood in the stools and hemorrhoids due to blood heat. In addition, it can

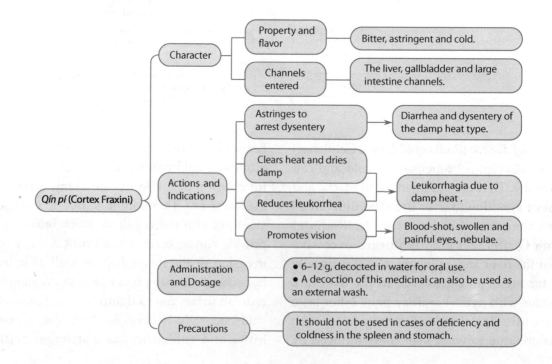

kill parasites and is used for abdominal pain due to roundworms, scabies, tinea and pruritus.

⑥ *Kǔ shēn* (苦参, Radix Sophorae Flavescentis, Lightyellow Sophora Root) ★ ★

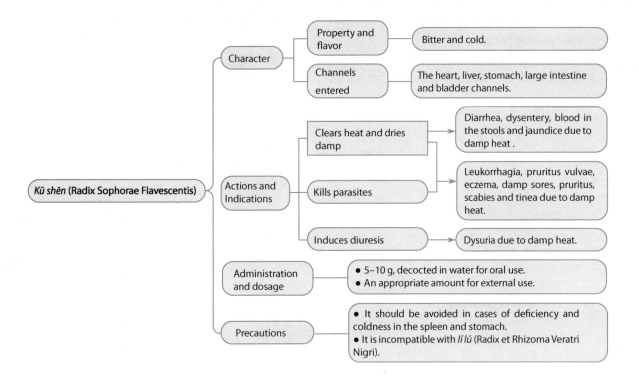

⑦ *Bái xiān pí* (白鲜皮, Cortex Dictamni, Dictamnus Root Bark) ★

Kǔ shēn (Radix Sophorae Flavescentis) and *bái xiān pí* (Cortex Dictamni) are bitter and cold, can clear heat, dry damp, and kill parasites to relieve itching. The two medicinals are combined

together in mutual reinforcement when used for pruritus vulvae, eczema, wet sores, pruritus, scabies, and tinea due to damp heat. They are also used to cure jaundice of the damp heat type.

Kǔ shēn (Radix Sophorae Flavescentis) has a strong action of clearing heat, drying damp, and killing

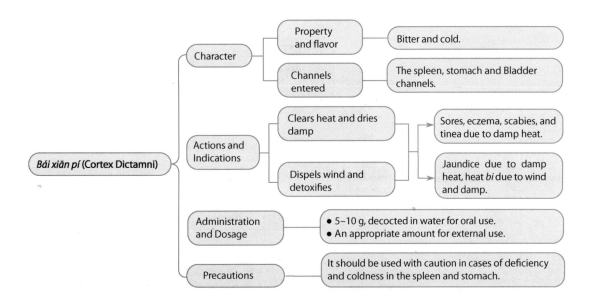

parasites to relieve itching, and can relieve diarrhea and dysentery as well as induce diuresis. It is indicated for diarrhea, dysentery, hemafecia, hemorrhoids with bleeding, hot stranguria and leukorrhagia due to damp heat, dysuria during pregnancy.

Bái xiān pí (Cortex Dictamni) can clear heat and detoxify, and is especially suitable for sores, ulcerated skin with yellow exudation due to damp heat. In addition, it can dispel wind to relieve *bi* and is used for heat *bi* due to wind damp with red swelling pain in the joints.

⑧ *Kǔ dòu zǐ* (苦豆子, Sophora Alopecuroides, All-grass of Foxtail-like Sophora)

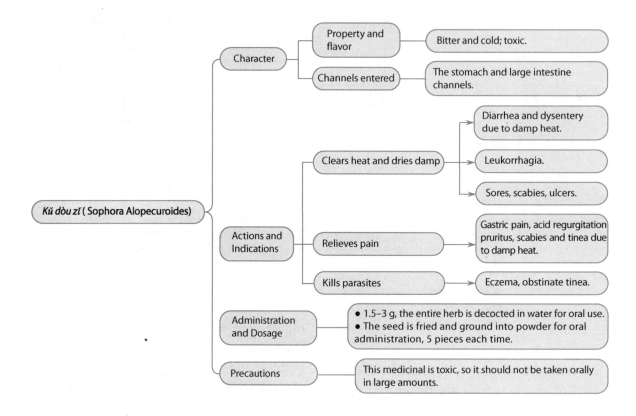

⑨ *Sān kē zhēn* (三颗针, Radix Berberidis, Barberry Root)

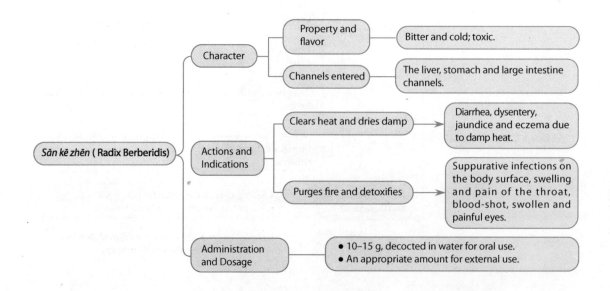

⑩ *Mǎ wěi lián* (马尾连, Radix et Rhizoma Thalictri Baicalensis, Manyleaf Meadowure Rhizome and Root)

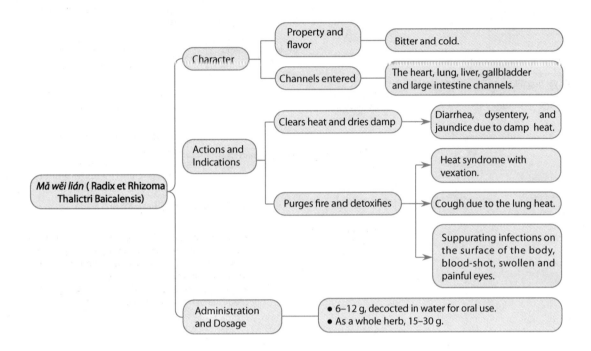

Section 3   Medicinals that Clear Heat and Detoxify

Medicinals of this kind are cold or cool and can clear fire heat toxins. They are indicated for suppurating infections on the surface of the body, erysipelas, maculae due to epidemic febrile diseases, mumps, throat swelling and pain, dysentery due to heat toxin, insect or snake bites, carcinoma, scalds, burns, or other acute heat syndromes.

① *Jīn yín huā* (金银花, Flos Lonicerae Japonicae, Honeysuckle Flower) ★ ★ ★

Addition   *Rěn dōng téng* (忍冬藤, **Caulis Lonicerae Japonicae, Honeysuckle Stem**) is similar to *jīn yín huā* (Flos Lonicerae Japonicae) in action, but is inferior in its ability to detoxify. However, it can clear heat, expel wind and activate collaterals to relieve pain. Therefore it is often used for epidemic febrile disease with fever and heat *bi* due to wind dampness with red, swollen, painful, and inflexible joints.

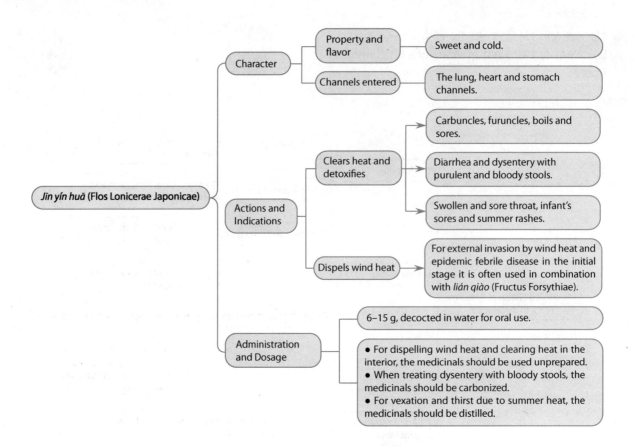

② *Lián qiào* (连翘, Fructus Forsythiae, Forsythia Fruit) ★ ★ ★

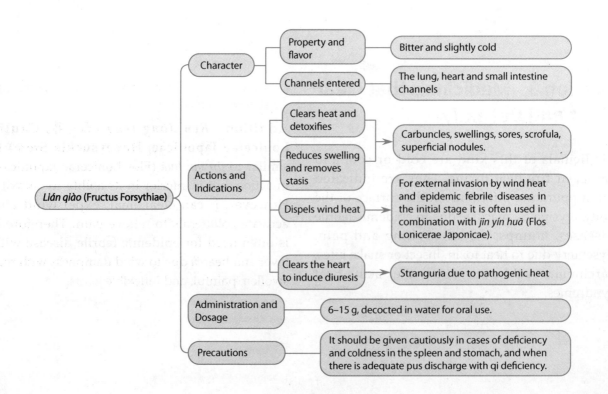

Jīn yín huā (Flos Lonicerae Japonicae) and *lián qiào* (Fructus Forsythiae) are cold and can clear heat, detoxify, and dispel wind heat. They are often chosen for treating skin diseases of the excessive heat type. They are usually indicated for suppurating infections on the surface of the body due to heat toxin exuberance; fever with slight aversion to cold and headache due to invasion by external pathogenic wind heat or epidemic febrile disease in the initial stage. The two medicinals are used in combination to treat strong fever with vexation and thirst due to heat entering the *qi* level; a crimson tongue with coma, and insomnia with vexation due to heat entering the *ying* blood. They can be used throughout the course of epidemic febrile diseases.

Jīn yín huā (Flos Lonicerae Japonicae) is sweet and cold, and has a strong action of dispelling wind heat. It can also cool blood and relieve dysentery, and is indicated for diarrhea and dysentery with purulent and bloody stools, abdominal pain with fever and tenesmus.

Lián qiào (Fructus Forsythiae) is bitter and slightly cold, and is effective for clearing the heart, detoxifying, reducing swellings, and dissolving lumps. It is called the most effective medicinal in treating infections on the surface of the body. It is used for scrofula, and superficial nodules due to phlegm and fire congealing. It can clear the heart to induce diuresis, and is used for hot stranguria.

③ *Chuān xīn lián* (穿心莲, Herba Andrographis, Andrographis) ★★

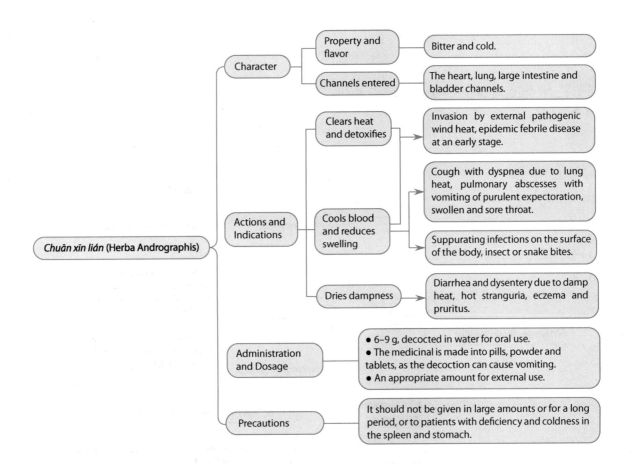

④ *Dà qīng yè* (大青叶, Folium Isatidis, Dyers Woad Leaf) ★★

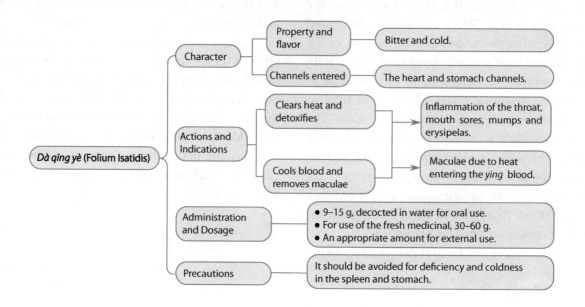

⑤ *Bǎn lán gēn* (板蓝根, Radix Isatidis, Isatis Root) ★★★

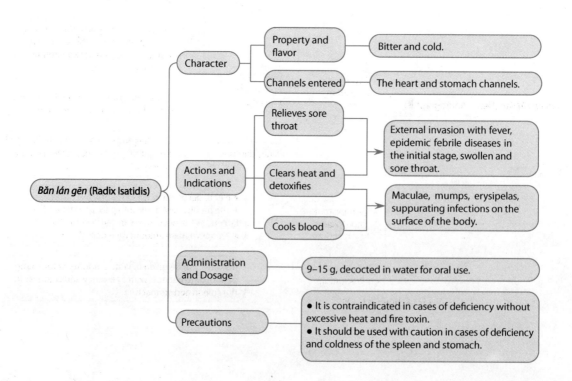

⑥ *Qīng dài* (青黛, Indigo Naturalis, Natural Indigo) ★★

Dà qīng yè (Folium Isatidis), *bǎn lán gēn* (Radix Isatidis) and *qīng dài* (Indigo Naturalis) originate from the same plant, they are cold, and can clear heat, detoxify, cool blood and remove maculae. They are indicated for maculae due to epidemic febrile toxins, hematemesis, epistaxis, mumps, inflammation of the throat, suppurating infections on the surface of the body, and erysipelas.

Both *dà qīng yè* (Folium Isatidis) and *bǎn lán gēn* (Radix Isatidis) are bitter and cold, and are effective for clearing heat toxin in the heart and stomach channels so as to relieve sore throat. They are indicated for swollen and sore throat and mouth sores due to heat toxin invading upwards in the heart and stomach channels; fever, headache, thirst and sore throat due to

invasion by external pathogenic wind heat or epidemic febrile disease in the initial stage. *Dà qīng yè* (Folium Isatidis) is effective for cooling blood and removing maculae, so it is often used for maculae, skin rashes, hematemesis and epistaxis due to enduring blood heat toxin. *Bǎn lán gēn* (Radix Isatidis) is effective for detoxifying, relieving sore throat and removing stasis, so it is often used for craniofacial infection characterized by a swollen head, a flushing swollen face and sore throat.

Qīng dài (Indigo Naturalis) is able to clear the liver, purge fire and extinguish wind so as to relieve convulsions. It is often used for cough with chest pain and bloody phlegm due to the liver fire invading the lung, and epilepsy due to fright and convulsions due to summer heat.

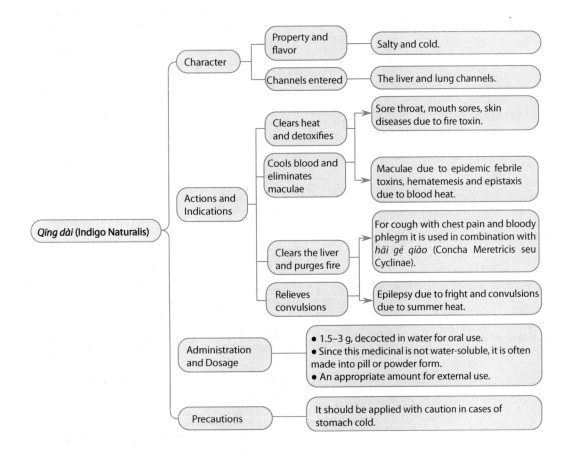

⑦ *Guàn zhòng* (贯众, Rhizoma Cyrtomii, Cyrtomium Rhizome) ★★

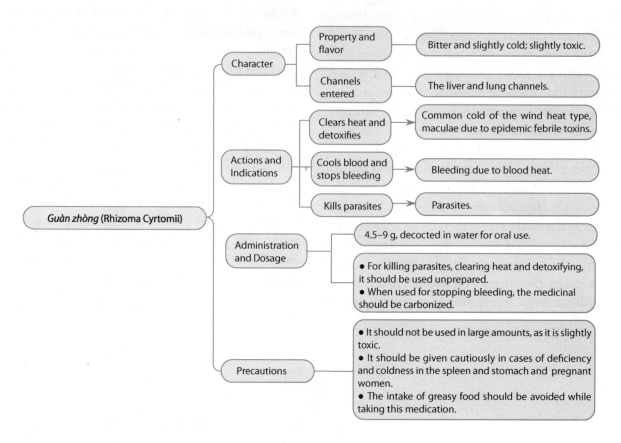

⑧ *Pú gōng yīng* (蒲公英, Herba Taraxaci, Dandelion) ★★★

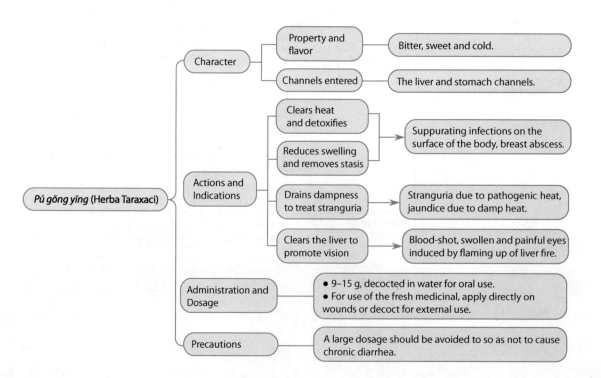

⑨ *Zǐ huā dì dīng* (紫花地丁, Herba Violae, Tokyo
Violet Herb) ★

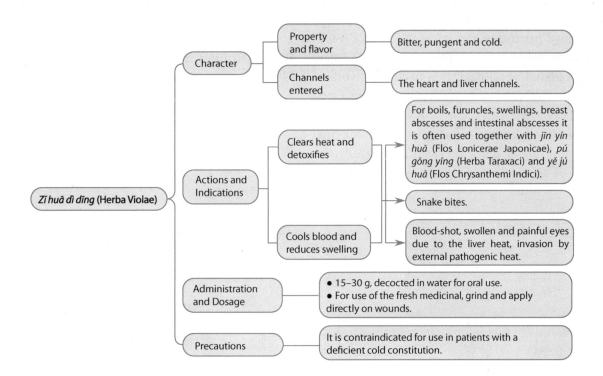

⑩ *Yě jú huā* (野菊花, Flos Chrysanthemi Indici,
Wild Chrysanthemum Flower) ★★

Pú gōng yīng (Herba Taraxaci), *zǐ huā dì dīng* (Herba Violae) and *yě jú huā* (Flos Chrysanthemi Indici) can clear heat, detoxify, reduce swelling and remove stasis, and are used for treating carbuncles, sores, boils and furuncles, swellings, erysipelas, breast abscesses, intestinal abscesses, snake bites and blood-shot, swollen and painful eyes due to liver heat. *Pú gōng yīng* (Herba Taraxaci) is able to activate the channels and promote lactation, and is an important medicinal

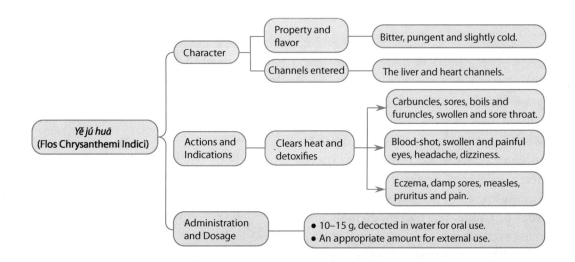

for treating breast abscesses. It can also drain dampness and relieve stranguria, and is indicated for stranguria, and jaundice due to damp heat. *Zǐ huā dì dīng* (Herba Violae) is used especially to detoxify furuncles and sores. *Yě jú huā* (Flos Chrysanthemi Indici) can clear and purge liver fire and dispel wind heat. It is used for swollen and sore throat due to wind heat invading upwards.

In addition, both *yě jú huā* (Flos Chrysanthemi Indici) and *jú huā* (Flos Chrysanthemi) are from the same species, and both can clear heat and detoxify. However, *yě jú huā* (Flos Chrysanthemi Indici) is bitter and cold and effective for detoxifying and relieving infections on the surface of the body. *Jú huā* (Flos Chrysanthemi) has a stronger action of dispelling wind and clearing heat, so it is often used for headache, and blood-shot and swollen eyes caused by wind heat.

⑪ *Chóng lóu* (重楼, Rhizoma Paridis, Paris Rhizome) ★

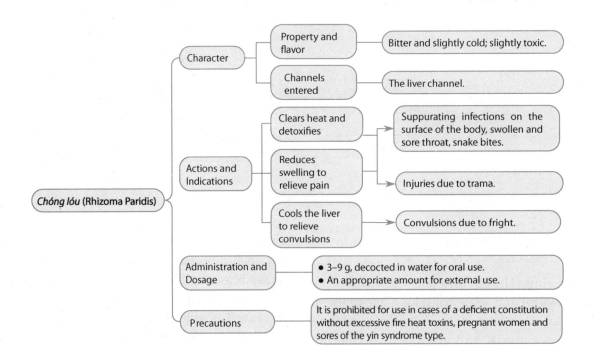

⑫ *Quán shēn* (拳参, Rhizoma Bistortae, Bistort Rhizome)

Both *chóng lóu* (Rhizoma Paridis) and *quán shēn* (Rhizoma Bistortae) can clear heat, detoxify, subdue swelling, cool the liver to extinguish wind, and relieve convulsion. They can be used for carbuncles, swellings, snake bites, scrofula, superficial nodules, and epilepsy due to fright. In some areas of China, the two medicinals are substituted for each other.

Chóng lóu (Rhizoma Paridis) is effective for clearing heat, detoxifying and reducing swelling to relieve pain. Therefore it is used for carbuncles, swellings, and snake bites. It can also transform stasis to relieve pain, and is used for bleeding due to trauma.

Quán shēn (Rhizoma Bistortae) can cool blood, stop bleeding, and drain dampness. Therefore it is used for diarrhea and dysentery of the heat type, bleeding due to blood heat, edema, and dysuria.

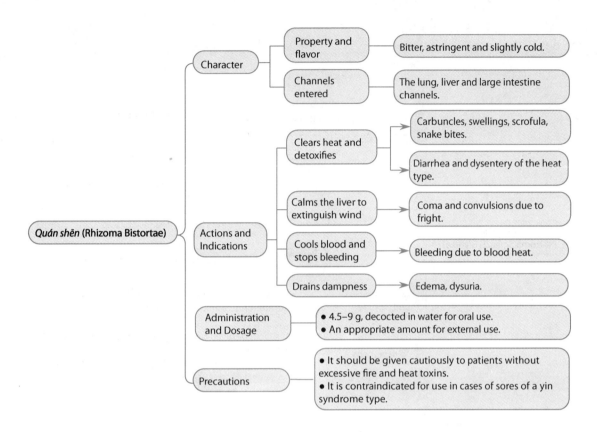

⑬ *Lòu lú* (漏芦, Radix Rhapontici, Rhaponticum Root)

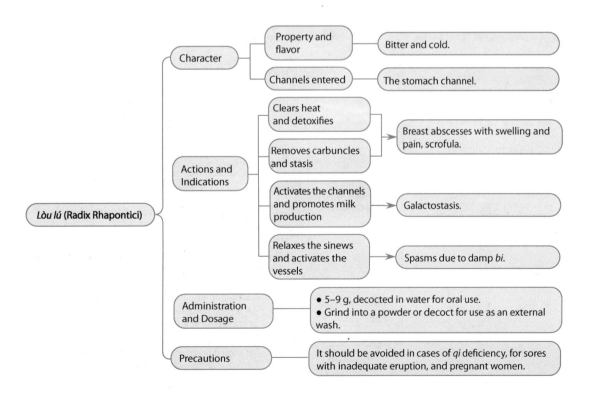

⑭ *Tǔ fú líng* (土茯苓, Rhizoma Smilacis Glabrae, Glabrous Greenbrier Rhizome) ★★

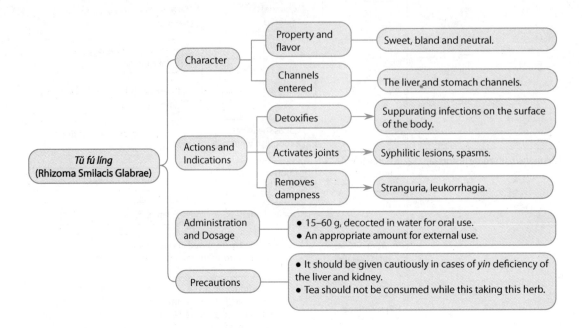

⑮ *Yú xīng cǎo* (鱼腥草, Herba Houttuyniae, Heartleaf Houttuynia Herb) ★★★

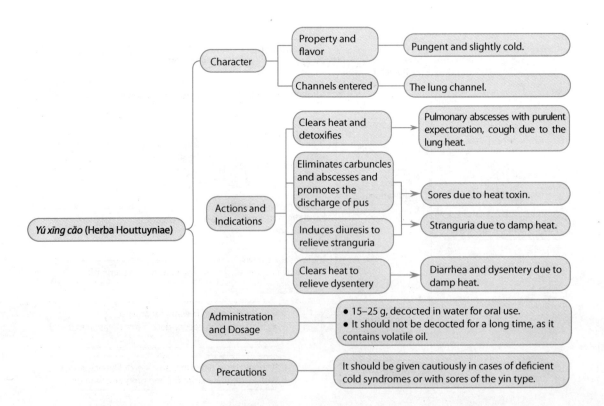

⑯ *Jīn qiáo mài* (金荞麦, Rhizoma Fagopyri Dibotryis, Wild Buckwheat)

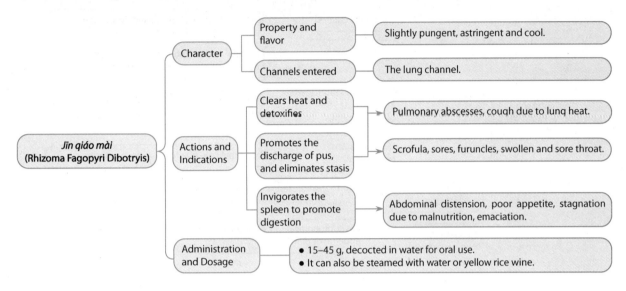

⑰ *Dà xuè téng* (大血藤, Caulis Sargentodoxae, Sargentgloryvine)

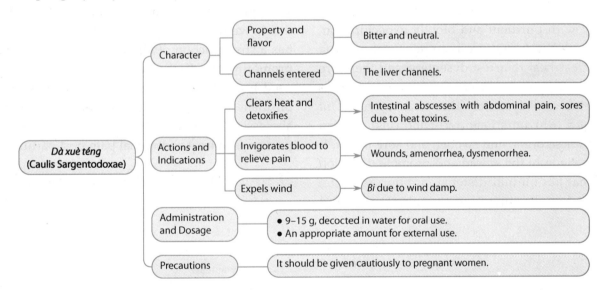

⑱ *Bài jiàng cǎo* (败酱草, Herba Patriniae, Patrinia) ★

Yú xīng cǎo (Herba Houttuyniae), *jīn qiáo mài* (Rhizoma Fagopyri Dibotryis), *dà xuè téng* (Caulis Sargentodoxae) and *bài jiàng cǎo* (Herba Patriniae) can clear heat, and detoxify to remove carbuncles and abscesses. Therefore they are indicated for both carbuncles on the surface of the body and abscesses of the internal organs, and are especially effective for curing abscesses of the internal organs.

Yú xīng cǎo (Herba Houttuyniae) and *jīn qiáo mài* (Rhizoma Fagopyri Dibotryis) mainly treat pulmonary abscesses with chest pain and cough with purulent and foul expectoration, as well as cough due to lung heat. *Dà xuè téng* (Caulis Sargentodoxae) and *bài jiàng cǎo* (Herba Patriniae) are indicated for intestinal abscesses with abdominal pain. They are important medicinals

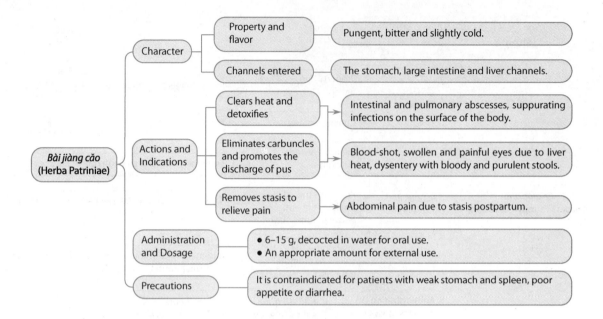

in the treatment of intestinal abscesses.

In addition, *yú xīng cǎo* (Herba Houttuyniae) can promote the discharge of pus, and is effective in treating pulmonary abscesses with cough along with purulent and bloody expectoration. It can also induce diuresis to relieve stranguria and clear heat to arrest dysentery, and therefore is used for stranguria of a heat type, as well as diarrhea and dysentery due to damp heat. *Jīn qiáo mài* (Rhizoma Fagopyri Dibotryis) is often used for scrofula, and swollen and sore throat. It can invigorate the spleen and promote digestion to treat abdominal distension, poor appetite, distended abdomen due to malnutrition and

emaciation. *Dà xuè téng* (Caulis Sargentodoxae) can activate blood and expel wind to relieve pain, and is used for wounds, swelling and pain due to static blood, amenorrhea, dysmenorrhea, and *bi* due to wind damp. *Bài jiàng cǎo* (Herba Patriniae) has a strong action of eliminating abscesses and promoting the discharge of pus. Therefore, it is used for pulmonary abscesses with cough and purulent and bloody expectoration, and hepatic abscesses. It can also eliminate stasis to relieve pain so as to treat abdominal pain post partum.

⑲ *Shè gān* (射干, Rhizoma Belamcandae, Blackberrylily Rhizome) ★★★

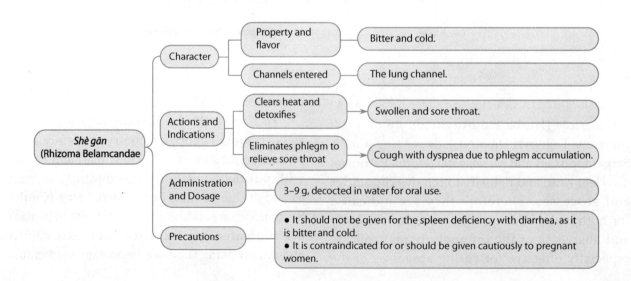

20 *Shān dòu gēn* (山豆根, Radix et Rhizoma Sophorae Tonkinensis, Vietnamese Sophora Root) ★ ★

Addition **Bĕi dòu gēn (北豆根, Rhizoma Menispermi, Asiatic Moonseed Rhizome)** is bitter in flavor and cold in property and slightly toxic. It can clear heat, detoxify and expel wind to relieve pain. It is used for swollen and sore throat, diarrhea, dysentery due to heat toxin exuberance, and *bi* due to wind dampness.

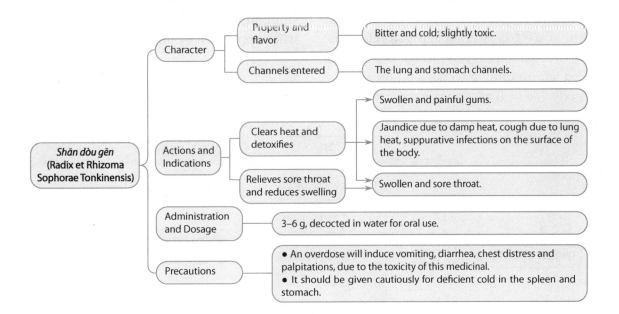

21 *Mă bó* (马勃, Lasiosphaera seu Calvatia, Puffball)

Shè gān (Rhizoma Belamcandae), *shān dòu gēn* (Radix et Rhizoma Sophorae Tonkinensis) and *mă bó* (Lasiosphaera seu Calvatia) act to clear heat and detoxify to relieve sore throats. They are very effective medicinals used in laryngology.

Shè gān (Rhizoma Belamcandae) is bitter, cold and descending. It can dispel phlegm, scatter blood and reduce swelling. It is especially suitable for a swollen and sore throat due to blood stasis with heat accumulation or phlegm heat exuberant congestion. It is also used for

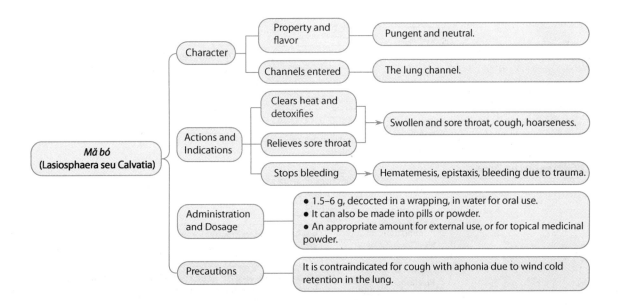

cough with dyspnea due to phlegm exuberance of either a cold or heat type, when combined with other proper medicinals. *Shān dòu gēn* (Radix et Rhizoma Sophorae Tonkinensis) is severely bitter and cold and has a stronger action in purging fire, detoxifying and reducing swelling. It is suitable to treat a swollen and sore throat caused by fire toxin exuberance in the lung and stomach, as well as swollen and painful gums, jaundice of a damp heat type, cough due to lung heat, and suppurating infections on the surface of the body. *Mǎ bó* (Lasiosphaera seu Calvatia) is

pungent and neutral, and can dispel wind heat in the lung channel. It is indicated for swollen and sore throat, cough and aphonia due to wind heat invasion of the lung or depressed heat in the lung. In addition it is able to stop bleeding. When taken orally, it can treat hematemesis and epistaxis due to blood heat. It has the effect of stopping bleeding due to injuries from trauma when applied on wounds.

㉒ *Qīng guǒ* (青果, Fructus Canarii, Chinese White Olive)

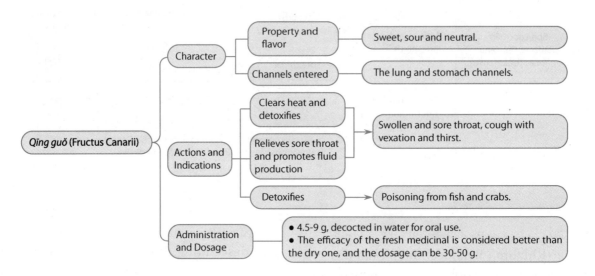

㉓ *Jǐn dēng lóng* (锦灯笼, Calyx seu Fructus Physalis, Franchet Groundcherry Fruit)

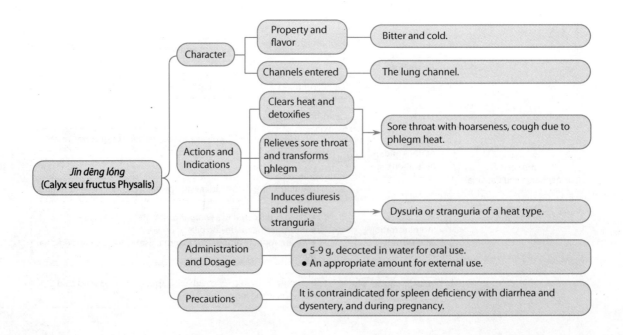

㉔ *Jīn guǒ lǎn* (金果榄, Radix Tinosporae, Tinospora Root)

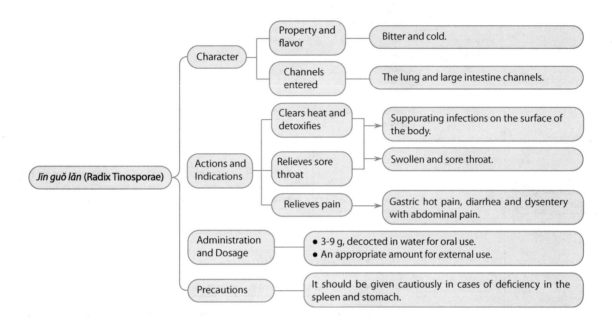

㉕ *Mù hú dié* (木蝴蝶, Semen Oroxyli, Indian Trumpetflower Seed)

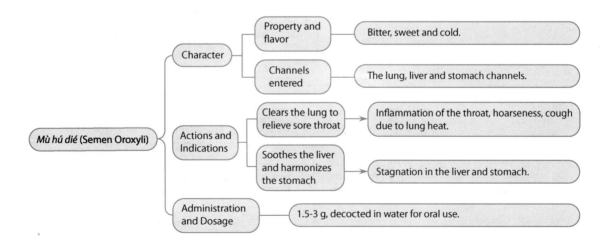

㉖ *Bái tóu wēng* (白头翁, Radix Pulsatillae, Pulsatilla Root) ★★★

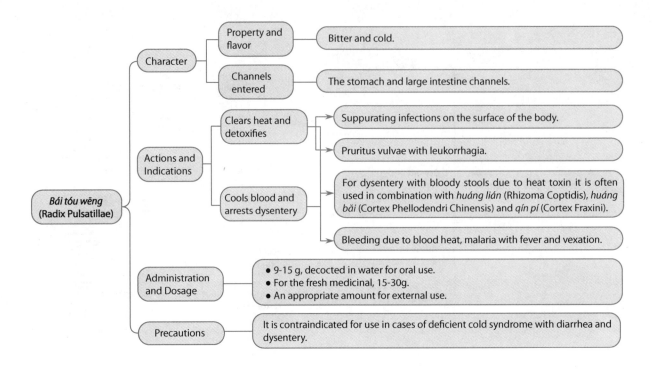

㉗ *Mǎ chǐ xiàn* (马齿苋, Herba Portulacae, Purslane Herb)

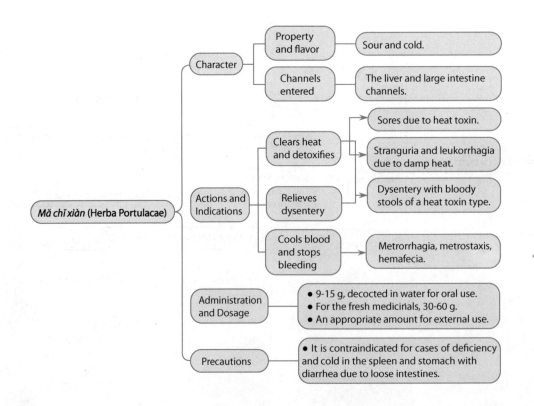

㉘ *Yā dǎn zǐ* (鸦胆子, Fructus Bruceae, Java Brucea Fruit)

Bái tóu wēng (Radix Pulsatillae), *mǎ chǐ xiàn* (Herba Portulacae) and *yā dǎn zǐ* (Fructus Bruceae) can clear heat, and detoxify as well as cool blood to relieve dysentery. Therefore they are indicated for dysentery with bloody and purulent stools, fever, abdominal pain, and tenesmus due to heat toxins. *Bái tóu wēng* (Radix Pulsatillae) is bitter and cold with a descending action, and can clear damp heat in the stomach and large intestine, as well as heat toxin in the *xue* level. It is used for suppurating infections on the surface of the body, pruritus vulvae and malaria. *Mǎ chǐ xiàn* (Herba Portulacae) is able to cool blood and arrest bleeding, and is used for metrorrhagia, metrostaxis, and hemafecia due to blood heat, as well as skin diseases, and stranguria due to pathogenic heat and hematuria. *Yā dǎn zǐ* (Fructus Bruceae) is bitter, cold, and slightly toxic. It is used to treat chronic dysentery due to cold and food retention. It can also stop malaria of all kinds, as well as eliminate abnormal growths when used externally.

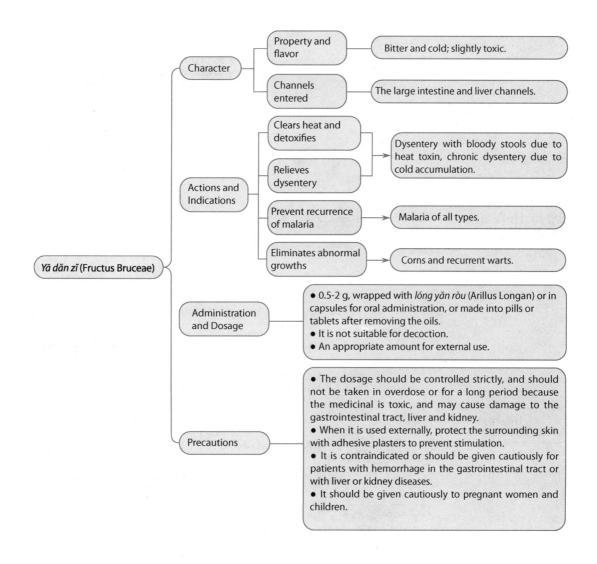

Yā dǎn zǐ (Fructus Bruceae)

- **Character**
  - **Property and flavor** → Bitter and cold; slightly toxic.
  - **Channels entered** → The large intestine and liver channels.

- **Actions and Indications**
  - **Clears heat and detoxifies**
  - **Relieves dysentery** → Dysentery with bloody stools due to heat toxin, chronic dysentery due to cold accumulation.
  - **Prevent recurrence of malaria** → Malaria of all types.
  - **Eliminates abnormal growths** → Corns and recurrent warts.

- **Administration and Dosage**
  - 0.5-2 g, wrapped with *lóng yǎn ròu* (Arillus Longan) or in capsules for oral administration, or made into pills or tablets after removing the oils.
  - It is not suitable for decoction.
  - An appropriate amount for external use.

- **Precautions**
  - The dosage should be controlled strictly, and should not be taken in overdose or for a long period because the medicinal is toxic, and may cause damage to the gastrointestinal tract, liver and kidney.
  - When it is used externally, protect the surrounding skin with adhesive plasters to prevent stimulation.
  - It is contraindicated or should be given cautiously for patients with hemorrhage in the gastrointestinal tract or with liver or kidney diseases.
  - It should be given cautiously to pregnant women and children.

㉙ *Dì jǐn cǎo* (地锦草, Herba Euphorbiae Humifusae, Humifuse Euphorbia Herb)

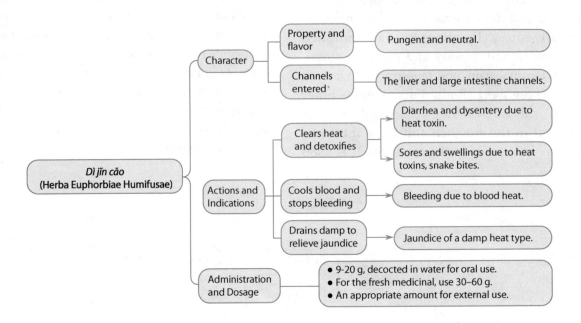

㉚ *Wěi líng cài* (委陵菜, Herba Potentillae Chinensis, Chinese Cinquefoil)

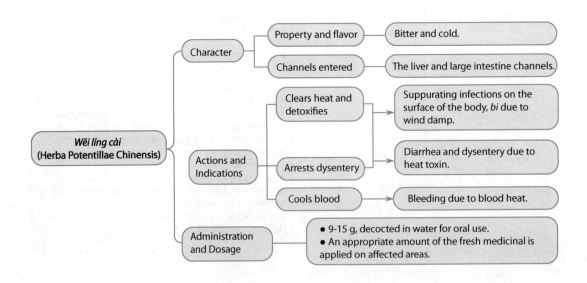

㉛ *Fān bái cǎo* (翻白草, Herba Potentillae Discoloris, Descolor Cinquefoil Herb)

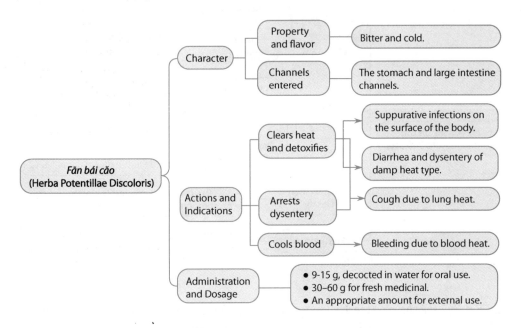

㉜ *Bàn biān lián* (半边莲, Herba Lobeliae Chinensis, Chinese Lobelia)

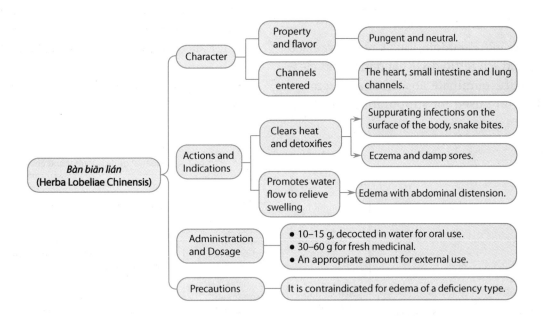

㉝ *Bái huā shé shé cǎo* (白花蛇舌草, Herba Hedyotis Diffusae, Spreading Hedyotis Herb) ★★

Both *bàn biān lián* (Herba Lobeliae Chinensis) and *bái huā shé shé cǎo* (Herba Hedyotis Diffusae) can clear heat, detoxify and drain damp to relieve stranguria, and are used for suppurating infections on the surface of the body, snake bites; stranguria of a heat type and dysuria. *Bàn biān lián* (Herba Lobeliae Chinensis) has a stronger action in draining damp, and therefore can promote water flow to reduce swelling. Therefore it is used for edema, dropsy, and jaundice with

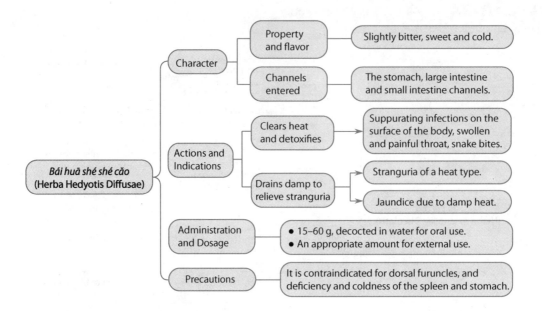

reddish urine. *Bái huā shé shé cǎo* (Herba Hedyotis Diffusae) is able to treat swollen and sore throat, intestinal abscesses with abdominal pain by clearing heat and detoxifying.

③④ *Shān cí gū* (山慈菇, Pseudobulbus Cremastrae seu Pleiones, Common Pleione Pseudobulb)

Both *shān cí gū* (Pseudobulbus Cremastrae seu Pleiones) and *lòu lú* (Radix Rhapontici) can clear heat, detoxify, eliminate abscesses and remove stasis. They are used for suppurating infections on the surface of the body, scrofula and obstinate ulcers. *Shān cí gū* (Pseudobulbus Cremastrae seu Pleiones) has a stronger action in removing stasis, and in recent years has been used extensively to treat abdominal masses and various tumors. *Lòu lú* (Radix Rhapontici) is most effective in activating channels to induce lactation, so it is used for stagnation of the breast collaterals with such manifestations as lack of lactation, breast distending pain, and swelling pain due to breast abscesses.

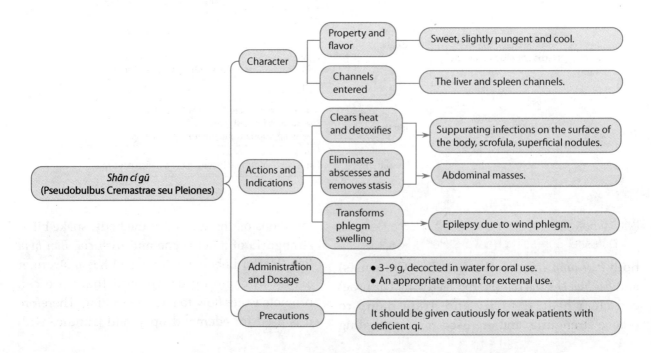

㉟ *Xióng dăn* (熊胆, Ursi Fel, Bear Gall) ★★

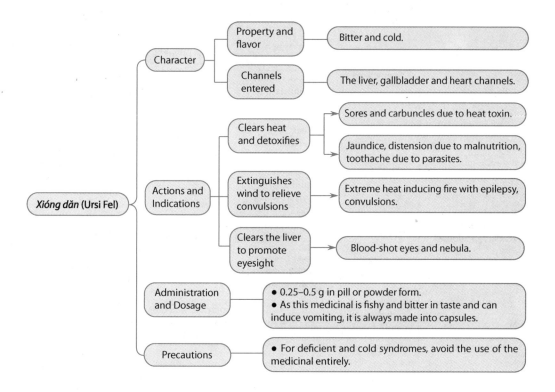

㊱ *Qiān lǐ guāng* (千里光, Herba Senecionis Scandentis, Climbing Groundsel Herb)

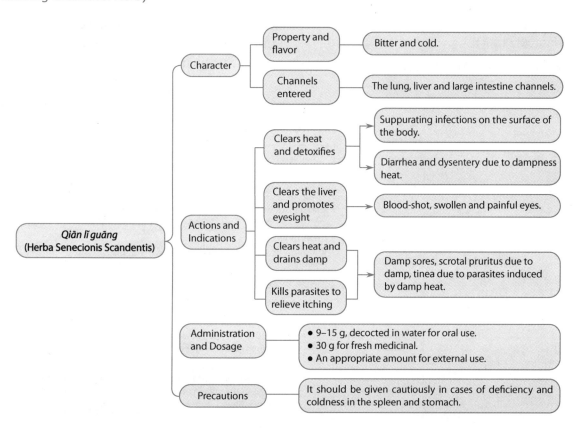

㊲ *Bái liǎn* (白蔹, Radix Ampelopsis, Radix Ampelopsis, Ampelopsis)

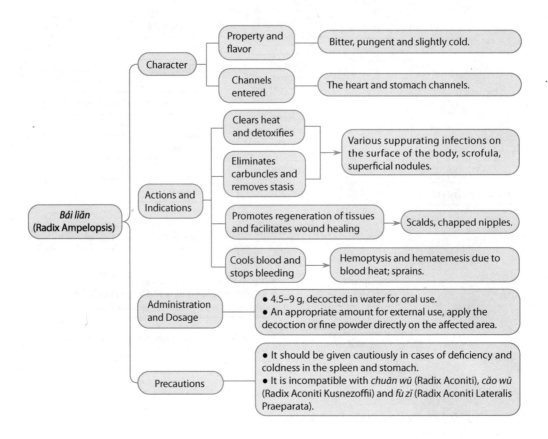

㊳ *Sì jì qīng* (四季青, Folium Illics Purpureae, Purple Flower Holly Leaf)

Both *bái liǎn* (Radix Ampelopsis) and *sì jì qīng* (Folium Illics Purpureae) can clear heat, detoxify and promote wound healing, and are used for suppurating infections on the surface of the

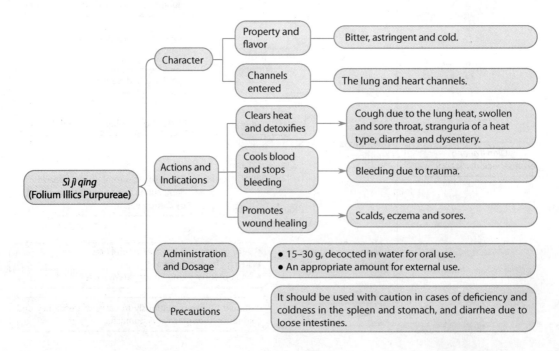

body and scalds. *Bái liǎn* (Radix Ampelopsis) is effective for eliminating carbuncles and removing stasis, and promoting regeneration of tissues to relieve pain. Therefore it is able to eliminate sores without pus, promote the discharge of pus and encourage wound healing. *Sì jì qīng* (Folium Illics Purpureae) is effective for cooling blood and promoting wound healing, and is the most effective in treating scalds, eczema, damp sores,

and ulcers in the lower limbs. It can also astringe to stop bleeding, and is used for bleeding due to trauma. In addition, it is used for the common cold due to wind cold, cough due to lung heat, swollen and sore throat, stranguria of a heat type, and diarrhea and dysentery of a damp heat type.

㊴ *Lǜ dòu* (绿豆, Semen Phaseoli Radiati, Mung Bean)

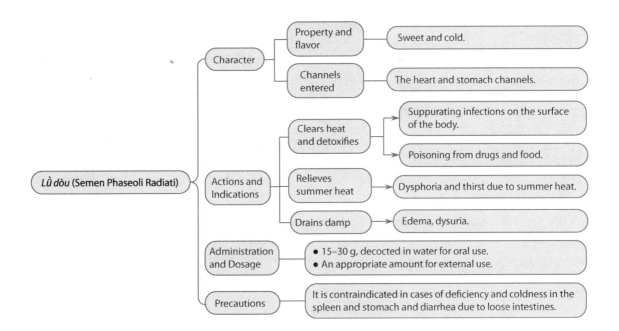

Section 4   Medicinals that Clear Heat and Cool Blood

Medicinals of this kind are usually bitter and cold or salty and cold. They are able to enter the *xue* level to clear heat, and therefore are often attributed to the heart and kidney channels. They are used for heat syndrome of an excess type in the *ying* level and the *xue* level, such as heat entering the *ying* level, consuming yin and disturbing the mind due to epidemic febrile disease, with symptoms like a crimson tongue, fever that worsens at night, insomnia with vexation, a thready and rapid pulse, or even

coma, delirium and visible ecchymoses and rash. In cases of heat invading the pericardium, there are manifestations of coma, delirium, dysphagia, dysfunction of the limbs, and a red crimson tongue. For cases of exuberant heat disturbing the blood and the mind, there are symptoms such as a deep crimson tongue, hematemesis, epistaxis, hematuria, hemafecia, dark purplish ecchymoses and rash, restlessness, or even coma and madness. They are also used for bleeding of a blood heat type induced by other diseases.

① *Shēng dì huáng* (生地黄, Radix Rehmanniae, Rehmannia Root) ★★★

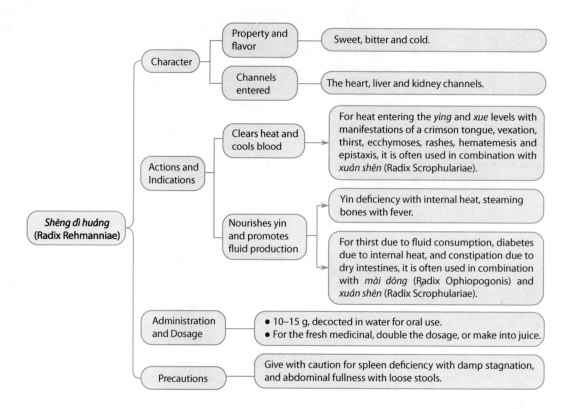

② *Xuán shēn* (玄参, Radix Scrophulariae, Figwort Root) ★ ★ ★

Both *shēng dì huáng* (Radix Rehmanniae Recens)

and *xuán shēn* (Radix Scrophulariae) are sweet and bitter in flavor and cold in property, and can clear heat to cool blood and nourish yin to

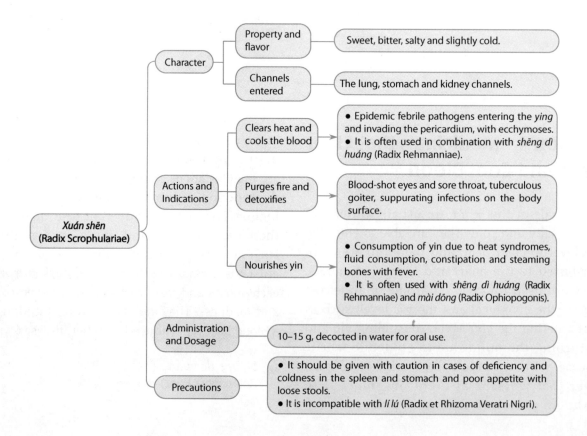

promote fluid production. Both medicinals are used for heat pathogens entering the *ying* and *xue* levels with manifestations such as general fever, ecchymoses, restlessness, dry mouth, a crimson tongue, or even coma, and delirium. They are also used for consumption due to heat syndrome with diabetes, manifesting as vexation, thirst and polydypsia; as well as internal heat due to yin deficiency with steaming bones and fever, night sweats and seminal emission; and the depletion of yin due to severe heat with constipation. The two medicinals are used in combination for heat syndromes of either an excess or deficient type. *Shēng dì huáng* (Radix Rehmanniae Recens) can clear heat to cool the blood, nourish yin to promote fluid production, and is often used for yin consumption due to heat syndrome with vexation, thirst and polydypsia, as well as for internal heat due to yin deficiency with diabetes. It is also used in the later stages of epidemic

febrile diseases with inadequate elimination of heat, yin consumption and pathogens retained in the yin, with symptoms such as night fever and cool skin in the morning, a red tongue and a rapid pulse; as well as hematemesis, epistaxis, hemafecia, hematuria, metrorrhagia and metrostaxis due to blood heat. *Xuán shēn* (Radix Scrophulariae) has a salty flavor, and is effective for purging fire, detoxifying and removing stasis. It is often used for swollen and sore throat induced by heat toxin exuberance, craniofacial infections characterized by a swollen and sore throat, swelling and redness of the head, diphtheria induced by fire hyperactivity due to yin deficiency; scrofula and superficial nodules due to mingling of phlegm and fire, and skin diseases.

③ *Mǔ dān pí* (牡丹皮, Cortex Moutan, Tree Peony Bark) ★ ★ ★

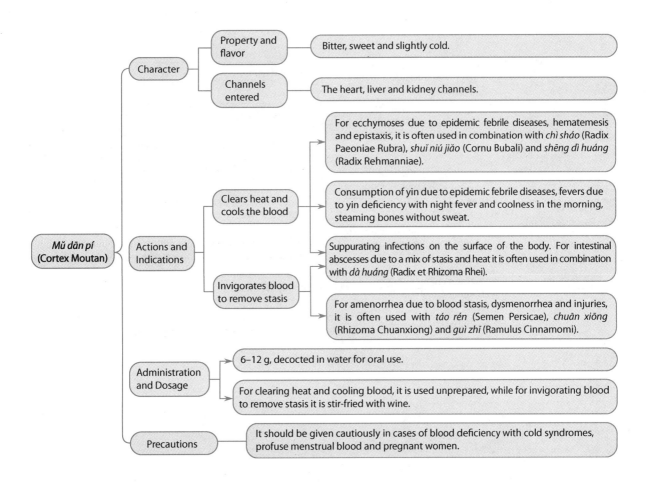

④ *Chì sháo* (赤芍, Radix Paeoniae Rubra, Red Peony Root) ★ ★ ★

Both *mǔ dān pí* (Cortex Moutan) and *chì sháo* (Radix Paeoniae Rubra) are bitter in flavor and slightly cold in nature, and are attributed to the liver channel. They can clear heat and cool blood, invigorate blood to remove stasis, and are used for diseases caused by blood heat and blood stasis, and especially a mix of blood heat with blood stasis. The two medicinals are indicated for general fever with ecchymoses, dry mouth and crimson tongue due to heat invading the *ying* and *xue*; hematemesis, epistaxis, metrorrhagia, metrostaxis, profuse menstruation due to blood heat; amenorrhea due to blood stasis, dysmenorrhea, abdominal pain post partum, abdominal masses due to blood stasis, injuries due to trauma, swelling pain due to blood stasis, and suppurating infections on the surface of the body. However, *mǔ dān pí* (Cortex Moutan) has a pungent flavor, and has a stronger action of clearing heat and cooling blood, and therefore is effective in clearing and dispelling heat retention in the yin and blood, in the later stage of epidemic febrile disease, with manifestations of night fever with cool body in the morning, fever receding without sweat; steaming bones with fever, night sweats, and seminal emission due to yin deficiency. *Mǔ dān pí* (Cortex Moutan) can clear heat, cool blood, invigorate blood to remove stasis so as to eliminate organ abscesses, and is often used for intestinal abscesses in the initial stage of mingling of stasis and heat type, with fever and abdominal pain. It has a strong action of invigorating blood to remove stasis and relieve pain, and therefore is often used for diseases induced by blood stagnation. In addition, it can clear and purge liver fire, and is indicated for blood-shot and painful eyes and nebulae due to upwardly flaring liver fire.

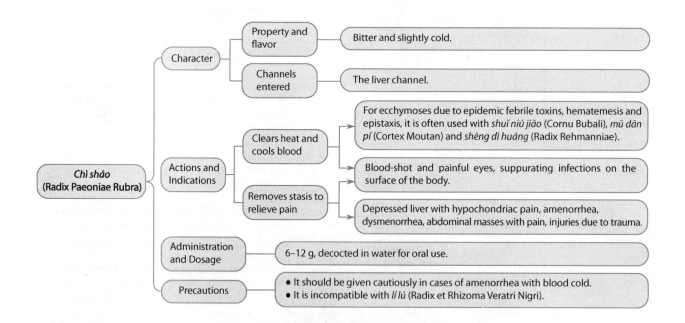

Chì sháo (Radix Paeoniae Rubra)

- Character
  - Property and flavor — Bitter and slightly cold.
  - Channels entered — The liver channel.
- Actions and Indications
  - Clears heat and cools blood — For ecchymoses due to epidemic febrile toxins, hematemesis and epistaxis, it is often used with *shuǐ niú jiǎo* (Cornu Bubali), *mǔ dān pí* (Cortex Moutan) and *shēng dì huáng* (Radix Rehmanniae).
  - Removes stasis to relieve pain
    - Blood-shot and painful eyes, suppurating infections on the surface of the body.
    - Depressed liver with hypochondriac pain, amenorrhea, dysmenorrhea, abdominal masses with pain, injuries due to trauma.
- Administration and Dosage — 6–12 g, decocted in water for oral use.
- Precautions
  - It should be given cautiously in cases of amenorrhea with blood cold.
  - It is incompatible with *lí lú* (Radix et Rhizoma Veratri Nigri).

⑤ *Zǐ cǎo* (紫草, Radix Arnebiae, Arnebia Root) ★★

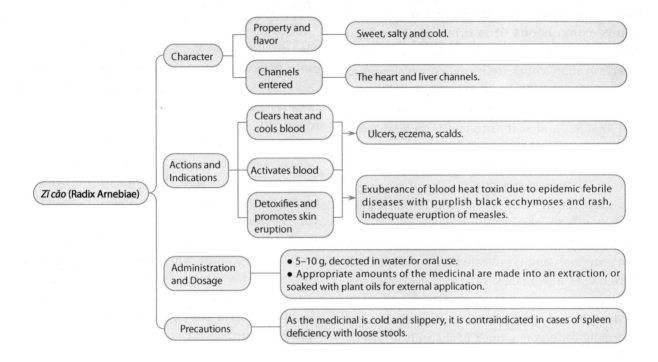

⑥ *Shuǐ niú jiǎo* (水牛角, Cornu Bubali, Buffalo Horn) ★★

Shuǐ niú jiǎo (Cornu Bubali) and *zǐ cǎo* (Radix Arnebiae) are cold and attributed to the heart and liver channels. Both medicinals can clear heat, cool blood and detoxify, and are indicated for purplish black ecchymoses and rashes, as well as carbuncles and skin diseases. However,

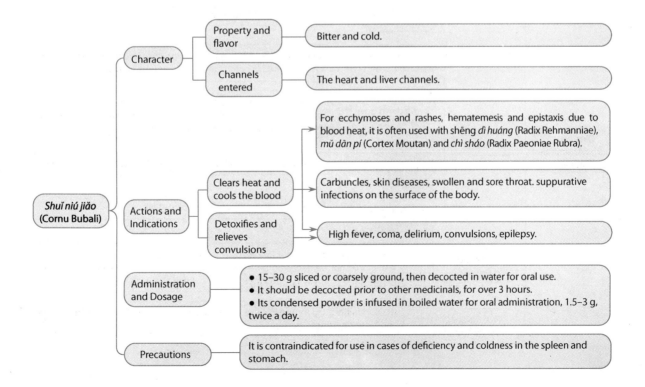

shuǐ niú jiǎo (Cornu Bubali) has a stronger action in clearing heat, cooling blood and detoxifying than *zǐ cǎo* (Radix Arnebiae), and it is able to relieve convulsions. It is often used for heat invading the *ying* and *xue* levels with general fever, vexation, coma, delirium, convulsions and epilepsy induced by epidemic febrile diseases; hematemesis and epistaxis due to blood heat; and swollen and sore throat due to heat toxin exuberance. In addition, it has the same action as *xī jiǎo* (Cornu Rhinocerotis) but is milder in efficacy. Therefore currently it is frequently used as a substitution for *xī jiǎo* (Cornu Rhinocerotis). *Zǐ cǎo* (Radix Arnebiae) is effective for cooling and activating the blood, detoxifying and promoting skin eruptions, and is indicated for purplish black ecchymoses and rashes, purplish dark measles and inadequate eruption of measles due to blood heat exuberance. In addition, it is often used externally for eczema, tinea of the vulvae, scalds and burns.

Section 5   Medicinals that Clear Deficient Heat

Medicinals of this kind are usually cold or cool, enter the *yin* level, and have actions of clearing deficient fever and steaming bones. They are mainly indicated for steaming bones with tidal fever, tidal fever, or feverish sensation in the palms and soles, insomnia with vexation, night sweats, seminal emissions, a red tongue with a scanty coating, a thready and rapid pulse due to deficient fire invading the interior caused by yin deficiency in the liver and kidney; deficient syndrome with symptoms such as nocturnal fever, fever receding without sweat, a red crimson tongue, and a thready and rapid pulse due to consumption of yin fluids caused by inadequate clearance of heat pathogens in the later stages of epidemic febrile diseases.

① *Qīng hāo* (青蒿, Herba Artemisiae Annuae, Sweet Wormwood Herb) ★ ★ ★

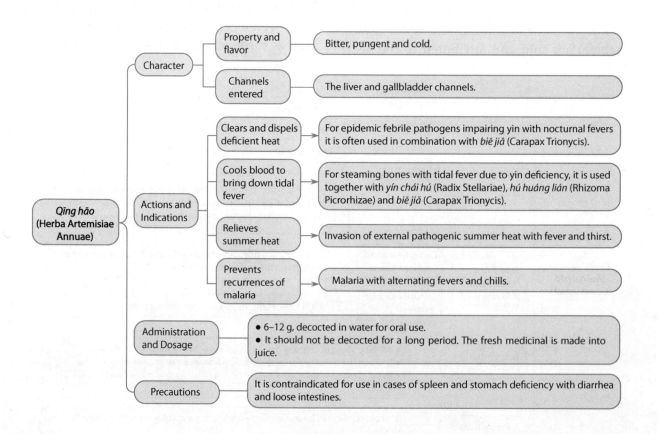

Qīng hāo (Herba Artemisiae Annuae)	Character	Property and flavor → Bitter, pungent and cold.
		Channels entered → The liver and gallbladder channels.
	Actions and Indications	Clears and dispels deficient heat → For epidemic febrile pathogens impairing yin with nocturnal fevers it is often used in combination with *biē jiǎ* (Carapax Trionycis).
		Cools blood to bring down tidal fever → For steaming bones with tidal fever due to yin deficiency, it is used together with *yín chái hú* (Radix Stellariae), *hú huáng lián* (Rhizoma Picrorhizae) and *biē jiǎ* (Carapax Trionycis).
		Relieves summer heat → Invasion of external pathogenic summer heat with fever and thirst.
		Prevents recurrences of malaria → Malaria with alternating fevers and chills.
	Administration and Dosage	• 6–12 g, decocted in water for oral use. • It should not be decocted for a long period. The fresh medicinal is made into juice.
	Precautions	It is contraindicated for use in cases of spleen and stomach deficiency with diarrhea and loose intestines.

② *Bái wēi* (白薇, Radix et Rhizoma Cynanchi Atrati, Cynanchi Root and Rhizome) ★

Qīng hāo (Herba Artemisiae Annuae) and *bái wēi* (Radix et Rhizoma Cynanchi Atrati) are bitter in flavor and cold in nature, and can clear heat, cool blood and remove steaming bones by simultaneously clearing and dispelling heat. They are indicated for febrile diseases in the later stages, with accumulation of heat, marked by nocturnal fever, fever receding without sweat, or lingering low fever after febrile diseases; yin deficiency with fever and steaming bones; and invasion by external pathogens due to yin deficiency with fever, dry throat, thirst, and vexation. The differences between these herbs are that: *Qīng hāo* (Herba Artemisiae Annuae) is pungent and aromatic; it has a strong effect in clearing heat and relieving steaming bones; it is effective for clearing heat in the *ying* level; and is an essential medicinal for clearing deficient heat. It can also relieve summer-heat and prevent the recurrence of malaria, it is often used for external invasion by summer heat, dizziness, headache, fever, thirst, and alternating fever and chills due to malaria, and is an effective medicinal to treat malaria. *Bái wēi* (Radix et Rhizoma Cynanchi Atrati) is salty and enters the *xue* level, it can clear deficient heat and can clear excessive heat in the *xue* level. It is also used for post-partum fever due to blood-deficiency and pathogenic heat invasion in the *ying* level due to febrile disease. It can induce diuresis and relieve stranguria, can detoxify and treat sores, and is used for stranguria due to heat, and for hematuria and inflamed sores.

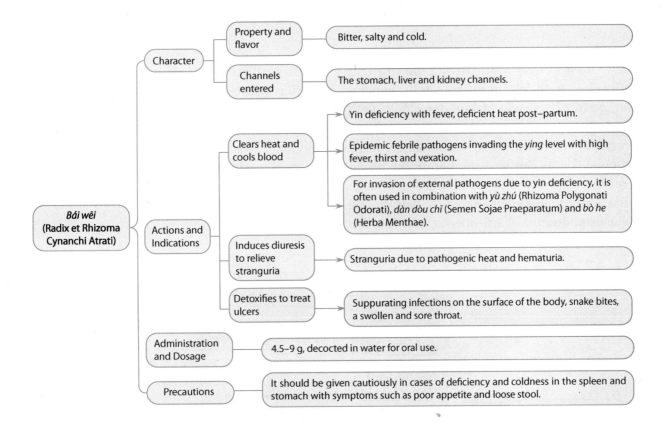

③ *Dì gǔ pí* (地骨皮, Cortex Lycii, Chinese Wolfberry Root-bark) ★ ★ ★

Both *mǔ dān pí* (Cortex Moutan) and *dì gǔ pí* (Cortex Lycii) can cool blood to clear blood heat, and are indicated for yin deficiency with fever, hematemesis, epistaxis and hematuria due to blood heat. *Mǔ dān pí* (Cortex Moutan) has actions of clearing heat and cooling blood, and is

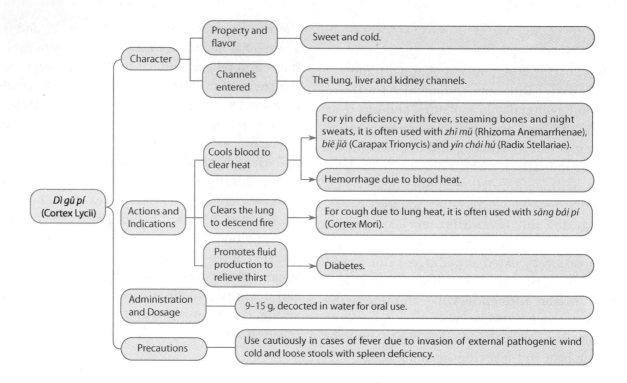

usually used to treat heat entering the *ying* and *xue* levels due to febrile diseases with general fever, ecchymoses, skin rashes, dry mouth with a crimson tongue, and heat syndrome of the excessive type manifesting with hematemesis and epistaxis. It can also invigorate the blood to remove stasis and is used for amenorrhea, dysmenorrhea, abdominal pain post-partum due to stasis, abdominal hard masses, and injuries

and intestinal abscesses with abdominal pain. *Dì gǔ pí* (Cortex Lycii) can clear deficient heat to relieve steaming bones, and therefore is used for yin deficiency with tidal fever, steaming bones and night sweating. It is also used for cough with dyspnea by clearing lung heat.

④ *Yín chái hú* (银柴胡, Radix Stellariae, Starwort Root) ★★

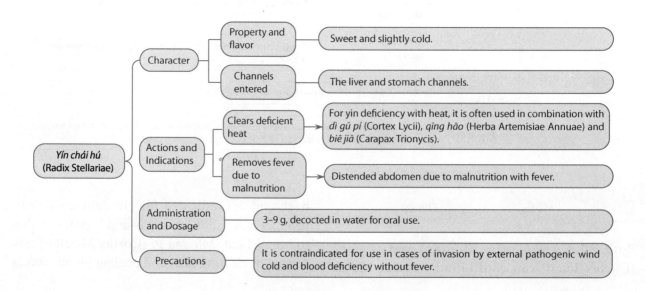

⑤ *Hú huáng lián* (胡黄连, Rhizoma Picrorhizae, Figwortflower Picrorhiza Rhizome) ★ ★ ★

Dì gǔ pí (Cortex Lycii), *yín chái hú* (Radix Stellariae) and *hú huáng lián* (Rhizoma Picrorhizae) can clear deficient heat and remove steaming bones, and are used for yin deficiency with fever, steaming bones with tidal fever, night sweats and vexation. *Dì gǔ pí* (Cortex Lycii) and *yín chái hú* (Radix Stellariae) are most effective in bringing down deficient fever and removing steaming bones. *Yín chái hú* (Radix Stellariae) and *hú huáng lián* (Rhizoma Picrorhizae) can clear fever caused by a distended abdomen due to malnutrition with an enlarged abdomen, and emaciation and withered hair. *Dì gǔ pí* (Cortex Lycii) is sweet and cold, and can cool blood, stop bleeding and clear the lungs to descend fire. It is used for hematemesis, epistaxis, and hematuria due to blood heat, and cough with dyspnea due to lung heat. *Yín chái hú* (Radix Stellariae) is sweet and slightly cold, and has a strong action of clearing fever due to a distended abdomen from malnutrition. *Hú huáng lián* (Rhizoma Picrorhizae) is bitter and cold with a descending nature, and is used for diarrhea and dysentery due to damp heat, and hemorrhoids.

Hú huáng lián (Rhizoma Picrorhizae) and *huáng lián* (Rhizoma Coptidis) have a bitter flavor and cold nature, and can clear heat and dry dampness. They are used for diarrhea and dysentery of a damp heat type, manifesting as abdominal pain with fever, tenesmus, and purulent and bloody stool. *Hú huáng lián* (Rhizoma Picrorhizae) can be a substitute for *huáng lián* (Rhizoma Coptidis) if *huáng lián* (Rhizoma Coptidis) is not available. However, there are differences. *Hú huáng lián* (Rhizoma Picrorhizae) is bitter and cold with a descendant action, and has an inferior action in clearing damp heat. It is mainly used for damp heat syndrome in the lower *jiao* with symptoms such as diarrhea, dysentery, and hemorrhoids. It can also bring down deficient fever and clear fever caused by distended abdomen due to malnutrition, and therefore is indicated for fever of a yin deficiency type with steaming bones, tidal fever, night sweating and vexation; fever due to distended abdomen from malnutrition in infants, an enlarged abdomen, emaciation, and withered hair. *Huáng lián* (Rhizoma Coptidis) has strong heat-clearing and drying actions and is especially effective for clearing damp heat in the lower *jiao*. Therefore it is used for all diseases induced by damp heat such as diarrhea, dysentery, jaundice, stranguria due to chyluria, leukorrhagia, and damp sores. It can relieve vexation and vomiting, and detoxify through clearing heart and stomach

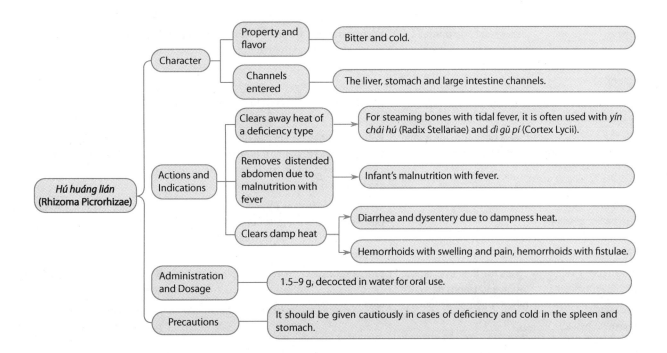

fire of an excessive type. Therefore it is often used for fire exuberance of febrile diseases with manifestations such as high fever, vexation, or even coma and delirium; heart fire hyperactivity with vexation, insomnia and mouth sores; vomiting due to stomach fire hyperactivity; disharmony between the liver and stomach with hypochondriac distending pain, vomiting and sour regurgitation; as well as symptoms such as ear pain with pustular discharge, blood-shot, swollen and painful eyes, and sepsis.

Actions of medicinals that clear heat are summarized as follows (Tables 9-2~9-7, see p.128~133):

Table 9-2: Summary of Medicinals that Clear Heat and Purge Fire:

Medicinal	Actions in Common	Individual Characteristics	
		Characteristic Actions	Other Actions
Shí gāo (Gypsum Fibrosum)	Clears heat and purges fire to relieve vexation and thirst	Pungent, sweet and severely cold, it has a strong action in clearing heat and purging fire, clearing heat as well as dispelling pathogens from superficial muscles. It can mainly clear fire in the lung and stomach.	The calcined one is used for promoting regeneration of the tissue and wound healing, removing dampness, stopping blood
Zhī mǔ (Rhizoma Anemarrhenae)		Bitter, sweet and cold with a moist texture, it is effective for nourishing the yin to moisten dryness as well as clearing heat. It can mainly nourish dryness in the lung and stomach	Effective for nourishing the kidney to bring down fire
Hán shuǐ shí (Glauberitum)	Clears heat and purges fire		
Lú gēn (Rhizoma Phragmitis)	Clears heat and purges fire to relieve vexation and thirst	With a stronger action in clearing heat than *tiān huā fěn* (Radix Trichosanthis)	Clears the lung, removes phlegm and promotes the discharge of pus, clears the stomach to relieve vomiting, clears heat and induces diuresis
Tiān huā fěn (Radix Trichosanthis)		Effective for promoting fluid production	Clears the lung and moistens dryness, reduces swelling and promotes the discharge of pus
Zhú yè (Folium Phyllostachydis Henonis)	Clears heat and purges fire to relieve vexation and induces diuresis	With a stronger action in clearing heart fire to relieve vexation than *dàn zhú yè* (Herba Lophatheri)	Promotes the production of fluid
Dàn zhú yè (Herba Lophatheri)		Effective for clearing heat to induce diuresis	
Zhī zǐ (Fructus Gardeniae)	Clears heat and purges fire, detoxifies and drains damp	With a strong action in clearing heat, it can purge fire and detoxify, it is effective for clearing and purging fire in the heart, lung, stomach and *san jiao* to relieve vexation	Cools blood, stops bleeding, reduces swelling to relieve pain
Yā zhí cǎo (Herba Commelinae)		Clears heat as well as dispels external pathogens from the exterior. It has a strong action in promoting water flow to relieve edema	Dispels pathogenic factors from the exterior
Xià kū cǎo (Spica Prunellae)	Clears the liver to promote vision and brings down blood pressure	With a strong action in clearing liver fire	Removes stasis and reduces swelling
Jué míng zǐ (Semen Cassiae)		With a strong action in promoting vision	Moistens intestines to promote defecation

Table 9-2: Summary of Medicinals that Clear Heat and Purge Fire:

continued

Medicinal	Actions in Common	Individual Characteristics		Other Actions
		Characteristic Actions		**Other Actions**
Gǔ jīng cǎo (Flos Eriocauli)	Relieves exterior syndrome, promotes skin eruptions	It can mainly dispel wind heat to promote vision and remove nebula		
Mì méng huā (Flos Buddlejae)		It can mainly clear the liver to promote vision and remove nebula	Nourishes the liver, suitable for eye diseases of both excess and deficiency type	
Qīng xiāng zǐ (Semen Celosiae)			It has a strong action in clearing liver fire	

Table 9-3: Summary of Medicinals that Clear Heat and Dry Dampness:

Medicinal	Action in Common	Individual Character		Other Actions
		Characteristic Actions		**Other Actions**
Huáng qín (Fructus Gardeniae)	Clears heat and dries dampness, purges fire and detoxifies	Effective for clearing damp heat in the upper *jiao*, clearing lung fire, cooling blood, stopping bleeding, clearing heat to prevent miscarriage		
Huáng lián (Rhizoma Coptidis)		It has a strong action in clearing damp heat in the middle *jiao*. It is effective for clearing fire of an excess type in the heart and stomach, and relieving vomiting		
Huáng bǎi (Cortex Phellodendri Chinensis)		Effective for clearing damp heat in the lower *jiao*, purging kidney fire to remove steaming bones		
Lóng dǎn cǎo (Radix et Rhizoma Gentianae)	Clears heat and dries dampness, particularly effective for clearing damp heat in the lower *jiao* by clearing excessive fire in the liver and gallbladder			
Kǔ shēn (Radix Sophorae Flavescentis)	Clears heat and dries damp, kills parasites to relieve itching, indicated for skin diseases	It has a strong action.		Clears heat and dries damp to relieve diarrhea and dysentery and promotes diuresis
Bái xiān pí (Cortex Dictamni)				Clears heat and detoxifies, dispels wind to relieve *bi*
Qín pí (Cortex Fraxini)	Clears heat and dries damp, relieves dysentery and diarrhea by astringing, reduces leukorrhagia, promotes vision			
Sān kē zhēn (Radix Berberidis)	Clears heat and dries damp, purges fire, detoxifies			
Mǎ wěi lián (Radix et Rhizoma Thalictri Baicalensis)				
Kǔ dòu zǐ (Sophora Alopecuroides)	Clears heat and dries damp, kills parasites to relieve pain			

Table 9-4: Summary of Medicinals that Clear Heat and Detoxify (one):

Medicinal	Action in Common		Individual Character	
			Characteristic Actions	Other Actions
Jīn yín huā (Flos Lonicerae Japonicae)	Clears heat and detoxifies, dispels wind heat, commonly used for clearing heat and detoxifying, effective for treating sores of an excess type		It has a strong action in dispelling wind heat	Cools blood and relieves dysentery
Lián qiào (Fructus Forsythiae)			It has a strong action in clearing the heart and detoxifying, is effective for relieving carbuncles and removing stasis, known as "*the most effective medicinal to treat ulcers*"	Induces diuresis
Pú gōng yīng (Herba Taraxaci)	Clears heat and detoxifies, reduces swelling and removes stasis		Activates channels to promote milk production, activates channels to induce lactation, especially effective for treating breast abscesses with swelling pain	
Zǐ huā dì dīng (Herba Violae)			Specializes in detoxifying, effective for treating sores and boils	
Yě jú huā (Flos Chrysanthemi Indici)				Clears and purges liver fire, dispels wind heat
Dà qīng yè (Folium Isatidis)	Clears heat and detoxifies, cools blood to remove ecchymoses		Effective for clearing fire toxin in the heart and stomach channels to relieve sore throat	Effective for cooling blood to remove ecchymoses
Bǎn lán gēn (Radix Isatidis)				Effective for detoxifying to relieve sore throat and for removing stasis
Qīng dài (Indigo Naturalis)			With a stronger wind heat dispelling action than *yě jú huā* (Flos Chrysanthemi)	Clears the lung to moisten dryness, cools blood and stops bleeding
Chóng lóu (Rhizoma Paridis)	Clears heat and detoxifies, removes carbuncles and reduces swelling, cools the liver and extinguishes wind to relieve convulsions		It has a strong action in clearing heat and detoxifying, reducing swelling to relieve pain	Transforms stasis to stop bleeding
Quán shēn (Rhizoma Bistortae)				Cools blood, stops bleeding, drains damp
Yú xīng cǎo (Herba Houttuyniae)	Clears heat and detoxifies, removes visceral abscesses, indicated for both visceral abscess and carbuncles	Mainly indicated for pulmonary abscesses	Promotes the discharge of pus, effective for treating pulmonary abscesses	Induces diuresis and relieves stranguria, clears heat and relieves dysentery
Jīn qiáo mài (Rhizoma Fagopyri Dibotryis)				Invigorates the spleen to promote digestion
Dà xuè téng (Caulis Sargentodoxae)		Mainly indicated for intestinal abscesses		Activates the blood, dispels wind to relieve pain
Bài jiàng cǎo (Herba Patriniae)			It has a strong action in eliminating abscesses and promoting the discharge of pus, indicated for pulmonary and hepatic abscesses	Removes stasis to relieve pain

Table 9-4: Summary of Medicinals that Clear Heat and Detoxify (one):

continued

Medicinal	Action in Common	Individual Character	
		Characteristic Actions	Other Actions
Shè gān (Rhizoma Belamcandae)	Clears heat and detoxifies to relieve sore throat, indicated for swollen and sore throat	Eliminates phlegm, removes stasis and reduces swelling, especially indicated for swollen and sore throat due to heat and blood accumulation, or phlegm heat exuberance	
Shān dòu gēn (Radix et Rhizoma Sophorae Tonkinensis)		It has a strong action in purging fire, and detoxifying, and is effective for treating a swollen and sore throat	
Mǎ bó (Lasiosphaera seu Calvatia)		It has a mild action in clearing heat, but can dispel wind heat in the lung channel. It is indicated for sore throat with loss of voice due to wind heat invading the lung or depressed heat in the lung	Stops bleeding
Bái tóu wēng (Radix Pulsatillae)	Clears heat and detoxifies, effective for cooling blood and relieving dysentery, indicated for dysentery with bloody stool due to heat toxin	Effective for clearing damp heat in the stomach and large intestine, effective for treating dysentery with bloody stool due to heat toxins	
Mǎ chǐ xiàn (Herba Portulacae)			Cools blood and stops bleeding
Yā dǎn zǐ (Fructus Bruceae)			Prevents the recurrence of malaria, removes abnormal growths
Bàn biān lián (Herba Lobeliae Chinensis)	Clears heat and detoxifies, drains damp to relieve dysuria	It has a strong action in draining damp	Promotes water flow to relieve edema
Bái huā shé shé cǎo (Herba Hedyotis Diffusae)			Drains damp to relieve jaundice

Table 9-5: Summary of Medicinals that Clear Heat and Detoxify (two):

Medicinal	Action in Common	Individual Character	
		Characteristic Actions	Other Actions
Shān cí gū (Pseudobulbus Cremastrae seu Pleiones)	Clears heat and detoxifies, removes abscesses and stasis	Has a strong action in removing stasis, indicated for hard abdominal masses	
Lòu lú (Radix Rhapontici)		Effective for activating channels to induce lactation	
Bái liǎn (Radix Ampelopsis)	Clears heat and detoxifies, promotes wound healing	Effective for cooling blood and removing damp, especially effective for treating scalds	Astringes to stop blood when used externally
Sì jì qīng (Folium Illics Purpureae)		Effective for removing abscesses and stasis, promotes regeneration of the tissue to relieve pain	

Table 9-5: Summary of Medicinals that Clear Heat and Detoxify (two):

continued

Medicinal	Action in Common	Individual Character	
		Characteristic Actions	Other Actions
Qīng guǒ (Fructus Canarii)	Clears heat and detoxifies to relieve sore throat		Promotes fluid production
Jǐn dēng lóng (Calyx seu Fructus Physalis)			Transforms phlegm, induces diuresis to relieve stranguria
Jīn guó lán (Radix Tinosporae)			Relieves pain
Mù hú dié (Semen Oroxyli)		It can mainly clear the lung to relieve sore throat	Soothes the liver to harmonize the stomach
Dì jǐn cǎo (Herba Euphorbiae Humifusae)	Clears heat and detoxifies, cools blood and relieves dysentery, stops bleeding		
Wěi líng cài (Herba Potentillae Chinensis)			
Fān bái cǎo (Herba Potentillae Discoloris)			
Xióng dǎn (Ursi Fel)	Clears heat and detoxifies, clears the liver to promote vision	Extinguishes wind to relieve convulsions	
Qiān lǐ guāng (Herba Senecionis Scandentis)		Clears heat and drains dampness, kills parasites to relieve itching	
Chuān xīn lián (Herba Andrographis)	Clears heat and detoxifies	Cools blood, reduces swelling, dries damp	
Guàn zhòng (Rhizoma Cyrtomii)		Stops bleeding, kills parasites	
Tǔ fú líng (Rhizoma Smilacis Glabrae)		Removes damp, activates the joints, effective in treating syphilis	
Lǜ dòu (Semen Phaseoli Radiati)		Removes summer heat, promotes the flow of water	

Table 9-6: Summary of Medicinals that Clear Heat and Cool Blood:

Medicinal	Action in Common	Individual Character	
		Characteristic Actions	Other Actions
Shēng dì huáng (Radix Rehmanniae)	Clears heat and cools blood, nourishes yin to promote fluid production	It has a strong action in clearing heat and cooling blood, nourishing yin to promote fluid production, and is most effective for cooling blood and nourishing yin	
Xuán shēn (Radix Scrophulariae)		Effective for purging fire, detoxifying and removing stasis	
Mǔ dān pí (Cortex Moutan)	Clears heat and cools blood, activates blood to remove stasis, characterized by cooling blood without leaving stasis and activating blood without causing bleeding	Has a strong action in clearing heat and cooling blood, is effective for clearing and dispelling heat retention in the blood	Removes visceral abscesses
Chì sháo (Radix Paeoniae Rubra)		It has a strong action in activating blood to remove stasis and relieve pain	Clears and purges fire

Table 9-6: Summary of Medicinals that Clear Heat and Cool Blood:

continued

Medicinal	Action in Common	Individual Character	
		Characteristic Actions	Other Actions
Shuǐ niú jiǎo (Cornu Bubali)	Cools blood and detoxifies	It has a stronger action in clearing heat, cooling blood and detoxifying than *zǐ cǎo* (Radix Arnebiae), used as a substitution for *xī jiǎo* (Cornu Rhinocerotis)	Relieves convulsions
Zǐ cǎo (Radix Arnebiae)		It can mainly cool blood, activate blood, detoxify and promote skin eruptions, indicated for purplish black ecchymoses and skin rashes, as well as purplish dark measles due to fire toxin exuberance in the *xue* level	

Table 9-7: Summary of Medicinals that Clear Deficient Heat:

Medicinal	Action in Common	Individual Character	
		Characteristic Actions	Other Actions
Qīng hāo (Herba Artemisiae Annuae)	Clears heat and cool blood to remove steaming bones, characterized by clearing heat as well as dispersing	With a strong action, it is effective for clearing and dispelling heat retention, and is most effective in treating deficient heat	Removes summer heat, prevents recurrence of malaria
Bái wēi (Radix et Rhizoma Cynanchi Atrati)		Reduces fever of a deficient type as well as clears blood heat of an excessive type	Induces diuresis to relieve stranguria, detoxifies to relieve ulcers
Dì gǔ pí (Cortex Lycii)	Clears deficient heat, relieves steaming bones			Cools blood, stops bleeding, clears the lung to descend fire
Yín chái hú (Radix Stellariae)		Reduces fever due to distention from malnutrition	It has a strong action in clearing fever due to distention from malnutrition	
Hú huáng lián (Rhizoma Picrorhizae)				Clears damp heat

Tables to test your herbal knowledge of the actions and indications of medicinals that clear heat are as follows (Tables 9-8~9-19, see p.133~142):

Table 9-8: Test your Herbal Knowledge of the Actions of Medicinals that Clear Heat and Purge Fire:

Actions \ Medicinal	Shí gāo	Hán shuǐ shí	Zhī mǔ	Lú gēn	Tiān huā fěn	Zhú yè	Dàn zhú yè	Yā zhí cǎo	Zhī zǐ	Xià kū cǎo	Jué míng zǐ	Gǔ jīng cǎo	Mì méng huā	Qīng xiāng zǐ
Clears heat														
Opens the orifices and reduces swelling														
Relieves vomiting														
Relieves thirst														
Promotes wound healing and tissue regeneration														

Table 9-8: Test your Herbal Knowledge of the Actions of Medicinals that Clear Heat and Purge Fire:

continued

Medicinal / Actions	Shí gāo	Hán shuǐ shí	Zhī mǔ	Lú gēn	Tiān huā fěn	Zhú yè	Dàn zhú yè	Yā zhí cǎo	Zhī zǐ	Xià kū cǎo	Jué míng zǐ	Gǔ jīng cǎo	Mì méng huā	Qīng xiāng zǐ
Purges fire														
Nourishes yin to moisten dryness														
Promotes fluid production														
Removes vexation														
Induces diuresis														
Promotes skin eruption														
Disperses wind heat														
Detoxifies														
Clears liver fire														
Promotes the flow of water to reduce edema														
Clears heat and drains damp														
Cools blood														
Subdues swelling to relieve pain														
Promotes the discharge of pus														
Removes carbuncles														
Removes depressed stasis														
Moistens intestines to promote defecation														
Clears the lung and moistens dryness														
Improves visual acuity														
Nourishes liver blood														

Table 9-9: Test your Herbal Knowledge of the Actions of Medicinals that Clear Heat and Dry Damp:

Actions　　　　Medicinal	Huáng qín	Huáng lián	Huáng bǎi	Lóng dǎn cǎo	Qín pí	Kǔ shēn	Bái xiǎn pí	Chūn pí
Clears heat and dries damp								
Purges fire								
Induce diuresis								
Cools blood and stops bleeding								
Clears heat and prevents miscarriage								
Stops diarrhea								
Purges fire in the liver and gallbladder								
Arrests dysentery								
Reduces leukorrhea								
Improves visual acuity								
Kills parasites								
Detoxifies								
Dispels wind								
Removes steaming bones								
Stops bleeding by astringing								

Table 9-10: Test your Herbal Knowledge of the Actions of Medicinals that Clear Heat and Detoxify (one):

Actions　　　　Medicinal	Jīn yín huā	Rěn Dōng Téng	Lián qiào	Pú gōng yīng	Zǐ huā dì dīng	Yě jú huā	Chuān xīn lián	Dà qīng yè	Bǎn lán gēn	Qīng dài	Tǔ fú líng	Xióng dǎn
Clears heat and detoxifies												
Disperses wind heat												
Clears the liver to improve visual acuity												
Clears summer-heat												
Activates the channels and collaterals												
Relieves sore throat												
Clears heat to induce diuresis												
Drains damp to relieve stranguria												
Dries damp to reduce edema												
Cools blood												
Removes carbuncles												
Clears the liver to purge fire												
Relieves convulsions												
Cools blood and arrests dysentery												
Detoxifies and removes damp												
Activates the joints												

Table 9-11: Test your Herbal Knowledge of the Actions of Medicinals that Clear Heat and Detoxify (two):

Medicinal / Actions	Guàn Zhòng	Yú xīng cǎo	Jīn qiáo mài	Dà xuè téng	Bài jiàng cǎo	Shè gān	Shān dòu gēn	Lòu lú	Shān cí gū	Bái liǎn
Clears heat and detoxifies										
Activates the channels to induce lactation										
Cools blood and stops bleeding										
Promotes tissue regeneration and wound healing										
Induces diuresis to relieve stranguria										
Clears the lung to transform phlegm										
Invigorates blood to relieve pain										
Reduces leukorrhea										
Eliminates phlegm										
Relieves sore throat										
Reduces swelling										
Kills parasites										
Eliminates carbuncles and promotes the discharge of pus										
Relieves carbuncles										

Table 9-12: Test your Herbal Knowledge of the Actions of Medicinals that Clear Heat and Detoxify (three):

Medicinal / Actions	Mǎ bó	Bái tóu wēng	Mǎ chǐ xiàn	Yā dǎn zǐ	Dì jǐn cǎo	Chóng lóu	Quán shēn	Bàn biān lián	Bái huā shé shé cǎo
Promotes the flow of water to reduce edema									
Relieves sore throat									
Stops bleeding									
Reduces swelling to relieve pain									
Arrests dysentery									
Prevents the recurrence of malaria									
Remove abnormal growths									
Drains damp to relieve jaundice									
Cools blood									
Cools the liver to relieve convulsions									
Calms the liver to extinguish wind									
Clears heat and detoxifies									
Drains damp to relieve stranguria									

Table 9-13: Test your Herbal Knowledge of the Actions of Medicinals that Clear Heat and Cool Blood, and Medicinals that Clear Deficient Fire:

Medicinal / Actions	Shēng dì huáng	Xuán shēn	Mǔ dān pí	Chì sháo	Zǐ cǎo	Shuǐ niú jiǎo	Qīng hāo	Bái wēi	Dì gǔ pí	Yín chái hú	Hú huáng lián
Clears heat											
Cools blood											
Prevents the recurrence of malaria											
Promotes fluid production											
Nourishes yin											
Induce diuresis to relieve stranguria											
Invigorates blood											
Removes stasis											
Relieves pain											
Promotes skin eruptions											
Clears liver fire											
Clears deficient fire											
Removes steaming bones											
Relieves summer-heat											
Cultivates yin											
Detoxifies											
Detoxifies to treat ulcers											
Clears the lung to descend fire											
Removes heat due to malnutrition											

Table 9-14: Test your Herbal Knowledge of the Indications of Medicinals that Clear Heat and Purge Fire:

Medicinal / Indications	Shí gāo	Hán shuǐ shí	Zhī mǔ	Lú gēn	Tiān huā fěn	Zhú yè	Dàn zhú yè	Yā zhí cǎo	Zhī zǐ	Xià kū cǎo	Jué míng zǐ	Gǔ jīng cǎo	Mì méng huā	Qīng xiāng zǐ
Strong fever, vexation and thirst														
Vomiting due to stomach heat														
Toothache due to stomach fire														
Slow–healing skin diseases														
Pulmonary abscesses with purulent discharge														
Scalds and burns														

Table 9-14: Test your Herbal Knowledge of the Indications of Medicinals that Clear Heat and Purge Fire:

continued

Medicinal / Indications	Shí gāo	Hán shuǐ shí	Zhī mǔ	Lú gēn	Tiān huā fěn	Zhú yè	Dàn zhú yè	Yā zhí cǎo	Zhī zǐ	Xià kū cǎo	Jué míng zǐ	Gǔ jīng cǎo	Mì méng huā	Qīng xiāng zǐ
Infant's bacterial skin infections														
Dry cough due to yin deficiency														
Steaming bones with tidal fever														
Diabetes due to yin deficiency														
Constipation due to dry intestines														
Cough and panting due to lung heat														
Eczema with water effusion														
Carbuncles, skin diseases														
Mouth sores, reddish urine														
Edema due to pathogenic wind and water														
Hypertension														
Mumps, inflammation of the throat														
Scrofula, goiter														
Hematemesis and epistaxis due to blood heat														
Injuries due to trauma														
Blood-shot, swollen and painful eyes														
Headaches, dizziness														
Dim vision														
Stranguria due to pathogenic heat														
Hyperlipidemia														
Jaundice due to damp heat														

Table 9-15: Test your Herbal Knowledge of the Indications of Medicinals that Clear Heat and Dry Damp:

Medicinal / Indications	Huáng qín	Huáng lián	Huáng bǎi	Lóng dǎn cǎo	Qín pí	Kǔ shēn	Bái xiān pí	Chūn pí
Damp warmth, summer-heat damp								
Jaundice due to damp heat								
Diarrhea and dysentery due to damp heat								
Cough due to lung heat								
Bi due to damp heat								
Carbuncles, skin diseases								
Sore and swollen throat								
Hematemesis and epistaxis due to blood heat								
Swelling or pruritus of the vulvae								
Eczema, damp sores								
Blood-shot, swollen and painful eyes								
Leukorrhagia due to damp heat								
Stranguria due to pathogenic heat								
Beriberi								
Fire hyperactivity due to yin deficiency								
Threatened miscarriage due to heat								
Flaring up of liver fire								
Extreme heat generating wind								
Nebula								
Scabies, tinea								
Vexation and thirst due to febrile diseases								
Chronic diarrhea and dysentery								
Metrorrhagia, metrostaxis, hemafecia								

Table 9-16: Test your Herbal Knowledge of the Indications of Medicinals that Clear Heat and Detoxify (one):

Medicinal / Indications	Jīn yín huā	Lián qiào	Pú gōng yīng	Zǐ huā dì dīng	Yě jú huā	Chuān xīn lián	Dà qīng yè	Bǎn lán gēn	Qīng dài	Xióng dǎn	Lí lú
Carbuncles, furuncles, boils											
Breast abscesses with swelling and pain											
Epidemic febrile diseases in the initial stages											
Scrofula, superficial nodules											
Vexation and thirst due to summer-heat											
Infant's summer rashes											
Dysentery with bloody discharge due to heat toxin											
Stranguria due to pathogenic heat											
External invasion of wind heat											
Jaundice due to damp heat											
Convulsions, spasms											

Table 9-16: Test your Herbal Knowledge of the Indications of Medicinals that Clear Heat and Detoxify (one):

continued

Medicinal / Indications	Jīn yín huā	Lián qiào	Pú gōng yīng	.Zǐ huā dì dīng	Yě jú huā	Chuān xīn lián	Dà qīng yè	Bǎn lán gēn	Qīng dài	Xióng dǎn	Lí lú
Poisonous snake bites											
Swollen and sore throat											
Hematemesis and epistaxis due to blood heat											
Pulmonary abscesses with purulent expectoration											
Diarrhea and dysentery due to damp heat											
Eczema with itching											
Maculae caused by warm toxin											
Mumps, inflammation of the throat											
Cough and panting due to lung heat											
Hemoptysis due to chest pain											
Convulsions due to summer-heat											
Blood-shot, swollen and painful eyes											
Hemorroids with swelling and pain											
Breast distending pain											
Delactation											

Table 9-17: Test your Herbal Knowledge of the Indications of Medicinals that Clear Heat and Detoxify (two):

Medicinal / Indications	Guàn Zhòng	Yú xīng cǎo	Jīn qiáo mài	Dà xuè téng	Bài jiàng cǎo	Shè gān	Shān dòu	Mǎ bó	Bái tóu wēng
Scrofula, sores, boils									
Maculae due to warmth toxin									
Mumps									
Intestinal parasites									
Bi due to wind damp									
Pulmonary abscesses with purulent expectoration									
Cough due to lung heat									
Skin diseases due to heat toxin									
Stranguria due to damp heat									
Common cold of a wind heat type									
Swollen and sore throat									
Abdominal pain due to intestinal abscesses									
Hematemesis and epistaxis due to blood heat									

Table 9-17: Test your Herbal Knowledge of the Indications of Medicinals that Clear Heat and Detoxify (two):
continued

Indications \ Medicinal	Guàn Zhòng	Yú xīng cǎo	Jīn qiáo mài	Dà xuè téng	Bài jiàng cǎo	Shè gān	Shān dòu	Mǎ bó	Bái tóu wēng
Injuries due to trauma									
Amenorrhea, dysmenorrhea									
Hemorrhage due to trauma									
Pruritic vulvae									
Swollen and painful gums									
Jaundice due to damp heat									
Dysentery with bloody discharge due to heat toxin									
Cough and panting due to phlegm exuberance									

Table 9-18: Test your Herbal Knowledge of the Indications of Medicinals that Clear Heat and Detoxify (three):

Indications \ Medicinal	Mǎ chǐ xiàn	Yā dǎn zǐ	Dì jǐn cǎo	Chóng lóu	Quán shēn	Bàn biān lián	Bái huā shé shé cǎo	Shān cí gū	Tǔ fú líng	Bái liǎn
Diarrhea and dysentery due to damp heat										
Poisonous snake bites										
Metrorrhagia and metrostaxis due to blood heat										
Hemafecia and hemorrhoids with blood										
Dysentery with bloody discharge due to heat toxin										
Hemorrhage due to trauma										
Malaria of various kinds										
Thickening of the skin, abnormal growths										
Skin diseases due to heat toxin										
Jaundice due to damp heat										
Convulsions, spasms										
Injuries due to trauma										
Chronic dysentery due to cold food retention										
Scrofula										
Tetanus										
Syphilitic lesions										
Jaundice with ascites										
Swollen and sore throat										
Stranguria due to pathogenic heat										
Abdominal pain due to blood stasis										
Breast abscesses with swelling and pain										

Table 9-18: Test your Herbal Knowledge of the Indications of Medicinals that Clear Heat and Detoxify (three):

continued

Indications \ Medicinal	Mă chĭ xiàn	Yā dăn zĭ	Dì jĭn căo	Chóng lóu	Quán shēn	Bàn biān lián	Bái huā shé shé căo	Shān cí gū	Tŭ fú líng	Bái liăn
Leukorrhagia with pruritic vulvae										
Eczema										
Ulcers on the lower limbs										
Scalds and burns										
Hemorrhage due to trauma										

Table 9-19: Test your Herbal Knowledge of the Indications of Medicinals that Clear Heat and Cool Blood, and Medicinals that Clear Deficient Heat:

Indications \ Medicinal	Shēng dì huáng	Xuán shēn	Mŭ dān pí	Chì sháo	Zĭ căo	Shuĭ niú jiăo	Qīng hāo	Bái wēi	Dì gŭ pí	Yín chái hú	Hú huáng lián
Scrofula, superficial nodules											
Bleeding due to blood heat											
Yin consumption due to pathogenic warmth											
Heat invading the pericardium											
Thirst due to fluid consumption											
Diabetes due to internal heat											
Constipation due to dry intestines											
Swollen and sore throat											
Heat invading the *ying* and *xue* levels											
Carbuncles, sores											
Fever due to yin deficiency											
Amenorrhea and dysmenorrhea due to blood stagnation											
Injuries due to trauma											
Stranguria due to pathogenic heat, hematuria											
Blood-shot eyes, nebula											
Inadequate eruption of measles											
Cough due to lung heat											
Eczema, pruritic vulvae											
Scalds											
Headache due to summer-heat											
Alternate chills and fever due to malaria											
Abdominal pain due to intestinal abscesses											
Poisonous snake bites											
Convulsions, spasms											
External invasion due to yin deficiency											
Fever due to malnutrition causing distention											
Diarrhea and dysentery due to damp heat											
Hemorrhoids with swelling and pain											

Chapter 10
Medicinals that Drain Downwards

Concept

Medicinals that can induce diarrhea and moisten the intestines to promote defecation are defined as medicinals that drain downwards.

Character and Actions

Medicinals of this type have a sinking or descending action, and mainly enter the large intestine channel. They can relax the bowels to remove stagnation and dry stools in the stomach and intestines, clear heat and purge fire to remove heat, dispel fluid retention, and relieve edema.

Indications

They are indicated for interior syndromes of an excess type, manifesting with dry stools, constipation, food stagnation in the stomach and intestines, accumulation of excess heat in the interior, edema, or fluid retention.

Combinations

Medicinals with the action of draining downwards should be used on the basis of an interior excess syndrome in combination with the patient's constitution, and should be chosen based on compatibility with other medicinals. As for interior excess accompanied by an external pathogen, the exterior should be resolved first and then the interior can be treated. If it is necessary, the interior and exterior can be resolved simultaneously so as to prevent the external pathogen falling inward. As for patients with an external pathogen and right qi deficiency, supplementing and nourishing medicinals can also be used so that there is simultaneous attacking and supplementing. In this way there is an attack on the pathogen but no damage to the right qi. This type of medicinal can also be combined with qi moving herbs, to strengthen the descending and purging effects. In cases of heat accumulation, one should combine the medicinals with those that clear heat. In cases of cold accumulation one should combine the medicinals with those that warm the interior.

Precautions

Medicinals of this kind are violent or toxic, and can cause impairment to the spleen and stomach, so they should be used cautiously in the elderly, the weak, and patients with deficiency of the spleen and stomach. They are prohibited for women during pregnancy, post-partum, or during the menstrual period. Due to their strength, they should be discontinued as soon as symptoms are relieved. When using drastic and toxic medicinals, processing standards should be specified and dosages controlled so as to prevent poisoning and ensure the safety of the medication.

Classification

These medicinals are divided into three types: Medicinals that promote defecation by purgation, medicinals that promote defecation by moistening the intestines, and medicinals that drastically promote defecation and purge fluids.

Section 1   Medicinals that Promote Defecation by Purgation

Medicinals of this type are usually bitter in flavor and cold in nature with a descending action, and mainly enter the stomach and large intestine channels. They have strong actions of promoting defecation as well as clearing heat and purging fire. They are indicated for dry stools, constipation, and accumulation of excess heat. They are often used in combination with medicinals that promote the flow of qi, so as to reinforce the action of purging downwards and eliminating distension and fullness. For cases of constipation due to coldness and food accumulation, medicinals that warm the interior should be used simultaneously.

Medicinals with a strong action for clearing heat and purging fire are also used for heat syndromes with high fever, coma and delirium, headache, blood-shot eyes, swollen and sore throat and gums due to fire heat flaring upwards, as well as hemorrhaging in the upper part of the body including hematemesis, epistaxis and hemoptysis induced by fire heat exuberance. For the above mentioned symptoms and signs, medicinals of this type can be taken to clear excess heat or guide heat downwards to eliminate symptoms, regardless of whether or not there is also constipation.

① *Dà huáng* (大黄, Radix et Rhizoma Rhei, Rhubarb Root and Rhizome) ★ ★ ★

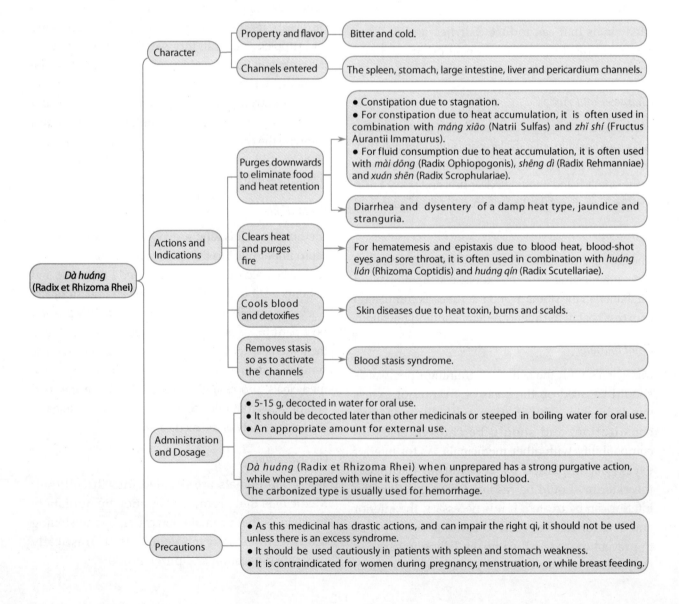

② *Máng xiāo* (芒硝, Natrii Sulfas, Sodium Sulfate)
★ ★ ★

Both *dà huáng* (Radix et Rhizoma Rhei) and *máng xiāo* (Natrii Sulfas) are bitter and cold with a descending action. They enter the stomach and large intestine channels and can purge fire to promote defecation. These two medicinals are indicated for excess heat accumulation in the stomach and large intestine manifesting as dry stool and constipation, abdominal distending pain and fullness, or even unrelieved high fever, coma and delirium. At the same time, they can clear heat and reduce swelling when used externally, and therefore can be used to treat suppurating infections that are red swollen and painful. However, they have some different actions. *Dà huáng* (Radix et Rhizoma Rhei) also enters the spleen, liver and heart channels. It has a strong effect of purging food and heat retention in the stomach and large intestine to promote the generation of new substances, and therefore is known as the "General". With correct combination with other medicinals, it can treat dry stools, constipation, and food retention in the stomach and large intestine of various types

such as constipation with heat accumulation accompanied by qi and blood deficiency, and constipation with cold and cold retention due to spleen yang deficiency. It can also be used for dysentery of a damp heat kind in the initial stage with tenesmus, or unsmooth defecation, due to food retention. In addition, *dà huáng* (Radix et Rhizoma Rhei) enters the *xue* level so as to purge excess heat and remove stasis. Therefore, it has the effects of clearing heat and purging fire, stopping bleeding, cooling blood, detoxifying, activating blood to remove stasis, and draining damp heat. It is often used for hematemesis, epistaxis and hemoptysis due to blood heat, blood-shot eyes, swollen and painful eyes, mouth sores, swollen and sore gums due to ascendant hyperactivity of fire heat; abdominal pain due to intestinal abscesses, burns and scalds (applied externally), amenorrhea and postpartum abdominal pain due to blood stasis, lochia, abdominal masses, injuries due to trauma, swelling and pain due to blood stasis, jaundice, and dysuria of the damp heat type. *Máng xiāo* (Natrii Sulfas) has a salty flavor and is effective for moistening dryness and softening masses so

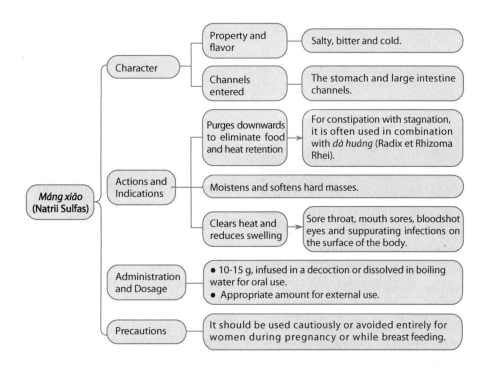

as to purge downwards and promote defecation. It is used to treat dry stools and constipation due to excess heat retention. When applied externally, it can clear heat and reduce swellings, so it is often used for swollen and sore throats, mouth sores, blood-shot eyes, and swollen and painful eyes. According to different processing methods, three products can be obtained: *Pí xiāo (pò xiāo)* (Mirabilitum), *máng xiāo* (Natrii Sulfas) and *xuán míng fěn* (玄明粉, Natrii Sulfas Exsiccatus, Exsiccated Sodium Sulfate). There are slight differences between them. *Pí xiāo* (Mirabilitum) contains more impurities than *máng xiāo* (Natrii

Sulfas) and is usually used externally. *Máng xiāo* (Natrii Sulfas) is also often used externally. *Xuán míng fěn* (Natrii Sulfas Exsiccatus) is pure and dehydrated, and therefore is convenient to be made into a powder form. In addition to oral administration, it is often used as an external agent for mouth and eye diseases. In pharmacies of some areas in China, *máng xiāo* (Natrii Sulfas) and *xuán míng fěn* (Natrii Sulfas Exsiccatus) are considered the same medicinal.

③ *Fān xiè yè* (番泻叶, Folium Sennae, Senna Leaf) ★★

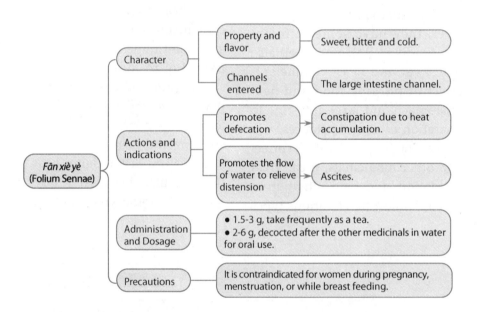

④ *Lú huì* (芦荟, Aloe, Aloe) ★★

Both *fān xiè yè* (Folium Sennae) and *lú huì* (Aloe) have a bitter flavor and a cold nature with a descending action. They can purge downwards to promote defecation. They are often used for constipation due to heat accumulation, habitual constipation, and constipation in the elderly. *Fān xiè yè* (Folium Sennae) has a similar action to *dà huáng* (Radix et Rhizoma Rhei) in purging heat and promoting defecation. It can moderately promote defecation in small dosages, while in larger dosages it can promote defecation more drastically. In addition, it can promote the flow

of water to relieve distension and is used for ascites, and edema of a yang excess type. *Lú huì* (Aloe) can promote defecation as well as clear liver fire, so it is frequently used for dizziness, headache, vexation, agitation and anger, epilepsy, and convulsions dues to fire hyperactivity in the liver channel accompanied by dry stools and constipation. It can also kill parasites and relieve abdominal distension due to malnutrition. Therefore, it is used for infant's abdominal distension due to malnutrition, abdominal pain due to parasite accumulation, scabies, and tinea (used externally).

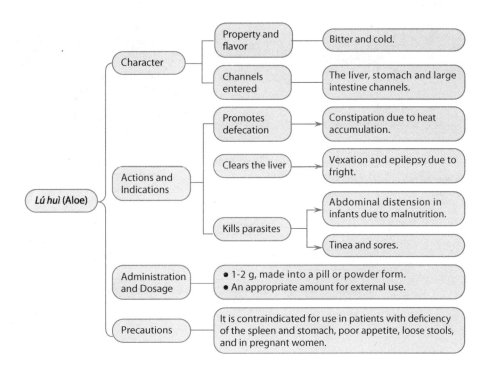

Section 2   Medicinals that Promote Defecation by Moistening Intestines

Medicinals of this type are usually seeds and kernels that are rich in fats. They are sweet in flavor with a moist texture and they enter the spleen and large intestine channels so as to moisten the large intestine to gently promote defecation. They are indicated for constipation with dry intestines caused by old age with fluid consumption, postpartum blood deficiency, heat syndrome with fluid consumption, or blood loss.

① *Huǒ má rén* (火麻仁, Fructus Cannabis, Hemp Seed) ★

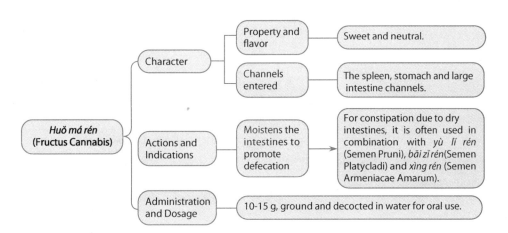

② *Yù lǐ rén* (郁李仁, Semen Pruni, Chinese Dwarf Cherry Seed) ★

Both *huǒ má rén* (Fructus Cannabis) and *yù lǐ rén* (Semen Pruni) are neutral in property with a moist texture, and can moisten the intestines to promote defecation. They are used for constipation due to

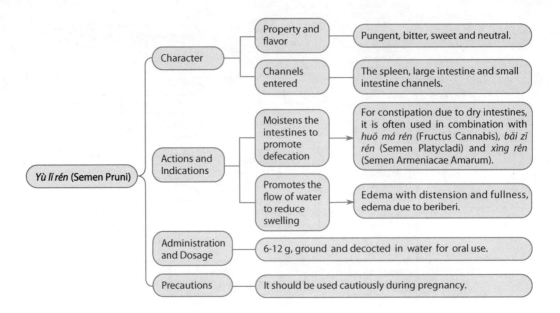

dry intestines. The two medicinals are often used in combination to increase their efficacy. *Huǒ má rén* (Fructus Cannabis) is sweet and neutral with a moist texture, and can nourish blood to treat constipation with dry intestines, in the elderly, as well as in pregnant women and weak patients with blood deficiency and fluid consumption. *Yù lǐ rén* (Semen Pruni) is bitter in flavor and has a stronger action than *huǒ má rén* (Fructus Cannabis) in moistening the bowels in order to

promote defecation. It can promote qi flow in the large intestine, and is indicated for constipation with dry intestines and qi stagnation in the large intestine. In addition, it can promote the flow of water to reduce swelling, and is used for edema with distension and fullness, and edema due to beriberi.

③ *Sōng zǐ rén* (松子仁, Semen Pini Koraiensis, Pine Nut) ★

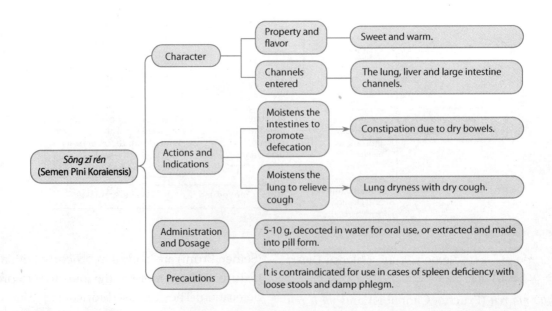

Section 3 Medicinals that Drastically Promote Defecation and Purge Fluids

Medicinals of this kind are usually bitter, cold and slightly toxic. They have drastic actions and can cause intense diarrhea or induce diuresis to discharge fluid retention via the stools or urine. These medicinals are indicated for general edema, distension and fullness in the abdomen, and fluid retention.

① *Gān suì* (甘遂, Radix Kansui, Gansui Root) ★★

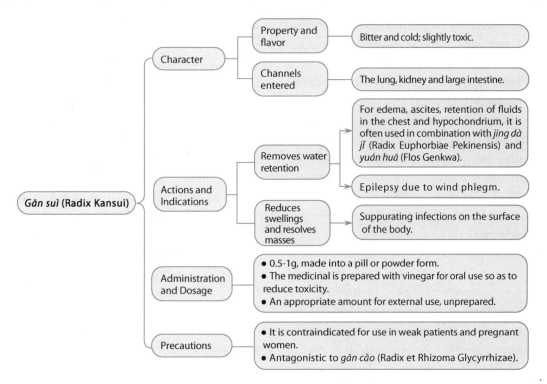

② *Jīng dà jǐ* (京大戟, Radix Euphorbiae Pekinensis, Peking Euphorbia Root) ★

Addition: **Hóng dà jǐ (红大戟, Radix Knoxiae, Knoxia Root)** is bitter and cold, has similar

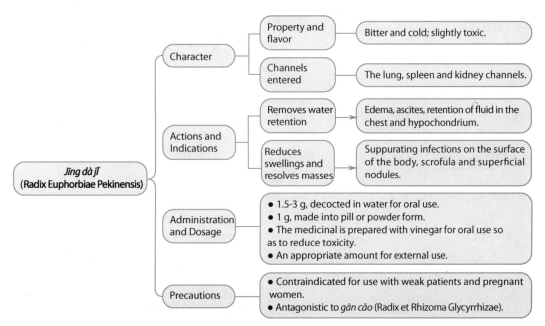

actions to *jīng dà jǐ* (Radix Euphorbiae Pekinensis). *Jīng dà jǐ* (Radix Euphorbiae Pekinensis) has a stronger action in removing water retention, while *hóng dà jǐ* (Radix Knoxiae) is more effective in reducing swellings and resolving masses.

③ *Yuán huā* (芫花, Flos Genkwa, Lilac Daphne Flower Bud) ★

Gān suì (Radix Kansui), *jīng dà jǐ* (Radix Euphorbiae Pekinensis) and *yuán huā* (Flos Genkwa) enter the lung, kidney and large intestine channels, are toxic, and have drastic actions in removing water retention through defecation and urination. They are often used in combination for cases of edema, and edema and fluid retention in the chest and hypochondrium without debilitated right qi. When used externally, *gān suì* (Radix Kansui) and *jīng dà jǐ* (Radix Euphorbiae Pekinensis) can reduce swellings and remove stasis to treat suppurating infections on the surface of the body, scrofula, and superficial nodules. *Gān suì* (Radix Kansui) is bitter in flavor and cold in property, and is effective for removing water retention in the channels. Therefore, of the three medicinals, it has the strongest action in removing water retention and promoting defecation and diuresis. It is inferior to *jīng dà jǐ* (Radix Euphorbiae Pekinensis) in

reducing swellings and removing stasis. It is less toxic than *yuán huā* (Flos Genkwa). In addition, *gān suì* (Radix Kansui) is used to treat epilepsy induced by wind phlegm. *Jīng dà jǐ* (Radix Euphorbiae Pekinensis) specializes in removing water retention in the *zang* and *fu* organs, and therefore has a stronger action of reducing swellings and removing stasis than *gān suì* (Radix Kansui). It has the least toxicity of the three medicinals. *Jīng dà jǐ* (Radix Euphorbiae Pekinensis) and *hóng dà jǐ* (Radix Knoxiae) have similar actions and indications. However, *jīng dà jǐ* (Radix Euphorbiae Pekinensis) comes from the root of *Euphorbia pekinensis Rupr.* (family Euphorbiaceae), and has a stronger action in removing water retention; while *hóng dà jǐ* (Radix Knoxiae) is the root of *Knoxia valerianoides Thorel et Pitard* (family Euphorbiaceae), and has a stronger action in reducing swellings and removing stasis. *Yuán huā* (Flos Genkwa) has the mildest action in removing water retention but is the most toxic. It is effective for purging water retention in the chest and hypochondrium, eliminating phlegm, relieving cough, and killing parasites so as to treat ulcers. It can also be used for cough with dyspnea due to cold fluid retention, tinea capitis, tinea tonsure, and obstinate tinea.

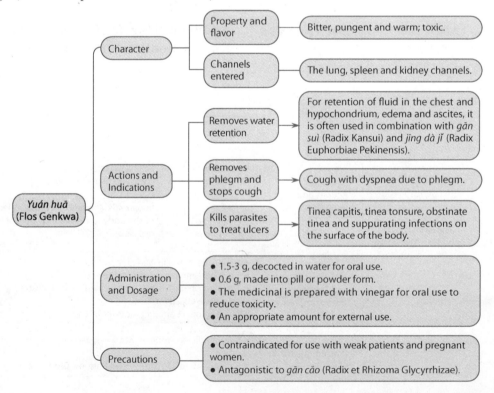

④ *Shāng lù* (商陆, Radix Phytolaccae, Pokeberry Root) ★

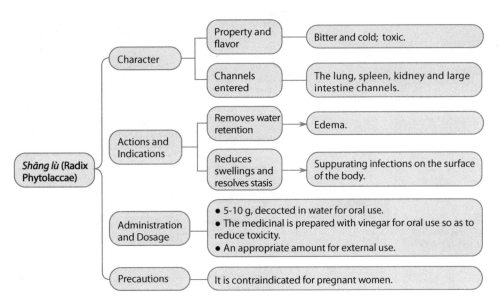

⑤ *Qiān niú zǐ* (牵牛子, Semen Pharbitidis, Pharbitidis Seed) ★

Both *qiān niú zǐ* (Semen Pharbitidis) and *shāng lù* (Radix Phytolaccae) are bitter, cold, and toxic, with a descending action. They can remove water retention through the stools and urine. The two medicinals have similar but milder actions than *gān suí* (Radix Kansui), *jīng dà jǐ* (Radix Euphorbiae Pekinensis) and *yuán huā* (Flos Genkwa). They are used in cases of edema, and edema with difficulty in defecation and urination but without right qi debilitation. *Qiān niú zǐ* (Semen Pharbitidis) can remove food retention and kill parasites. It is used for cough with dyspnea due to phlegm-fluids, heat accumulation of an excess type in the stomach and large intestine, constipation with abdominal distension, damp heat accumulation with dysentery, abdominal pain and tenesmus, and abdominal pain due to the accumulation of parasites. Used externally, *shāng lù* (Radix Phytolaccae) can reduce swellings and remove stasis, and therefore

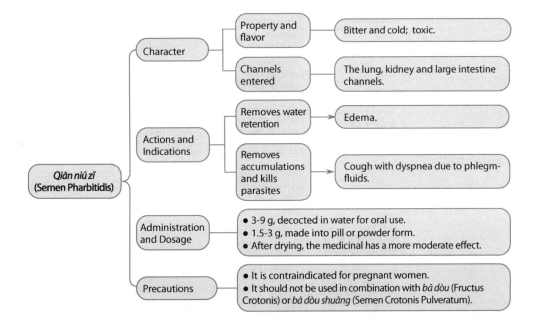

is used for early stage suppurating infections on the surface of the body.

⑥ *Bā dòu* (巴豆, Semen Crotonis, Croton Seed) ★★

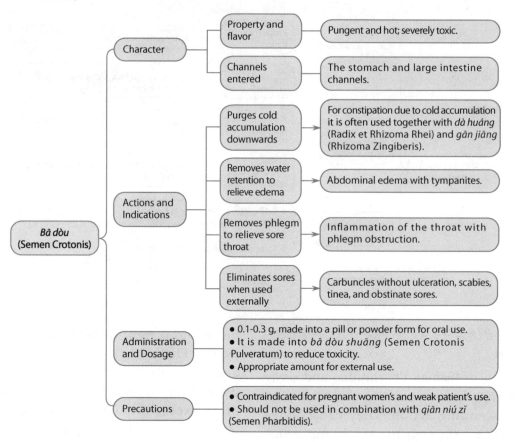

⑦ *Qiān jīn zǐ* (千金子, Semen Euphorbiae, Caper Euphorbia Seed)

Both *bā dòu* (Semen Crotonis) and *qiān jīn zǐ* (Semen Euphorbiae) are pungent in flavor, warm

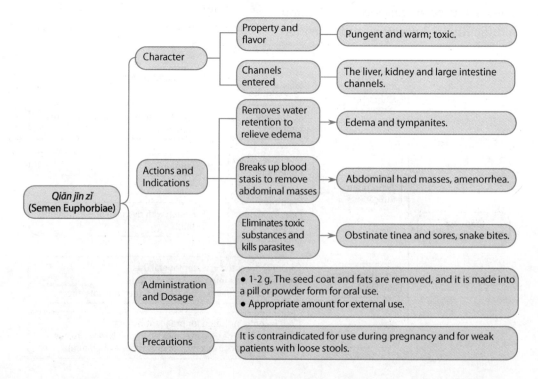

in property, and toxic. They can remove water retention to reduce edema. They are used for edema, tympanites, and difficulty in defecation and urination without right qi debilitation. *Bā dòu* (Semen Crotonis) is hot and very toxic, with a drastic action to remove cold accumulation. Therefore, it is often used for constipation due to cold accumulation. It can remove phlegm to relieve sore throat, and when used externally it can eliminate sores. It is indicated for inflammation of the throat with phlegm obstruction, cold excess congealed in the chest, carbuncles with pus that fails to ulcerate, scabies, tinea, and obstinate sores. *Qiān jīn zǐ* (Semen Euphorbiae) is warm, with a moderate action. It can break up stasis and remove abdominal masses, eliminate toxic substances, and kill parasites. Therefore it is used for amenorrhea due to blood stasis, abdominal masses, obstinate tinea, sores, and snake bites.

Actions of medicinals that purge downwards are summarized as follows (Table 10-1).

Table 10-1: Summary of Medicinals that Purge Downwards:

Medicinal	Action in Common		Individual Character	
			Characteristic Actions	Other Actions
Dà huáng (Radix et Rhizoma Rhei)	Promotes defecation by purgation	Purges heat by promoting defecation, clears heat to reduce swelling	It has a strong action in purging downwards, and is a most effective medicinal	Clears heat and purges fire, stops bleeding, cools blood and detoxifies, activates the channels to remove stasis, clears and drains damp heat
Máng xiāo (Natrii Sulfas)			Effective for moistening the bowels and softening hard masses to promote defecation	
Fān xiè yè (Folium Sennae)		Promotes defecation	Moderately promotes defecation in small dosages, and strongly promotes defecation in large dosages	Promotes the flow of water to relieve edema
Lú huì (Aloe)			Promotes defecation as well as clears liver fire, it is especially indicated for dry stool and constipation accompanied by fire exuberance in the liver channel	Kills parasites to relieve distended abdomen due to malnutrition.
Huǒ má rén (Semen Cannabis)	Promotes defecation by moistening the bowels		Replenishes deficiency, especially suitable for the elderly, pregnant women, and weak patients with constipation due to dry intestines and fluid consumption	
Yù lǐ rén (Semen Pruni)			Removes qi stagnation in the large intestine, indicated for constipation with dry intestines due to fluid consumption accompanied by qi stagnation in the large intestine	Promotes the flow of water to reduce edema
Sōng zǐ rén (Semen Pini Koraiensis)				Moistens the lung to relieve cough

Table 10-1: Summary of Medicinals that Purge Downwards:

continued

Medicinal	Action in Common			Individual Character	
				Characteristic Actions	Other Actions
Gān suì (Radix Kansui)	Toxic, drastically promotes defecation and purges fluids	Removes water retention, promotes defecation and urination	Relieves edema and removes stasis	Has the strongest action in purging water retention and promoting defecation and urination, inferior to *jīng dà jǐ* (Radix Euphorbiae Pekinensis), less toxic than *yuán huā* (Flos genkwa)	
Jīng dà jǐ (Radix Euphorbiae Pekinensis)				Has the least toxicity among the three medicinals	
Yuán huā (Flos Genkwa)				Has the largest toxicity	
Shāng lù (Radix Phytolaccae)	Drastically promotes defecation and purges fluids	Removes water retention through the stool and urine. Has a similar but milder action compared with *gān suí* (Radix Kansui), *jīng dà jǐ* (Radix Euphorbiae Pekinensis) and *yuán huā* (Flos genkwa)			Reduces swelling and removes stasis
Qiān niú zǐ (Semen Pharbitidis)					Removes stagnation, kills parasites
Bā dòu (Semen Crotonis)		Removes water retention through stool and urine to relieve edema		Has a hot property, severe toxicity and drastic actions, it is effective for removing cold stagnation by purgation, often used for constipation with cold retention	Removes phlegm to relieve sore throat, eliminates sores (used externally)
Qiān jīn zǐ (Semen Euphorbiae)				With a warm property, has a more moderate action compared to *bā dòu* (Semen Crotonis)	Breaks up blood stasis to remove abdominal masses, kills parasites and removes toxic substances

Tables to test your herbal knowledge of medicinals that purge downwards are as follows (Table 10-2 and Table 10-3):

Table 10-2: Test your Herbal Knowledge of Actions of Medicinals that Purge Downwards:

Medicinal / Actions	Dà huáng	Máng xiāo	Fān xiè yè	Lú huì	Huǒ má rén	Yù lǐ rén	Gān suì	Jīng dà jǐ	Hóng dà jǐ	Yuán huā	Shāng lù	Qiān niú zǐ	Bā dòu	Qiān jīn zǐ
Purges downwards														
Removes stagnation														
Clears heat														
Moistens bowels to promote defecation														
Stops bleeding														
Reduces swelling and removes stasis														
Activates blood to remove stasis														
Softens hard masses														
Clears the liver														
Kills parasites														
Purges fire														
Promotes the flow of water to reduce edema														
Purges cold retention														
Detoxifies														
Removes phlegm to relieve cough														
Eliminates sores														
Removes food retention														
Removes water retention														
Removes phlegm to relieve sore throats														
Eliminates scabies														
Breaks up blood stasis in the abdomen														

Table 10-3: Test your Herbal Knowledge of Indications of Medicinals that Purge Downwards:

Indication \ Medicinal	Dà huáng	Máng xiāo	Fān xiè yè	Lú huì	Huŏ má rén	Yù lĭ rén	Gān suì	Jīng dà jĭ	Hóng dà jĭ	Yuán huā	Shāng lù	Qiān niú zĭ	Bā dòu	Qiān jīn zĭ
Constipation with heat accumulation														
Constipation in the elderly														
Damp heat dysentery														
Abdominal pain due to food retention														
Excess fire in the liver channel														
Blood-shot, swollen, and painful eyes														
Swollen sore throat														
Burns and scalds														
Blood stasis syndrome														
Damp heat syndrome														
Intestinal and breast abscesses in the initial stage														
Habitual constipation														
Constipation with cold retention														
Hemorrhage due to blood heat														
Infant's abdominal distention due to malnutrition														
Tinea and sores														
Suppurating infections on the surface of the body														
Edema														
Beriberi														
Tinea tonsure														
Fluid retention in the chest and hypochondrium														
Epilepsy due to wind phlegm														
Constipation due to dry bowels														
Scrofula and superficial nodules														
Cough with dyspnea due to phlegm-fluids														
Scabies, tinea, and obstinate sores														
Tympanites														
Obstinate tinea														
Abdominal pain due to parasites														
Cold retention in the chest														
Inflammation of the throat with phlegm obstruction														
Tinea capitis														
Abdominal masses, amenorrhea														
Abnormal growths														
Poisoning snake bites														

Chapter 11
Medicinals that Expel Wind and Damp

Concept

Medicinals whose principal effect is to expel pathogenic wind, cold and damp and treat *bi* are called medicinals that dispel wind and damp.

Character and Actions

Medicinals of this kind are mostly pungent and bitter with a warm or cool property, and can eliminate pathogenic wind and damp in the muscles, bones, sinews, channels, and collaterals. Some of them have the effects of relaxing muscles and sinews, activating channels and collaterals, relieving pain, and nourishing the liver and kidney so as to strengthen bones and sinews.

Indications

They are indicated for pain in the body and limbs, inflexible and enlarged joints, and spasms. Some of them are also used for aching and weakness in the waist and knees, and flaccidity of the lower limbs.

Combinations

Medicinals that dispel wind and damp should be selected according to the different types and locations of *bi*, and the specific disease process. They should be used in combination with other kinds of medicinals. For example, for wind pathogen exuberance, select anti-rheumatics with good wind-dispelling actions, in combination with medicinals with actions of activating and nourishing the blood. For *zhuo bi* (着痹), anti-rheumatics that are warm and dry should be selected, assisted by medicinals with actions of invigorating the spleen to drain damp. In cases of *xing bi* (行痹) due to cold pathogen exuberance, select warm anti-rheumatics combined with medicinals that have actions of invigorating yang and warming the channels and collaterals. For *tong bi* due to cold pathogen exuberance, select warm anti-rheumatics with appropriate medicinals for activating yang and warming the channels. For *re bi* of a heat type induced by external pathogens invading the interior and transforming into heat, or chronic depression transforming into heat, select cold or cool anti-rheumatics with appropriate medicinals for cooling blood, clearing heat, and detoxifying. For external attack in the early stage, medicinals that relieve the exterior by dispersing wind and removing damp are selected; while for external pathogens invading the interior of the body, medicinals with actions of activating blood to dredge collaterals should also be used. For cases with phlegm-turbidity or blood stasis, medicinals for eliminating phlegm and removing stasis should be used simultaneously. For patients with a weak constitution due to chronic diseases with liver and kidney deficiency and weakened body resistance, anti-rheumatics that can strengthen the bones and sinews should be selected, in combination with medicinals for nourishing the liver and kidney and replenishing qi and blood. This combination can strengthen body resistance and eliminate pathogens.

Precautions

Since *bi* is a chronic disease, medicinals can be made into wines, pill or powder forms for convenient administration. In addition, wine can reinforce their therapeutic effects. The medicinals can also be processed so as to be directly applied to the affected areas. As medicinals of this kind are always pungent, warm and dry, and can consume yin and blood, they should be prescribed cautiously in cases of yin and blood deficiency.

Classification

According to their characters and functions, medicinals that dispel pathogenic wind and damp can be divided into three categories: medicinals that dispel wind, cold and damp; medicinals that dispel wind heat and damp; and medicinals that dispel wind damp and strengthen bones and sinews.

Section 1　Medicinals that Expel Wind, Cold and Damp

Medicinals in this section are usually pungent, bitter and warm, and enter the liver, spleen and kidney channels. They are effective for dispelling wind, eliminating damp, scattering cold, stopping pain and activating the channels and collaterals. They are especially effective at relieving pain and are mainly indicated for *bi* of a wind cold damp type, manifesting as body and joint aches, spasms, and fixed pain which can be aggravated by exposure to cold. They can also be used for *bi* of a wind heat damp type if they are properly combined with other types of medicinals.

① *Dú huó* (独活, Radix Angelicae Pubescentis, Doubleteeth Pubescent Angelica Root) ★ ★ ★

Both *qiāng huó* (Rhizoma et Radix Notopterygii) and *dú huó* (Radix Angelicae Pubescentis) are pungent, bitter and warm, and can dispel wind and damp, stop pain, and resolve the exterior. They are used in combination to treat *bi* of a wind cold type with aching joints all over the body, and external invasion of wind cold complicated by pathogenic damp in the interior. *Qiāng huó* (Rhizoma et Radix Notopterygii) has a strong odor and a powerful action to scatter. It mainly acts in the upper body and the exterior, and is indicated for external contraction of wind cold, headache and general aching, and *bi* of a wind cold type in the upper part of body with aching in the shoulders and back. *Dú huó* (Radix Angelicae Pubescentis) has a moderate action, and is inferior to *qiāng huó* (Rhizoma et Radix Notopterygii) in resolving the exterior. It is effective for expelling wind and damp in the interior and lower part of the body, and

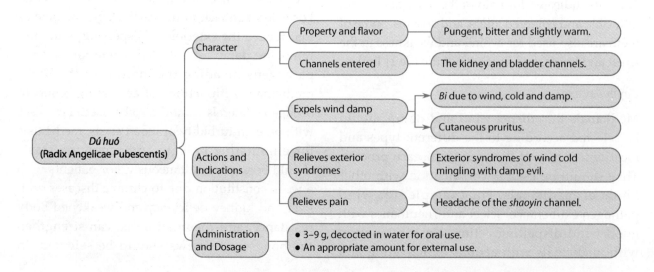

is indicated for *bi* of a wind cold type in the lower part of body with aching joints all over the body and headache due to wind retention in the *shaoyin* channel. It is said that *qiāng huó* (Rhizoma et Radix Notopterygii) is effective for expelling wind in the upper part of the body and on the surface of the body, while *dú huó* (Radix

Angelicae Pubescentis) is effective for removing wind retention in the lower part of the body and in the interior of the body.

② *Wēi líng xiān* (威灵仙, Radix et Rhizoma Clematidis, Chinese Clematis Root) ★★★

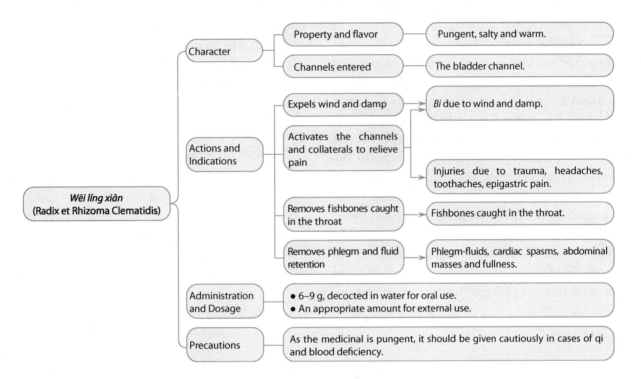

③ *Xú cháng qīng* (徐长卿, Radix et Rhizoma Cynanchi Paniculati, Paniculate Swallowwort Root) ★★★

Dú huó (Radix Angelicae Pubescentis), *wēi líng*

xiān (Radix et Rhizoma Clematidis) and *xú cháng qīng* (Radix et Rhizoma Cynanchi Paniculati) are pungent and warm, and can dispel wind damp to stop pain. They are indicated for *bi*

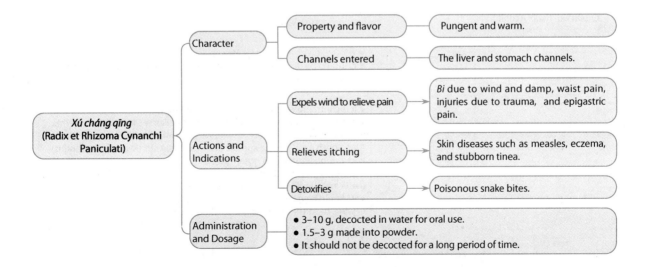

due to wind cold with aching joints all over the body, heaviness, and numbness. *Dú huó* (Radix Angelicae Pubescentis) is pungent, bitter and slightly warm, with a strong action to dispel wind damp. It is regarded as the main medicinal in treating *bi* due to wind damp. It mainly enters the kidney channel and is effective for treating aching joints in the lower part of the body caused by wind-damp *bi*. In addition, it can resolve the exterior, and is used for invasion of external pathogenic wind cold complicated by pathogenic damp, and headache due to wind retention in the *shaoyin* channel. *Wēi líng xiān* (Radix et Rhizoma Clematidis) has a drastic action and tends to encourage movement. It can expel wind damp, stop pain and activate the channels and collaterals. It is said to "activate all twelve channels", therefore it is indicated for *bi* of a wind cold type manifesting as numbness, spasms, inflexible joints, and fish bones caught in the throat. It can also treat injuries due to trauma, headaches, toothaches, and gastric pain. It is used to treat phlegm-fluids, cardiac spasm,

abdominal masses and fullness by eliminating phlegm and removing fluid retention. *Xú cháng qīng* (Radix et Rhizoma Cynanchi Paniculati) has a strong action in relieving pain, and therefore is used extensively to relieve various pains induced by wind damp, cold congealing, qi stagnation, and blood stasis, such as *bi* due to wind damp, pain of the midsection, injuries due to trauma, epigastric pain, toothaches, post-operative pain, and pain due to cancer. At the same time, it can dispel wind to relieve pain as well as detoxify, and therefore is used to treat eczema, measles, stubborn tinea, and poisonous snake bites.

④ *Chuān wū* (川乌, Radix Aconiti, Common Monkshood Mother Root) ★★

Addition: *Cǎo wū* (草乌, **Radix Aconiti Kusnezoffii, Kusnezoff Monkshood Root)** is the same as *chuān wū* (Radix Aconiti) in character, actions, indications, administration, dosage and precautions. However, it has a stronger toxicity than *chuān wū* (Radix Aconiti).

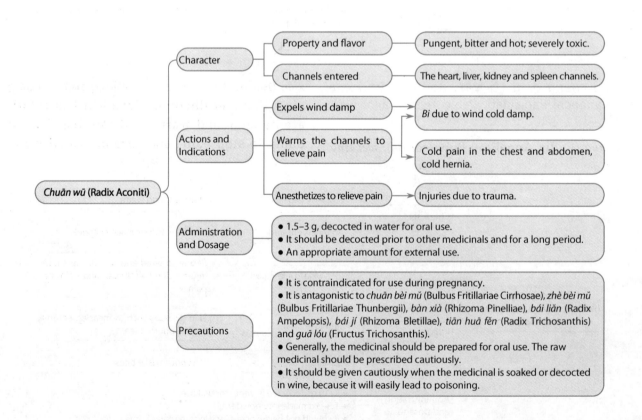

⑤ *Qí shé* (蕲蛇, Agkistrodon, Agkistrodon)

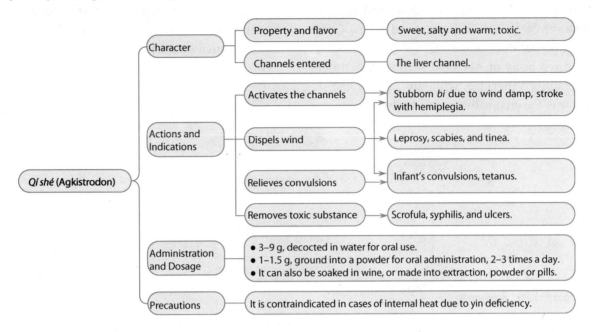

⑥ *Wū shāo shé* (乌梢蛇, Zaocys, Black-tail Snake)

Qí shé (Agkistrodon) and *wū shāo shé* (Zaocys) enter the liver channel, and can travel between the exterior and the interior of the body. In the interior they reach to the bowels and viscera, on the exterior they reach to the flesh and muscles, in this way they *"penetrate the bones to course wind"*. The two medicinals can dispel wind and activate the channels and collaterals to relieve convulsions. They are indicated for *bi* due to wind damp with numbness and spasm; stroke with facial distortion or hemiplegia; leprosy, scabies, tinea and pruritus; convulsions in infants, and tetanus. They are especially used to treat chronic and stubborn diseases caused by both internal and external wind toxin retention. *Qí shé* (Agkistrodon) is warm, dry and toxic, and has a strong action in treating stubborn *bi* of a wind damp type. *Wū shāo shé* (Zaocys) has a neutral property with a moderate action. The type of

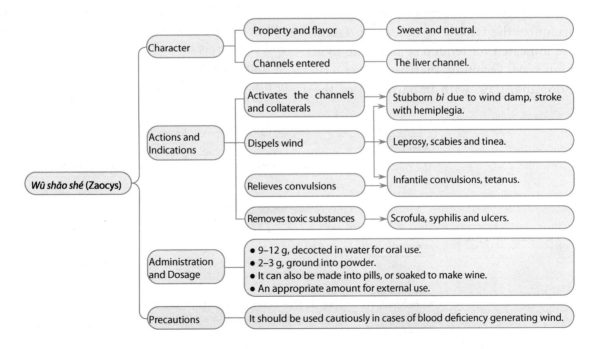

bái huā shé that is used in the clinic comes from two species: *Qí shé* (Agkistrodon) and *jīn qián bái huā shé* (金钱白花蛇, Bungarus Parvus, Coin-like White-banded Snake). *Qí shé* (Agkistrodon) is the dried body of *Agkistrodon acutus* Guenther., of the family Viperidae, while *jīn qián bái huā shé* (Bungarus Parvus) is the young body of *Bungarus*

multicinctus Blyth., of the family Elapidae. The two have similar actions and indications, but the latter one has stronger actions and should be used in a smaller dosage.

⑦ *Mù guā* (木瓜, Fructus Chaenomelis, Common Flowering Quince Fruit) ★ ★ ★

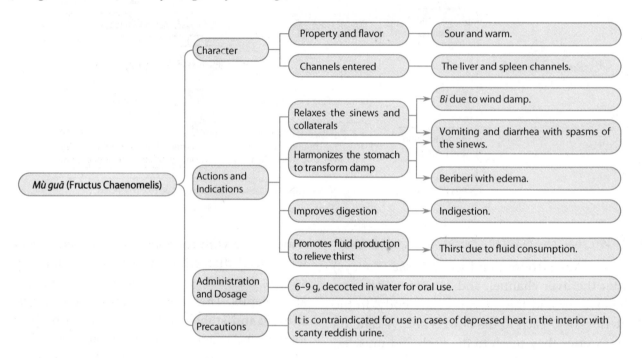

⑧ *Cán shā* (蚕沙, Faeces Bombycis, Silkworm Feces)

Mù guā (Fructus Chaenomelis) and *cán shā* (Faeces Bombycis) are warm in property, and can harmonize the middle to transform damp. They are indicated for tendon spasms due to *bi* of a damp type, vomiting, diarrhea, dysentery, and abdominal pain with impairment of the

sinews caused by a dysfunction of ascending and descending due to damp turbidity retention in the middle. However, *mù guā* (Fructus Chaenomelis) has a sour flavor, and therefore can relax the sinews and activate the channels and collaterals as well as harmonize the stomach to transform damp. It is frequently used to treat *bi* due to wind damp with tendon spasms, and

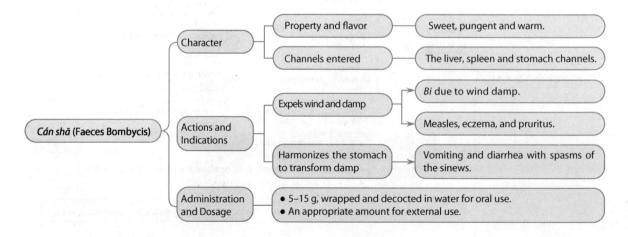

beriberi with swelling pain. In addition, it can promote digestion and fluid production so as to relieve thirst, and is also used for indigestion. *Cán shā* (Faeces Bombycis) can moderately expel wind and damp, and is used for *bi* due to wind and damp. It can relieve itching and treat German measles, eczema, and general pruritus.

⑨ *Shēn jīn cǎo* (伸筋草, Herba Lycopodii, Common Clubmoss Herb)

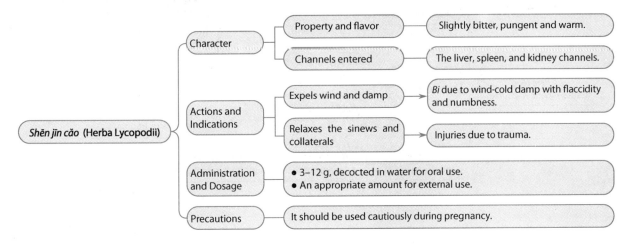

⑩ *Xún gǔ fēng* (寻骨风, Herba Aristolochiae Mollissimae, Wooly Dutchmanspipe Herb)

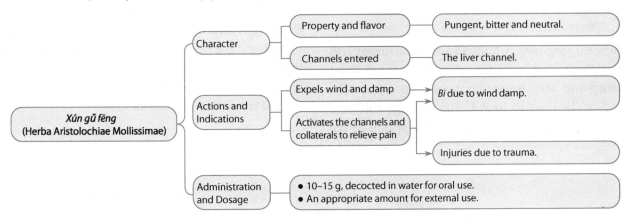

⑪ *Sōng jié* (松节, Lignum Pini Nodi, Chinese Pine Node)

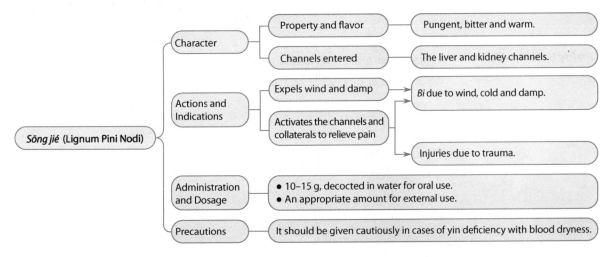

⑫ *Hǎi fēng téng* (海风藤, Caulis Piperis Kadsurae, Kadsura Pepper Stem)

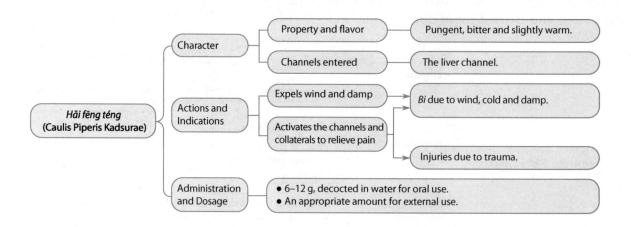

⑬ *Qīng fēng téng* (青风藤, Caulis Sinomenii, Orientvine Stem)

Both *hǎi fēng téng* (Caulis Piperis Kadsurae) and *qīng fēng téng* (Caulis Sinomenii) can expel wind damp and activate the channels and collaterals, and can be used to treat *bi* due to wind, cold and damp with aching joints and limbs, spasm of the sinews and vessels, and a lack of flexibility. *Hǎi fēng téng* (Caulis Piperis Kadsurae) is capable of relieving pain and can treat injuries due to trauma and pain with blood stasis. *Qīng fēng téng* (Caulis Sinomenii) is able to induce diuresis and is used for edema and beriberi.

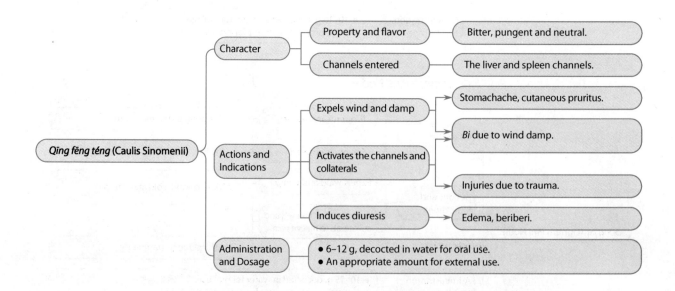

⑭ *Dīng gōng téng* (丁公藤, Caulis Erycibes, Obtuseleaf Erycibe Stem)

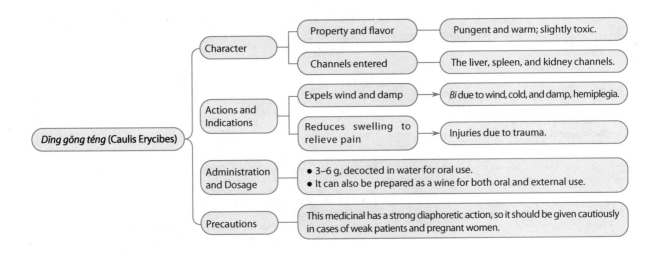

⑮ *Kūn míng shān hǎi táng* (昆明山海棠, Radix Tripterygium Hypoglaucum, Tripterygium Hypoglaucum Root)

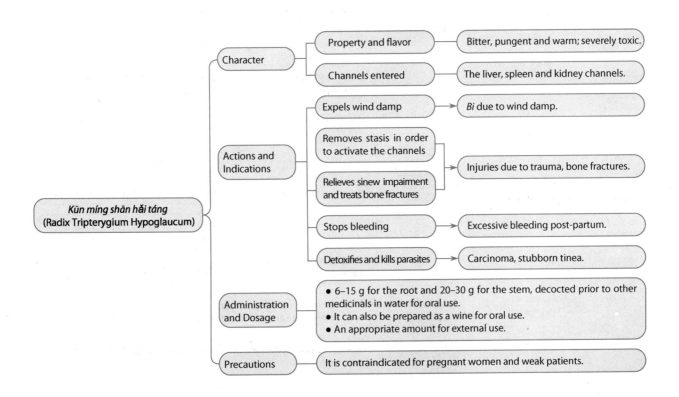

⑯ *Xuě shàng yī zhī hāo* (雪上一枝蒿, Radix Aconiti
Brachypodi, Shortstalk Monkshood Root)

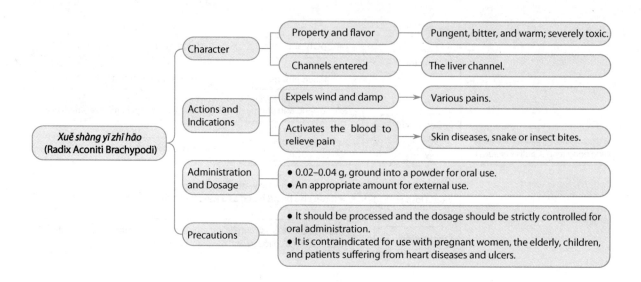

⑰ *Lù lù tōng* (路路通, Fructus Liquidambaris,
Liquidambar Fruit)

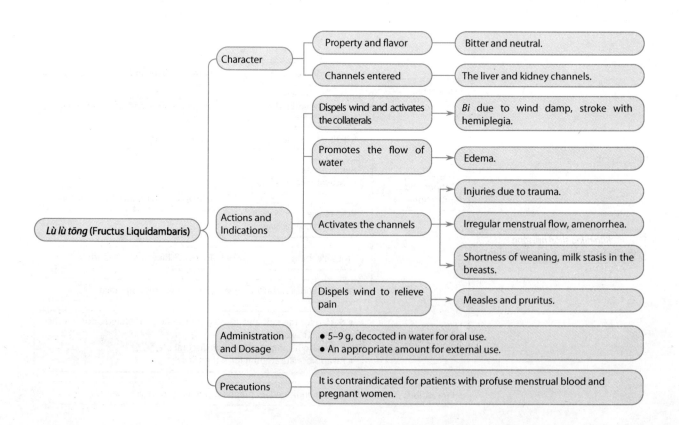

Section 2   Medicinals that Expel Wind, Heat and Damp

Medicinals in this section are usually pungent, bitter and cold, and enter the liver, spleen and kidney channels. They are effective for expelling wind and damp, activating the channels and collaterals to relieve pain, and clearing heat to reduce swelling. They are mainly indicated for *bi* due to wind, heat and damp with red, swollen, and painful joints. When properly combined with medicinals of other types, they can also be used to treat *bi* of a wind cold damp type.

① *Qín jiāo* (秦艽, Radix Gentianae Macrophyllae, Largeleaf Gentian Root) ★ ★ ★

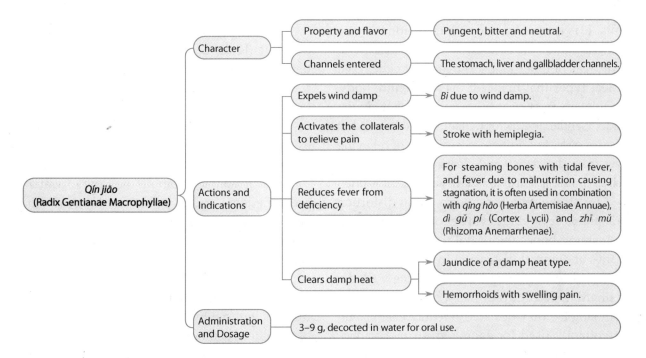

② *Fáng jǐ* (防己, Radix Stephaniae Tetrandrae, Fourstamen Stephania Root) ★ ★ ★

Qín jiāo (Radix Gentianae Macrophyllae) and *fáng jǐ* (Radix Stephaniae Tetrandrae) are pungent, bitter and cold. They can expel wind damp and relieve *bi*. They are indicated for *bi* due to wind, heat and

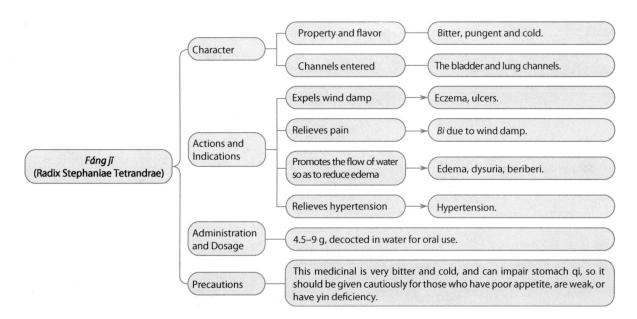

damp, manifesting as redness, swelling and pain in the joints and limbs. *Qín jiāo* (Radix Gentianae Macrophyllae) has a moist texture and is known as the "*moist agent in the group of medicinals that dispel pathogenic wind*". It can expel wind damp, relieve *bi*, and relax sinews and collaterals. Therefore it is indicated for *bi* due to wind damp, manifesting with numbness in the limbs, spasms of sinews and vessels, aching joints and bones, and inflexible joints. It is especially effective in treating *bi* of a heat type, and can be used in combination with medicinals of other kinds to treat *bi* of either cold or heat types that manifest over the entire body. Practitioners in ancient times believed that *qín jiāo* (Radix Gentianae Macrophyllae) was to be used in all cases of *bi*. In addition, it is capable of relieving fever from deficiency and clearing damp heat, as well as draining damp to relieve jaundice. It is often used for stroke with hemiplegia, facial distortion and aphasia; fever due to yin deficiency manifesting as steaming bones with tidal fever, fever due to infant's abdominal distension from malnutrition, and jaundice of a damp heat type. *Fáng jǐ* (Radix Stephaniae Tetrandrae) has a strong action in promoting the flow of water to reduce edema, and is frequently used for edema, dysuria, beriberi, eczema, and ulcers. The medicinal that we call *fáng jǐ* includes two types: *Hàn fáng jǐ* (汉防己, Radix Stephaniae Tetrandrae, Stephania Tetrandra) and *mù fáng jǐ* (木防己, Radix Cocculi Trilobi, Southern Fangji Root). Both medicinals have the actions of expelling wind damp, relieving pain, and promoting the flow of water to reduce edema. *Hàn fáng jǐ* (Radix Stephaniae Tetrandrae) comes from the root of *Stephania tetrandra S. Moore* (family *Menispermaceae*), while *mù fáng jǐ* (Radix Trilobi) is the root of *Aristolochia fangchi Wu* (family *Aristolochiaceae*). The former can mainly promote the flow of water to reduce edema, while the latter can expel wind to relieve pain.

Both *fáng jǐ* (Radix Stephaniae Tetrandrae) and *fáng fēng* (Radix Saposhnikoviae) can expel wind damp and relieve *bi*. They are indicated for *bi* due to wind damp with aching joints and limbs. *Fáng jǐ* (Radix Stephaniae Tetrandrae) is pungent, bitter and cold, and can mainly expel damp to relieve pain, as well as dispel wind and clear heat. Therefore, it is most effective in treating *bi* due to wind heat damp. It is able to promote the flow of water to reduce edema and is used for edema, dysuria, beriberi with swollen feet, eczema, and sores. *Fáng fēng* (Radix Saposhnikoviae) is pungent, sweet and slightly warm, and is capable of dispelling wind and cold to remove damp, therefore it is indicated for *bi* due to wind, cold and damp. It can treat all diseases induced by pathogenic wind. It is capable of dispelling pathogenic wind from the exterior of the body and relieving convulsions. Therefore, it is used for exterior wind cold, wind heat or wind cold complicated by pathogenic damp, as well as tetanus.

③ *Sāng zhī* (桑枝, Ramulus Mori, Mulberry Twig)

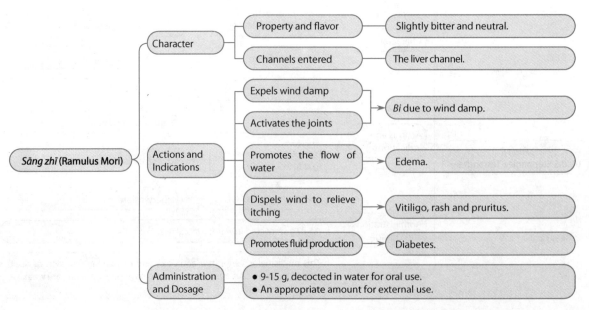

④ *Xī xiān cǎo* (豨莶草, Herba Siegesbeckiae, Siegesbeckia Herb) ★

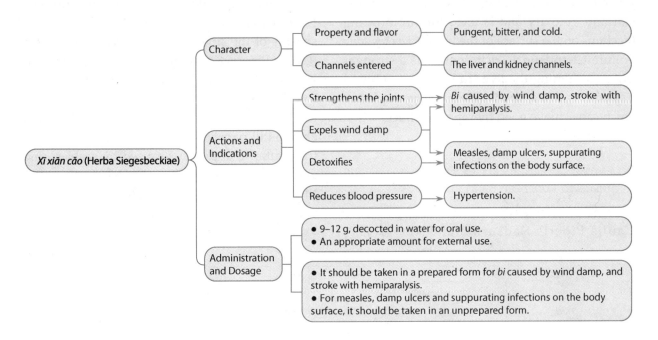

⑤ *Chòu wú tóng* (臭梧桐, Folium Clerodendri Trichotomi, Harlequin Glorybower Leaf)

Both *xī xiān cǎo* (Herba Siegesbeckiae) and *chòu wú tóng* (Folium Clerodendri Trichotomi) are pungent, bitter, and cold or cool. They can expel wind damp and activate the channels and collaterals. They are often used for *bi* due to wind damp, aching joints and bones, numb limbs, and spasms of the sinews and muscles. Due to their cold or cool property, they are especially suitable for *bi* caused by pathogenic wind, heat and damp. The two medicinals are also used for stroke with hemiparalysis, measles, eczema and damp ulcers. Modern research shows that both of the medicinals are capable of reducing blood pressure, and therefore are indicated for

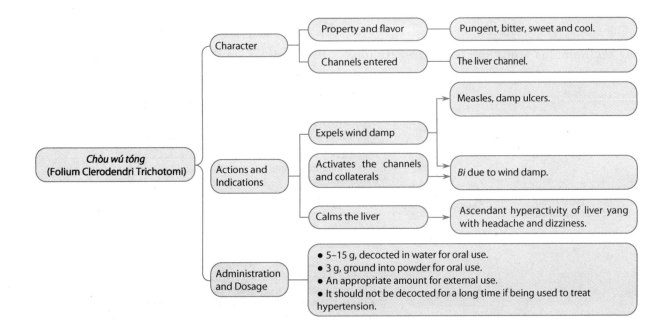

hypertension with headache and dizziness. However, there are differences between them. *Xī xiān cǎo* (Herba Siegesbeckiae) can clear heat and detoxify and is used for suppurating infections on the surface of the body. *Chòu wú tóng* (Folium Clerodendri Trichotomi) has a stronger action in calming the liver to bring down blood pressure than *xī xiān cǎo* (Herba Siegesbeckiae), which can achieve good therapeutic effects when used alone.

⑥ *Hǎi tóng pí* (海桐皮, Cortex Erythrinae, Oriental Variegated Coralbean Bark)

Hǎi tóng pí (Cortex Erythrinae), *hǎi fēng téng* (Caulis Piperis Kadsurae) and *xún gǔ fēng*

(Herba Aristolochiae Mollissimae) have actions of expelling wind damp and activating the channels and collaterals. They are indicated for *bi* caused by wind damp, numbness, and spasms of the sinews and muscles. *Hǎi fēng téng* (Caulis Piperis Kadsurae) and *xún gǔ fēng* (Herba Aristolochiae Mollissimae) are also used for injuries due to trauma, swelling, and pain due to blood stasis. *Hǎi tóng pí* (Cortex Erythrinae) is able to kill parasites to relieve itching in order to treat cutaneous pruritus caused by scabies, tinea and eczema. *Xún gǔ fēng* (Herba Aristolochiae Mollissimae) is capable of relieving pain and is used to treat stomachache and toothache.

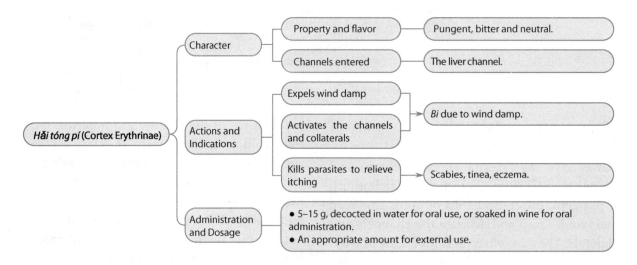

⑦ *Luò shí téng* (络石藤, Caulis Trachelospermi, Chinese Starjasmine Stem) ★

Sāng zhī (Ramulus Mori) and *luò shí téng* (Caulis

Trachelospermi) have the effect of dispelling wind to activate the collaterals, and are mainly indicated for *bi* due to wind damp (especially of a

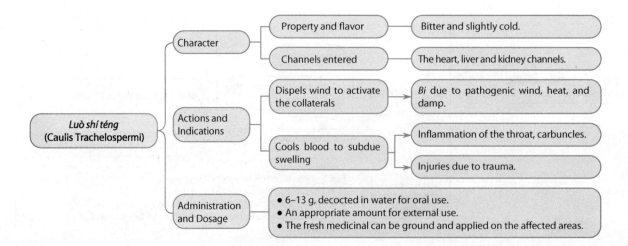

heat type), numbness, spasms of the sinews and muscles, and inflexible joints. *Sāng zhī* (Ramulus Mori) has a neutral property, and therefore is suitable for *bi* caused by wind damp of either a cold or a heat type. It is especially effective in treating *bi* of a heat type in the upper part of the body. In addition, it can promote the flow of water to alleviate edema. *Luò shí téng* (Caulis Trachelospermi) is cold and can cool blood to reduce swellings. It can be used for inflammation of the throat, carbuncles, ulcers, injuries due to trauma, and swelling with pain due to blood stasis.

⑧ *Léi gōng téng* (雷公藤, Radix Tripterygii Wilfordii, Tripterygium Wilfordii Root) ★

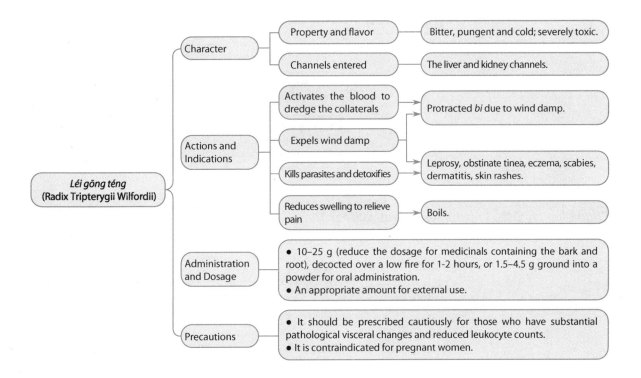

⑨ *Lǎo guàn cǎo* (老鹳草, Herba Erodii, Cranesbill) ★

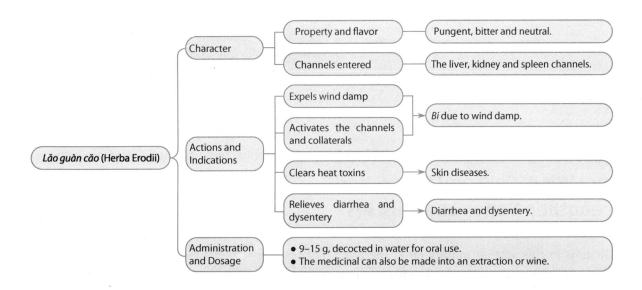

⑩ *Chuān shān lóng* (穿山龙, Rhizoma Dioscoreae Nipponicae, Japanese Dioscorea Rhizome)

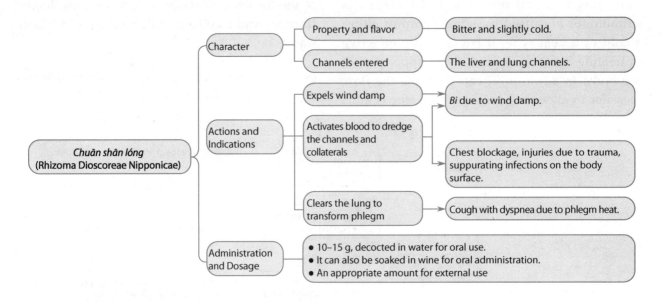

⑪ *Sī guā luò* (丝瓜络, Fructus Retinervus Luffae, Luffa Vegetable Sponge)

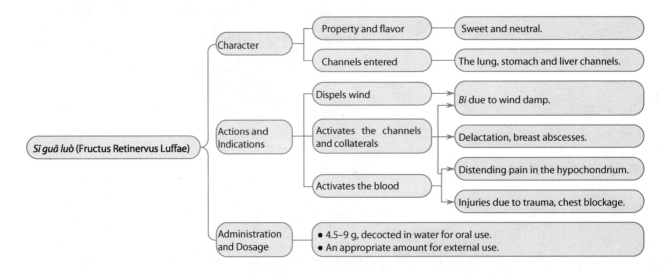

Section 3　Medicinals that Expel Wind, Cold and Damp, and Strengthen Bones and Muscles

Medicinals in this section mainly enter the liver and kidney channels, and in addition to expelling wind damp, have the actions of nourishing the liver and kidney and strengthening the bones and muscles. They are often used for aching loins and knees, and flaccidity caused by deficiencies of the liver and kidney due to chronic rheumatic diseases. They are also used to treat lumbago due to kidney deficiency, flaccidity, and weakness.

① *Wǔ jiā pí* (五加皮, Cortex Acanthopanacis, Slenderstyle Acanthopanax Bark) ★★

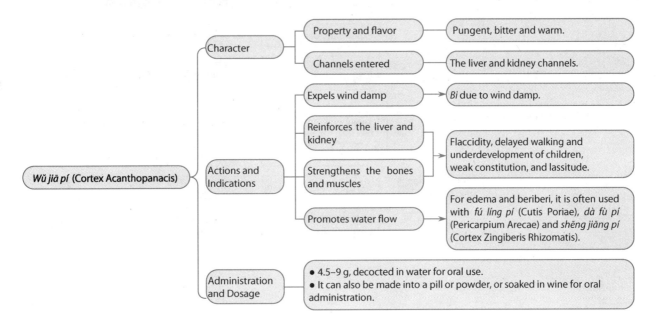

② *Sāng jì shēng* (桑寄生, Herba Taxilli, Chinese Taxillus Herb) ★★★

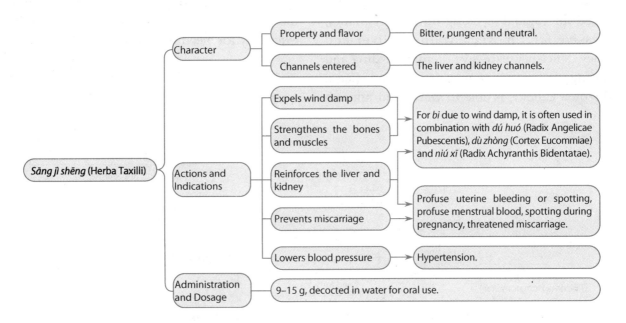

③ *Gǒu jǐ* (狗脊, Rhizoma Cibotii, Cibot Rhizome) ★★
Wǔ jiā pí (Cortex Acanthopanacis), *sāng jì shēng* (Herba Taxilli) and *gǒu jǐ* (Rhizoma Cibotii) enter the liver and kidney channels, and can nourish the liver and kidney and strengthen the bones

and muscles. They can be used for chronic *bi* due to wind damp complicated by liver and kidney deficiency, manifesting with aching waist and knees and flaccidity, and underdevelopment of children due to liver and kidney deficiency. *Wǔ*

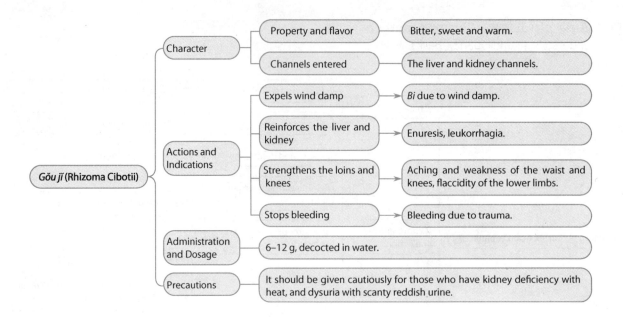

jiā pí (Cortex Acanthopanacis) can promote the flow of water and is used for edema, dysuria, and beriberi. *Sāng jì shēng* (Herba Taxilli) is capable of nourishing blood to prevent miscarriage, and is used for vaginal bleeding during pregnancy, excessive fetal movement due to liver and kidney deficiency, excessive uterine bleeding and spotting, and excessive menstrual blood. *Gŏu jǐ* (Rhizoma Cibotii) is able to warm and nourish

so as to consolidate essence, and therefore is used to treat enuresis, frequent urination and leukorrhagia caused by kidney deficiency. In addition, the hair of *gŏu jǐ* (Rhizoma Cibotii) has the effect of stopping bleeding, and is applied externally for bleeding due to trauma.

④ *Qiān nián jiàn* (千年健, Rhizoma Homalomenae, Obscured Homalomena Rhizome)

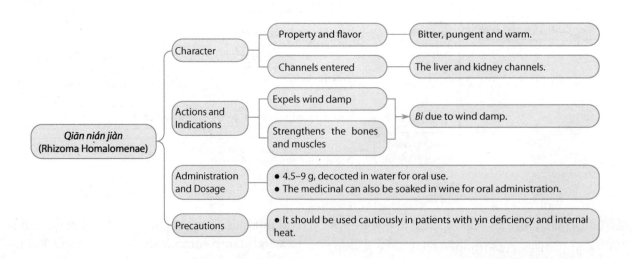

⑤ *Xuě lián huā* (雪莲花, Herba Saussureae Lanicepsis, Snow Lotus Herb)

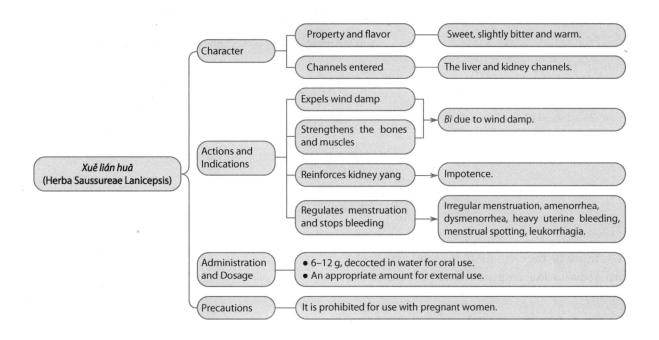

⑥ *Lù xián cǎo* (鹿衔草, Herba Pyrolae, Pyrola)

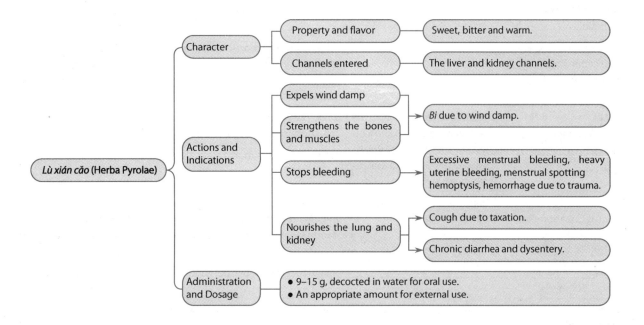

⑦ *Shí nán yè* (石楠叶, Folium Photiniae, Chinese Photinia Leaf)

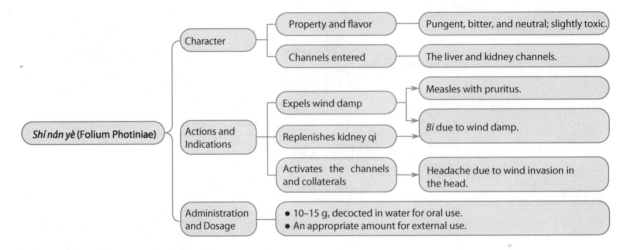

Actions of medicinals that expel wind and damp are summarized in the following tables (Tables 11-1~11-3):

Table 11-1: Summary of Medicinals that Expel Wind, Cold and Damp:

Medicinal	Action in Common	Individual Character	
		Characteristic Actions	**Other Actions**
Dú huó (Radix Angelicae Pubescentis)	Expels wind damp, alleviates pain	It has a strong action in expelling wind damp, is effective for treating *bi* due to wind cold in the lower part of body.	Relieves exterior syndromes
Wēi líng xiān (Radix et Rhizoma Clematidis)		It has a drastic action, activates the channels and collaterals.	Relieves fishbones caught in the throat
Xú cháng qīng (Radix et Rhizoma Cynanchi Paniculati)		It has a strong action in relieving pain, extensively used for various kinds of pain caused by wind damp, cold congealing, qi stagnation and blood stasis.	Dispels wind to relieve itching, detoxifies poisoning from snake bites
Qí shé (Agkistrodon)	Acts both on the exterior of the body and in the interior, dispels wind to activate the collaterals, relieves convulsions, specializes in removing wind	Toxic, has a strong action, commonly used for stubborn *bi* due to wind damp	
Wū shāo shé (Zaocys)		Non-toxic, with a moderate action	
Mù guā (Fructus Chaenomelis)	Harmonizes the middle to transform damp	It is effective for relaxing sinews and muscles, it is used for *bi* due to wind damp, spasm of the sinews and muscles	Improves digestion, promotes fluid production to relieve thirst
Cán shā (Faeces Bombycis)		Moderates action to expel wind and damp	Relieves itching
Chuān wū (Radix Aconiti)	Severely toxic, it can dispel wind and remove damp, warm channels to dispel cold, relieve pain		
Cǎo wū (Radix Aconiti Kusnezoffii)			

Table 11-1: Summary of Medicinals that Expel Wind, Cold and Damp:

continued

Medicinal	Action in Common	Individual Character	
		Characteristic Actions	**Other Actions**
Hǎi fēng téng (Caulis Piperis Kadsurae)	Expels wind damp, activates the channels and collaterals	Relieves pain	
Qīng fēng téng (Caulis Sinomenii)		Induces diuresis	
Xún gǔ fēng (Herba Aristolochiae Mollissimae)	Expels wind damp, activates the collaterals to relieve pain		
Sōng jié (Lignum Pini Nodi)			
Shēn jīn cǎo (Herba Lycopodii)	Expels wind damp	Relaxes the sinews and muscles	
Dīng gōng téng (Caulis Erycibes)		Reduces swelling to relieve pain	
Kūn míng shān hǎi táng (Radix Tripterygium Hypoglaucum)		Removes stasis to activate the collaterals, heals bone fractures	
Xuě shàng yī zhī hāo (Radix Aconiti Brachypodi)		Activates the blood to relieve pain	
Lù lù tōng (Fructus Liquidambaris)		Activates the channels and collaterals, promotes the flow of water	

Table 11-2: Summary of Medicinals that Expel Wind, Heat and Damp:

Medicinal	Action in Common	Individual Character	
		Characteristic Actions	**Other Actions**
Qín jiāo (Radix Gentianae Macrophyllae)	Expels wind damp, relieves *bi*	Known as *"the moist that can remove pathogenic wind"*, it is able to relax the sinews and muscles, suitable for *bi* due to wind damp of either a cold or heat type all over the body, especially effective for *bi* of the heat type	Reduces deficient heat, clears damp heat
Fáng jǐ (Radix Stephaniae Tetrandrae)			Promotes the flow of water to reduce edema
Sāng zhī (Ramulus Mori)	Dispels wind to activate collaterals	Suitable for *bi* due to wind-heat damp in the upper limbs	Promotes the flow of water to reduce edema
Luò shí téng (Caulis Trachelospermi)			Cools blood to reduce swelling
Xī xiān cǎo (Herba Siegesbeckiae)	Expels wind damp, activates the channels and collaterals, decreases blood pressure		Clears heat and detoxifies
Chòu wú tóng (Folium Clerodendri Trichotomi)		It has a stronger action in calming the liver to decrease blood pressure than *xī xiān cǎo* (Herba Siegesbeckiae)	

Table 11-2: Summary of Medicinals that Expel Wind, Heat and Damp:

continued

Medicinal	Action in Common	Individual Character	
		Characteristic Actions	**Other Actions**
Hǎi tóng pí (Cortex Erythrinae)	Expels wind damp, activates the channels and collaterals to relieve pain, kills parasites to relieve itching	Usually indicated for skin diseases	
Léi gōng téng (Radix Tripterygii Wilfordii)		Severely toxic, suitable for stiff and deformed joints	Activates blood to reduce swelling, detoxifies
Lǎo guàn cǎo (Herba Erodii)	Expels wind damp, activates the channels and collaterals		Clears heat and detoxifies, stops diarrhea and dysentery
Chuān shān lóng (Rhizoma Dioscoreae Nipponicae)			Clears the lung to transform phlegm
Sī guā luò (Fructus Retinervus Luffae)			Activates blood, promotes lactation

Table 11-3: Summary of Medicinals that Expel Wind and Damp, Strengthen Bones and Muscles:

Medicinal	Action in Common		Individual Character
Wǔ jiā pí (Cortex Acanthopanacis)	Expels damp and strengthens bones and muscles	Nourishes the liver and kidney	Promotes the flow of water
Sāng jì shēng (Herba Taxilli)			Prevents miscarriage
Gǒu jǐ (Rhizoma Cibotii)			Warms and nourishes to consolidate essence, stops bleeding
Qiān nián jiàn (Rhizoma Homalomenae)			Especially suitable for the elderly
Xuě lián huā (Herba Saussureae Lanicepsis)			Reinforces kidney yang, regulates menstruation to stop bleeding
Lù xián cǎo (Herba Pyrolae)			Stops bleeding, relieves cough
Shí nán yè (Folium Photiniae)			Activates the channels and collaterals, replenishes kidney qi

Tables to test your herbal knowledge of the actions and indications of medicinals that expel wind and damp follow (Tables 11-4~11-9):

Table 11-4: Test your Herbal Knowledge of the Actions of Medicinals that Expel Wind and Damp (one):

Actions \ Medicinal	*Dú huó*	*Wēi líng xiān*	*Chuān wū*	*Cǎo wū*	*Qí shé*	*Wū shāo shé*	*Léi gōng téng*	*Wǔ jiā pí*	*Sāng jì shēng*	*Gǒu jǐ*	*Qiān nián jiàn*
Expels wind damp											
Relieves *bi*											
Reduces swelling to relieve pain											
Activates the channels and collaterals											
Relieves fishbones caught in the throat											

Table 11-4: Test your Herbal Knowledge of the Actions of Medicinals that Expel Wind and Damp (one):

continued

Actions \ Medicinal	Dú huó	Wēi líng xiān	Chuān wū	Cǎo wū	Qí shé	Wū shāo shé	Léi gōng téng	Wǔ jiā pí	Sāng jì shēng	Gǒu jǐ	Qiān nián jiàn
Kills parasites and detoxifies											
Relieves convulsions											
Relieves itching											
Removes nebula											
Activates the blood to dredge collaterals											
Relieves exterior syndromes											
Dispels cold to relieve pain											
Strengthens bones and muscles											
Induces diuresis											
Nourishes the liver and kidney											
Prevents miscarriage											
Benefits the waist and knees											

Table 11-5: Test your Herbal Knowledge of the Actions of Medicinals that Expel Wind and Damp (two):

Actions \ Medicinal	Mù guā	Cán shā	Shēn jīn cǎo	Xún gǔ fēng	Sōng jié	Hǎi fēng téng	Lǎo guàn cǎo	Lù lù tōng
Relaxes sinews								
Activates collaterals								
Relaxes the sinews and activates channels and collaterals								
Expels wind damp								
Dispels wind and activates the collaterals								
Activates the collaterals to relieve pain								
Activates the channels and collaterals								
Removes damp to harmonize the stomach								
Relieves diarrhea and dysentery								
Harmonizes the middle to transform damp								
Promotes the flow of water								
Promotes lactation								

Table 11-6: Test your Herbal Knowledge of the Actions of Medicinals that Expel Wind and Damp (three):

Actions \ Medicinal	Qín jiāo	Fáng jǐ	Sāng zhī	Xī xiān cǎo	Chòu wú tóng	Hǎi tóng pí	Luò shí téng	Chuān shān lóng	Sī guā luò
Expels wind damp									
Dispels wind									
Reduces deficiency fever									
Clears damp heat									

Table 11-6: Test your Herbal Knowledge of the Actions of Medicinals that Expel Wind and Damp (three):

continued

Medicinal / Actions	Qín jiāo	Fáng jǐ	Sāng zhī	Xī xiān cǎo	Chòu wú tóng	Hǎi tóng pí	Luò shí téng	Chuān shān lóng	Sī guā luò
Clears heat and detoxifies									
Promotes the flow of water and reduces edema									
Relieves *bi*									
Dredges the collaterals									
Activates the joints									
Cools the blood to reduce swelling									
Relieves pain									
Reduces blood pressure									
Activates the collaterals									
Kills parasites to relieve itching									
Activates the channels and collaterals									
Activates the blood to dredge collaterals									
Clears the lung to transform phlegm									
Detoxifies to transform phlegm									

Table 11-7: Test your Herbal Knowledge of the Indications of Medicinals that Expel Wind and Damp (one):

Medicinal / Indications	Dú huó	Wēi líng xiān	Chuān wū	Cǎo wū	Qí shé	Wū shāo shé	Léi gōng téng	Mù guā	Cán shā
Bi due to wind, cold and damp									
Exterior syndrome of a wind cold type complicated by pathogenic damp									
Leprosy									
Various pains due to cold syndromes									
Infant's convulsions									
Anesthetizes so as to relieve pain									
Stubborn *bi* due to wind damp									
Post-stroke syndrome									
Bones caught in the throat									
Injuries due to trauma									
Tetanus									
Bi due to wind damp									
Vomiting and diarrhea with spasms of the sinews									
Herpes zoster									
Cutaneous pruritus									
Beriberi									
Boils and ulcers									

Table 11-8: Test your Herbal Knowledge of the Indications of Medicinals that Expel Wind and Damp (two):

Medicinal Indications	Shēn jīn cǎo	Xún gǔ fēng	Sōng jié	Hǎi fēng téng	Lǎo guàn cǎo	Lù lù tōng	Wǔ jiā pí	Sāng jì shēng	Gǒu jǐ	Qiān nián jiàn
Bi due to wind damp										
Pruritus due to measles										
Diarrhea and dysentery due to damp heat										
Edema, dysuria										
Weakness in the waist and knees										
Distending pain in breast										
Injuries due to trauma										
Insufficiency of the liver and kidney										
Galactostasis										
Underdevelopment and delayed walking in infants										
Leukorrhagia										
Excessive fetal movement										
Frequent urination, enuresis										
Vaginal bleeding during pregnancy										

Table 11-9: Test your Herbal Knowledge of the Indications of Medicinals that Expel Wind and Damp (three):

Medicinal Indications	Qín jiāo	Fáng jǐ	Sāng zhī	Xī xiān cǎo	Chòu wú tóng	Hǎi tóng pí	Luò shí téng	Chuān shān lóng	Sī guā luò
Bi due to wind damp									
Stroke with flaccidity									
Edema									
Phlegm-fluids									
Steaming bones with tidal fever									
Skin diseases									
Chest blockage									
Hypertension									
Scabies and tinea									
Hypochondriac pain									
Joint sprains									
Pain in the waist and lower limbs									
Cough due to phlegm heat									
Eczema with itching									
Inflammation of the throat									
Breast abscesses									

Chapter 12
Aromatic Medicinals that Transform Damp

Concept

"Aromatic medicinals" refers to medicinals that are aromatic in flavor, warm and dry in nature, and have the effect of transforming damp to invigorate the spleen.

Character and Actions

Medicinals in this chapter are pungent and aromatic in flavor, and warm and dry in property. They mainly enter the spleen and stomach channels so as to promote the spleen to transform and transport and resolve damp. They can also promote qi circulation in the middle *jiao*, and therefore can relieve qi stagnation in the spleen and stomach induced by obstruction of damp in the middle *jiao*.

Indications

Medicinals with the effect of transforming damp are indicated for obstruction of damp in the middle *jiao*, and dysfunction of the spleen and stomach in their ability to transform and transport. This can manifest as epigastric and abdominal distention and fullness, nausea, vomiting, sour regurgitation, loose stools, poor appetite, fatigue, salivation, and a white and greasy tongue coating. In addition, they can also clear summer-heat, and are indicated for syndromes of a damp-warm or summer-heat-damp type.

Combinations

Damp-transforming medicinals should be used in combination with medicinals of other kinds according to different types of damp obstruction and their complications. For qi stagnation due to damp obstruction with symptoms such as epigastric and abdominal distention and fullness, medicinals for promoting qi circulation should also be used. For cold-damp with epigastric and abdominal cold pain, combine with medicinals that have actions of warming the interior to dispel cold. For spleen deficiency manifesting as epigastric fullness, poor appetite, low spirit, and flaccidity, combine with medicinals that have actions of replenishing qi and invigorating the spleen. In cases of damp-warmth, damp-heat, or summer-heat damp, combine with medicinals that have actions of clearing heat and drying damp, clearing summer heat, or draining damp.

Precautions

Aromatic medicinals in this chapter usually contain volatile oils and can achieve good therapeutic results when made into a powdered form. They should be decocted after other medicinals and should not be decocted for a long period of time. The medicinals are mostly pungent and aromatic in flavor, and warm and dry in property, and can consume qi and yin, therefore they should be used with caution in cases of yin deficiency, blood dryness, and qi deficiency.

① *Huò xiāng* (藿香, Herba Agastachis, Ageratum) ★ ★ ★

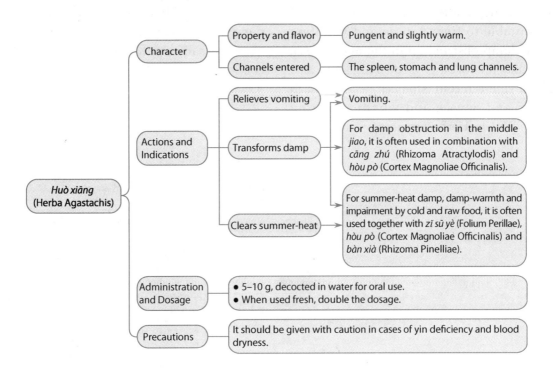

② *Pèi lán* (佩兰, Herba Eupatorii, Eupatorium) ★

Huò xiāng (Herba Agastachis) and *pèi lán* (Herba Eupatorii) are pungent and aromatic, and enter the spleen, stomach and lung channels. They can transform damp, clear summer-heat and relieve exterior syndromes. The two medicinals are indicated for epigastric and abdominal distension and fullness, poor appetite, nausea, vomiting, low spirits, and lassitude caused by damp obstruction in the middle *jiao*, invasion of summer-heat damp in the exterior, and damp-warmth in the initial stage. They are often used together. *Huò xiāng* (Herba Agastachis) has a pungent flavor and a slightly warm property. It is a commonly used medicinal for transforming damp turbidity. It has a stronger action in relieving exterior syndromes than *pèi lán* (Herba Eupatorii), so it is often used for exterior syndromes due to external pathogens. It is also used for external invasion of wind cold during the summer, with impairment by cold

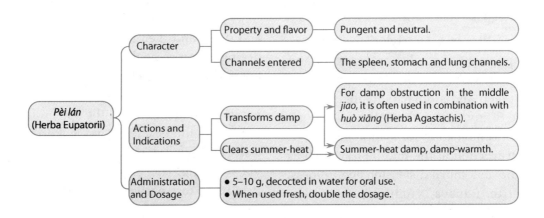

and raw food. This manifests as aversion to cold, fever, headache, epigastric fullness, vomiting, diarrhea, and dysentery. It can transform damp to harmonize the middle to relieve vomiting, and is most suitable to treat nausea and vomiting caused by damp obstruction in the middle *jiao*. When combined with other medicinals, it can also be used for stomach cold, stomach heat, stomach deficiency, and nausea and vomiting during pregnancy. *Pèi lán* (Herba Eupatorii) is neutral in property, but is less strong than *huò xiāng* (Herba Agastachis) to release the exterior. It is good for transforming damp and repelling foulness and turbidity. In addition, it is used for spleen channel damp heat, sweet and greasy tastes in the mouth, excessive saliva, putrid breath, and a dirty tongue coating.

③ *Cāng zhú* (苍术, Rhizoma Atractylodis, Atractylodes Rhizome) ★ ★ ★

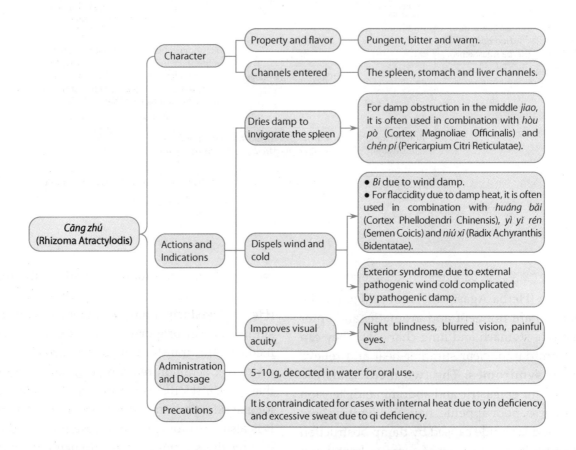

④ *Hòu pò* (厚朴, Cortex Magnoliae Officinalis, Officinal Magnolia Bark) ★ ★ ★

Both *cāng zhú* (Rhizoma Atractylodis) and *hòu pò* (Cortex Magnoliae Officinalis) are pungent and bitter in flavor, warm and dry in property, and enter the spleen and stomach channels to dry damp so as to invigorate the spleen. They are often used in combination for symptoms caused by damp obstruction in the middle *jiao*, such as epigastric and abdominal distension and fullness, poor appetite, nausea, vomiting, lassitude, diarrhea, and a turbid greasy tongue coating. *Cāng zhú* (Rhizoma Atractylodis) is warmer and drier, and therefore has a stronger action in drying damp so as to invigorate the spleen. It is known as the most effective medicinal for drying damp to invigorate the spleen, and is indicated for damp exuberance in the spleen manifesting as phlegm-fluids, edema and leukorrhagia. It can also expel wind damp, relieve exterior syndrome via sweating, and brighten the eyes. Therefore, it is used to treat *bi* due to pathogenic wind,

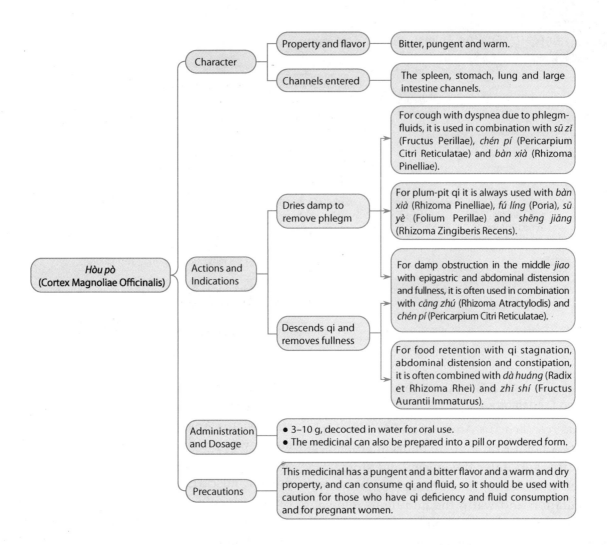

Hòu pò (Cortex Magnoliae Officinalis)

- Character
  - Property and flavor — Bitter, pungent and warm.
  - Channels entered — The spleen, stomach, lung and large intestine channels.

- Actions and Indications
  - Dries damp to remove phlegm
    - For cough with dyspnea due to phlegm-fluids, it is used in combination with sū zǐ (Fructus Perillae), chén pí (Pericarpium Citri Reticulatae) and bàn xià (Rhizoma Pinelliae).
    - For plum-pit qi it is always used with bàn xià (Rhizoma Pinelliae), fú líng (Poria), sū yè (Folium Perillae) and shēng jiāng (Rhizoma Zingiberis Recens).
  - Descends qi and removes fullness
    - For damp obstruction in the middle jiao with epigastric and abdominal distension and fullness, it is often used in combination with cāng zhú (Rhizoma Atractylodis) and chén pí (Pericarpium Citri Reticulatae).
    - For food retention with qi stagnation, abdominal distension and constipation, it is often combined with dà huáng (Radix et Rhizoma Rhei) and zhǐ shí (Fructus Aurantii Immaturus).

- Administration and Dosage
  - 3–10 g, decocted in water for oral use.
  - The medicinal can also be prepared into a pill or powdered form.

- Precautions
  - This medicinal has a pungent and a bitter flavor and a warm and dry property, and can consume qi and fluid, so it should be used with caution for those who have qi deficiency and fluid consumption and for pregnant women.

cold and damp with aching joints and limbs. It is especially effective for *bi* due to damp. It is also used for swelling pain in the feet and knees, flaccidity, leukorrhagia with foul and turbid discharge, damp ulcers and eczema caused by damp invasion in the lower *jiao*; exterior syndromes due to external invasion of wind cold complicated by damp; night blindness, dry and painful eyes, blurred vision, and so on. *Hòu pò* (Cortex Magnoliae Officinalis) enters the lung and large intestine channels, and therefore is able to activate qi circulation, promote digestion and remove fullness. It is indicated for disharmony between the spleen and stomach with epigastric

and abdominal distension and fullness caused by damp obstruction, food stagnation, or qi stasis. *Hòu pò* (Cortex Magnoliae Officinalis) is capable of eliminating both food retention and damp obstruction. It can also dry damp to eliminate phlegm, descend counterflow of qi to relieve asthma, and is indicated for cough with dyspnea due to phlegm-fluids, counterflow qi with excessive sputum; seven-emotions binding depression, phlegm and qi obstructed together, and plum pit qi causing a feeling of something blocking in the throat so that one cannot swallow and sound cannot come out.

⑤ *Shā rén* (砂仁, Fructus Amomi, Villous Amomum Fruit) ★★

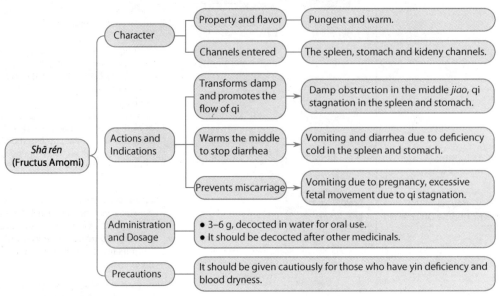

Character
- Property and flavor — Pungent and warm.
- Channels entered — The spleen, stomach and kideny channels.

Shā rén (Fructus Amomi)

Actions and Indications
- Transforms damp and promotes the flow of qi — Damp obstruction in the middle *jiao*, qi stagnation in the spleen and stomach.
- Warms the middle to stop diarrhea — Vomiting and diarrhea due to deficiency cold in the spleen and stomach.
- Prevents miscarriage — Vomiting due to pregnancy, excessive fetal movement due to qi stagnation.

Administration and Dosage
- 3–6 g, decocted in water for oral use.
- It should be decocted after other medicinals.

Precautions — It should be given cautiously for those who have yin deficiency and blood dryness.

⑥ *Bái dòu kòu* (白豆蔻, Fructus Amomi Kravanh, Round Cardamon) ★★

Both *shā rén* (Fructus Amomi) and *bái dòu kòu* (Fructus Amomi Kravanh) are pungent aromatic and warm, and enter the spleen and stomach channels in order to transform damp, promote qi circulation and warm the middle to relieve vomiting. They are often used together and are indicated for epigastric and abdominal distending pain, poor appetite, vomiting and diarrhea caused by damp obstruction in the middle *jiao*, qi stagnation in the spleen and stomach, and deficient cold in the spleen and stomach. They are especially suitable for cold and damp in the spleen and stomach with qi stagnation. *Shā rén* (Fructus Amomi) mainly acts in the middle and lower *jiao* to warm the spleen to relieve diarrhea as well as promote qi circulation to prevent miscarriage. Therefore it is often used for spleen cold with diarrhea, vomiting due to pregnancy, and excessive fetal movement due to qi stagnation. *Bái dòu kòu* (Fructus Amomi Kravanh) mainly acts in the upper and middle *jiao* to remove qi stagnation in the lung and spleen, and therefore can warm the stomach to relieve vomiting. It is often used for vomiting

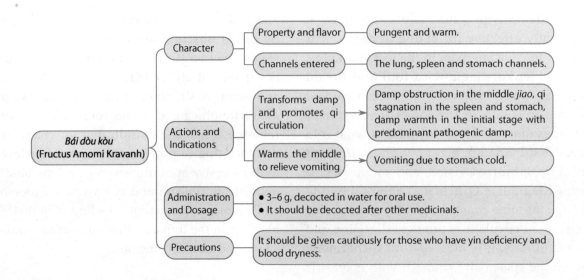

Character
- Property and flavor — Pungent and warm.
- Channels entered — The lung, spleen and stomach channels.

Bái dòu kòu (Fructus Amomi Kravanh)

Actions and Indications
- Transforms damp and promotes qi circulation → Damp obstruction in the middle *jiao*, qi stagnation in the spleen and stomach, damp warmth in the initial stage with predominant pathogenic damp.
- Warms the middle to relieve vomiting → Vomiting due to stomach cold.

Administration and Dosage
- 3–6 g, decocted in water for oral use.
- It should be decocted after other medicinals.

Precautions — It should be given cautiously for those who have yin deficiency and blood dryness.

caused by stomach cold, damp obstruction and qi stagnation, and damp warmth in the initial stage with chest distension, no appetite and a turbid and greasy tongue coating.

⑦ *Cǎo dòu kòu* (草豆蔻, Semen Alpiniae Katsumadai, Katsumade Galangal Seed)

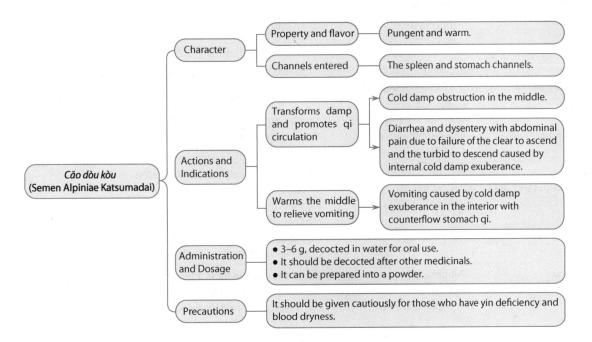

⑧ *Cǎo guǒ* (草果, Fructus Tsaoko, Tsaoko Fruit) ★

Both *cǎo dòu kòu* (Semen Alpiniae Katsumadai) and *cǎo guǒ* (Fructus Tsaoko) are pungent and warm, and enter the spleen and stomach channels to dry damp and warm the middle to dispel cold. They are indicated for epigastric and abdominal distending pain, vomiting, diarrhea, and a turbid and greasy tongue coating caused by cold damp obstruction in the middle. *Cǎo dòu kòu* (Semen Alpiniae Katsumadai) can warm the stomach to relieve vomiting and can be used as a substitute for *bái dòu kòu* (Fructus Amomi Kravanh) to treat vomiting of a stomach-cold type. It is capable of activating qi circulation, and is used for qi stagnation in the spleen and stomach. *Cǎo guǒ* (Fructus Tsaoko) has a particular odor and an acrid taste. It has a drastic action and is superior to *cǎo dòu kòu* (Semen Alpiniae Katsumadai) in the

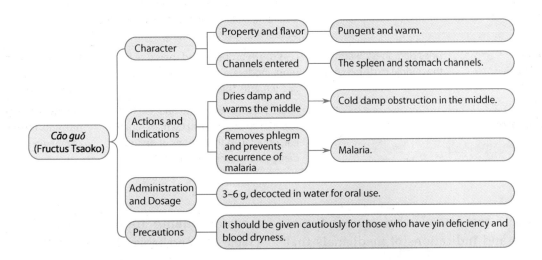

actions of drying damp and warming the middle. It can remove phlegm and prevent the recurrence of malaria. Therefore, it is used for malaria of a cold damp exuberance type, and malignant malaria caused by epidemic pathogenic factors from mountains, or foul and turbid pathogenic damp.

Actions of medicinals that transform damp are summarized in the following table (Table 12-1):

Table 12-1: Summary of Medicinals that Transform Damp:

Medicinal	Action in Common	Individual Character	
		Characteristic Actions	**Other Actions**
Huò xiāng (Herba Agastachis)	Transforms damp, clears away summer-heat	Slightly warm, transforms damp without consuming body fluids, releases the exterior moderately	Relieves vomiting
Pèi lán (Herba Eupatorii)		Inferior to huò xiāng (Herba Agastachis) in releasing the exterior, is effective for transforming internal damp and removing foul and turbid substances, especially indicated for damp-warmth in the spleen with heat.	
Cāng zhú (Rhizoma Atractylodis)	Pungent, bitter, warm and dry, dries damp to manipulate the spleen	Warm and dry, the most important medicinal in drying damp to invigorate the spleen. Indicated for spleen damp exuberance manifesting as phlegmatic fluid, edema and leukorrhagia.	Dispels wind and cold, brightens the eyes
Hòu pò (Cortex Magnoliae Officinalis)		Descends counterflow qi flow, removes food stagnation and fullness. Indicated for disharmony between the spleen and stomach with epigastric and abdominal distension and fullness caused by damp obstruction, food retention or qi stagnation	Eliminates phlegm to relieve asthma
Shā rén (Fructus Amomi)	Transforms damp, promotes qi circulation, warms the middle to relieve vomiting	It mainly acts in the middle and lower jiao to relieve qi stagnation in the spleen and stomach, and is effective for warming the spleen to relieve diarrhea.	Prevents miscarriage
Bái dòu kòu (Fructus Amomi Kravanh)		It mainly acts in the upper and middle jiao to relieve qi stagnation in the spleen and lung, and is effective for warming the stomach to relieve vomiting	
Cǎo dòu kòu (Semen Alpiniae Katsumadai)	Dries dampness, warms the middle to dispel cold	Less dry in property and therefore has a more moderate action compared to cǎo guǒ (Fructus Tsaoko)	Warms the stomach to relieve vomiting, promotes qi circulation
Cǎo guǒ (Fructus Tsaoko)		It has a distinct odor and an acrid taste, is superior to cǎo dòu kòu (Semen Alpiniae Katsumadai) in the actions of drying damp and warming the middle.	Removes phlegm and prevents the recurrence of malaria

Tables to test your herbal knowledge of the actions and indications of medicinals that transform damp are demonstrated as follows (Table 12-2 and Table 12-3, see p.189):

Table 12-2: Test your Herbal Knowledge of the Actions of Medicinals that Transform Damp:

Actions / Medicinal	Huò xiāng	Pèi lán	Cāng zhú	Hòu pò	Shā rén	Bái dòu kòu	Cǎo dòu kòu	Cǎo guǒ
Transforms damp								
Removes food retention								
Relieves vomiting								
Dries dampness								
Relieves asthma								
Expels wind damp								
Brightens the eyes								
Promotes qi circulation								
Clears summer-heat								
Invigorates the spleen								
Soothes the chest								
Warms the middle								
Relieves diarrhea								
Prevents miscarriage								
Dispels cold								
Removes phlegm and prevents the recurrence of malaria								

Table 12-3: Test your Herbal Knowledge of the Indications of Medicinals that Transform Damp:

Indications / Medicinal	Huò xiāng	Pèi lán	Cāng zhú	Hòu pò	Shā rén	Bái dòu kòu	Cǎo dòu kòu	Cǎo guǒ
Damp obstruction in the middle *jiao*								
Summer-heat damp								
Damp warm the in the early stages								
Vomiting due to pregnancy								
Bi due to wind damp								
External invasion by wind cold complicated by pathogenic damp								
Night blindness								
Cold congealing with damp								
Cough with dyspnea due to phlegm-fluids								
Qi stagnation in the spleen and stomach								
Vomiting and diarrhea due to deficiency cold in the spleen and stomach								
Vomiting								
Excessive fetal movement due to qi stagnation								
Cold damp obstruction in the middle								
Food retention in the stomach and large intestine								
Chronic diarrhea due to spleen deficiency								
Malaria								

Chapter 13
Medicinals that Promote Water Flow and Drain Damp

Concept

Medicinals whose principal effect is to drain damp through urination and remove water retention in the interior are called medicinals that promote water flow and drain damp.

Character and Actions

Most medicinals in this chapter are sweet, bland or bitter in flavor, and enter the bladder and small intestine channels. They mainly have a downward action, and therefore have the actions of promoting water flow to reduce edema, inducing diuresis to relieve stranguria and draining damp to relieve jaundice.

Indications

These herbs are indicated for various diseases caused by water retention, such as dysuria, edema, diarrhea, phlegm-fluids, stranguria, jaundice, damp ulcers, leukorrhagia and damp-warmth.

Combinations

Medicinals for promoting water flow and draining damp should be used in combination with medicinals of other types according to different pathological conditions. For edema accompanied by an exterior syndrome, combine with medicinals for diffusing the lung and inducing sweating. For protracted edema associated with yang deficiency of the spleen and kidney, combine with medicinals for warming and nourishing the spleen and kidney.

For cases of heat mingling with damp, it is better to combine with medicinals that have the action of clearing heat, while for cold and damp, it is best to combine with medicinals for warming the interior and dispelling cold. In cases of hematuria due to impairment of blood by heat, combine with medicinals for cooling blood and stopping bleeding. For cases with diarrhea, phlegm-fluids, damp warmth and jaundice, combine with medicinals for invigorating the spleen, transforming damp, or clearing heat and drying damp. In addition, qi circulation can promote water flow, while qi stagnation leads to water retention. Therefore, medicinals for promoting water flow and draining damp are often used in combination with medicinals for activating qi circulation to enhance their therapeutic effects.

Precautions

Medicinals for promoting water flow and draining damp can cause impairment to the body fluids. Therefore they should be given cautiously or prohibited entirely for those who have yin and fluid deficiency, or in cases of kidney deficiency with seminal emission and enuresis. Some of the medicinals that have a comparatively strong diuretic action should be used with caution in pregnant women.

Classification

According to their action characteristics and different applications in the clinic, these medicinals can be divided into three categories: Medicinals for promoting water flow to reduce edema, medicinals for inducing diuresis to relieve stranguria and medicinals for draining damp to relieve jaundice.

Section 1 Medicinals that Promote Water Flow to Reduce Edema

Medicinals in this section are mostly sweet and bland in flavor, and neutral or slightly cold in property. The bland flavor can drain damp, so medicinals with such a nature are capable of dispersing and abating edema through urination. They are indicated for water retention in the interior of the body, manifesting as edema, dysuria, diarrhea and phlegm-fluids.

① *Fú líng* (茯苓, Poria, Indian Bread) ★ ★ ★

Addition: 1. *Fú líng pí* (茯苓皮, **Cutis Poriae, Indian Bread Exodermis)** promotes water flow

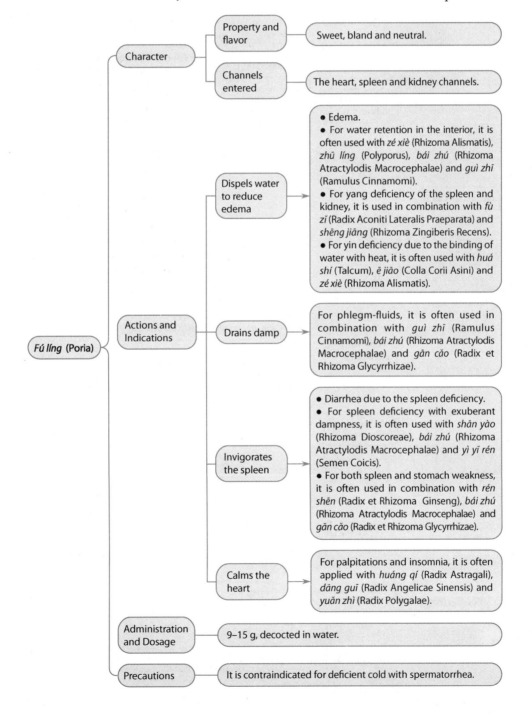

Character
- Property and flavor → Sweet, bland and neutral.
- Channels entered → The heart, spleen and kidney channels.

Fú líng (Poria)

Actions and Indications
- Dispels water to reduce edema →
  - Edema.
  - For water retention in the interior, it is often used with *zé xiè* (Rhizoma Alismatis), *zhū líng* (Polyporus), *bái zhú* (Rhizoma Atractylodis Macrocephalae) and *guì zhī* (Ramulus Cinnamomi).
  - For yang deficiency of the spleen and kidney, it is used in combination with *fù zǐ* (Radix Aconiti Lateralis Praeparata) and *shēng jiāng* (Rhizoma Zingiberis Recens).
  - For yin deficiency due to the binding of water with heat, it is often used with *huá shí* (Talcum), *ē jiāo* (Colla Corii Asini) and *zé xiè* (Rhizoma Alismatis).
- Drains damp → For phlegm-fluids, it is often used in combination with *guì zhī* (Ramulus Cinnamomi), *bái zhú* (Rhizoma Atractylodis Macrocephalae) and *gān cǎo* (Radix et Rhizoma Glycyrrhizae).
- Invigorates the spleen →
  - Diarrhea due to the spleen deficiency.
  - For spleen deficiency with exuberant dampness, it is often used with *shān yào* (Rhizoma Dioscoreae), *bái zhú* (Rhizoma Atractylodis Macrocephalae) and *yì yǐ rén* (Semen Coicis).
  - For both spleen and stomach weakness, it is often used in combination with *rén shēn* (Radix et Rhizoma Ginseng), *bái zhú* (Rhizoma Atractylodis Macrocephalae) and *gān cǎo* (Radix et Rhizoma Glycyrrhizae).
- Calms the heart → For palpitations and insomnia, it is often applied with *huáng qí* (Radix Astragali), *dāng guī* (Radix Angelicae Sinensis) and *yuǎn zhì* (Radix Polygalae).

Administration and Dosage → 9–15 g, decocted in water.

Precautions → It is contraindicated for deficient cold with spermatorrhea.

to reduce edema. It is effective for transforming water retention under the skin, and is indicated for edema.

2. *Fú shén* (茯神, **Sclerotium Poriae Pararadicis, Indian Bread with Hostwood)** calms the heart to tranquilize the mind. It is especially effective for treating restlessness, palpitations, and forgetfulness.

② *Yì yǐ rén* (薏苡仁, Semen Coicis, Coix Seed) ★ ★ ★

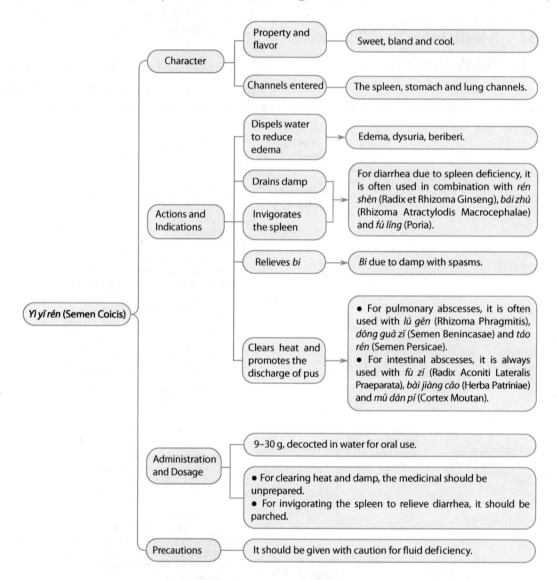

③ *Zhū líng* (猪苓, Polyporus, Chuling) ★ ★

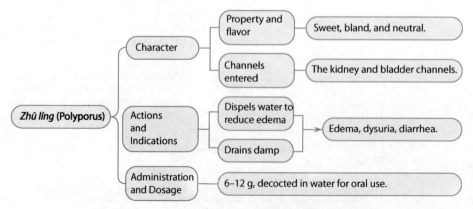

④ *Zé xiè* (泽泻, Rhizoma Alismatis, Oriental Waterplantain Rhizome) ★ ★ ★

Fú líng (Poria), *yì yǐ rén* (Semen Coicis), *zhū líng* (Polyporus) and *zé xiè* (Rhizoma Alismatis) are sweet and bland in flavor, and can promote water flow to reduce edema and drain damp. They are indicated for edema, dysuria, diarrhea, leukorrhagia and stranguria. *Fú líng* (Poria) and *yì yǐ rén* (Semen Coicis) can promote water flow to reduce edema and drain damp as well as invigorate the spleen. Their actions are characterized by drainage with tonification. They are especially suitable for spleen deficiency with damp exuberance. *Fú líng* (Poria) is neutral in property with a moderate action, and can drain water retention without impairing the right qi, and strengthen the body's resistance without drastically tonifying. It is considered as an essential medicinal for promoting water flow and draining damp. Its actions in promoting water flow, draining damp and invigorating the spleen are stronger than that of *yì yǐ rén* (Semen Coicis). It can be used for edema of various types if combined properly with other medicinals. It is also used for phlegm-fluids, manifesting as dizziness, palpitations, and cough (from water retention due to spleen deficiency). It is capable of calming the heart to tranquilize the mind, and therefore is used to treat deficiency syndromes manifesting with palpitations, insomnia and amnesia; and qi deficiency in both the spleen and stomach with poor appetite, sluggish digestion, and lassitude. *Yì yǐ rén* (Semen Coicis), is slightly

cold, and can relieve *bi*, clear heat and promote the discharge of pus. It is often used for *bi* due to pathogenic wind, cold and damp with spasms and convulsions, especially of the damp type; damp-warmth in the initial stages or summer-heat damp in the qi level, manifesting with fever, aversion to cold, headache, chest oppression and heaviness of the body; pulmonary abscesses with chest pain, cough with purulent expectoration, and intestinal abscesses with abdominal pain. *Zhū líng* (Polyporus) is neutral in property. It has a strong action for draining damp and is mainly used for water retention. Modern research has shown that its grifola polysaccharide has the effect of resisting tumors and preventing hepatitis. *Zé xiè* (Rhizoma Alismatis) is cold in property, and has a similar action to *zhū líng* (Polyporus) in promoting water flow. It specializes in purging heat from both the kidney and the bladder, and especially heat in the lower *jiao*. It is also used for dizziness due to failure of the clear yang to ascend, with phlegm-fluids accumulation; seminal emissions, night sweating, and steaming bones with tidal fever caused by kidney yin deficiency with hyperactivity of kidney fire.

In addition, *fú líng* (Poria) comes from the sclerotium of *Poria cocos* (schw) Wolf, family Polyporaceae. *Fú líng pí* (Cutis Poriae) is the exodermis of the same plant, which is also effective for promoting water flow to reduce edema. The pink layer under the exodermis is *chì fú líng* (赤茯苓, Poria Rubra, Indian Bread

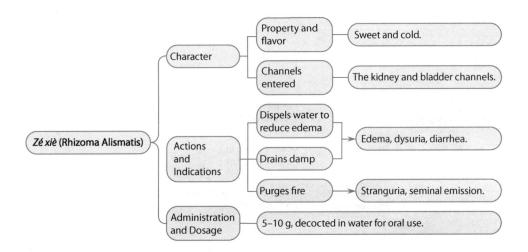

Pink Epidermis), which is effective for clearing and draining damp heat and is indicated for water retention of a heat type. The white part of the sclerotium is called *fú líng* (Poria), which can invigorate the spleen and drain damp, and is indicated for spleen deficiency with damp exuberance. Pieces containing pine root are known as *fú shén* (Sclerotium Poriae Pararadicis), and are also called *bào mù shén*. It is effective for calming the heart to tranquilize the mind and is used for restlessness, palpitations, and forgetfulness. The pine root is called *fú shén mù*

(Radix Pini in Poria), which specializes in calming the liver to tranquilize the mind.

⑤ *Dōng guā pí* (冬瓜皮, Exocarpium Benincasae, Chinese Waxgourd Peel)

Addtion: *Dōng guā zǐ* (冬瓜子, **Semen Benincasae, Chinese Waxgourd Seed)** clears the lung to transform phlegm, drains damp and promotes the discharge of pus. It is indicated in cases of cough due to lung heat, pulmonary abscesses, intestinal abscesses, leukorrhagia, and stranguria with white turbid discharge.

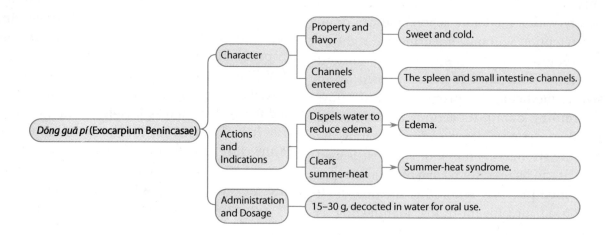

⑥ *Yù mǐ xū* (玉米须, Stigma Maydis, Stigmata Maydis) ★★★

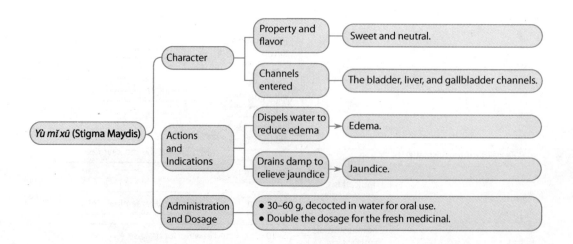

⑦ *Hú lu* (葫芦, Fructus Lagenariae, Bottle Gourd)

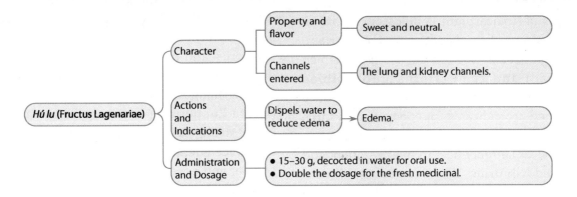

⑧ *Xiāng jiā pí* (香加皮, Cortex Periplocae, Chinese Silkvine Root-bark) ★

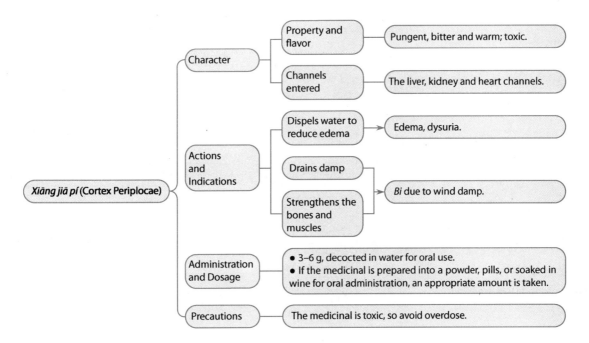

⑨ *Zhǐ jù zǐ* (枳椇子, Semen Hoveniae, Raisin Tree Seed)

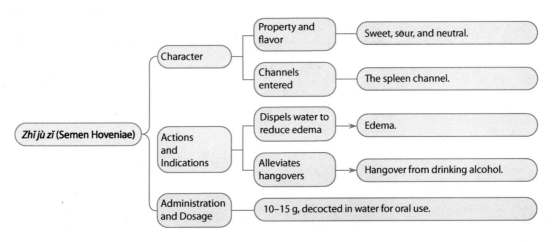

⑩ *Zé qī* (泽漆, Herba Euphoribiae Helioscopiae, Sun Euphorbia Herb)

Dōng guā pí (Exocarpium Benincasae), *yù mǐ xū* (Stigma Maydis), *hú lu* (Fructus Lagenariae), *xiāng jiā pí* (Cortex Periplocae), *zhǐ jù zǐ* (Semen Hoveniae) and *zé qī* (Herba Euphoribiae Helioscopiae) can promote water flow to reduce edema, and are indicated for edema and dysuria. *Dōng guā pí* (Exocarpium Benincasae) is cool, and can clear summer-heat to treat vexation, and scanty reddish urine. When combined with the right medicinals, *yù mǐ xū* (Stigma Maydis) can drain damp to relieve jaundice of both the yang and yin types. It is also used for scanty reddish urine and stranguria. *Hú lu* (Fructus Lagenariae) is neutral and cool, and is able to drain damp to

relieve jaundice. *Xiāng jiā pí* (Cortex Periplocae) is toxic, and it can strengthen the heart to induce diuresis in order to treat cardiogenic edema. In addition, it can expel wind damp, and strengthen the bones and muscles to treat *bi* due to wind damp. *Zhǐ jù zǐ* (Semen Hoveniae) is effective for treating hangovers from drinking alcohol. *Zé qī* (Herba Euphoribiae Helioscopiae) is toxic, and has a strong action for promoting water flow to reduce edema. It is indicated for abdominal edema, and edema of the face and limbs. It can also transform phlegm to relieve cough, detoxify, and remove stasis, and is used for cough with dyspnea due to phlegm-fluids, scrofula, tinea, and ulcers with itching.

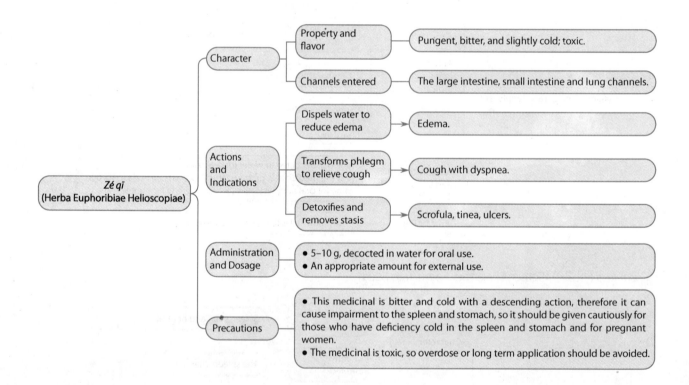

⑪ *Lóu gū* (蝼蛄, Gryllotalpa, Chinese Mole Cricket)

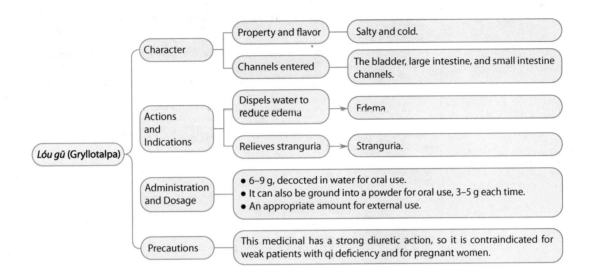

⑫ *Jì cài* (荠菜, Herba Capsellae, Shepherdspurse Herb)

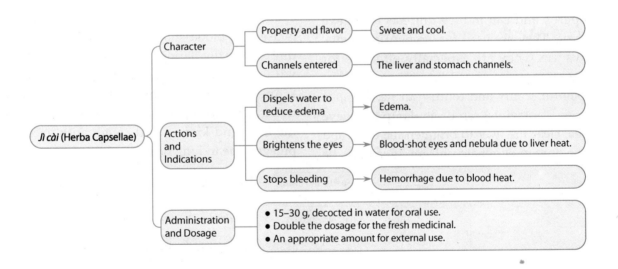

Section 2 Medicinals that Induce Diuresis to Relieve Stranguria

Medicinals of this kind are usually bitter, sweet or bland in flavor and cold in property. The bitter flavor acts to descend and purge, while the cold flavor can clear heat. Medicinals with such characters mainly act in the lower *jiao* to clear damp heat, and have the principal effects of inducing diuresis to relieve stranguria. They are indicated for stranguria caused by pathogenic heat, hematuria, urolithiasis or chyluria.

① *Chē qián zǐ* (车前子, Semen Plantaginis, Plantain Seed) ★★★

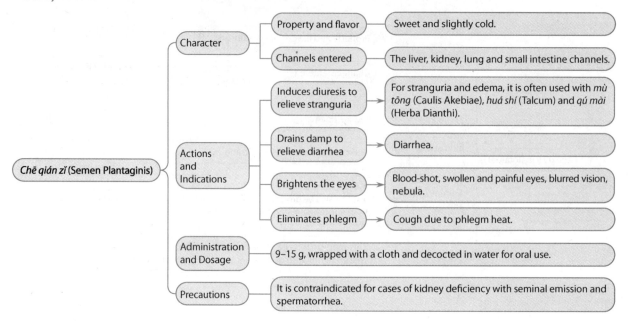

② *Huá shí* (滑石, Talcum, Talc) ★★

Both *chē qián zǐ* (Semen Plantaginis) and *huá shí* (Talcum) are sweet in flavor and cold or cool in property, and can induce diuresis to relieve stranguria. They are used for stranguria, edema, and dysuria. They are especially effective for treating stranguria caused by pathogenic heat with painful scanty and reddish urine. *Chē qián zǐ* (Semen Plantaginis) can drain damp to relieve diarrhea, clear the liver to brighten the eyes, and clear the lung to eliminate phlegm. It can also be used to treat diarrhea due to summer-heat damp. It can induce diuresis to relieve diarrhea, and therefore is suitable for dysuria caused by damp exuberance in the large intestine with diarrhea. It is used for blood-shot, swollen and painful eyes due to liver fire flaring upwards. When combined with medicinals for nourishing the liver and kidney to brighten the eyes, it is capable of treating blurred eyes due to yin deficiency in both the liver and kidney, and cough with excessive phlegm due to lung heat. In addition, *chē qián cǎo*

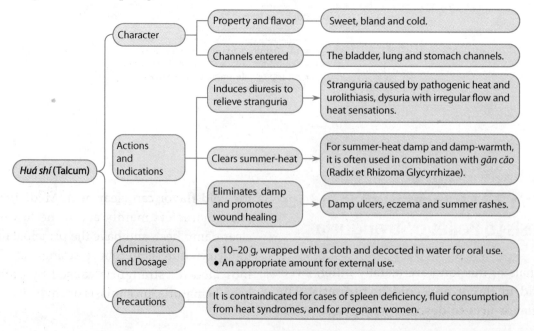

(车前草, Herba Plantaginis, Plantain Herb) is the whole herb of *Plantago asiatica* L. or *P. depressa* Willa., of the family Plantaginaceae. It has the same actions and indications as *chē qián zǐ* (Semen Plantaginis), and can clear heat and detoxify to treat suppurating infections on the surface of the body. *Huá shí* (Talcum) can clear summer-heat, eliminate damp and promote wound healing. It is used for vexation and thirst caused by summer-

heat; headache, aversion to cold, heaviness of the body, and chest oppression due to damp-warmth or summer-heat damp in the early stage; diarrhea and dysentery due to damp heat; eczema, damp ulcers, and prickly heat.

③ *Guān mù tōng* (关木通, Caulis Aristolochiae Manshuriensis, Manchurian Dutchmanspipe Stem) ★★

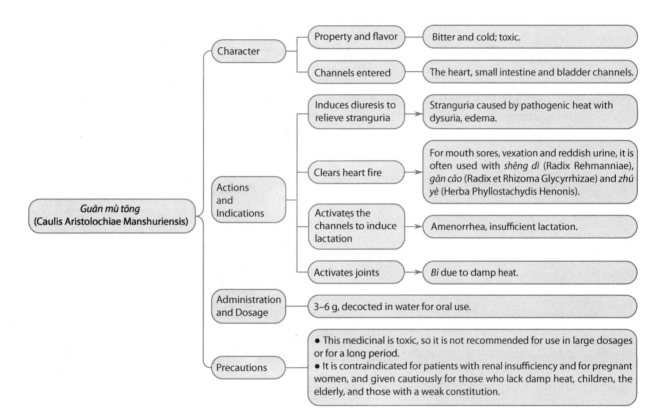

Addition: ***Chuān mù tōng* (川木通, Caulis Clematidis Armandii, Armand Clematia Stem)** has similar actions to *guān mù tōng* (Caulis Aristolochiae Manshuriensis) but with fewer side effects.

④ *Tōng cǎo* (通草, Medulla Tetrapanacis, Ricepaperplant Pith)

Guān mù tōng (Caulis Aristolochiae Manshuriensis) and *tōng cǎo* (Medulla Tetrapanacis) are cold or cool in property, and can clear heat and induce diuresis to relieve stranguria as well as induce lactation. The two medicinals are used together to treat stranguria of a heat type with painful urination, scanty and

reddish urine, edema, beriberi, and stasis of milk in the mammary glands after delivery. *Guān mù tōng* (Caulis Aristolochiae Manshuriensis) is bitter and cold with a strong heat-purging action, and is effective for clearing and purging fire in both the heart and small intestine through urination. It is used for mouth sores due to heart fire flaring upwards, or vexation and reddish urine caused by heart fire invading the small intestine. It can also enter the *xue* level to activate the channels, vessels and joints, as well as to induce lactation, and is used for amenorrhea due to blood stagnation and *bi* due to damp heat. *Tōng cǎo* (Medulla Tetrapanacis) is sweet and bland in flavor and slightly cold in

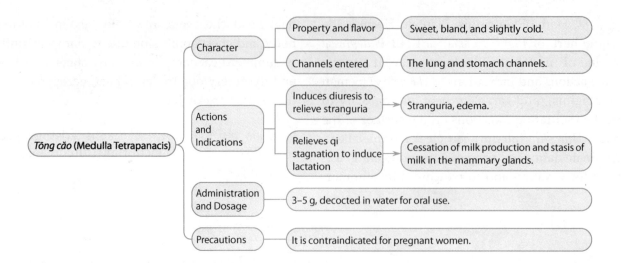

property, and therefore has moderate purgative and descending actions. It is effective for clearing lung heat, and can enter the qi level to remove qi stagnation in order to induce lactation. It is also used for damp warmth in the early stage with fever and chest oppression.

⑤ *Qú mài* (瞿麦, Herba Dianthi, Lilac Pink Herb) ★

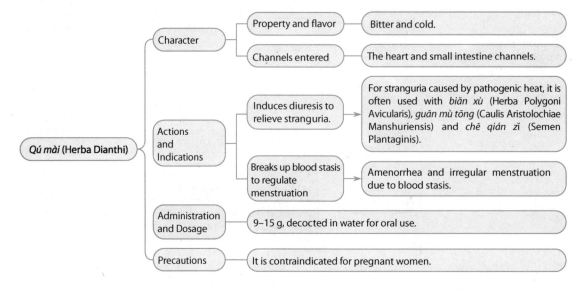

⑥ *Biǎn xù* (萹蓄, Herba Polygoni Avicularis, Knotgrass)

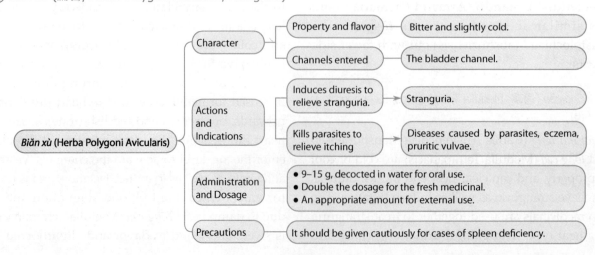

⑦ *Dì fū zǐ* (地肤子, Fructus Kochiae, Belvedere Fruit) ★

Biǎn xù (Herba Polygoni Avicularis) and *dì fū zǐ* (Fructus Kochiae) are bitter in flavor and cold or cool in property, and can clear heat and induce diuresis to relieve stranguria, and kill parasites to relieve itching. They are used in combination for stranguria caused by pathogenic heat with dysuria, scanty and reddish urine, stranguria due to hematuria or urolithiasis and skin diseases such as eczema, damp ulcers, pruritic vulvae, and general itching. *Biǎn xù* (Herba Polygoni Avicularis) has a strong action for inducing diuresis to relieve stranguria and is frequently used for this. It can also treat abdominal pain due to the accumulation of parasites. *Dì fū zǐ* (Fructus Kochiae) is effective for killing parasites to relieve itching, and is used mostly for various skin diseases.

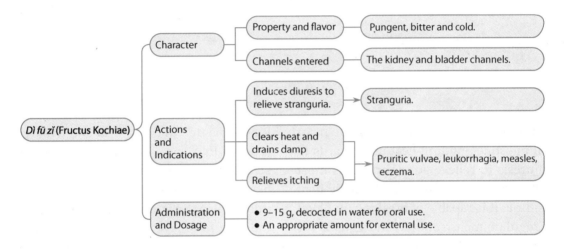

⑧ *Hǎi jīn shā* (海金沙, Spora Lygodii, Japanese Climbing Fern Spore) ★

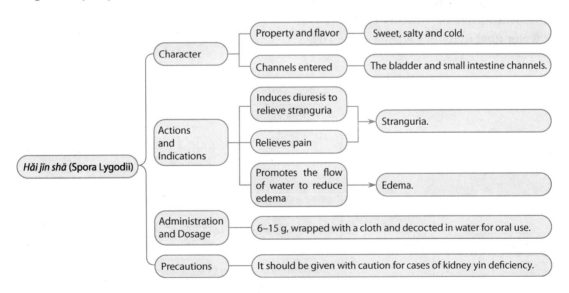

⑨ *Shí wéi* (石韦, Folium Pyrrosiae, Shearer's Pyrrosia Leaf) ★★

Qú mài (Herba Dianthi), *hǎi jīn shā* (Spora Lygodii) and *shí wéi* (Folium Pyrrosiae) are cold or cool in property, and can induce diuresis to relieve stranguria. They are indicated for stranguria caused by pathogenic heat, urolithiasis, or hematuria and dysuria, and are always used in combination.

Qú mài (Herba Dianthi) has a bitter flavor and

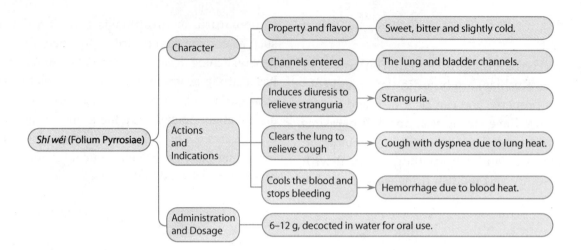

cold property and can clear fire in both the heart and small intestine, guiding heat downwards to induce diuresis to relieve stranguria. It is most suitable for stranguria due to pathogenic heat and hematuria. It is capable of breaking up blood stasis to regulate menstruation, and is used for amenorrhea and irregular menstruation caused by blood heat and stasis.

Hǎi jīn shā (Spora Lygodii) specializes in relieving pain in the urinary tract, and is effective in treating stranguria of various types. It can promote water flow to reduce edema, and is used for edema due to damp heat and dysuria. *Shí wéi* (Folium Pyrrosiae) can induce diuresis to relieve stranguria as well as cool the blood and stop bleeding; therefore it is suitable to treat stranguria due to hematuria. In addition, it is able to clear the lung to relieve cough, and is used for cough with dyspnea due to lung heat, and hemorrhage due to blood heat.

⑩ *Dōng kuí zǐ* (冬葵子, Fructus Malvae, Cluster Mallow Seed)

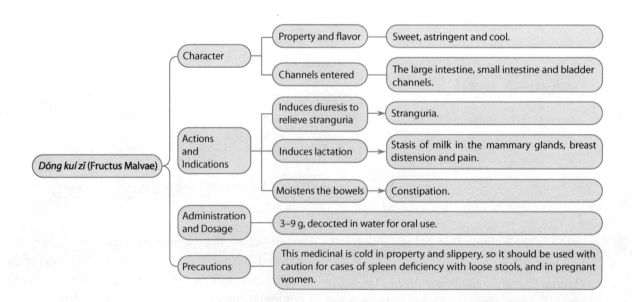

⑪ *Dēng xīn cǎo* (灯心草, Medulla Junci, Juncus)

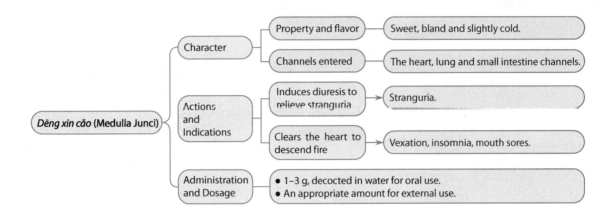

⑫ *Bì xiè* (萆薢, Rhizoma Dioscoreae Hypoglaucae, Hypoglaucous Collett Yam Rhizome) ★

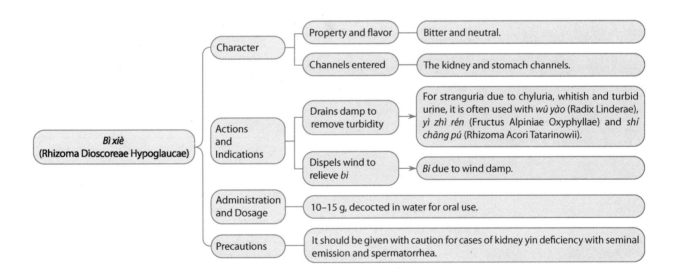

Section 3   Medicinals that Drain Damp to Relieve Jaundice

Medicinals in this section are mostly bitter in flavor and cold in property, and mainly enter the spleen, stomach, liver and gallbladder channels.

The bitter flavor and cold property have the actions of clearing and purging damp heat. Therefore medicinals with these characters have the principal action of draining damp to relieve jaundice, and are mainly used for jaundice of a damp heat type, manifesting as yellow eyes and skin, and reddish urine.

① *Yīn chén* (茵陈, Herba Artemisiae Scopariae, Virgate Wormwood Herb) ★ ★ ★

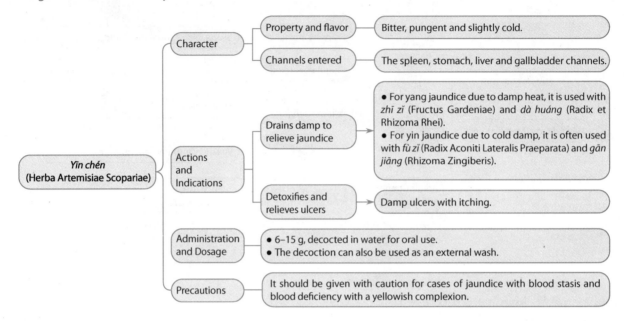

② *Jīn qián cǎo* (金钱草, Herba Lysimachiae, Christina Loosestrife) ★ ★ ★

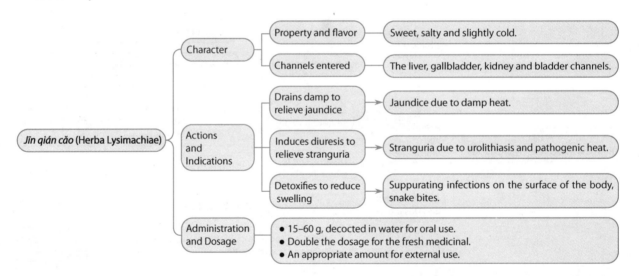

③ *Hǔ zhàng* (虎杖, Rhizoma Polygoni Cuspidati, Giant Knotweed Rhizome) ★ ★ ★

Both *hǔ zhàng* (Rhizoma Polygoni Cuspidati) and *dà huáng* (Radix et Rhizoma Rhei) belong to the family Polygonaceae. They are bitter in flavor and cold in property, and can invigorate blood to remove stasis, clear and purge damp heat, promote defecation, clear heat, and detoxify. The two medicinals are used in combination for blood stasis manifesting as amenorrhea, dysmenorrhea, postpartum abdominal pain, and injuries due to trauma; constipation due to heat accumulation in the interior; jaundice of damp heat type, stranguria due to chyluria; suppurating infections on the surface of the body, and scalds. Differences: *Hǔ zhàng* (Rhizoma Polygoni Cuspidati) has effective actions for activating the blood to relieve pain. It can transform phlegm to relieve cough in order to treat cough with excessive phlegm due to lung heat. It is also used for *bi* due to wind

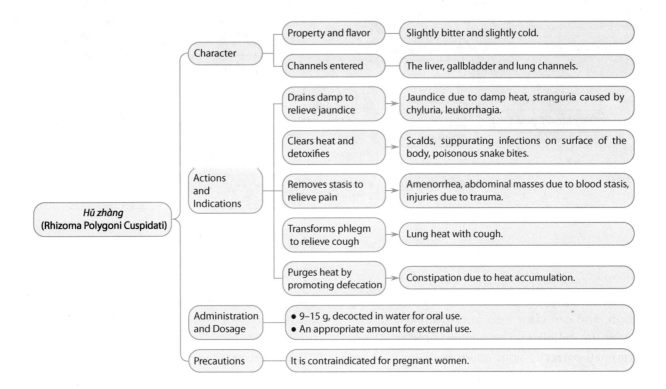

damp, poisonous snake bites, and leukorrhagia due to damp heat. *Dà huáng* (Radix et Rhizoma Rhei) has a strong action in purging downwards, and can be used for dry stools and constipation of various types if combined properly with other medicinals. It can also clear heat, purge fire, cool blood, and stop bleeding. It is often used for hematemesis, epistaxis due to blood heat, blood-shot eyes, swollen and painful gums and throat due to fire flaring upwards, and intestinal abscesses with abdominal pain.

④ *Dì ěr cǎo* (地耳草, Herba Hyperici Japonici, Japanese St. John's Wort Herb)

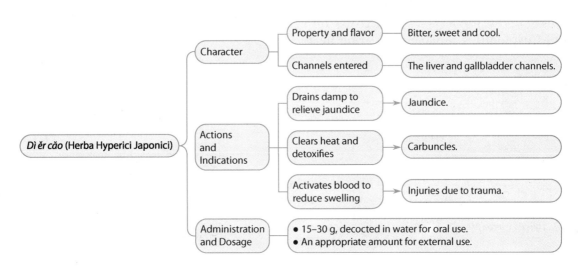

⑤ *Chuí pén cǎo* (垂盆草, Herba Sedi, Hanging Stonecrop)

Yīn chén (Herba Artemisiae Scopariae), *jīn qián cǎo* (Herba Lysimachiae), *hǔ zhàng* (Rhizoma Polygoni Cuspidati) and *chuí pén cǎo* (Herba Sedi) are cold or cool in property, and can drain damp to relieve jaundice. They are indicated for jaundice of a damp heat type. Differences: *Yīn chén* (Herba

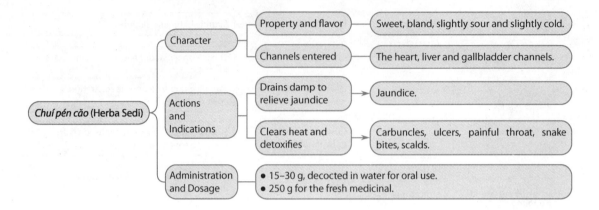

Artemisiae Scopariae) is bitter with a descending action, and can clear heat and drain damp, and benefit the gallbladder to relieve jaundice. When combined correctly with other medicinals, it can be used to treat jaundice of either a yin or yang type. It can also detoxify to treat ulcers, and is used for eczema, itching due to damp ulcers, and diseases caused by damp-warmth. *Jīn qián cǎo* (Herba Lysimachiae) is sweet, bland and slightly cold, and is effective for inducing diuresis to relieve stranguria, removing lithiasis, and detoxifying to reduce swelling. It is often used for stranguria caused by pathogenic heat, hematuria, or urolithiasis, gallstones, chronic ulcers, and poisonous snake bites. *Hǔ zhàng* (Rhizoma Polygoni Cuspidati) is capable of clearing heat,

detoxifying, activating blood to remove stasis and relieve pain, transforming phlegm to relieve cough, purging heat, and loosening the bowels. It is therefore used mainly for stranguria due to chyluria, leukorrhagia, scalds, suppurating infections on the surface of the body, poisonous snake bites; amenorrhea, abdominal hard masses and injuries due to blood stasis; and cough with lung heat and constipation due to heat accumulation. *Chuí pén cǎo* (Herba Sedi) can clear heat and detoxify to treat suppurating infections on the surface of the body, swollen and sore throat, poisonous snake bites and scalds.

⑥ *Jī gǔ cǎo* (鸡骨草, Herba Abri, Canton Love-pea Vine)

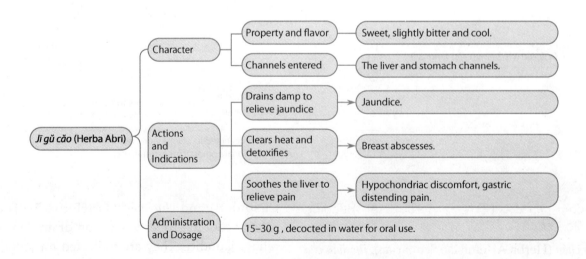

⑦ *Zhēn zhū cǎo* (珍珠草, Herba Phyllanthi Urinariae, Common Leafflower Herb)

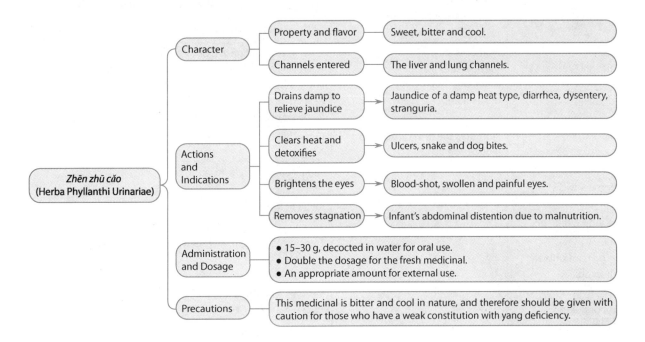

Actions of medicinals that promote the flow of water and drain damp are summarized in the following tables (Tables 13-1~13-3):

Table 13-1: Summary of Medicinals that Induce Diuresis to Subside Swelling:

Medicinal	Action in Common		Individual Character	
			Characteristic Actions	**Other Actions**
Fú líng (Poria)	Promotes the flow of water and drains damp	Invigorates the spleen, characterized by simultaneous drainage with tonification, suitable for spleen deficiency with damp exuberance	It has a neutral property and moderate action, it can promote the flow of water without impairment of the right qi, and strengthen the body's resistance without strong tonification. It is regarded as the most important medicinal in this chapter. It has a stronger action in promoting the flow of water and draining damp than *yì yǐ rén* (Semen Coicis)	Calms the heart to tranquilize the mind
Yì yǐ rén (Semen Coicis)			It has a moderate action in promoting the flow of water, draining damp and invigorating the spleen compared to *fú líng* (Poria)	Relieves *bi*, clears heat to promote the discharge of pus
Zhū líng (Polyporus)			It has singular and comparatively strong actions in promoting the flow of water and draining damp	

Table 13-1: Summary of Medicinals that Induce Diuresis to Subside Swelling:

continued

Medicinal	Action in Common		Individual Character	
			Characteristic Actions	Other Actions
Zé xiè (Rhizoma Alismatis)	Promotes the flow of water and drains damp		It has a similar action in promoting the flow of water to zhū líng, it purges heat, and is especially effective for purging heat in the kidney and bladder, suitable for damp heat in the lower jiao	
Dōng guā pí (Exocarpium Benincasae)	Promotes the flow of water to reduce edema		Clears heat and detoxifies	
Yù mǐ xū (Stigma Maydis)			Drains damp to relieve jaundice	
Zhǐ jù zǐ (Semen Hoveniae)			Relieves hangover from alcohol	
Zé qī (Herba Euphoribiae Helioscopiae)			Transforms phlegm to relieve cough, detoxifies to remove stasis	
Lóu gū (Gryllotalpa)			Relieves stranguria	
Jì cài (Herba Capsellae)			Brightens the eyes, stops bleeding	
Hú lu (Fructus Lagenariae)			Drains damp to relieve stranguria	
Xiāng jiā pí (Cortex Periplocae)			Expels wind damp, strengthens the bones and muscles	

Table 13-2: Summary of Medicinals that Induce Diuresis to Relieve Stranguria:

Medicinal	Action in Common		Individual Character	
			Characteristic Actions	Other Actions
Chē qián zǐ (Semen Plantaginis)	Induces diuresis to relieve stranguria		Drains damp to relieve diarrhea, clears the liver to brighten the eyes, clears the lung to transform phlegm	
Huá shí (Talcum)			Clears summer-heat, transforms damp to promote the healing of wounds	
Guān mù tōng (Caulis Aristolochiae Manshuriensis)		Induces lactation	It has a strong descending action and is good at purging heat, especially from the heart and small intestine. It also enters the xue level to activate the channels in order to induce lactation, and activates the vessels and joints.	
Tōng cǎo (Medulla Tetrapanacis)			It has a moderate action. It is effective for clearing lung heat, and enters the qi level to remove qi stagnation to induce lactation.	
Qú mài (Herba Dianthi)			Suitable for stranguria caused by pathogenic heat or hematuria	Breaks up blood stasis to activate the channels

Table 13-2: Summary of Medicinals that Induce Diuresis to Relieve Stranguria:

continued

Medicinal	Action in Common		Individual Character	
			Characteristic Actions	Other Actions
Biǎn xù (Herba Polygoni Avicularis)	Induces diuresis to relieve stranguria	Kills parasites to relieve itching	It has a strong action in inducing diuresis to relieve stranguria.	
Dì fū zǐ (Fructus Kochiae)			It has a strong action in killing parasites to relieve itching, so is often used for skin diseases	
Hǎi jīn shā (Fructus Kochiae)			Especially effective for relieving pain in the urinary tract. It is regarded as an essential medicinal for stranguria of various types	Promotes the flow of water to reduce edema
Shí wéi (Folium Pyrrosiae)			Cools blood, stops bleeding, effective for treating stranguria due to hematuria	Clears the lung to relieve cough
Dōng kuí zǐ (Fructus Malvae)				Induces lactation, moistens the bowels
Dēng xīn cǎo (Medulla Junci)				Clears the heart to descend fire
Bì xiè (Rhizoma Dioscoreae Hypoglaucae)			Effective for draining damp to ascend the clear and descend the turbid. It is considered an essential medicinal for stranguria due to chyluria.	Dispels wind to relieve *bi*

Table 13-3: Summary of Medicinals that Drain Damp to Relieve Jaundice:

Medicinal	Action in Common		Individual Character	
			Characteristic Actions	Other Actions
Yīn chén (Herba Artemisiae Scopariae)	Drains damp to relieve jaundice		It has a strong action in clearing damp heat, and benefiting the gallbladder to relieve jaundice of either a yang or yin type	Detoxifies to relieve ulcers
Jīn qián cǎo (Herba Lysimachiae)			It can induce diuresis to relieve stranguria, and is regarded as an important medicinal for treating lithiasis.	Detoxifies to relieve swellings
Hǔ zhàng (Rhizoma Polygoni Cuspidati)		Clears heat and detoxifies	Removes stasis to relieve pain, transforms phlegm to relieve cough, purges fire and promotes defecation	
Dì ěr cǎo (Herba Hyperici Japonici)			Activates blood to reduce swellings	
Chuí pén cǎo (Herba Sedi)			Relieves carbuncles	
Jī gǔ cǎo (Herba Abri)			Soothes the liver to relieve pain	
Zhēn zhū cǎo (Herba Phyllanthi Urinariae)			Brightens the eyes, removes stagnation	

Tables to test herbal knowledge of actions and indications of medicinals that promote the flow of water and drain damp are as follows (Tables 13-4~13-8):

Table 13-4: Test your Herbal Knowledge of the Actions of Medicinals that Promote the Flow of Water and Drain Damp (one):

Actions \ Medicinal	Fú líng	Yì yǐ rén	Zhū líng	Zé xiè	Dōng guā pí	Yù mǐ xū	Hú lu	Xiāng jiā pí	Zé qī
Promotes the flow of water and drains damp									
Invigorates the spleen									
Expels wind damp									
Removes water retention from the skin									
Calms the heart									
Removes stasis									
Clears heat and promotes the discharge of pus									
Purges heat									
Promotes the flow of water to reduce edema									
Drains damp to relieve jaundice									
Tranquilizes the mind									
Relieves pain									
Transforms phlegm to relieve cough									
Relieves bi									
Cools blood and stops bleeding									

Table 13-5: Test your Herbal Knowledge of the Actions of Medicinals that Promote the Flow of Water and Drain Damp (two):

Actions \ Medicinal	Chē qián zǐ	Chē qián cǎo	Huá shí	Guān mù tōng	Tōng cǎo	Qú mài	Biǎn xù	Dì fū zǐ	Hǎi jīn shā
Induces diuresis to relieve stranguria									
Removes qi stagnation									
Clears the liver to brighten the eyes									
Clears the lung to transform phlegm									
Kills parasites									
Clears summer-heat									
Removes damp to promote the healing of wounds									
Activates the channels									
Induces lactation									
Drains damp to relieve diarrhea									
Clears heat and drains damp									
Activates blood									
Clears heat and detoxifies									
Alleviates itching									

Table 13-6: Test your Herbal Knowledge of the Actions of Medicinals that Promote
the Flow of Water and Drain Damp (three):

Actions \ Medicinal	Shí wéi	Dōng kuí zǐ	Dēng xīn cǎo	Bì xiè	Yīn chén	Jīn qián cǎo	Hǔ zhàng	Chuí pén cǎo	Dì ěr cǎo
Induces diuresis to relieve stranguria									
Clears the lung to relieve cough									
Detoxifies to reduce swellings									
Induces lactation									
Moistens the bowels to promote defecation									
Eliminates phlegm to relieve cough									
Drains damp									
Dispels wind damp									
Clears heat damp									
Benefits the gallbladder to relieve jaundice									
Cools blood and stops bleeding									
Invigorates the blood to remove phlegm									
Clears the heart to relieve vexation									
Purges downwards									

Table 13-7: Test your Herbal Knowledge of the Indications of Medicinals that Promote
the Flow of Water and Drain Damp (one):

Indications \ Medicinal	Fú líng	Yì yǐ rén	Zhū líng	Zé xiè	Dōng guā pí	Xiāng jiā pí	Yīn chén	Jīn qián cǎo	Hǔ zhàng
Edema									
Various symptoms caused by spleen deficiency									
Damp warmth									
Bi due to damp, with spasms									
Pulmonary abscesses, intestinal abscesses									
Hemorrhage due to blood heat									
Stranguria caused by chyluria									
Damp heat in the lower jiao									
Palpitations, insomnia									
Cough with dyspnea due to phlegm-fluids									
Stranguria caused by pathogenic heat or urolithiasis									
Diarrhea and dysentery due to water retention									
Jaundice of a cold damp type									
Jaundice of a damp heat type									

Table 13-7: Test your Herbal Knowledge of the Indications of Medicinals that Promote the Flow of Water and Drain Damp (one):

continued

Indications \ Medicinal	Fú líng	Yì yǐ rén	Zhū líng	Zé xiè	Dōng guā pí	Xiāng jiā pí	Yīn chén	Jīn qián cǎo	Hǔ zhàng
Eczema, damp ulcers									
Chronic ulcers									
Burns and scalds									
Amenorrhea due to blood stasis									
Injuries due to trauma									
Cough due to the lung heat									
Poisonous snake bites									

Table 13-8: Test your Herbal Knowledge of the Indications of Medicinals that Promote the Flow of Water and Drain Damp (two)

Indications \ Medicinal	Chē qián zǐ	Chē qián cǎo	Huá shí	Guān mù tōng	Tōng cǎo	Qú mài	Biǎn xù	Dì fū zǐ	Hǎi jīn shā
Edema									
Diarrhea and dysentery due to damp heat									
Stranguria caused by pathogenic heat									
Blurred eyes									
Cough due to phlegm heat									
Bi due to damp heat									
Damp warmth									
Eczema and damp ulcers									
Blood-shot, dry and painful eyes									
Beriberi with swelling pain									
Amenorrhea, decreased lactation									
Carbuncles due to heat toxin									
Amenorrhea due to blood heat obstruction									
Abdominal pain due to the accumulation of parasites									

Chapter 14
Medicinals that Warm the Interior

Concept

Medicinals that have the action to warm the interior and dispel cold to relieve internal cold syndrome are known as interior-warming medicinals.

Character and Actions

Medicinals in this chapter are pungent in flavor, and warm or hot in property. The pungent flavor has the actions of dispelling, promoting qi and blood circulation and warming. Therefore medicinals that are pungent are capable of warming the interior and dispelling cold, warming the channels to relieve pain, and are indicated for excess cold in the interior. Some of these medicinals can also reinforce and revive yang in order to treat the syndrome of deficient cold or yang depletion.

Medicinals that enter different channels have different actions, e.g. medicinals that mainly enter the spleen and stomach channels can warm the middle and dispel cold to relieve pain, and are used for external pathogenic cold invasion in the spleen and stomach or deficient cold in the spleen and stomach, manifesting as cold pain in the epigastrium, vomiting, diarrhea, dysentery, and a pale tongue with a whitish coating. Medicinals that mainly enter the lung channel can warm the lung to dissolve fluid to treat phlegm-fluids due to lung cold, with symptoms such as cough with dyspnea, wheezing and phlegm, whitish and thin expectoration, and a pale-colored tongue with a whitish and slippery coating. Medicinals that mainly enter the liver channel have the actions of warming the liver and dispelling cold to relieve pain, and are indicated for pain in the lower abdomen, cold hernia with abdominal pain or *jueyin* headache caused by cold invasion in the liver channel. Medicinals mainly attributed to the kidney channel can warm the kidney to reinforce yang, and are used for deficiency of kidney yang, manifesting as impotence, cold uterus, cold pain in the loins and knees, frequent urination, spermatorrhea and enuresis. Medicinals that enter both the heart and kidney channels can warm yang to activate the vessels to treat yang deficiency in both the heart and kidney, manifesting as palpitations, aversion to cold, cold limbs, dysuria, puffiness of the limbs. They can also rescue depleted yang in order to resuscitate with symptoms such as aversion to cold, sweating with a diminished spirit, cold limbs, and an indistinct and faint pulse.

Combinations

Medicinals for warming the interior should be combined properly with other medicinals according to different syndromes. For external pathogenic cold invasion with unrelieved exterior syndrome of a cold type, they should be used in combination with pungent and warm medicinals for releasing the exterior. For qi stagnation and blood stasis due to cold congealing in the channels and collaterals, they should be combined with medicinals for promoting both qi and blood circulation. For cold damp obstruction in the interior, add aromatic medicinals for transforming damp or warm and dry medicinals for removing damp. For yang deficiency in both the spleen and kidney, combine with medicinals for warming and invigorating the spleen and kidney. For yang depletion with sinking qi, they should be used in combination with medicinals for strongly replenishing the original qi.

Precautions

Since medicinals of this category are mostly pungent, hot and dry in nature, and can consume yin, the dosage should be cut down during hot days or for patients with a fire hyperactivity constitution. They should not be used for heat syndromes with false-cold symptoms. They are prohibited for excessive heat, fire hyperactivity due to yin deficiency with fluid and blood deficiency. These medicinals should be used with caution with pregnant women.

① *Fù zǐ* (附子, Radix Aconiti Lateralis Praeparata, Aconite Root) ★★★

Fù zǐ (Radix Aconiti Lateralis Praeparata), *chuān wū* (Radix Aconiti) and *cǎo wū* (Radix Aconiti Kusnezoffii) are pungent, hot, and toxic. They

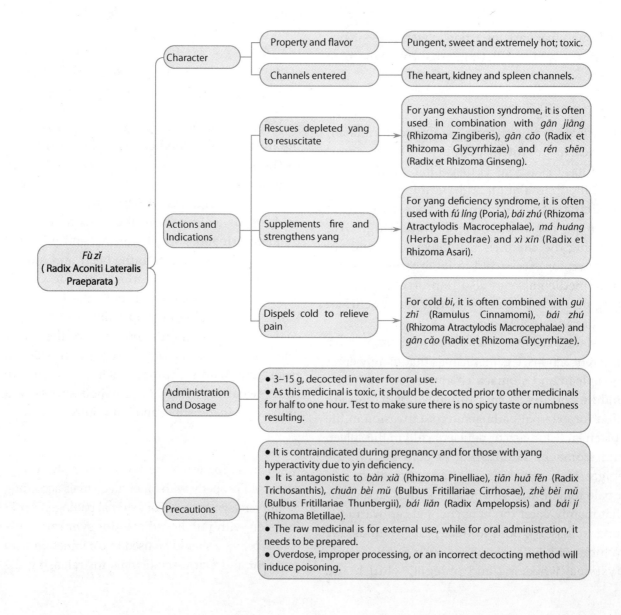

can dispel wind to relieve pain and are used for cold pain in the chest and abdomen, as well as for *bi* due to wind damp. However, the three medicinals have different actions because they are from different parts of the plant and of differing varieties. *Fù zǐ* (Radix Aconiti Lateralis Praeparata) is part of the buttercup family and is a perennial plant. It is the processed product of the daughter root of *Aconitum carmichaeli* Debx., of the family Raunuculaceae. It has actions of rescuing depleted yang, supplementing fire, and reinforcing yang. It is often used for yang depletion syndrome and deficiency of the kidney, spleen and heart yang. It can be used for the syndrome of yin hyperactivity with yang depletion. *Chuān wū* (Radix Aconiti) is from the root tuber of *Aconitum carmichaeli* Debx., of the family Raunuculaceae. It is effective for dispelling wind, cold and damp, and has stronger actions for warming channels to dispel cold and relieving *bi* than *fù zǐ* (Radix Aconiti Lateralis Praeparata). Therefore it is commonly used for *bi* due to cold damp, cold pain in chest and abdomen, injuries due to trauma, and pain. *Cǎo wū* (Radix Aconiti Kusnezoffii) is the tuber root of *Aconitum*

kusnezoffii Reichb., family Raunuculaceae. It has similar actions to *chuān wū* (Radix Aconiti) but with a stronger toxicity. The two medicinals are often used for mutual reinforcement.

② *Gān jiāng* (干姜, Rhizoma Zingiberis, Dried Ginger Rhizome) ★★★

Fù zǐ (Radix Aconiti Lateralis Praeparata) and *gān jiāng* (Rhizoma Zingiberis) are pungent and hot. They can warm the middle to dispel cold, and rescue depleted yang in order to resuscitate. They are used for cold exuberance in the interior, inactivity of spleen yang with epigastric and abdominal cold pain and loose stools; yang depletion with cold extremities, an indistinct and faint pulse due to yang deficiency in both the heart and kidney, and cold exuberance in the interior. *Fù zǐ* (Radix Aconiti Lateralis Praeparata) is toxic, with strong actions for warming the interior to dispel cold and rescuing depleted yang in order to resuscitate. It is considered the first choice for reviving yang in order to resuscitate. It can supplement fire so as to reinforce yang, and is used for impotence, cold pain in the waist and knees, seminal emission, spermatorrhea,

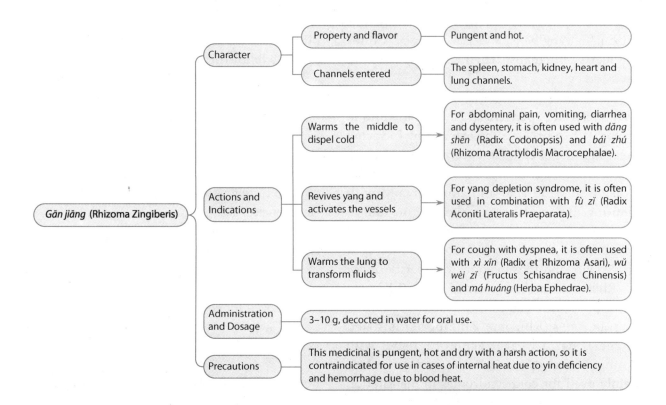

enuresis and frequent urination due to kidney yang deficiency and decline of *mingmen* fire; edema and dysuria due to water retention in the interior caused by yang deficiency in both the spleen and kidney; chest blockage with cardiac pain due to heart yang decline; external invasion of wind cold due to yang deficiency with aversion to cold, fever and a deep pulse; and *bi* due to cold damp. *Fù zǐ* (Radix Aconiti Lateralis Praeparata) is commonly used for cold syndromes in the interior in the middle and lower *jiao*. *Gān jiāng* (Rhizoma Zingiberis) is inferior to *fù zǐ* (Radix Aconiti Lateralis Praeparata) in warming the interior to dispel cold and reviving yang to activate the vessels, however, it can warm the lung to transform fluids. It is often used for cough with dyspnea due to cold fluids, chills and general feeling of coldness, a cold feeling in the back, and profuse and thin sputum. It is mainly used for cold syndromes in the upper and middle *jiao*.

Ginger is commonly used for cooking in daily life. According to different requirements in treatments, it is processed into various medicinals, which are known as "six ginger medicinals". They include *shēng jiāng* (Rhizoma Zingiberis Recens), *gān jiāng* (Rhizoma Zingiberis), *páo jiāng* (blast-fried Rhizoma Zingiberis), *wèi jiāng* (roasted Rhizoma Zingiberis), *shēng jiāng zhī* (Succus Rhizomatis Zingiberis) and *shēng jiāng pí* (Cortex Zingiberis Officinalis). Their characteristics are discussed below.

Shēng jiāng (Rhizoma Zingiberis Recens) is fresh ginger. It is pungent in flavor and warm in property. It can relieve the exterior by inducing sweating, dispel cold, and warm the middle to relieve vomiting. It is often used for external invasion of wind cold and stomach cold with vomiting. It can also warm the lung to relieve cough and detoxify, and therefore is used for cold syndromes in the spleen and stomach, lung cold with cough, and to counteract the toxicity of *bàn xià* (Rhizoma Pinelliae), *tiān nán xīng* (Rhizoma Arisaematis), fish, and crabs.

Gān jiāng (Rhizoma Zingiberis) is dried ginger. It has a weaker action to dispel with a pungent flavor, but is hotter and drier. It is mainly used for cold syndromes in the interior,

and can warm the middle, dispel cold, revive yang to activate the vessels, and warm the lung to dissolve fluids. It is indicated for cold syndrome in the spleen and stomach, yang depletion, and cough with dyspnea due to cold fluids. If *gān jiāng* (Rhizoma Zingiberis) is parched to the extent that the surface of the medicinal is black, then it is called *páo jiāng* (blast-fried Rhizoma Zingiberis).

Páo jiāng (Blast-fried Rhizoma Zingiberis) is able to warm the channels to stop bleeding, and is indicated for hemorrhage in the middle *jiao* of a deficiency cold type. It can also warm the middle to relieve pain and diarrhea, and is used for abdominal pain and diarrhea due to deficiency cold in the spleen and stomach. Ancient physicians regarded *shēng jiāng* (Rhizoma Zingiberis Recens) as being able to encourage movement but without guarding the middle, and *gān jiāng* (Rhizoma Zingiberis) as being able to encourage movement as well as guarding the middle; while *páo jiāng* (blast-fried Rhizoma Zingiberis) was regarded as only being able to guard the middle.

They regarded *wèi jiāng* (roasted Rhizoma Zingiberis) as being able to disperse to a lesser extent than *shēng jiāng* (Rhizoma Zingiberis Recens), and less dry compared to *gān jiāng* (Rhizoma Zingiberis), it has a similar character to *páo jiāng* (blast-fried Rhizoma Zingiberis), but has a more moderate action; it can warm the middle to relieve vomiting and diarrhea.

Shēng jiāng zhī (Succus Rhizomatis Zingiberis) is fresh ginger juice. It has similar actions to *shēng jiāng* (Rhizoma Zingiberis Recens), but has a stronger action in dispersing. It can remove phlegm to relieve vomiting, and is prescribed for emergencies.

Shēng jiāng pí (Cortex Zingiberis Officinalis) is ginger peel. It is pungent in flavor and cool in property. It can harmonize the spleen and promote the flow of water to reduce edema. It is mainly used for edema and dysuria.

③ *Ròu guì* (肉桂, Cortex Cinnamomi, Cassia Bark) ★★★

Both *fù zǐ* (Radix Aconiti Lateralis Praeparata)

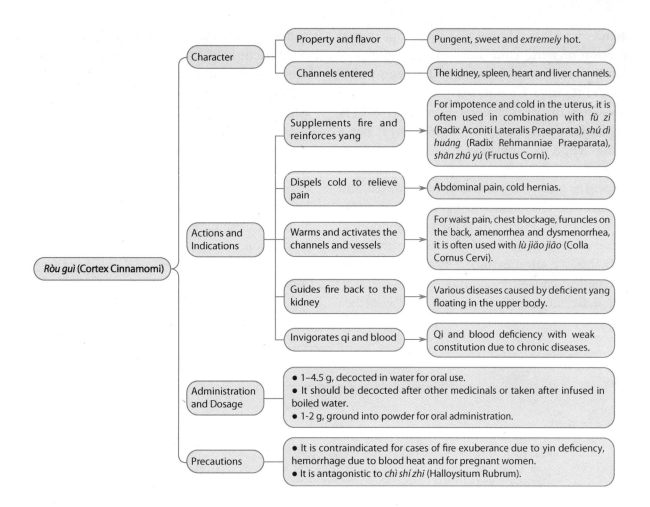

and *ròu guì* (Cortex Cinnamomi) are pungent and sweet in flavor, and extremely hot in property. They enter the heart, kidney and spleen channels and can supplement fire in order to reinforce yang, and dispel cold to relieve pain. The two medicinals have the actions of strengthening heart yang in the upper, warming spleen yang in the middle, and reinforcing kidney yang in the lower. Both medicinals can be used for kidney yang deficiency and declining fire at the *mingmen*, with manifestations such as impotence, cold in the uterus, cold pain in the waist and knees, seminal emission, spermatorrhea, enuresis and frequent urination; cold damp accumulation in the interior due to yang depletion of both the spleen and kidney, with symptoms such as epigastric and abdominal cold pain and loose stools; chest blockage with cardiac cold pain due to heart yang decline or inactivity of the chest yang; and *bi* due to cold damp. However, there are differences between the two medicinals. *Fù zǐ*

(Radix Aconiti Lateralis Praeparata) is pungent in flavor, hot and dry in property and has drastic actions and strong toxicity. It powerfully supplements fire so as to reinforce yang, and dispels cold to relieve pain. It can warm and nourish both the spleen and kidney as well as rescue the depleted yang in order to resuscitate. It can be used for all symptoms caused by yin cold hyperactivity in the interior with insufficient yang qi. Ancient physicians believed that *fù zǐ* (Radix Aconiti Lateralis Praeparata) could treat all diseases caused by excessive cold pathogens. It is the most important medicinal with actions of warming the interior to dispel cold and rescuing depleted yang in order to resuscitate. It is often used for syndromes of yang depletion manifesting as aversion to cold, sleeping curled up in a ball, sweating, low spirits, cold limbs, and an indistinct and faint pulse. It is also used for yang deficiency in both the spleen and kidney with water retention and symptoms such as edema of a yin cold type and dysuria; external invasion of wind cold due to yang deficiency with aversion to cold, fever, and a deep pulse. *Ròu guì* (Cortex Cinnamomi) is not toxic and also enters the liver channel. Compared with *fù zǐ* (Radix Aconiti Lateralis Praeparata) it has a milder action in supplementing fire to reinforce yang and dispelling cold to relieve pain. It can warm and nourish the kidney, warm and activate the channels and vessels, and guide fire back to the kidney. It is used for abdominal pain due to cold hernia, furuncles on the back of the body caused by blood stasis and phlegm obstruction caused by cold congealing due to yang deficiency; amenorrhea and dysmenorrhea

caused by cold congealing with blood stasis due to deficient cold in the *chong* and *ren*; deficient yang floating due to kidney yang depletion, with manifestations such as flushing, deficient asthma, sweating, palpitations, insomnia, and a faint pulse. In addition, for patients with weak constitutions, and qi and blood deficiency due to chronic diseases, a small dosage of *ròu guì* (Cortex Cinnamomi) can be added into their prescription. This is in order to boost actions of replenishing qi and nourishing blood to promote qi and blood production.

④ *Wú zhū yú* (吴茱萸, Fructus Evodiae, Medicinal Evodia Fruit) ★ ★ ★

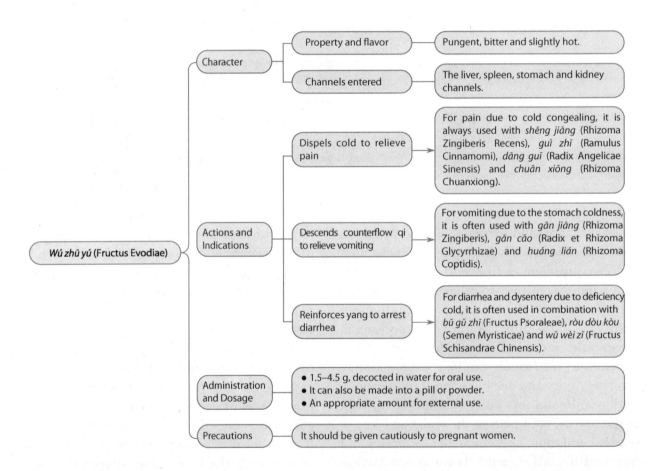

⑤ *Xiǎo huí xiāng* (小茴香, Fructus Foeniculi, Fennel) ★ ★

Wú zhū yú (Fructus Evodiae) and *xiǎo huí xiāng* (Fructus Foeniculi) are pungent in flavor, warm or hot in property, and enter the liver, kidney, spleen and stomach channels. They can warm

the middle to dispel cold and alleviate pain. The two medicinals are used in combination to treat cold stagnation in the liver channel manifesting as cold hernia with abdominal pain, cold pain in the abdomen, amenorrhea and dysmenorrhea; and lower abdominal pain due to stomach cold.

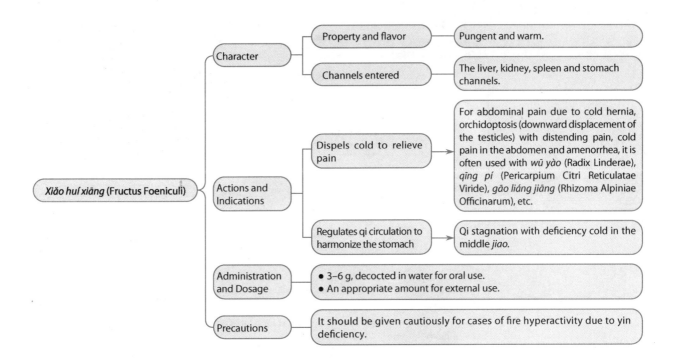

Xiǎo huí xiāng (Fructus Foeniculi)

Character

- **Property and flavor** — Pungent and warm.
- **Channels entered** — The liver, kidney, spleen and stomach channels.

Actions and Indications

- **Dispels cold to relieve pain** — For abdominal pain due to cold hernia, orchidoptosis (downward displacement of the testicles) with distending pain, cold pain in the abdomen and amenorrhea, it is often used with *wū yào* (Radix Linderae), *qīng pí* (Pericarpium Citri Reticulatae Viride), *gāo liáng jiāng* (Rhizoma Alpiniae Officinarum), etc.
- **Regulates qi circulation to harmonize the stomach** — Qi stagnation with deficiency cold in the middle *jiao*.

Administration and Dosage

- 3–6 g, decocted in water for oral use.
- An appropriate amount for external use.

Precautions — It should be given cautiously for cases of fire hyperactivity due to yin deficiency.

Wú zhū yú (Fructus Evodiae) is pungent and bitter, slightly toxic, and has strong actions. It can soothe liver depression, descend counterflow qi to relieve vomiting, and reinforce yang to relieve diarrhea. It is an essential medicinal to treat various pains due to qi stagnation caused by cold in the liver. It is used for headache at the top of the head, retching and spitting of saliva due to counterflow of turbid yin caused by deficiency cold in the liver and stomach; beriberi with swollen and painful feet, or counterflow qi into the abdomen due to cold damp; vomiting due to stomach cold, hypochondriac pain, bitter taste in the mouth, vomiting and sour regurgitation from disharmony between the liver and stomach caused by liver depression transforming into fire; and diarrhea before dawn due to yang deficiency in both the spleen and kidney. *Xiǎo huí xiāng* (Fructus Foeniculi) can regulate qi activity in the spleen and stomach to improve appetite and relieve vomiting; therefore it is used for qi stagnation with deficiency cold in the middle *jiao* with manifestations such as poor appetite and vomiting.

In addition, there are two medicinals called *huí xiāng*: One is *xiǎo huí xiāng* (Fructus Foeniculi) and the other is *dà huí xiāng* (大茴

香, Fructus Anisi Stellati, Chinese Star Anise). *Xiǎo huí xiāng* (Fructus Foeniculi) is the mature fruit of *Foeniculum Vulgare* Mill., of the family Umbelliferae, which is also known as *gǔ huí xiāng*. *Dà huí xiāng* (Fructus Anisi Stellati) comes from the mature fruit of Illcium verum Hook., of the family Magnoliaceae, and is known as *bā jiǎo huí xiāng* or *bā jiǎo*. These two medicinals have similar actions. However, *xiǎo huí xiāng* (Fructus Foeniculi) has a stronger action than *dà huí xiāng* (Fructus Anisi Stellati), which is used both medicinally and in cooking. *Dà huí xiāng* (Fructus Anisi Stellati) is mainly used as a flavoring spice.

⑥ *Dīng xiāng* (丁香, Flos Caryophylli, Clove) ★★

Dīng xiāng (Flos Caryophylli) and *xiǎo huí xiāng* (Fructus Foeniculi) are pungent and aromatic in flavor and warm in property. They can dispel cold and regulate qi to relieve pain, and can be used for unsmooth qi flow due to cold congealing. *Dīng xiāng* (Flos Caryophylli) is effective for warming the middle and descending counterflow qi, and is used for hiccups and vomiting due to stomach cold. It is an essential medicinal to treat vomiting due to the stomach cold. In addition, it can warm the kidney and reinforce yang, and therefore is used for cold pain in the epigstrium

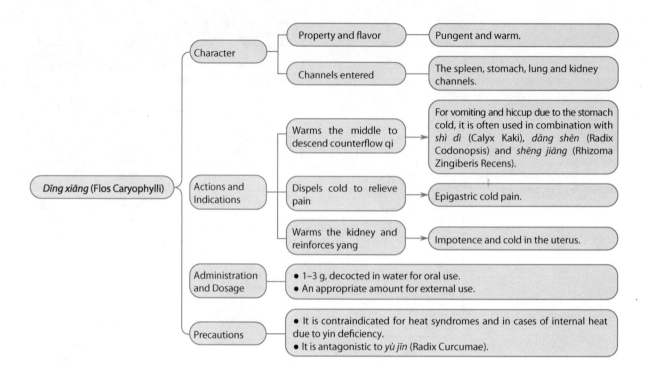

due to stomach cold, impotence, and cold in the uterus due to kidney yang deficiency. *Xiǎo huí xiāng* (Fructus Foeniculi) is capable of warming the kidney and liver to dispel cold and relieve pain, and is used for various pains due to cold stagnation in the liver channel, manifesting as cold hernia with abdominal pain, orchidoptosis (downward displacement of the testicles) cold pain in the lower abdomen, and dysmenorrhea.

In addition, *dīng xiāng* (Flos Caryophylli), which is a flower bud, is also known as *gōng dīng xiāng*. The mature fruit of the same origin is called *mǔ dīng xiāng* (Fructus Caryophylli), and is also known as *jī xiāng shé*. These two medicinals have similar actions. However, *gōng dīng xiāng* (Flos

Caryophylli) has a potent odor and a stronger action compared to that of *mǔ dīng xiāng* (Fructus Caryophylli).

⑦ *Gāo liáng jiāng* (高良姜, Rhizoma Alpiniae Officinarum, Lesser Galangal Rhizome) ★★

Both *gān jiāng* (Rhizoma Zingiberis) and *gāo liáng jiāng* (Rhizoma Alpiniae Officinarum) are pungent in flavor and hot in property. They enter the spleen and stomach channels, and can warm the middle to dispel cold. They are considered important medicinals to warm the middle so as to dispel cold. They are indicated for cold syndromes of the spleen and stomach manifesting as epigastric cold pain, vomiting,

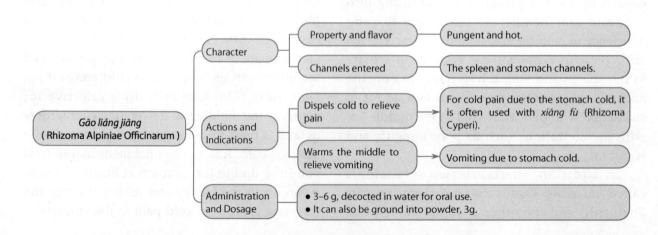

diarrhea, and dysentery. They can be added to formulas that treat excess syndrome due to external pathogenic cold invasion becoming internal, or for deficiency syndromes of a yang qi deficiency type. In clinical practice, the two medicinals are used in combination for mutual reinforcement. *Gān jiāng* (Rhizoma Zingiberis) can warm the middle to dispel cold, and therefore is effective for warming the spleen yang. It is mainly used for abdominal pain, diarrhea and dysentery due to cold in the spleen. It also enters the kidney, heart and lung channels, and can activate the vessels to revive yang, and warm the lung to dissolve fluids. It is used to treat yang depletion syndrome, manifesting as cold limbs, and an indistinct and faint pulse. Compared to *fù zǐ* (Radix Aconiti Lateralis Praeparata), it has a more moderate action to rescue depleted yang in order to resuscitate. It can be used for cough with dyspnea due to cold fluids, with a cold appearance and cold back, and profuse and thin sputum. *Gāo liáng jiāng* (Rhizoma Alpiniae Officinarum) is effective for dispelling cold in the stomach to relieve pain and vomiting. It can be used for cold pain, vomiting and hiccup due to cold in the stomach.

⑧ *Hú jiāo* (胡椒, Fructus Piperis, Pepper Fruit) ★

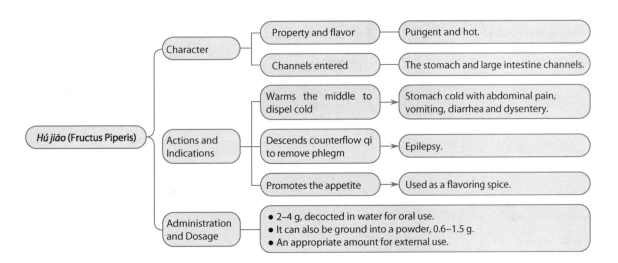

⑨ *Huā jiāo* (花椒, Pericarpium Zanthoxyli, Pricklyash Peel) ★ ★ ★

Huā jiāo (Pericarpium Zanthoxyli) and *hú jiāo* (Fructus Piperis) are pungent in flavor, warm or hot in property, and can warm the middle to dispel cold and relieve pain. They can be

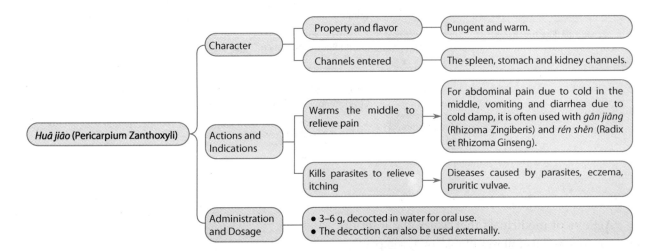

used in combination for cold syndromes of the spleen and stomach, with manifestations such as epigastric cold pain, poor appetite, vomiting and diarrhea. *Huā jiāo* (Pericarpium Zanthoxyli) can also kill parasites to relieve itching. It is often used for abdominal pain due to parasite accumulation, eczema and pruritic vulvae. It is used both medicinally and in cooking. *Hú jiāo* (Fructus Piperis) quickly dispels cold, and is often used as a flavoring spice in cooking. In addition, it can descend counterflow qi to remove phlegm and is used for epilepsy with profuse sputum due to stagnated phlegm invading the clear orifices.

⑩ *Bì bá* (荜茇, Fructus Piperis Longi, Long Pepper Fruit) ★

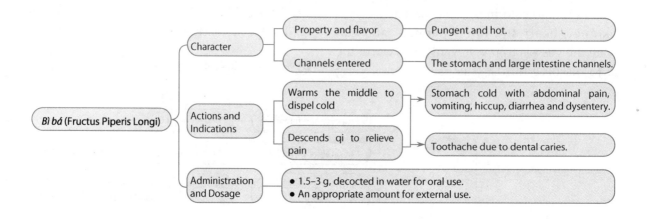

⑪ *Bì chéng qié* (荜澄茄, Fructus Litseae, Cubeb Fruit) ★

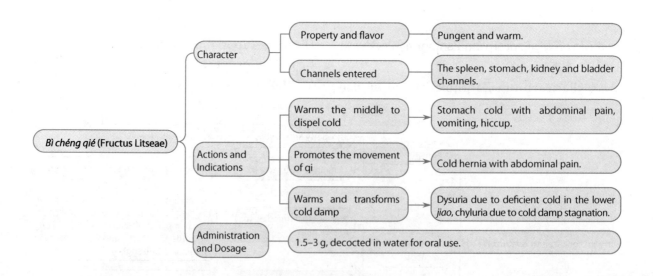

Actions of medicinals that warm the interior are summarized as follows (Table 14-1, see p.223):

Table 14-1: Summary of Medicinals that Warm the Interior:

Medicinal	Action in Common	Individual Character	
		Characteristic Actions	Other Actions
Fù zǐ (Radix Aconiti Lateralis Praeparata)	Supplements fire and strengthens yang, dispels cold to relieve pain	Toxic with a strong action, it mainly can warm and nourish the spleen and kidney, and is effective for rescuing depleted yang in order to resuscitate. Suitable for yin hyperactivity with yang depletion. It is an essential medicinal for warming the interior to dispel cold, and rescuing depletion in order to resuscitate.	
Ròu guì (Cortex Cinnamomi)		Non-toxic, it can mainly warm and nourish the kidney.	Warms and activates channels and vessels, guides fire back to the kidney, invigorates the production of qi and blood
Gān jiāng (Rhizoma Zingiberis)	Warms the middle to dispel cold	Effective for warming the spleen yang, indicated for abdominal pain, diarrhea and dysentery due to cold in the spleen	Revives yang, activates the vessels, warms the lung to transform fluids
Gāo liáng jiāng (Rhizoma Alpiniae Officinarum)		Effective for relieving pain and vomiting, indicated for cold pain in the stomach, stomach cold, vomiting, hiccup	
Wú zhū yú (Fructus Evodiae)	Dispels cold to relieve pain, effective for treating various pain due to cold stagnation in the liver channel	Slightly toxic, effective for soothing the liver to relieve depression, descending counterflow qi to relieve vomiting, regarded as an important medicinal to treat various pains from qi stagnation due to liver cold	Reinforces yang to arrest diarrhea
Xiǎo huí xiāng (Fructus Foeniculi)			Regulates qi to harmonize the stomach
Dīng xiāng (Flos Caryophylli)		Effective for warming the middle and descending counterflow qi, regarded as an essential medicinal to treat vomiting due to cold in the stomach	Warms the kidney to reinforce yang
Huā jiāo (Pericarpium Zanthoxyli)	Warms the middle to dispel cold and relieves pain	Commonly used both medicinally and for cooking	Kills parasites to relieve itching
Hú jiāo (Fructus Piperis)		Often used as a food	
Bì bá (Fructus Piperis Longi)			Descends stomach qi to relieve vomiting and hiccup
Bì chéng qié (Fructus Litseae)			Promotes qi circulation

Tables to test your herbal knowledge of the actions and indications of medicinals that warm the interior are as follows (Tables 14-2 and 14-3):

Table 14-2: Test your Herbal Knowledge of the Actions of Medicinals that Warm the Interior:

Actions \ Medicinal	Fù zǐ	Gān jiāng	Ròu guì	Wú zhū yú	Xiǎo huí xiāng	Dīng xiāng	Gāo liáng jiāng	Huā jiāo	Hú jiāo	Bì bá	Bì chéng qié
Relieves pain											
Warms the middle to dispel cold											
Supplements fire to strengthen yang											
Dispels cold											
Rescues depleted yang so as to resuscitate											
Warms the kidney to reinforce yang											
Warms the lung to transform fluids											
Descends qi to remove phlegm											
Relieves vomiting											
Descends qi to relieve asthma											
Regulates qi to harmonize the middle											
Kills parasites											
Relieves itching											
Promotes the flow of water to reduce edema											
Stops diarrhea											
Promotes qi circulation											
Warms and activates the channels and vessels											

Table 14-3: Test your Herbal Knowledge of the Indications of Medicinals that Warm the Interior:

Actions \ Medicinal	Fù zǐ	Gān jiāng	Ròu guì	Wú zhū yú	Xiǎo huí xiāng	Gāo liáng jiāng	Huā jiāo	Dīng xiāng	Bì bá	Bì chéng qié	Hú jiāo
Yang depletion syndrome											
Pain due to cold hernia											
Epigastric cold pain											
Edema of a yin cold type											
Qi stagnation due to deficient cold in the middle *jiao*											
Cold *bi*											
Cough with dyspnea due to cold fluid retention											
Cardiac cold pain											
Impotence and cold in the uterus											
Chest blockage, dorsal furuncles											
Amenorrhea and dysmenorrhea											
Various pains due to cold stagnation in the liver channel											
Epilepsy											
Diarrhea due to deficiency cold											
Jaundice of a yin type											
Abdominal pain due to the retention of parasites											
Eczema with itching											
Pruritic vulvae											
Hiccup of a deficiency cold type											
Vomiting due to cold in the stomach											
Diarrhea due to spleen cold											

Chapter 15
Medicinals that Regulate Qi

Medicinals that act to regulate qi activity, and are mainly used for qi stagnation or counterflow qi are defined as qi-regulating medicinals.

Character and Actions

Medicinals that regulate qi are mostly pungent, bitter and aromatic in flavor, and warm in property. The pungent flavor can disperse, the bitter flavor can purge, and the aromatic flavor can penetrate. The warm property has the actions of activating and promoting. Therefore, medicinals of this kind can smooth the qi, i.e. promote qi circulation, descend qi, relieve depression, and remove stasis. They can also relieve pain through promoting qi circulation and removing qi stagnation. Medicinals that regulate qi mainly enter the spleen, liver and lung channels. According to their differences, they have varied actions such as soothing the liver to relieve depression, regulating qi to soothe the chest, promoting qi circulation to relieve pain, and breaking up qi to remove stasis.

Indications

Medicinals in this chapter are indicated for epigastric and abdominal distending pain, belching, sour regurgitation, nausea, vomiting, diarrhea or constipation due to qi stagnation in the spleen and stomach; hypochondriac distending pain, depression, hernia with pain, breast distending pain and irregular menstruation due to liver qi constraint; chest distress and pain, and cough with dyspnea due to lung qi stagnation.

Combinations

When using these kinds of medicinals, doctors must select individual medicinals according to the pathological condition of their patient. Pertinent combinations should then be selected. For example, with qi stagnation of the spleen and stomach, select medicinals for regulating the qi of the spleen and stomach. For food stagnation, select medicinals for removing food retention. For qi deficiency in the spleen and stomach, add medicinals for nourishing the middle and replenishing qi. For damp heat obstruction, add medicinals for clearing heat and removing damp. For cold damp obstruction in the spleen, combine with medicinals for drying damp. For liver qi constraint, combine with medicinals for soothing the liver and regulating qi. For liver blood deficiency, combine with medicinals for nourishing blood and softening the liver. For cold invasion in the liver channel, add medicinals for warming the liver to dispel cold. In cases complicated by blood stasis, combine with medicinals for invigorating the blood to remove stasis. For lung qi stagnation, choose medicinals with the action of regulating qi to soothe the chest. For cases caused by external pathogens invading the lung, combine with medicinals for diffusing the lung to relieve exterior syndromes. For phlegm-fluids retention in the lung, add medicinals for removing phlegm and transforming fluid.

Precautions

Medicinals of this kind are pungent, aromatic, warm, and dry, which implies they can consume qi and yin. Therefore they should be used cautiously for those who have insufficient qi and yin.

① *Chén pí* (陈皮, Pericarpium Citri Reticulatae, Aged Tangerine Peel) ★ ★ ★

Addition: *Jú hé* (橘核, **Semen Citri Reticulatae, Tangerine Seed**) acts to regulate qi to remove stasis and relieve pain. It is indicated for pain due to hernia, testicular swelling and pain, and hard breast masses.

Jú luò (橘络, **Vascular Aurantii, Tangerine Pith**) has the actions of promoting qi circulation

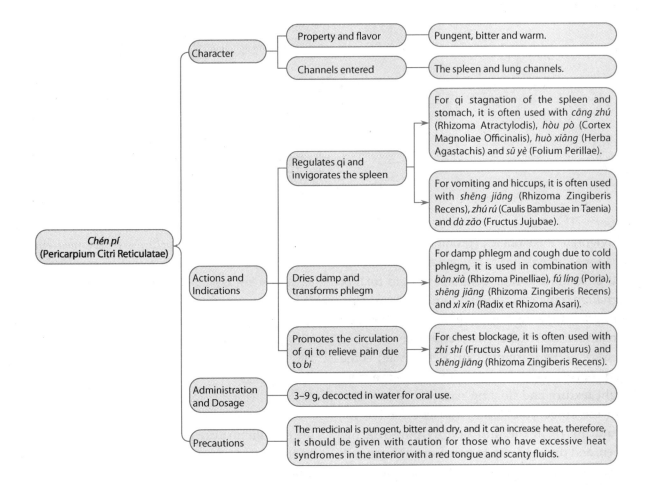

to dredge the collaterals and transforming phlegm to relieve cough. It is indicated for chest pain, and cough and profuse sputum due to phlegm retention in the channels and collaterals.

Jú yè (橘叶, **Folium Citri Reticulatae, Tangerine Leaf**) can soothe the liver and promote qi circulation to remove stasis and reduce swellings. It is indicated for hypochondriac pain, breast abscesses, and masses in the breast.

Huà jú hóng (化橘红, **Exocarpium Citri Grandis, Pummelo Peel**) can regulate qi to soothe the chest

and dry damp to transform phlegm. It is used for cough due to damp or cold phlegm, vomiting and nausea due to food retention, and chest oppression.

② *Qīng pí* (青皮, Pericarpium Citri Reticulatae Viride, Green Tangerine Peel) ★ ★

Chén pí (Pericarpium Citri Reticulatae) and *qīng pí* (Pericarpium Citri Reticulatae Viride) come from the dried peel of *Citrus reticuta* Blanco, of the family Rutaceae. Both of these medicinals are pungent and bitter in flavor, and warm in

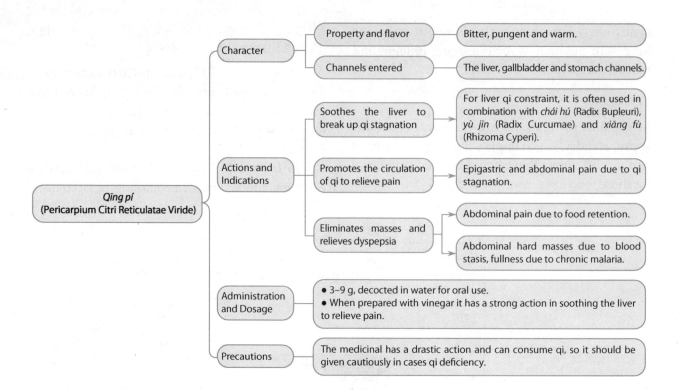

property. They can regulate qi in the middle *jiao* to invigorate the stomach (promote qi circulation to relieve distension). The two medicinals are used in combination for reinforcement to treat qi stagnation, epigastric and abdominal distending pain, poor appetite, vomiting, and diarrhea due to food retention in the spleen and stomach.

Chén pí (Pericarpium Citri Reticulatae) is the dried peel of mature fruit. It has a moderate action, a light texture and floating nature. It dominates qi in the spleen and lung, and is effective for regulating qi in the middle, invigorating the spleen, and drying damp to transform phlegm. It is indicated for epigastric and abdominal distending pain, belching, vomiting, nausea and no appetite due to qi stagnation in the spleen and stomach; epigastric and abdominal distension and fullness, poor digestion, lassitude, loose stools, and a thick and greasy coat due to damp turbid obstruction. It is most suitable for qi stagnation due to cold damp obstruction in the middle; vomiting and hiccup due to counterflow qi of the stomach; and shortness of breath due to chest blockage. As noted in the *Compendium of Materia Medica*: "*Chén pí (Pericarpium Citri Reticulatae) is used to treat a variety of diseases by regulating qi and drying damp.*

It can tonify when combined with tonic medicinals, purge when combined with purgative medicinals, ascend when combined with ascendant medicinals, and descend when combined with descendant medicinals. It is a medicinal for regulating qi activity in both the spleen and lung channels. However, it has a variety of actions when used in different combinations" (其治百病，总取其理气燥湿之功。同补药则补，同泻药则泻，同升药则升，同降药则降，……为肺脾二经气分药，但随所配而补泻升降也。).

Qīng pí (Pericarpium Citri Reticulatae Viride) is the dried immature peel or fruit. It has a relatively strong action in promoting qi circulation and has a descending nature. It regulates qi in the liver and gallbladder. It can soothe the liver, break up qi stagnation, eliminate masses, and relieve dyspepsia. It is indicated for hypochondriac distending pain, breast distending pain or masses, hernia with pain, and breast abscesses with swelling pain due to liver qi constraint; epigastric and abdominal distending pain due to qi stagnation caused by food retention; abdominal hard masses due to blood stasis, and masses due to chronic malaria caused by qi stagnation and blood stasis. Ancient physicians considered *chén pí* (Pericarpium Citri Reticulatae) to be ascending and floating in nature, and entering the spleen and lung to treat diseases in the upper body. Whereas *qīng pí* (Pericarpium Citri Reticulatae Viride) has a descending nature and enters the liver and gallbladder to purge to treat diseases in the lower. For diseases in the liver involving the spleen and stomach leading to disharmony between the liver and stomach, the two medicinals are used in combination for mutual reinforcement.

③ *Zhǐ shí* (枳实, Fructus Aurantii Immaturus, Immature Orange Fruit) ★ ★ ★

Addition: ***Zhǐ qiào* (枳壳, Fructus Aurantii, Orange Fruit)** is the same as *zhǐ shí* (Fructus Aurantii Immaturus) in character, channels entered and function, but it is moderate in action. It can promote qi circulation to soothe the chest and relieve distension.

Zhǐ shí (Fructus Aurantii Immaturus) and *zhǐ qiào* (Fructus Aurantii) come from the fruit of *Citrus aurantium* L., or *Citrus wilsonii* Tana ka, of the family Rutaceae. Li Shi-zhen thought that the two medicinals were bitter, pungent and sour in flavor, warm in property, and entered the spleen, stomach and large intestine channels. Both medicinals can promote qi circulation to treat qi stagnation. The larger one is called *zhǐ qiào* (Fructus Aurantii), while the smaller one is called *zhǐ shí* (Fructus Aurantii

Immaturus). They have different clinical uses. *Zhǐ shí* (Fructus Aurantii Immaturus) is the immature fruit, which has a drastic action in breaking up qi stagnation, eliminating masses, and transforming phlegm to relieve fullness. It is mainly used for epigastric and abdominal distending pain and fullness due to qi stagnation caused by food retention; constipation of a heat accumulation type, abdominal fullness and distending pain due to stagnation in the stomach and large intestine; diarrhea and dysentery with tenesmus due to food or damp heat retention; chest blockage due to phlegm obstruction caused by inactivity of chest yang, chest accumulations due to phlegm heat; chest and hypochondriac pain due to qi stagnation; abdominal pain post partum due to blood stasis. In addition, when used alone, *zhǐ shí* (Fructus Aurantii Immaturus) can treat gastric dilation, stomach prolapse, uterine prolapse, and anal prolapse. It is used in combination with medicinals that have the actions of tonifying the middle and replenishing qi so as to reinforce its therapeutic effect. *Zhǐ qiào* (Fructus Aurantii) is the mature fruit (with the inner part removed). It acts to promote qi circulation and soothe the chest to relieve distension. It is often used for distending pain in the chest, hypochondrium,

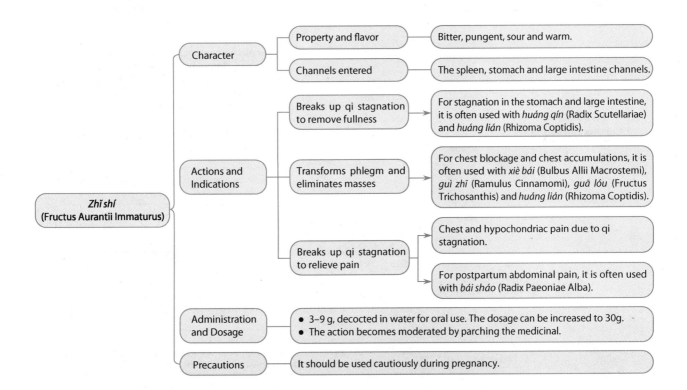

epigastrium, and abdomen due to qi stagnation as well as mild symptoms due to food retention with qi stagnation.

Zhǐ shí (Fructus Aurantii Immaturus) and *hòu pò* (Cortex Magnoliae Officinalis) are bitter and pungent in flavor, and warm in property. They have strong actions in promoting qi circulation and eliminating masses, and are considered essential medicinals to eliminate distension and fullness. The two medicinals are used for constipation due to heat accumulation or food retention, as well as damp obstruction in the middle. *Zhǐ shí* (Fructus Aurantii Immaturus) has a descending nature with a drastic action and is capable of breaking up qi stagnation and eliminating masses. It is suitable to relieve fullness of an excessive type by eliminating food retention and promoting defecation. It can also transform phlegm to remove fullness, and is used for diarrhea and dysentery with tenesmus

due to food or damp heat accumulation; chest blockage due to chest accumulations; abdominal pain post-partum due to blood stasis; and prolapse of the internal organs. *Hòu pò* (Cortex Magnoliae Officinalis) is bitter and dry in nature, and has a strong action to relieve fullness. It is effective for relieving fullness due to damp through drying damp and invigorating the spleen. It can be used for epigastric and abdominal distending pain due to disharmony between the spleen and stomach caused by damp obstruction, food retention or qi stagnation. It is able to dry damp to transform phlegm, and descend counterflow qi to relieve asthma. Therefore, it is used for cough with dyspnea due to phlegm-fluids; and plum pit qi due to binding obstruction of phlegm and qi caused by depression.

④ *Mù xiāng* (木香, Radix Aucklandiae, Common Aucklandia Root) ★★★

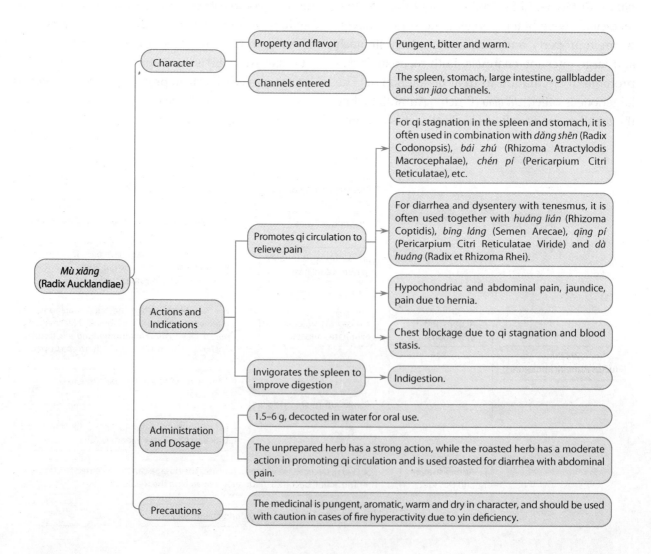

⑤ *Chén xiāng* (沉香, Lignum Aquilariae Resinatum, Aquilaria Wood) ★★

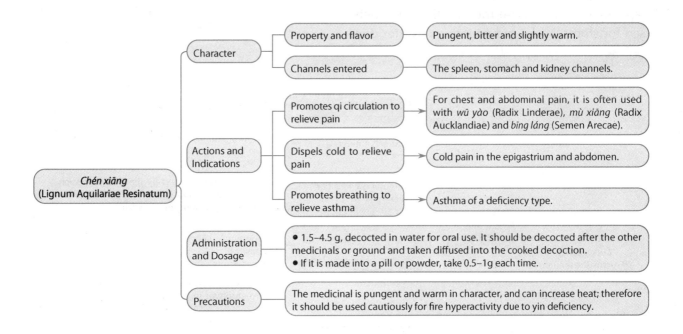

⑥ *Tán xiāng* (檀香, Lignum Santali Albi, Sandalwood) ★

Both *chén xiāng* (Lignum Aquilariae Resinatum) and *tán xiāng* (Lignum Santali Albi) are pungent and aromatic in flavor, and warm in property. Both medicinals can promote qi circulation and dispel cold to relieve pain. They are used in combination to treat chest and abdominal distending pain and distress due to cold congealing and qi stagnation. *Chén xiāng* (Lignum Aquilariae Resinatum) is bitter in flavor with a heavy texture and descending nature. It is effective for warming the middle, descending counterflow qi to relieve vomiting and promoting respiration to relieve asthma. It is often used for vomiting due to stomach cold, lower *jiao* deficiency cold, asthma of a deficiency type due to failure of the cold kidney to grasp qi. *Tán xiāng*

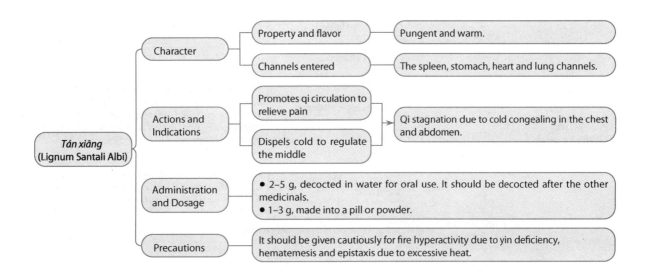

(Lignum Santali Albi) is effective for regulating the spleen and lung. It can soothe the chest and promote qi circulation to relieve pain, as well as dispel cold and regulate the middle. It is often used for stomachache and vomiting of water due to stomach cold; angina due to qi stagnation, and blood stasis from cold congealing.

⑦ *Chuān liàn zǐ* (川楝子, Fructus Toosendan, Sichuan Chinaberry Fruit) ★★

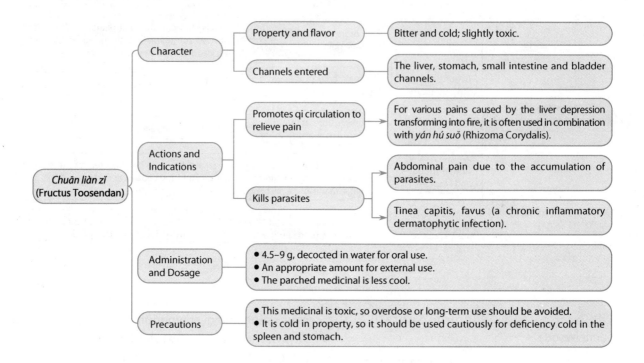

⑧ *Wū yào* (乌药, Radix Linderae, Combined Spicebush Root) ★

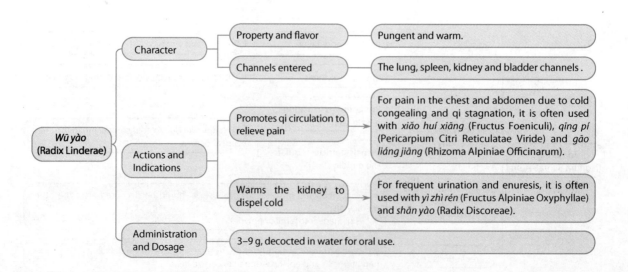

⑨ *Qīng mù xiāng* (青木香, Radix Aristolochiae, Slender Dutchmanspipe Root) ★

Mù xiāng (Radix Aucklandiae) and *qīng mù xiāng* (Radix Aristolochiae) can promote qi circulation to relieve pain. Both can be used for distending pain in the epigastrium, abdomen, chest and hypochondrium due to qi stagnation, poor appetite, vomiting and diarrhea; or diarrhea and dysentery with tenesmus due to damp heat. *Mù xiāng* (Radix Aucklandiae) comes from the root of *Aucklandia lappa* Decne., or *Vladimiria souliei* (Franch.) Ling, of the family Compositae. It is pungent and aromatic in flavor, warm and dry in property, and therefore can regulate the *san jiao*, especially to remove qi stagnation in the spleen, stomach and large intestine. It is an essential medicinal to promote qi circulation and regulate the middle to relieve pain. It is most suitable to treat diseases mentioned above which belong to the type of qi stagnation in the spleen, stomach and large intestine, complicated by cold. It can also invigorate the spleen to promote

digestion, and therefore is used for epigastric and abdominal distending pain, poor appetite and loose stools due to spleen deficiency with qi stagnation; chest and hypochondriac distending pain, jaundice and bitter taste in the mouth due to binding of damp heat with qi stasis caused by a failure of the spleen to transport and transform, and the liver to course; hernia with pain; and chest blockage and cardiac pain due to qi stagnation and blood stasis of cold congealing. *Qīng mù xiāng* (Radix Aristolochiae) is the dried root of *Aristolochia contorta* Bge., of the family Aristolochiaceae. It is pungent and bitter in flavor, and cold in property. It enters the liver and stomach channels and is used for qi stagnation in the liver and stomach complicated by heat. It can detoxify to reduce swellings. It can be used for abdominal pain, *sha zhang* (痧胀) (summerheat gastric disturbance) with vomiting and diarrhea due to improper diet during the summer days; poisonous snake bites, suppurating infections on the surface of the body and damp ulcers.

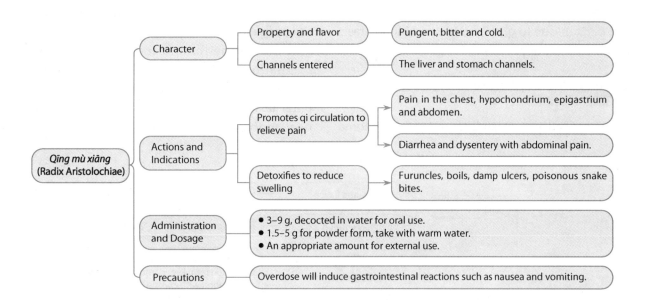

⑩ *Lì zhī hé* (荔枝核, Semen Litchi, Lychee Seed) ★
Chuān liàn zǐ (Fructus Toosendan) and *lì zhī hé* (Semen Litchi) can promote qi circulation to relieve pain, and are indicated for hypochondriac pain, epigastric and abdominal pain due to liver qi depression or disharmony between

the liver and stomach, and hernia pain. *Chuān liàn zǐ* (Fructus Toosendan) is bitter and cold with a descending nature, and can clear liver fire and purge depressed heat (soothe the liver to purge fire). Therefore it is suitable to treat the diseases mentioned above with heat

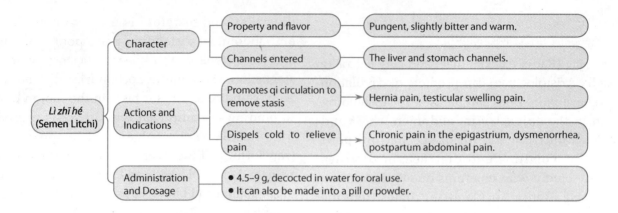

manifestations (various pains due to depressed liver qi transforming into fire). In addition, it can kill parasites and treat tinea, and is used for abdominal pain with accumulation of parasites, tinea capitis and favus. *Lì zhī hé* (Semen Litchi) is pungent and bitter in flavor and warm in property. It is effective for dispelling cold and eliminating stasis. It is indicated for hernia with pain due to cold congealing and qi stagnation in the liver channel and testicular swelling pain. It is also used for dysmenorrhea and abdominal pain post partum due to qi stagnation and blood stasis caused by liver depression.

⑪ *Xiāng fù* (香附, Rhizoma Cyperi, Nutgrass Galingale Rhizome) ★★★

Mù xiāng (Radix Aucklandiae), *xiāng fù* (Rhizoma Cyperi) and *wū yào* (Radix Linderae) are pungent and aromatic in flavor, and can promote qi circulation to relieve pain. They can be used to treat pain due to qi stagnation. The differences are as follows: *Mù xiāng* (Radix Aucklandiae) is pungent, bitter, warm and dry in nature, and can regulate the *san jiao*, and promote qi circulation in the spleen, stomach and large intestine. It is considered an essential medicinal to regulate the middle in order to relieve pain. It can invigorate the spleen to promote digestion and is used for epigastric and abdominal distending pain and poor appetite and loose stools due to qi stagnation with spleen deficiency; chest and hypochondriac distending pain, jaundice and bitter taste in the mouth due to binding of damp heat with qi stasis caused by a failure of the

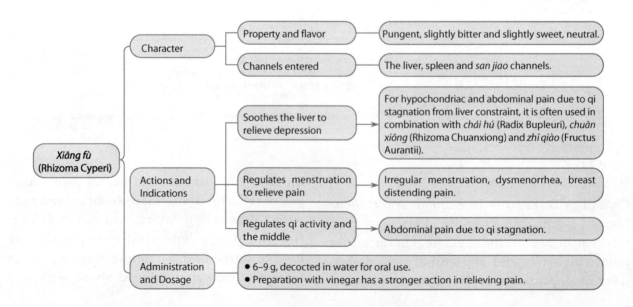

spleen to transport and transform and the liver to course; hernia with pain; and chest blockage and cardiac pain due to qi stagnation and blood stasis of cold congealing. *Xiāng fù* (Rhizoma Cyperi) is pungent, aromatic in flavor and neutral in property. It mainly soothes the liver to relieve depression, regulates menstruation to relieve pain and regulates qi movement and the middle. It is indicated for hypochondriac distending pain, epigastric and abdominal distending pain, irregular menstruation, dysmenorrhea, breast distending pain and hernia pain caused by liver qi constraint. It can also be used for epigastric and abdominal distending pain, poor appetite and digestion, belching, and sour regurgitation due to qi stagnation of the spleen and stomach. *Xiāng fù* (Rhizoma Cyperi) is a most effective medicinal to soothe the liver and regulate qi activity, and is an essential gynecological medicinal for regulating menstruation. Li Shi-zhen said: "*Xiāng fù*

(Rhizoma Cyperi) dominates all diseases induced by qi disturbance, and is the first choice in gynecology." (气病之总司，女科之主帅). *Wū yào* (Radix Linderae) has a very mild odor. It is pungent and aromatic in flavor and warm in property. Its actions can reach the lung and spleen in the upper as well as the kidney and bladder in the lower. It is effective for promoting qi circulation and dispelling cold to relieve pain, and therefore is used for distending pain in the chest, hypochondrium, epigastrium and abdomen due to cold congealing and qi stagnation, abdominal pain due to cold hernia or menstruation. In addition, it can warm the kidney to dispel cold, and is also used for enuresis and frequent urination due to kidney yang deficiency and deficient cold in the bladder.

⑫ *Fó shǒu* (佛手, Fructus Citri Sarcodactylis, Finger Citron) ★

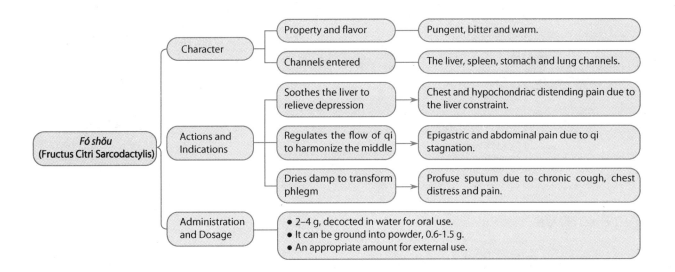

⑬ *Xiāng yuán* (香橼, Fructus Citri, Citron Fruit)

Fó shǒu (Fructus Citri Sarcodactylis) and *xiāng yuán* (Fructus Citri) are pungent, bitter and aromatic in flavor, and warm in property. They have moderate actions in soothing the liver to relieve depression, regulating qi flow to harmonize the middle and drying damp to transform phlegm. They can be used to treat distending pain in the chest, hypochondrium, epigastrium, and abdomen due to disharmony between the liver and stomach with liver qi constraint; epigastric and abdominal pain, vomiting, nausea and poor appetite due to qi stagnation in the spleen and stomach; and cough with profuse sputum and chest distress due to phlegm-damp accumulation. The two medicinals are always used together for mutual reinforcement. *Fó shǒu* (Fructus Citri

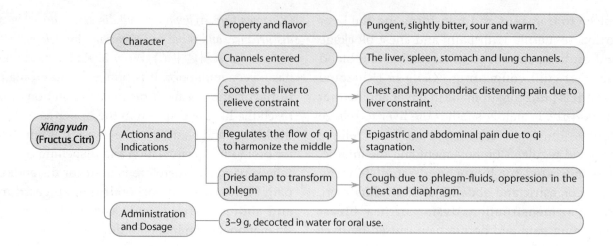

Sarcodactylis) mainly regulates qi in the liver and stomach to relieve pain, while *xiāng yuán* (Fructus Citri) has a strong action in transforming phlegm to relieve cough by regulating qi in the spleen and lung.

⑭ *Méi gui huā* (玫瑰花, Flos Rosae Rugosae, Rose Flower)

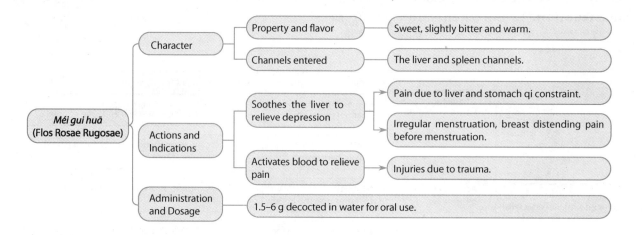

⑮ *Lǜ è méi* (绿萼梅, Flos Mume, Plum Flower)

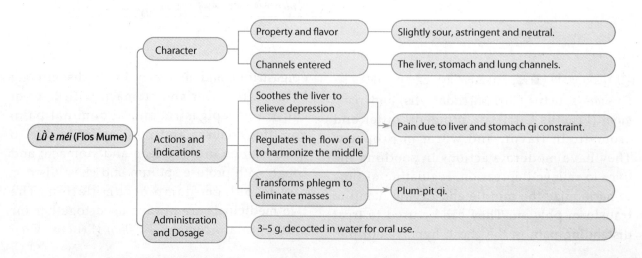

⑯ *Suō luó zǐ* (娑罗子, Semen Aesculi, Buckeye Seed)

Méi gui huā (Flos Rosae Rugosae), *lǜ è méi* (Flos Mume) and *suō luó zǐ* (Semen Aesculi) can soothe the liver to relieve depression and regulate qi to harmonize the stomach. They can be used for distending pain in the chest, hypochodrium, epigastrium and abdomen, vomiting, nausea and poor appetite due to liver qi constraint and disharmony between the liver and stomach. *Méi gui huā* (Flos Rosae Rugosae) can activate blood to relieve pain, and is used for irregular menstruation as well as breast distending pain before menstruation caused by qi stagnation and blood stasis from liver constraint; injuries due to trauma and swelling pain due to stagnation. *Lǜ è méi* (Flos Mume) is capable of transforming phlegm to eliminate masses, and can be used for plum pit qi due to binding of phlegm with qi. *Suō luó zǐ* (Semen Aesculi) is effective for regulating qi to soothe the middle and harmonize the stomach, and therefore is often used for diseases created by disharmony between the liver and stomach.

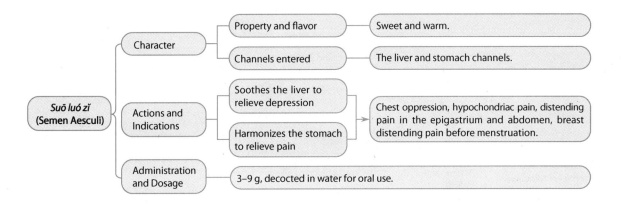

⑰ *Xiè bái* (薤白, Bulbus Allii Macrostemi, Longstamen Onion Bulb) ★★

Xiè bái (Bulbus Allii Macrostemi) and *cōng bái* (Bulbus Allii Fistulosi) have a similar Chinese name. Both originate from the family Liliaceae and can dispel cold, and activate yang to remove stasis. However, they have many differences in actions and indications. *Xiè bái* (Bulbus Allii Macrostemi) is pungent and bitter in flavor, warm in property with a slippery nature, and mainly acts in the interior of the body. It can activate chest yang to dispel cold, and is used for chest

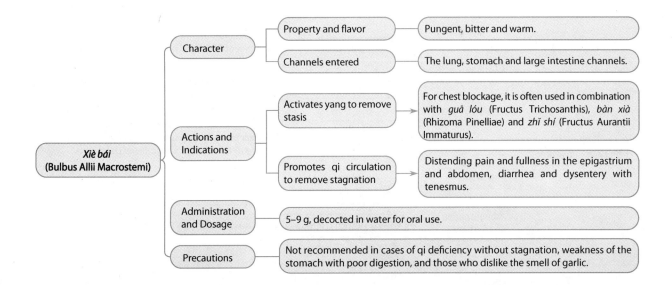

blockage and cardiac pain due to cold phlegm damp stagnating in the chest and blocking yang qi. It is an essential medicinal to treat chest blockage. It can also remove qi stagnation in the stomach and large intestine, and therefore can be used for distending pain and fullness in the epigastrium and abdomen, diarrhea and dysentery with tenesmus caused by qi stagnation in the stomach and large intestine. *Cōng bái* (Bulbus Allii Fistulosi) is pungent in flavor and warm in property, and can act both on the surface of the body and in the interior. It can relieve exterior syndromes by inducing sweating, and is used for mild cases of the common cold of a wind cold type. It is capable of dispelling cold and activating yang, and is used for hyperactive yin repelling yang. When used externally, it is able to detoxify to remove stasis, activate the collaterals to induce lactation, and therefore is used to treat suppurating infections on the surface of the body, brief lactation, and distending pain of the breasts.

⑱ *Tiān xiān téng* (天仙藤, Herba Aristolochiae, Dutchmanspipe Vine)

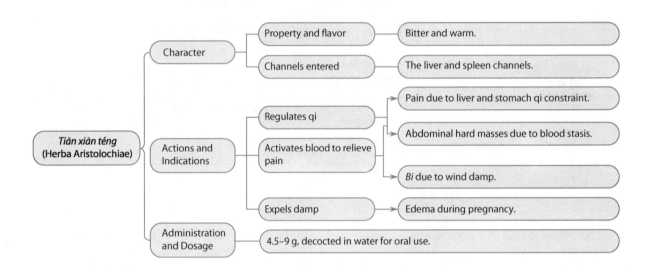

⑲ *Dà fù pí* (大腹皮, Pericarpium Arecae, Areca Peel)

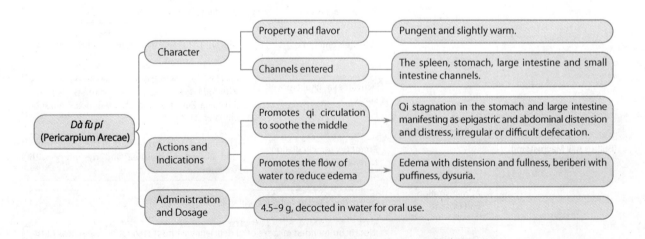

⑳ *Gān sōng* (甘松, Radix et Rhizoma Nardostachyos, Nardostachys Root)

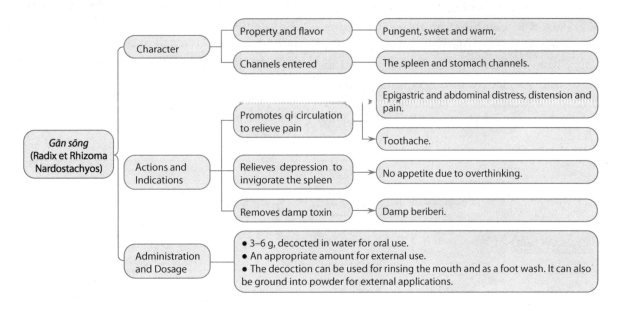

㉑ *Jiǔ xiāng chóng* (九香虫, Aspongopus, Stink-bug)

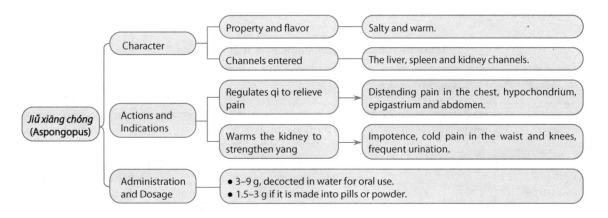

㉒ *Dāo dòu* (刀豆, Semen Canavaliae, Sword Bean)

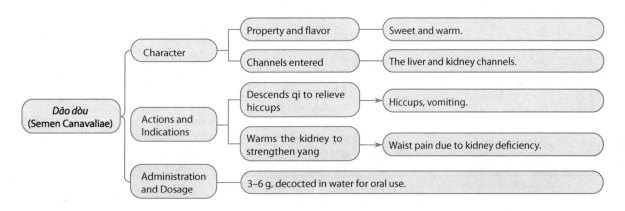

㉓ *Shì dì* (柿蒂, Calyx Kaki, Persimmon Calyx) ★

Both *shì dì* (Calyx Kaki) and *dāo dòu* (Semen Canavaliae) can descend qi to relieve hiccups. They are used in combination to treat hiccups and vomiting due to counterflow stomach qi. *Shì dì* (Calyx Kaki) is bitter in flavor and neutral in property, and specializes in descending stomach qi to relieve hiccups. It is therefore considered an essential medicinal to descend qi in order to relieve hiccups. It can be added for hiccups of different types caused by counterflow stomach qi. *Dāo dòu* (Semen Canavaliae) is sweet and warm, and mainly acts to warm the middle in order to harmonize the stomach and descend qi to relieve hiccups. It is indicated for hiccups and vomiting due to deficiency cold in the middle *jiao*. It can also warm the kidney to strengthen yang, hence is used for waist pain due to kidney deficiency.

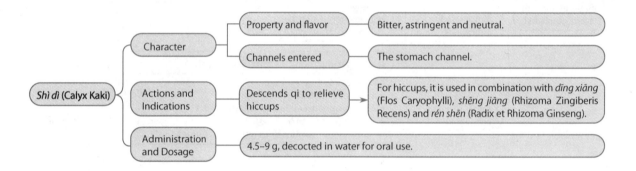

Actions of medicinals that regulate qi are summarized in the following table (Table 15-1):

Table 15-1: Summary of Medicinals that Regulate Qi:

Medicinal	Action in Common	Individual Character	
		Characteristic Actions	**Other Actions**
Chén pí (Pericarpium Citri Reticulatae)	Promotes qi circulation to relieve distension	It has a moderate action in promoting qi circulation, a light texture and a floating nature; it can mainly regulate qi in the spleen and lung, and is effective for regulating qi and the middle to invigorate the spleen and for drying damp to transform phlegm.	
Qīng pí (Pericarpium Citri Reticulatae Viride)		It has a drastic action in promoting qi circulation and has a descending nature, it can mainly course qi in the liver and gallbladder, soothe the liver and break up qi stagnation, eliminate masses and promote digestion.	
Zhǐ shí (Fructus Aurantii Immaturus)	With an acute action, it is good at breaking up qi stagnation to remove masses, transforming phlegm and eliminating food retention.		
Mù xiāng (Radix Aucklandiae)	Promotes qi circulation to relieve pain	It can regulate the *san jiao*, and is especially effective for removing qi stagnation in the spleen, stomach and large intestine. It is regarded as an essential medicinal to promote qi circulation and regulate the middle to relieve pain.	Invigorates the spleen to promote digestion
Xiāng fù (Rhizoma Cyperi)		With a neutral property, it can soothe the liver to relieve depression, regulate menstruation to relieve pain and regulate qi flow and the middle. It is effective for soothing the liver and regulating qi, and is regarded as an essential medicinal to regulate menstruation.	

Table 15-1: Summary of Medicinals that Regulate Qi:

continued

Medicinal	Action in Common	Individual Character	
		Characteristic Actions	Other Actions
Wū yào (Radix Linderae)	Promotes qi circulation to relieve pain	Acts on the spleen, lung, kidney and bladder, and is effective for promoting qi circulation and dispelling cold to relieve pain	Warms the kidney to dispel cold
Qīng mù xiāng (Radix Aristolochiae)			Detoxifies to reduce swelling
Chuān liàn zǐ (Fructus Toosendan)		It has a bitter flavor, cold property and descending nature, can clear liver fire, and purge depressed heat. It is suitable for treating various pains due to depressed liver transforming into fire	Kills parasites, cures tinea
Lì zhī hé (Semen Litchi)		It is effective for dispelling cold and removing stasis. Indicated for hernia pain, testicular swelling pain due to cold congealing and qi stagnation in the liver channel	
Fó shǒu (Fructus Citri Sarcodactylis)	Soothes the liver to relieve depression, regulates qi to harmonize the middle, dries damp to transform phlegm	Regulates qi in the liver and stomach to relieve pain	
Xiāng yuán (Fructus Citri)		Regulates qi in the spleen and lung to transform phlegm and relieves cough	
Tán xiāng (Lignum Santali Albi)	Promotes qi circulation and dispels cold to relieve pain	It is effective for regulating the spleen and lung, soothing the chest and diaphragm to promote qi circulation and relieve pain, dispelling cold and regulating the middle	Promotes skin eruption, eliminates infections on the surface of the body, stops bleeding
Chén xiāng (Lignum Aquilariae Resinatum)		With a heavy texture and descending nature, it is effective for warming the middle and descending counterflow qi to relieve vomiting, and promote respiration to relieve asthma	Removes damp to relieve pain, relieves convulsions
Xiè bái (Bulbus Allii Macrostemi)	It is effective for activating chest yang, removing congealing cold and promoting qi circulation to remove stagnation. It is regarded as an essential medicinal to treat chest blockage.		
Méi gui huā (Flos Rosae Rugosae)	Soothes the liver to relieve constraint, regulates qi to harmonize the stomach		Activates blood to relieve pain
Lǜ è méi (Flos Mume)			Transforms phlegm to remove stasis
Suō luó zǐ (Semen Aesculi)			Relieves pain
Dà fù pí (Pericarpium Arecae)	Promotes qi circulation to soothe the middle, promotes the flow of water to reduce edema		
Shì dì (Calyx Kaki)	Descends qi to relieve hiccups	An essential medicinal to descend qi to relieve hiccups. Suitable to treat hiccups of various kinds caused by counterflow stomach qi.	
Dāo dòu (Semen Canavaliae)		Warms the middle to harmonize the stomach, descends qi to relieve hiccups	Warms the kidney to reinforce yang
Tiān xiān téng (Herba Aristolochiae)			Expels damp and activates blood
Gān sōng (Radix et Rhizoma Nardostachyos)			Relieves depression to invigorate the spleen
Jiǔ xiāng chóng (Aspongopus)			Warms the kidney to reinforce yang

Tables to test herbal knowledge of actions and indications of medicinals that regulate qi are as follows (Tables 15-2~15-5):

Table 15-2: Test your Herbal Knowledge of the Actions of Medicinals that Regulate Qi (one):

Medicinal Actions	Chén pí	Qīng pí	Zhī shí	Mù xiāng	Chén xiāng	Tán xiāng	Xiāng fù	Chuān liàn zǐ	Wū yào	Xiè bái	Qīng mù xiāng	Lì zhī hé
Regulates qi												
Soothes the liver												
Dries damp												
Transforms phlegm												
Removes stasis												
Relieves stagnation												
Relieves cough												
Invigorates the spleen												
Removes food retention												
Relieves indigestion												
Breaks up qi stagnation												
Relieves pain												
Regulates menstruation												
Relieves vomiting												
Promotes respiration to relieve asthma												
Dispels cold												
Regulates the middle												
Warms the middle												
Kills parasites												
Treats tinea												
Repels pathogens												
Activates yang to remove stasis												
Promotes qi circulation to remove stagnation												
Detoxifies to reduce swelling												
Warms the kidney												

Table 15-3: Test your Herbal Knowledge of the Actions of Medicinals that Regulate Qi (two):

Medicinal Actions	Dà fù pí	Fó shǒu	Xiāng yuán	Méi gui huā	Lǜ è méi	Shì dì	Dāo dòu	Gān sōng	Jiǔ xiāng chóng
Promotes qi circulation									
Transforms phlegm									
Soothes the liver									
Promotes the flow of water to reduce edema									
Harmonizes the middle									
Dries damp									

Table 15-3: Test your Herbal Knowledge of the Actions of Medicinals that Regulate Qi (two):

continued

Actions \ Medicinal	Dà fù pí	Fó shǒu	Xiāng yuán	Méi gui huā	Lǜ è méi	Shì dì	Dāo dòu	Gān sōng	Jiǔ xiāng chóng
Relieves pain									
Soothes the middle									
Relieves cough									
Activates blood									
Relieves depression									
Descends qi									
Relieves hiccups									
Warms the kidney to reinforce yang									
Relieves depression to invigorate the spleen									

Table 15-4: Test your Herbal Knowledge of the Indications of Medicinals that Regulate Qi (one):

Indications \ Medicinal	Chén pí	Qīng pí	Zhǐ shí	Mù xiāng	Chén xiāng	Tán xiāng	Xiāng fù	Chuān liàn zǐ	Xiè bái	Qīng mù xiāng
Qi stagnation in the spleen and stomach										
Damp phlegm and cold phlegm										
Diseases caused by liver qi constraint										
Abdominal pain due to food retention										
Chest and abdominal distending pain										
Chest blockage with phlegm obstruction										
Chest accumulations with phlegm heat										
Irregular menstruation due to liver constraint										
Diarrhea and dysentery due to damp heat										
Hypochondriac pain, jaundice										
Qi stagnation with heat accumulation in the stomach and large intestine										
Vomiting due to stomach cold										
Deficient asthma										
Hypochondriac and abdominal pain due to qi stagnation										
Prolapse of internal organs										
Various pains due to liver depression transforming into fire										
Abdominal pain due to accumulation of parasites										
Chest blockage										
Distending pain and fullness in the epigastrium and abdomen										

Table 15-5: Test your Herbal Knowledge of the Indications of Medicinals that Regulate Qi (two):

Medicinal / Indications	Wū yào	Lì zhī hé	Fó shǒu	Xiāng yuán	Méi gui huā	Lǜ è méi	Tiān xiān téng	Dà fù pí	Shì dì	Dāo dòu	Gān sōng	Jiǔ xiāng chóng
Various pains in the chest and abdomen caused by cold congealing and qi stagnation												
Qi stagnation in the spleen and stomach												
Hernia pain, testicular swelling pain												
Suppurating infections												
Dysmenorrhea												
Postpartum abdominal pain												
Chest and hypochondriac distending pain due to liver constraint, pain due to liver and stomach qi stagnation												
Frequent urination, enuresis												
Chronic cough with profuse phlegm, chest oppression, hypochondriac pain												
Irregular menstruation, breast swelling and pain												
Plum-pit qi												
Chronic pain in the epigastrium												
Damp ulcers												
Poisonous snake bites												
Qi stagnation in the stomach and large intestine												
Edema, beriberi with swelling pain												
Impotence												
Vomiting												
Waist pain due to kidney deficiency												
Impairment of the spleen due to overthinking												
Hiccups												

Chapter 16
Medicinals that Eliminate Food Retention

Concept

Medicinals that have the principal effects of eliminating food retention and treating indigestion are called medicinals that eliminate food retention.

Character and Actions

Medicinals of this kind are mostly sweet in flavor and neutral in property. They mainly enter the spleen and stomach channels. They can remove food retention, invigorate the spleen, promote digestion, and harmonize the middle.

Indications

They are indicated for epigastric and abdominal distension and fullness, belching, sour regurgitation, nausea, vomiting, no appetite, irregular defecation due to food retention; and spleen and stomach weakness due to indigestion.

Combinations

Medicinals in this chapter have a gradual action to promote digestion. Therefore they should be properly combined with the other medicinals according to the patient's pathological condition. Medicinals for regulating qi should be added for cases of food retention with qi stagnation. Medicinals for clearing heat or gently purging should be added for cases of food retention transforming into heat. Aromatic medicinals with actions of transforming damp should be added for cases with cold damp obstruction in the spleen or damp turbidity in the stomach. Medicinals for warming the middle and invigorating the spleen should be added for deficient cold in the middle *jiao*. Medicinals for invigorating the spleen and replenishing qi should be added for cases of congenital weakness in the spleen and stomach and food retention, so as to treat both the root and branch.

Precautions

Although medicinals that eliminate food retention generally have moderate actions, they can consume qi. Therefore, they should be given cautiously to patients with qi deficiency without food retention.

① *Shān zhā* (山楂, Fructus Crataegi, Hawthorn Fruit) ★ ★ ★

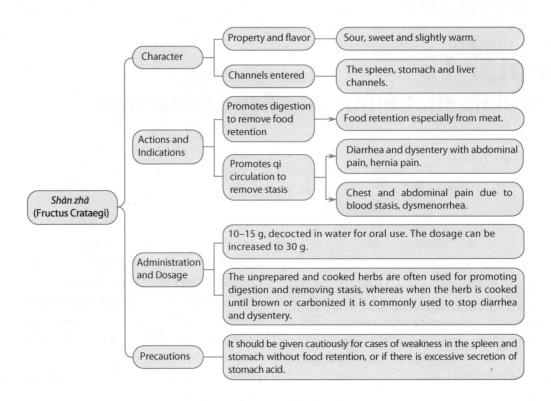

② *Shén qū* (神曲, Massa Medicata Fermentata, Medicated Leaven) ★ ★ ★

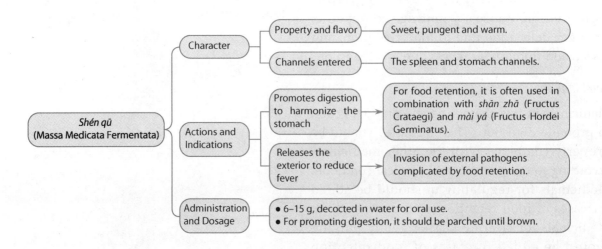

③ *Mài yá* (麦芽, Fructus Hordei Germinatus, Germinated Barley) ★★★

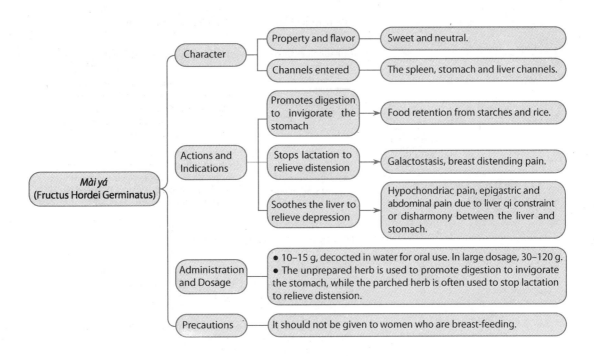

④ *Gǔ yá* (谷芽, Fructus Setariae Germinatus, Grain Sprout) ★

Addition: *Dào yá* (稻芽, **Fructus Oryzae Germinatus, Rice Grain Sprout)** is similar to *gǔ yá* (Fructus Setariae Germinatus) in the character, actions, indications, administration and dosage .

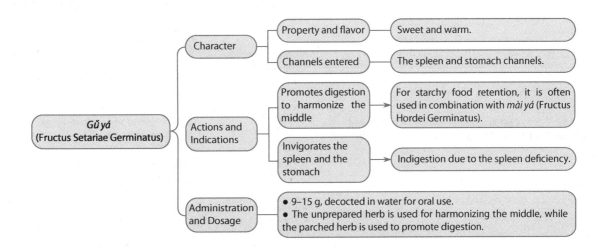

⑤ *Lái fú zǐ* (莱菔子, Semen Raphani, Radish Seed)
★★

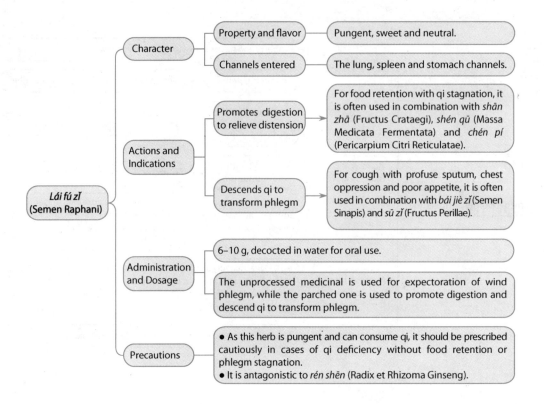

⑥ *Jī nèi jīn* (鸡内金, Endothelium Corneum Gigeriae Galli, Chicken's Gizzard-skin) ★★★

Shān zhā (Fructus Crataegi), *shén qū* (Massa Medicata Fermentata), *mài yá* (Fructus Hordei Germinatus), *dào yá* (Fructus Oryzae Germinatus), *gǔ yá* (Fructus Setariae Germinatus), *lái fú zǐ*

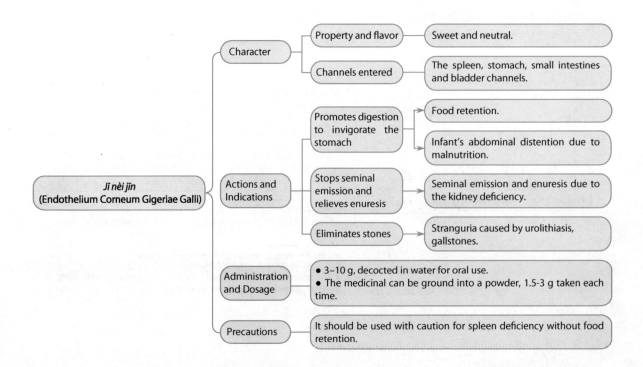

(Semen Raphani) and *jī nèi jīn* (Endothelium Corneum Gigeriae Galli) enter the spleen and stomach channels, and can promote digestion to remove food retention. They are used for food retention manifesting as distending pain in the epigastrium and abdomen, belching, sour regurgitation, nausea, vomiting, loss of appetite, irregular defecation, and indigestion due to weakness of the spleen and stomach.

Shān zhā (Fructus Crataegi) has a sour and sweet flavor and a slightly warm property, and can strengthen the spleen and stomach to promote digestion. It is considered an essential medicinal to eliminate food retention from meat, and is the first choice whenever there is meat or milk retention. It can also invigorate qi and blood to remove stasis, and is always used for food retention and qi stagnation manifesting as diarrhea or dysentery with abdominal pain, hernia with bearing-down distending pain, testicular swelling pain; chest and abdominal pain, dysmenorrhea, or abdominal pain post-partum due to blood stasis. *Shén qū* (Massa Medicata Fermentata) is sweet and pungent in flavor, and warm in property. It can promote digestion to remove food retention as well as invigorate the spleen and stomach to harmonize the middle. It is often selected for flour and grain retention, and impairment of the middle due to food retention. It can also relieve the exterior, and therefore is suitable to treat food retention complicated by an exterior syndrome. In addition, it can help the digestion and absorption of medicinals that are made of metal, stone, or shell, it can be used as a paste in pills with these type of medicinals. *Mài yá* (Fructus Hordei Germinatus) is sweet and neutral, and is effective for promoting the digestion of starches. It can strengthen the stomach to harmonize the middle, and therefore is suitable to treat indigestion due to weakness of the spleen and stomach. It can also stop lactation to relieve distention and soothe the liver to relieve depression. It is used for delactation of breast-feeding women or for distention and pain due to delactation; and liver qi constraint and disharmony between the liver and stomach. *Dào yá* (Fructus Oryzae

Germinatus) is similar to *mài yá* (Fructus Hordei Germinatus) in the action of promoting digestion and strengthening the stomach, but is more moderate. These two medicinals are often used in combination for mutual reinforcement. However, *dào yá* (Fructus Oryzae Germinatus) cannot stop lactation or soothe the liver. *Gǔ yá* (Fructus Setariae Germinatus) is usually used in the north area of China, and is similar to *dào yá* (Fructus Oryzae Germinatus). *Lái fú zǐ* (Semen Raphani), is pungent and sweet in flavor, and neutral in property. It is effective for promoting qi circulation and digestion to relieve distension. It is usually used for food retention and qi stagnation in the middle *jiao* with manifestations such as distending pain in the epigastrium and abdomen, belching, and sour regurgitation. It can also descend qi to transform phlegm, and is commonly used for phlegm-fluids retention in the lung, manifesting as cough with dyspnea, profuse sputum and chest oppression, complicated by food retention. *Jī nèi jīn* (Endothelium Corneum Gigeriae Galli) is sweet in flavor and neutral in property. It has strong actions for promoting digestion and removing food retention. It can also invigorate the spleen and stomach, and is used extensively for accumulation of various foods, indigestion, and a malnutrition induced distended abdomen in infants. It can also stop seminal emission, relieve enuresis, eliminate stones (relieve stranguria to eliminate stones), and is used for kidney deficiency with seminal emission, spermatorrhea, enuresis, and frequent urination; stranguria caused by urolithiasis, and gallstones.

⑦ *Jī shǐ téng* (鸡矢藤, Herba Paederiae, Chinese Fevervine Herb)

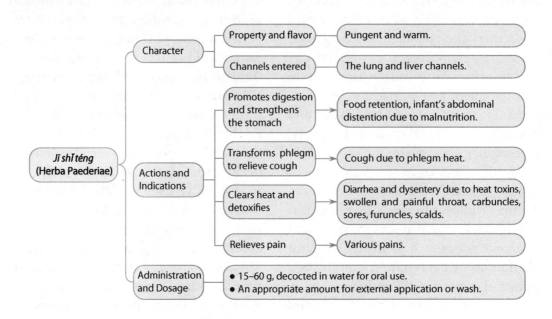

⑧ *Gé shān xiāo* (隔山消, Radix Cynanchi Wilfordii, Wilford Swallowwort Root)

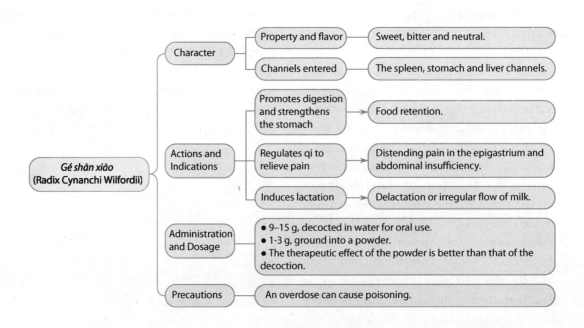

⑨ *Ā wèi* (阿魏, Resina Ferulae, Chinese Asafoetida)

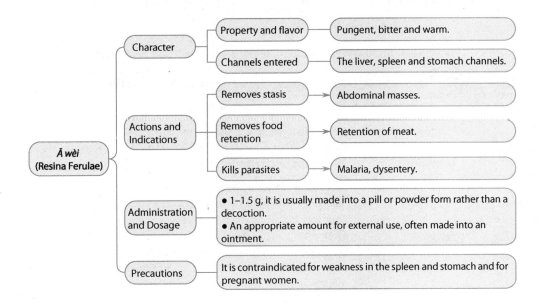

Actions of medicinals that eliminate food retention are summarized in the following table (Table 16-1):

Table 16-1: Summary of Medicinals that Eliminate Food Retention:

Medicinal	Action in Common	Individual Character	
		Characteristic Actions	Other Actions
Shān zhā (Fructus Crataegi)	Promotes digestion to remove food retention	Strengthens the spleen and stomach to promote digestion, effective and essential for eliminating food retention from meat.	Promotes qi circulation and activates blood to remove stasis
Shén qū (Massa Medicata Fermentata)		Invigorates the spleen and stomach to harmonize the middle, effective for eliminating flour and grain food retention. Relieves exterior syndromes, suitable to treat diseases caused by food retention complicated by exterior syndromes. Helps digestion and absorption of medicinals made of metal, stone and shell.	
Mài yá (Fructus Hordei Germinatus)		It is effective for eliminating starchy food retention. Strengthens the stomach to harmonize the middle, suitable to treat diseases caused by starchy food retention.	Stops lactation to relieve distension, soothes the liver to relieve depression
Dào yá (Fructus Oryzae Germinatus)		Similar action in promoting digestion and invigorating the spleen to *mài yá* (Fructus Hordei Germinatus).	
Gǔ yá (Fructus Setariae Germinatus)		With similar actions and indications to *dào yá* (Fructus Setariae Germinatus). Often used in North China.	
Lái fú zǐ (Semen Raphani)		It is effective for promoting qi circulation and promoting digestion to relieve distension, suitable for food digestion with qi stagnation in the middle *jiao*.	Descends qi to transform phlegm
Jī nèi jīn (Endothelium Corneum Gigeriae Galli)		It has a strong action in promoting digestion to remove food retention. Invigorates the spleen and stomach, extensively used for food retention. An essential medicinal to promote digestion and invigorate the spleen and to treat infant's abdominal distention due to malnutrition.	Stops seminal emission, relieves enuresis, eliminates stones
Jī shǐ téng (Herba Paederiae)			Strengthens the stomach, transforms phlegm to relieve cough, clears heat and detoxifies, relieves pain
Gé shān xiāo (Radix Cynanchi Wilfordii)			Strengthens the stomach, regulates qi to relieve pain, induces lactation
Ā wèi (Resina Ferulae)			Removes stasis, eliminates food retention, kills parasites

Tables for testing your herbal knowledge of the actions and indications of medicinals that eliminate food retention are as follows (Tables 16-2 and 16-3):

Table 16-2: Test your Herbal Knowledge of the Actions of Medicinals that Eliminate Food Retention:

Actions / Medicinal	Shān zhā	Shén qū	Mài yá	Gǔ yá	Jī nèi jīn	Jī shǐ téng	Lái fú zǐ
Promotes digestion to remove food retention							
Stops seminal emission and relieves enuresis							
Promotes qi circulation to remove stasis							
Induces lactation to relieve distention							
Descends qi to transform phlegm							
Promotes qi circulation to relieve distension							
Promotes digestion and strengthens the stomach							
Transforms phlegm to relieve cough							
Clears heat and detoxifies							
Relieves pain							

Table 16-3: Test your Herbal Knowledge of the Indications of Medicinals that Eliminate Food Retention:

Indications / Medicinal	Shān zhā	Shén qū	Mài yá	Gǔ yá	Jī nèi jīn	Jī shǐ téng	Lái fú zǐ
Food retention from meat							
Liver qi constraint							
Hernia with pain							
Chest pain, abdominal pain, and dysmenorrhea due to blood stasis							
Food accumulation							
Stranguria caused by urolithiasis, gallstones							
Delactation of breast-feeding, distending pain of the breasts							
Diarrhea and dysentery with abdominal pain							
Poor appetite due to spleen deficiency							
Food retention with qi stagnation							
Cough with dyspnea and profuse sputum, chest oppression, poor appetite							
Stomachache, intestinal pain, biliary colic							
Enuresis and seminal emission due to kidney deficiency							
Food retention of starches							
Cough due to phlegm heat							
Diarrhea and dysentery due to heat toxin, swollen and painful throat							
Suppurating infections on the surface of the body, scalds							
Infant's distended abdomen due to malnutrition							
Renal colic, dysmenorrhea, labor pain, neuralgia							

Chapter 17
Medicinals that Expel Worms

Concept

Medicinals whose principal effect is to expel or kill worms and treat worm induced syndromes are called medicinals that expel worms.

Character, effects, and indications

Medicinals in this chapter enter the spleen, stomach and large intestine channels. Some of the medicinals are toxic. This toxicity can kill or anesthetize worms inside the human body, especially in the intestines, and promote their discharge. They are used for various types of intestinal worms, such as ascariasis, enterobiasis, cestodiasis, ancylostomiasis and intestinal distomiasis. Some of the medicinals can even kill worms in other parts of the body, such as trichomonas vaginalis and schistosomiasis.

Combinations

Medicinals that expel worms should be chosen based upon the type of worm infestation, the patients' constitution, and other pathological conditions. They should be combined with medicinals that have actions to treat different complications. Medicinals for purging downwards should be added in cases with constipation. Medicinals for eliminating food retention should be added for cases complicated by food retention. Medicinals with the actions of invigorating the spleen and stomach should be added in cases of weakness of the spleen and stomach. If the patient has a weak constitution, one should use tonification or simultaneous tonification and purgation, rather than just purgation. Medicinals for expelling worms are often used in combination with medicinals for purging downwards so as to promote the discharge of worms.

Precautions

Medicinals that expel worms can often consume the right qi. Their dosage should be controlled to prevent poisoning or the consumption of right qi. They should be prescribed cautiously for those who have a weak constitution, are elderly, or are pregnant. Medicinals for expelling worms are generally taken on an empty stomach in order to ensure the best therapeutic effect. In cases with fever or acute abdominal pain, medicinals with the effect of expelling worms should be given after the primary accompanying symptoms are relieved.

① *Shǐ jūn zǐ* (使君子, Fructus Quisqualis, Rangooncreeper Fruit) ★★★

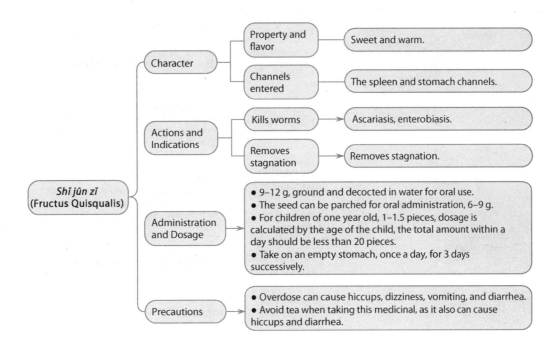

② *Kǔ liàn pí* (苦楝皮, Cortex Meliae, Szechwan Chinaberry Bark) ★★★

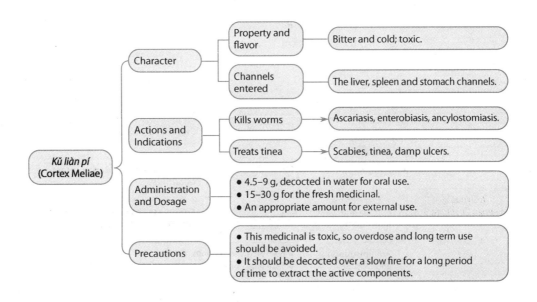

③ *Bīng láng* (槟榔, Semen Arecae, Betel Nut) ★ ★ ★

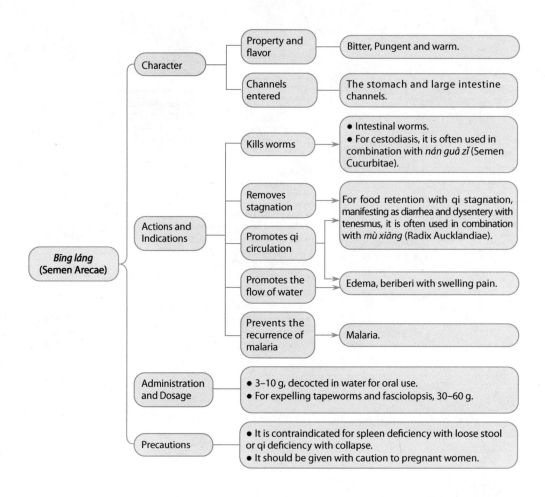

④ *Nán guā zǐ* (南瓜子, Semen Cucurbitae, Pumpkin Seed and Husk) ★ ★ ★

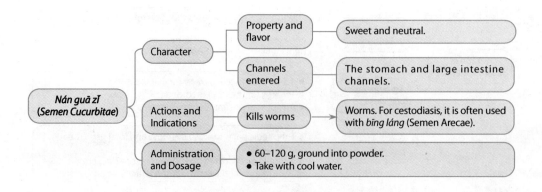

⑤ *Hè cǎo yá* (鹤草芽, Herba et Gemma Agrimoniae, Hairyvein Agrimonia Herb and Bud) ★★

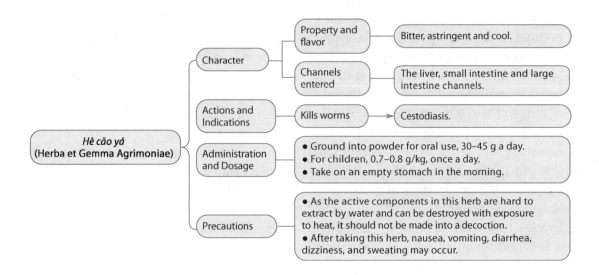

⑥ *Léi wán* (雷丸, Omphalia, Thunder Ball) ★★

Shǐ jūn zǐ (Fructus Quisqualis), *bīng láng* (Semen Arecae), *kǔ liàn pí* (Cortex Meliae), *léi wán* (Omphalia) and *guàn zhòng* (Rhizoma Cyrtomii) can kill roundworms, pinworms and hookworms, and are commonly used to treat infestations with these worms. *Shǐ jūn zǐ* (Fructus Quisqualis) has a sweet flavor and a warm property and can kill worms as well as invigorate the spleen and stomach and remove a malnutrition induced distended abdomen. It has a sweet taste and pleasant odor, so it is often used to treat ascariasis

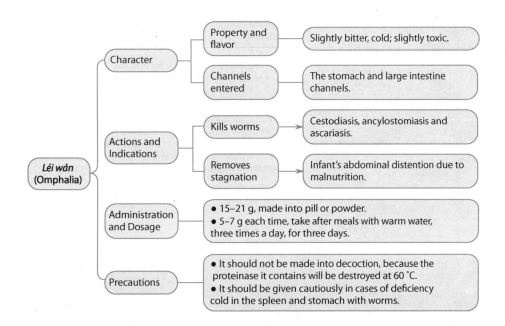

and enterobiasis in children. It is also used for a malnutrition induced distended abdomen in infants, manifesting in a yellowish complexion, abdominal pain due to worms, emaciation, and an enlarged abdomen. *Kǔ liàn pí* (Cortex Meliae) is bitter, cold, and toxic. It has a strong action to kill worms, and is effective for killing roundworms. It can treat tinea, scabies and damp ulcers when applied externally. *Bīng láng* (Semen Arecae) is pungent and bitter in flavor, warm in property, and has a descending action. It can kill worms, especially tapeworm, as well as promote defecation gradually, which helps with the discharge of worms. It can promote qi circulation, remove stagnation, promote the flow of water, and prevent the recurrence of malaria. Therefore, it is used for food retention with qi stagnation manifesting as abdominal pain and constipation; diarrhea, dysentery, tenesmus due to damp heat;

edema with distension and fullness, beriberi with swelling pain; and malaria. *Léi wán* (Omphalia) is the most effective in killing tapeworms even when used alone. It can also remove stagnation and is used for a malnutrition induced distended abdomen in infants. *Guàn zhòng* (Rhizoma Cyrtomii) is bitter in flavor and slightly cold in property. It can clear heat, detoxify, cool blood, and stop bleeding. It is often used for common cold of a wind heat type, maculae due to warmth toxin, mumps, and hemorrhage due to blood heat, manifesting as hematemesis, epistaxis, hematuria, metrorrhagia and metrostaxis. It is most effective in treating metrorrhagia and metrostaxis (abnormal uterine bleeding and menstrual spotting).

⑦ *Hè shī* (鹤虱, Fructus Carpesii, Common Carpesium Fruit) ★★

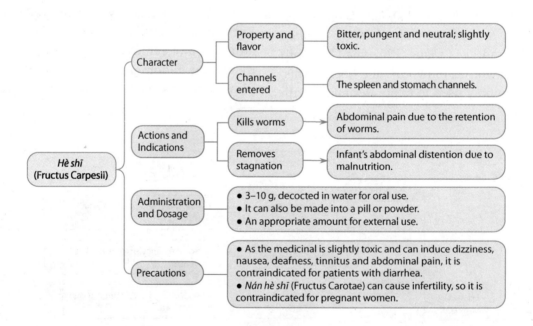

⑧ *Fěi zǐ* (榧子, Semen Torreyae, Grand Torreya
   Seed) ★★

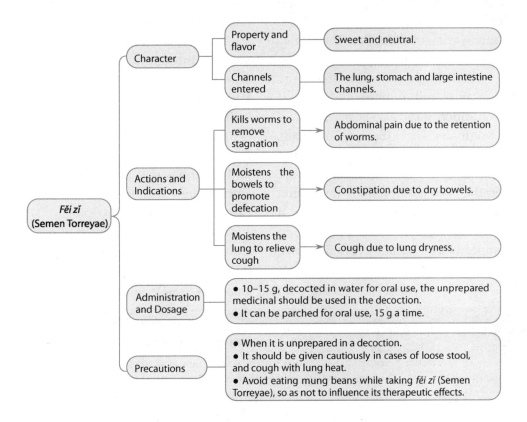

⑨ *Wú yí* (芜荑, Fructus Ulmi Macrocarpae
   Praeparata, Pasta Ulmi)

Nán guā zǐ (Semen Cucurbitae), *hè cǎo yá* (Radix

Agrimoniae Pilodae), *fěi zǐ* (Semen Torreyae), *hè
shī* (Fructus Carpesii) and *wú yí* (Fructus Ulmi
Macrocarpae Praeparata) can kill worms, and

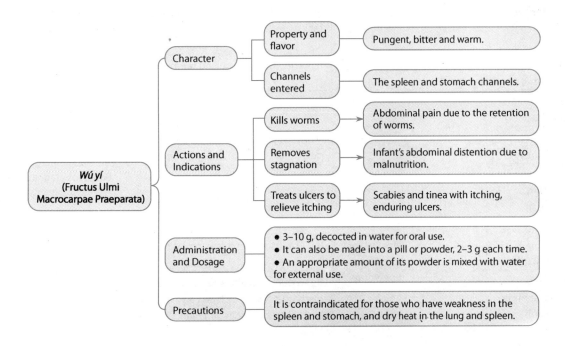

are used for intestinal worms. *Nán guā zǐ* (Semen Cucurbitae) is indicated for cestodiasis. If it is used in a large dosage (120-200g) over a long period of time, it can also treat schistosomiasis. *Hè cǎo yá* (Radix Agrimoniae Pilodae) is effective for killing tapeworms as well as purging downwards, which helps with the discharge of worms. It is an essential medicinal to treat cestodiasis. In addition, it can also be used to treat trichomonas vaginalis. *Fěi zǐ* (Semen Torreyae), is sweet in flavor and neutral in property, and can kill worms without consuming stomach qi. It can moisten the bowels to promote defecation in order to help with the discharge of worms. It is effective for treating abdominal pain due to various intestinal worms such as roundworms, hookworms, tapeworms, and fasciolopsis. It can also moisten the lung to relieve cough, and is used for cough with lung dryness, and constipation due to dryness in the intestines. *Hè shī* (Fructus Carpesii) can be used to treat various intestinal worms such as ascariasis, enterobiasis, ancylostomiasis and cestodiasis. It can remove stagnation to treat malnutrition induced distended abdomen in infants. *Wú yí* (Fructus Ulmi Macrocarpae Praeparata) is used for abdominal pain due to ascariasis, enteriobiasis and cestodiasis. It is ground into a powder for scabies, tinea with itching, and chronic ulcers on the surface of the body.

Actions of medicinals that expel worms are summarized in the following table (Table 17-1):

Table 17-1: Summary of Medicinals that Expel Worms:

Medicinal	Action in Common		Individual Character	
			Characteristic Actions	Other Actions
Shǐ jūn zǐ (Fructus Quisqualis)	Kills worms	Expels or kills worms in the intestines	Invigorates the spleen and stomach, removes abdominal distention due to malnutrition. The sweet taste and pleasant odor makes it easier for children to take. It is especially suitable to treat infant's ascariasis, enterobiasis, and infant's abdominal distention due to malnutrition.	
Kǔ liàn pí (Cortex Meliae)			It is toxic. It has a strong action in killing worms, especially roundworms.	Treats tinea
Bīng láng (Semen Arecae)			Promotes defecation moderately to help with the discharge of worms, especially tapeworms.	Promotes qi circulation, removes stagnation, promotes the flow of water, prevents the recurrence of malaria
Léi wán (Omphalia)			It is effective for expelling tapeworms	Relieves abdominal distention due to malnutrition
Hè shī (Fructus Carpesii)				
Fěi zǐ (Semen Torreyae)			Moistens intestines to promote defecation, helps discharge worms	Moistens the lung to relieve cough
Wú yí (Fructus Ulmi Macrocarpae Praeparata)				Removes stagnation
Nán guā zǐ (Semen Cucurbitae)		Effective for expelling tapeworms	It is also used for schistosomiasis.	
Hè cǎo yá (Herba et Gemma Agrimoniae)			It can purge downwards to promote the discharge of worms. It can also neutralise and kill trichomonas vaginalis.	

Tables to test your herbal knowledge of the actions and indications of medicinals that expel worms are summarized as follows (Tables 17-2 and 17-3):

Table 17-2: Test your Herbal Knowledge of the Actions of Medicinals that Expel Worms:

Actions \ Medicinal	*Shǐ jūn zǐ*	*Kǔ liàn pí*	*Bīng láng*	*Nán guā zǐ*	*Hè cǎo yá*	*Léi wán*	*Hè shī*	*Fěi zǐ*	*Wú yí*
Expels worms to remove retention									
Moistens the lung									
Promotes qi circulation and drains water									
Kills worms									
Loosens the bowels									
Treats tinea									

Table 17-3: Test your Herbal Knowledge of the Indications of Medicinals that Expel Worms:

Indications \ Medicinal	*Shǐ jūn zǐ*	*Kǔ liàn pí*	*Bīng láng*	*Nán guā zǐ*	*Hè cǎo yá*	*Léi wán*	*Hè shī*	*Fěi zǐ*	*Wú yí*
Cestodiasis									
Enterobiasis									
Infant's abdominal distention due to malnutrition									
Schistosomiasis									
Scabies, tinea, damp ulcers									
Ascariasis									
Food retention with qi stagnation, diarrhea and dysentery with tenesmus									
Edema									
Beriberi with swelling pain									
Ancylostomiasis									
Trichomonas vaginalis									
Constipation due to intestinal dryness									
Cough due to lung dryness									
Malaria									

Chapter 18
Medicinals that Stop Bleeding

Concept

Medicinals that stop various types of bleeding, internally or externally, and treat hemorrhage are called medicinals that stop bleeding.

Character and Actions

Medicinals of this kind enter the *xue* level and enter the heart, liver and spleen channels, but mainly the heart and liver channels. As such medicinals have different characteristics, they also have different actions of cooling blood and stopping bleeding, warming the channels to stop bleeding, transforming stasis to stop bleeding, or astringing to stop bleeding.

Classification

According to their different characters and actions, medicinals in this chapter are classified into four different categories: Medicinals for cooling blood and stopping bleeding, medicinals for warming the channels to stop bleeding, medicinals for transforming stasis to stop bleeding, and medicinals for astringing to stop bleeding.

Indications

Medicinals for stopping bleeding are indicated for various bleeding both internally and externally, such as hemoptysis, hematemesis, epistaxis, hematuria, hemafecia, metrorrhagia and metrostaxis, purpura and bleeding due to trauma.

Combinations

Medicinals that stop bleeding must be chosen based on the cause of bleeding, pathological conditions, and disease location. They should be used in combination with other medicinals if necessary, so as to treat both the root and branch. For example, for bleeding due to blood heat, medicinals for cooling blood and stopping bleeding should be used in combination with medicinals for clearing heat and purging fire or clearing heat and cooling blood. For bleeding due to fire hyperactivity with yin deficiency and yang hyperactivity with yin deficiency, the medicinals should be combined with those that nourish yin and descend fire or nourish yin to suppress yang. For bleeding due to failure of the blood to travel within the vessels resulting from blood stasis obstruction in the interior, these medicinals should be combined with those that transform blood to stop bleeding, and those that promote qi circulation, and activate the blood. For bleeding of a deficiency cold type, medicinals with the actions of warming the channels to stop bleeding, or astringing to stop bleeding should be combined with medicinals for replenishing qi, invigorating the spleen and warming yang. Ancient physicians believed that to treat hematuria and bloody stool, metrorrhagia and metrostaxis, the principle of lifting qi had to be used, whereas for hematemesis and epistaxis, the principle of descending the qi had to be used. Therefore, for bleeding in the lower part of the body, such as hematuria, metrorrhagia and metrostaxis, medicinals with the actions of elevating and ascending should be used; while for bleeding in the upper part of the body such as epistaxis and hematemesis, medicinals for descending qi should be added.

Precautions

When using medicinals that can stop bleeding, one must pay attention not to engender blood stasis while stopping bleeding. Medicinals for cooling blood and stopping bleeding, and astringing to stop bleeding, can also cause blood stasis, so they are not recommended to be used alone in cases of bleeding accompanied by stasis. For excessive bleeding followed by exhaustion of qi, medicinals for supplementing qi should be used for treating critical symptoms.

According to experiences handed down from ancient physicians, medicinals that are used to stop bleeding are often used after they have been carbonized. Generally speaking, after a medicinal is carbonized, it has a bitter and astringent flavor, which is believed to enhance its actions to stop blood. However, all medicinals for stopping bleeding do not necessarily need to be carbonized. Some of them may have a decreased effect of stopping bleeding when they are carbonized. Therefore, whether or not a medicinal should be carbonized depends on its character, function, and the disease it is used to treat. Simply put, the general principle is to enhance the therapeutic actions of the medicinal.

Section 1 Medicinals that Cool Blood and Stop Bleeding

Medicinals in this section are usually cold or cool in property, and sweet and bitter in flavor. They can clear and purge heat in the blood to stop bleeding, and are indicated for various types of bleeding due to blood heat.

① *Xiǎo jì* (小蓟, Herba Cirsii, Field Thistle Herb) ★ ★ ★

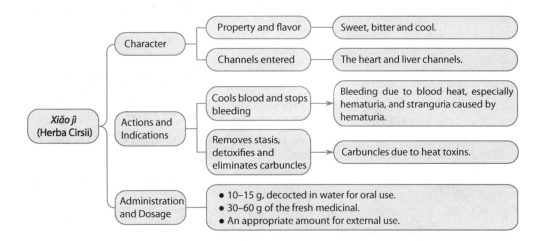

② *Dà jì* (大蓟, Herba seu Radix Cirsii Japonici, Japanese Thistle Herb and Root) ★ ★

Dà jì (Herba seu Radix Cirsii Japonici) and *xiǎo jì* (Herba Cirsii) were initially recorded in *Part* *Record of Famous Physicians.* At that time they were believed to be one medicinal because of their similar descriptions and functions. Then, in the period of the *Classified Materia Medica*

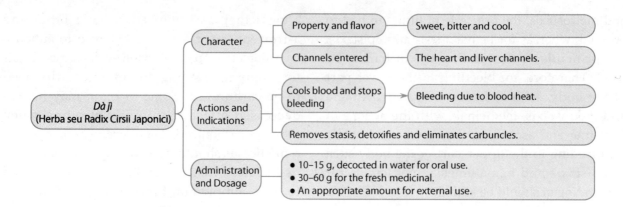

from *Historical Classics for Emergency*, the *Materia Medica for Famine Relief* and the *Compendium of Materia Medica*, they are distinguished separately and used as two different medicinals. *Dà jì* (Herba seu Radix Cirsii Japonici) and *xiǎo jì* (Herba Cirsii) are bitter and sweet in flavor, cool in property and enter the heart and liver channels. They can cool blood and stop bleeding, transform stasis, detoxify and eliminate carbuncles. They are used in combination for various types of bleeding due to blood heat, such as hemoptysis, hematemesis, epistaxis, hematuria, metrorrhagia and metrostaxis; and carbuncles resulting from heat toxins. Clinically, the two are commonly used for mutual reinforcement. *Dà jì* (Herba seu Radix Cirsii Japonici) has stronger actions in removing stasis, detoxifying and eliminating carbuncles compared with *xiǎo jì* (Herba Cirsii). It also has extensive hemostatic actions, so it is suitable to treat hematemesis, hemoptysis, metrorrhagia and metrostaxis. *Xiǎo jì* (Herba Cirsii) can induce diuresis, and it is often used to treat hematuria and stranguria caused by hematuria.

③ *Dì yú* (地榆, Radix Sanguisorbae, Garden Burnet Root) ★ ★ ★

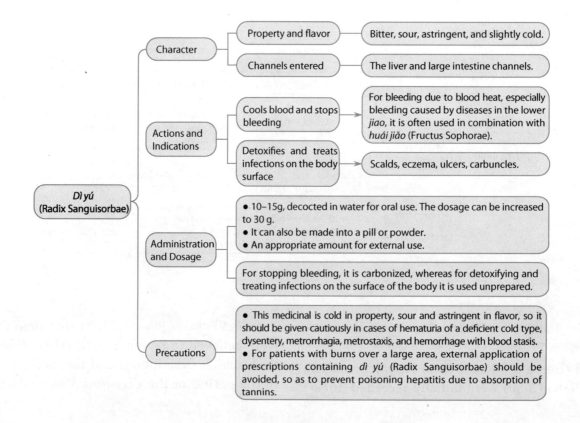

④ *Huái huā* (槐花, Flos Sophorae, Pagodatree Flower) ★ ★

Addition: ***Huái jiǎo*** (槐角, **Fructus Sophorae, Japanese Pagoda Tree Pod**) is similar to *huái huā* (Flos Sophorae) in the character, effects and indications, but it is inferior to *huái huā* (Flos Sophorae) in stopping blood. It has a stronger action in clearing and purging heat. It can moisten the intestines, and is mainly used for hemorrhoids with bleeding, hemafecia, and especially for hemorrhoids with bleeding and swelling pain.

Both *dì yú* (Radix Sanguisorbae) and *huái huā* (Flos Sophorae) are bitter in flavor and slightly cold in property. They enter the liver and large intestine channels, and can cool blood and stop bleeding. The two medicinals are used in combination for various types of bleeding due to blood heat manifesting as hemoptysis, hematemesis, epistaxis, bloody stools, hemorrhoids with bleeding, dysentery with bloody discharge, metrorrhagia, and metrostaxis. They are especially suitable to treat bleeding from blood heat in the lower *jiao*, such as bloody stools, hemorrhoids with bleeding, dysentery with bloody discharge, metrorrhagia, and metrostaxis. *Dì yú* (Radix Sanguisorbae) has a sour flavor, and can detoxify and treat infections on the surface of the body. It is used externally for scalds, burns, eczema, ulcerated skin, and skin diseases. It is an essential medicinal to treat scalds and burns. However, for patients with burns over a large area, external application of prescriptions containing *dì yú* (Radix Sanguisorbae) should be avoided, so as to prevent poisoning hepatitis due to the absorption of tannins. *Huái huā* (Flos Sophorae) is able to clear liver fire and reduce blood pressure. It can be used for blood-shot eyes, distension in the head, headache, dizziness, and hypertension from liver fire hyperactivity. Its character, effects and indications are similar to *huái huā* (Flos Sophorae), but it is inferior to *huái huā* (Flos Sophorae) in stopping blood. It has a stronger action in clearing and purging heat. It can moisten the intestines, and is mainly used for hemorrhoids with bleeding, bloody stools, and especially for hemorrhoids with bleeding and swelling pain.

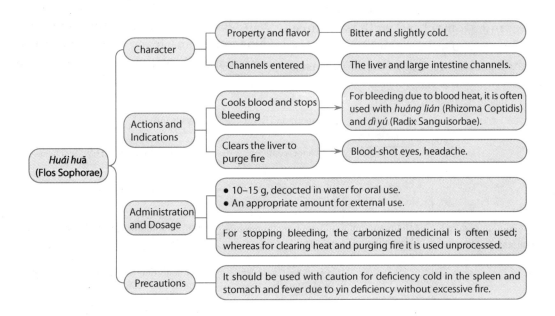

⑤ *Cè bǎi yè* (侧柏叶, Cacumen Platycladi, Oriental Arborvitae Leafy Twig) ★★

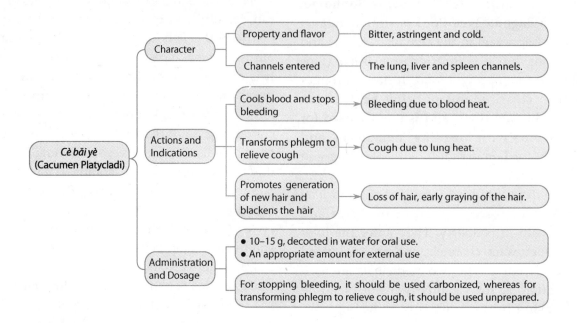

⑥ *Bái máo gēn* (白茅根, Rhizoma Imperatae, White Grass) ★★

Lú gēn (Rhizoma Phragmitis) and *bái máo gēn* (Rhizoma Imperatae) are sweet in flavor and cold in property. They enter the lung and stomach channels to clear and purge accumulated heat in the lung and stomach as well as induce diuresis. They are used in combination for mutual reinforcement to treat febrile diseases with vexation and thirst, cough due to lung heat, vomiting due to stomach heat and stranguria caused by pathogenic heat. *Lú gēn* (Rhizoma Phragmitis) mainly acts in the qi level, and is effective for clearing heat, purging fire and promoting fluid production to relieve thirst. It can clear and purge accumulated heat in the lung and stomach and therefore is considered an essential medicinal to treat pulmonary abscesses.

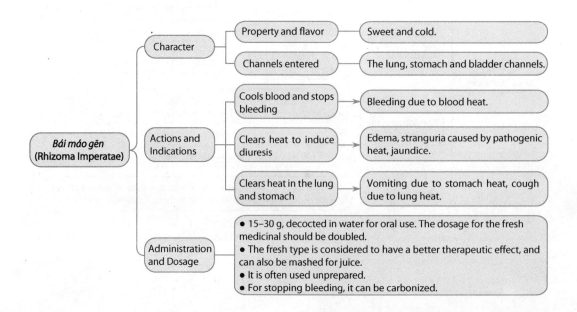

It is often used for pulmonary abscesses with purulent expectoration, cough due to lung heat and vomiting due to stomach heat. *Bái máo gēn* (Rhizoma Imperatae) acts mainly to remove heat in the blood to cool blood and stop bleeding. It also enters the bladder channel, and therefore has a better effect in clearing heat to induce diuresis than *lú gēn* (Rhizoma Phragmitis). It is often used for various types of bleeding due to blood heat, stranguria caused by pathogenic heat, edema, and jaundice of damp heat type.

⑦ *Zhù má gēn* (苎麻根, Radix Boehmeriae, Ramie Root) ★

Both *zhù má gēn* (Radix Boehmeriae) and *huáng qín* (Radix Scutellariae) are cold in property, and can clear heat to prevent miscarriage, cool blood, stop bleeding, and detoxify. They can be used for excessive fetal movement and vaginal bleeding during pregnancy due to heat accumulation; hemoptysis, hematemesis, epstaxis, hematuria,

metrorrhagia, metrostaxis and purpura due to blood heat and carbuncles caused by heat toxins. *Zhù má gēn* (Radix Boehmeriae), is sweet and cold, and has a more moderate action. It is effective for cooling blood and stopping bleeding, and is often used for bleeding due to blood heat, especially for vaginal bleeding during pregnancy, metrorrhagia, metrostaxis, and hematuria. *Huáng qín* (Radix Scutellariae), is bitter and cold and has a stronger action. It can clear heat and dry damp, purge fire, detoxify, and clear lung heat. It is often used for jaundice, diarrhea, dysentery, leukorrhagia, eczema, and damp ulcers due to damp heat; damp-warmth in the early stage with fever, chest oppression, no appetite, lung heat with cough; febrile diseases with vexation and thirst; and seasonal febrile disease with pathogenic invasion in the *shao yang*, manifesting as alternate chills and fever, chest and hypochondria discomfort, bitter taste in the mouth, dry throat and dizziness.

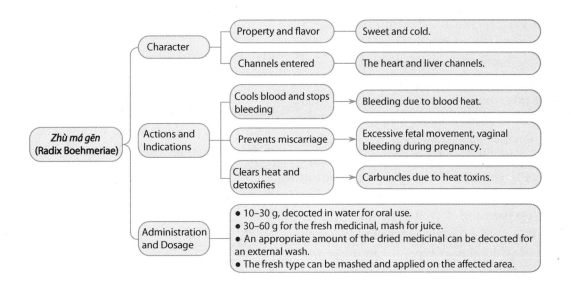

⑧ *Yáng tí* (羊蹄, Radix Rumicis Japonici, Japanese Dock Root)

Bái máo gēn (Rhizoma Imperatae), *zhù má gēn* (Radix Boehmeriae), *cè bǎi yè* (Cacumen Platycladi) and *yáng tí* (Radix Rumicis Japonici) are cold or cool in property, and can cool blood and stop bleeding. They can be used for various

types of bleeding due to blood heat such as hemoptysis, hematemesis, epistaxis, hematuria, bloody stools, metrorrhagia, and metrostaxis. *Bái máo gēn* (Rhizoma Imperatae), is sweet and cold, and can clear heat to induce diuresis to guide heat downwards. It is effective for treating hematuria and stranguria caused by pathogenic heat due to

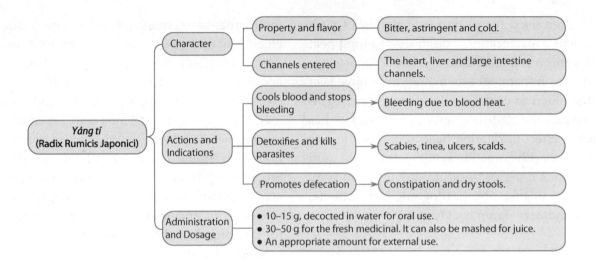

damp heat accumulated in the bladder. It is also used for stranguria due to heat, edema, dysuria, and jaundice due to damp heat. In addition, *bái máo gēn* (Rhizoma Imperatae) can clear and purge heat in the lung and stomach, and is used for febrile diseases with vexation and thirst, cough due to lung heat, and vomiting due to stomach heat. *Zhù má gēn* (Radix Boehmeriae) has a sweet flavor and a cold property, and is suitable for treating metrorrhagia, metrostaxis and excessive menstrual bleeding. It can clear heat to prevent miscarriage and detoxify, and is used for excessive fetal movement, vaginal bleeding during pregnancy caused by heat accumulation; and carbuncles due to heat toxins. *Cè bǎi yè* (Cacumen Platycladi) is bitter and astringent in flavor and slightly cold in property. It can cool blood to stop bleeding as well as astringe to stop bleeding. It is used for various types of bleeding especially of a blood heat type. It can transform phlegm to relieve cough, promote generation of hair and blacken the hair, and therefore is used for cough with excessive sputum due to lung heat; loss of hair and early graying of the hair due to blood heat. *Yáng tí* (Radix Rumicis Japonici) can detoxify to kill parasites and promotes defecation. It can be used to treat scabies, tinea, ulcers, scalds, constipation, and dry stools. Its action of promoting defecation to purge heat is similar to that of *dà huáng* (Radix et Rhizoma Rhei) but is more moderate, therefore it is also

known as "*tǔ dà huáng*".

Section 2   Medicinals that Transform Stasis to Stop Bleeding

Medicinals in this section cannot only stop bleeding, but can also transform stasis. They are characterized by being able to stop bleeding without retaining blood stasis. They are indicated for bleeding caused by blood stasis and obstruction in the interior leading to a failure of blood circulating within the vessels. They can also be used for bleeding of other types if combined properly in accordance with different syndromes.

① *Sān qī* (三七, Radix et Rhizoma Notoginseng, Sanchi) ★★★

Sān qī (Radix et Rhizoma Notoginseng), *jú yè sān qī* (菊叶三七, Radix Gynura, Gynura Root) and *jǐng tiān sān qī* (景天三七, Herba Sedi Aizoon, Aizoon Stonecrop Herb) can transform stasis to stop blood, and reduce swelling to relieve pain. They are used for hemoptysis, hematemesis, epistaxis, hematuria, bloody stools, metrorrhagia, metrostaxis, injuries due to trauma, and swelling pains due to stagnation. They are especially suitable to treat bleeding complicated by blood stasis. *Sān qī* (Radix et Rhizoma Notoginseng)

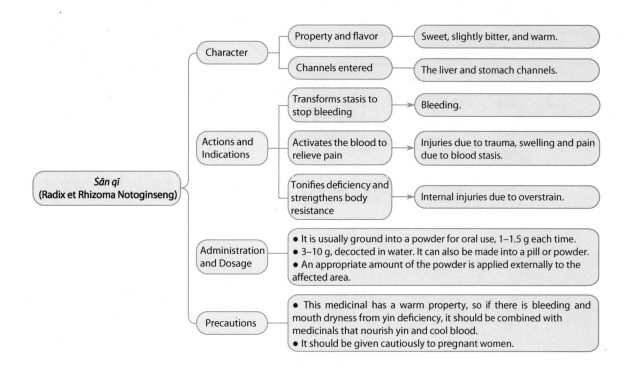

is the dried root of *Panax notoginseng* (Burk.) T. H. Chen, of the family Araliaceae. It has strong actions in transforming stasis to stop bleeding and activating blood to reduce swelling and relieve pain. It is commonly used in clinic to stop bleeding, treat injuries due to trauma, and alleviate pain. *Jú yè sān qī* (Radix Gynura) is the dried root and leaf of *Gynura segetum* (Lour.) Merr., of the family Compositae. It can detoxify to reduce swelling and is used for suppurating infections on the surface of the body, and breast abscesses. *Jǐng tiān sān qī* (Herba Sedi Aizoon) is the dried root or herb of *Sedum aizoon* L., or *S. kamtschaticum* Fisch., of the family Crassulaceae. It is capable of nourishing blood to tranquilize the mind, and is used to treat palpitations, insomnia, and restlessness.

② *Qiàn cǎo* (茜草, Radix et Rhizoma Rubiae, Indian Madder Root) ★ ★ ★

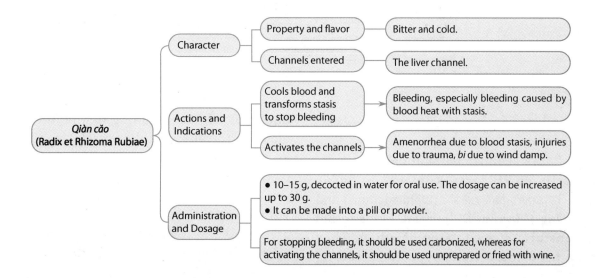

③ *Pú huáng* (蒲黄, Pollen Typhae, Cattail Pollen) ★ ★

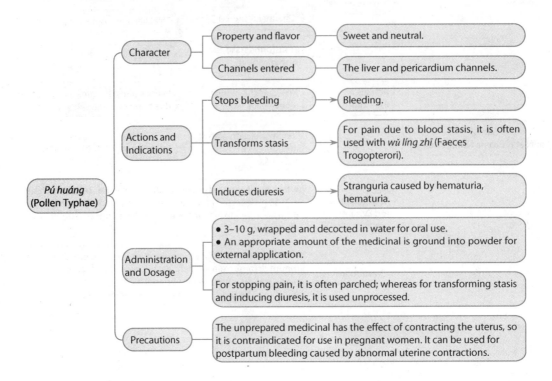

④ *Huā ruǐ shí* (花蕊石, Ophicalcitum, Ophicalcite)

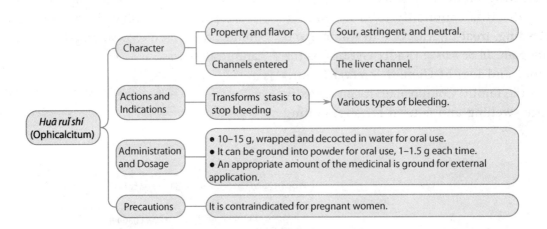

⑤ *Jiàng xiāng* (降香, Lignum Dalbergiae Odoriferae, Rosewood)

Sān qī (Radix et Rhizoma Notoginseng), *qiàn cǎo* (Radix et Rhizoma Rubiae), *pú huáng* (Pollen Typhae), *huā ruǐ shí* (Ophicalcitum) and *jiàng xiāng* (Lignum Dalbergiae Odoriferae) can transform stasis to stop bleeding. They can be used for various types of bleeding due to blood stasis leading to a failure of the blood to travel inside the vessels, manifesting as hemoptysis, hematemesis, epistaxis, metrorrhagia and metrostaxis. These medicinals are all characterized by stopping bleeding without retaining blood stasis, and therefore are suitable to treat bleeding accompanied by stasis and stagnation. *Sān qī* (Radix et Rhizoma

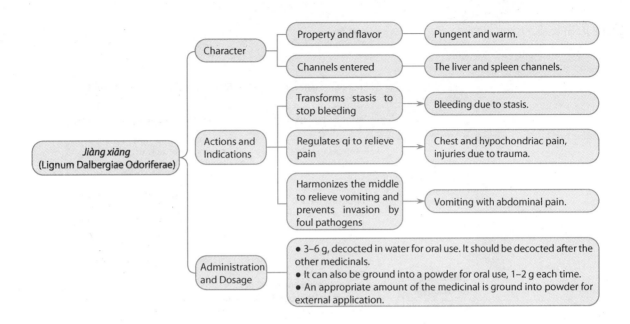

Notoginseng) is sweet and slightly bitter in flavor and warm in property. It has a strong action not only to stop bleeding, but to transform stasis. It is considered an essential medicinal to stop bleeding and is used extensively for bleeding, both internal and externally. It can be used alone to great effect. It is able to activate the blood to relieve pain, and is used for injuries due to trauma, swelling pain due to blood stasis, as well as chest blockage and angina due to blood stasis, and stroke with hemiparalysis. In addition, *sān qī* (Radix et Rhizoma Notoginseng) has the effect of tonifying deficiency, and it is often used for internal injury due to overstrain. *Qiàn cǎo* (Radix et Rhizoma Rubiae) is bitter in flavor and cold in property, and can transform stasis to stop bleeding, cool blood, and stop bleeding. Therefore it is suitable to treat bleeding due to blood heat with stasis. It can activate the channels and is also used for amenorrhea, injuries due to trauma, *bi* due to wind damp. In addition, it is considered an essential medicinal to regulate menstruation. *Pú huáng* (Pollen Typhae) is sweet in flavor and neutral in property. When it is used unprepared, it has a cool property and a slippery action, and can transform stasis to stop bleeding. When parched, it has a warm property, and is able to astringe to stop bleeding. It can be added for bleeding of any kind, but is most suitable

for an excess type with stasis. When it is used externally, it can treat bleeding from injuries due to trauma. It can also transform stasis to relieve pain and induce diuresis to relieve stranguria. It is used for injuries due to trauma, dysmenorrhea, postpartum abdominal pain, pain in the chest and abdomen, stranguria caused by hematuria. *Huā ruǐ shí* (Ophicalcitum) has a pure action in transforming stasis to stop bleeding. When used externally, it can treat bleeding from injuries due to trauma. *Jiàng xiāng* (Lignum Dalbergiae Odoriferae) is pungent in flavor and warm in property, and can regulate qi to relieve pain. It is used for pain in the chest, hypochondria and abdomen due to blood stasis and qi stagnation, injuries due to trauma, swelling pains due to stasis; vomiting, and abdominal pain due to foul turbidity obstruction in the spleen and stomach.

Section 3 Medicinals that Astringe to Stop Bleeding

Medicinals in this section often are astringent in flavor, carbonized or have a sticky nature. Therefore they can astringe to stop bleeding, and are indicated for various types of bleeding without blood stasis.

① *Bái jí* (白及, Rhizoma Bletillae, Bletilla Root) ★★★

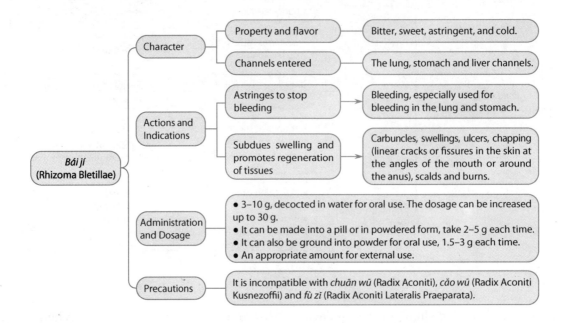

② *Xiān hè cǎo* (仙鹤草, Herba Agrimoniae, Hairy vein Agrimonia Herb) ★

Both *bái jí* (Rhizoma Bletillae) and *xiān hè cǎo* (Herba Agrimoniae) are astringent in flavor and can astringe to stop bleeding. They can be used for various types of bleeding without stasis. *Bái jí* (Rhizoma Bletillae) is astringent and sticky, and therefore has a strong action in stopping bleeding. It is considered an essential medicinal for astringing to stop bleeding. It is used for various types of bleeding internally and externally. Since it enters the lung and stomach channels, it is used especially for hemoptysis, and hematemesis due to pulmonary and stomach injuries. Meanwhile, *bái jí* (Rhizoma Bletillae) can be applied externally to reduce swellings

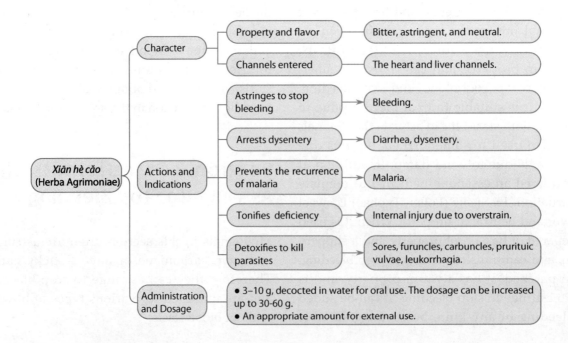

and promote the generation of tissues, and is used for carbuncles, swellings, ulcers, rhagades (linear cracks or fissures in the skin at the angles of the mouth or around the anus), scalds, and burns. *Xiān hè cǎo* (Herba Agrimoniae) is neutral in property, and is widely used for various types of bleeding all over the body of a cold, heat, excess or deficiency type, including hemoptysis, hematemesis, epistaxis, hematuria, hemafecia, metrorrhagia, and metrostaxis. It is able to relieve dysentery, prevent the recurrence of malaria, tonify deficiency, strengthen the body, and detoxify to kill parasites. It is therefore used for chronic diarrhea and dysentery, dysentery with blood; malaria, internal injury due to overstrain with symptoms such as low spirit, lassitude, a yellowish complexion, but with normal appetite; sores, furuncles, carbuncles, and pruritic vulvae due to trichomonas vaginitis.

③ *Zǐ zhū* (紫珠, Folium Callicarpae Formosanae, Taiwan Beautyberry Leaf)

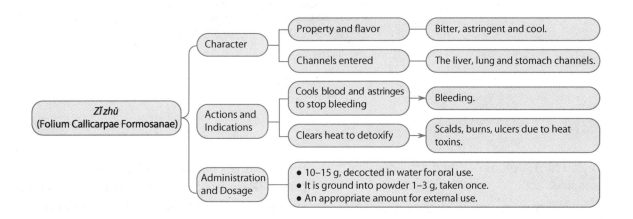

④ *Zōng lǚ tàn* (棕榈炭, Petiolus Trachycarpi, Fortune Windmillpalm Petiole) ★

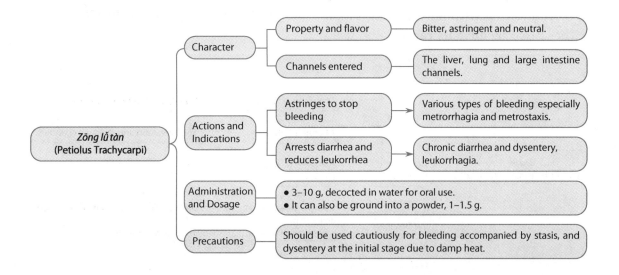

⑤ *Xuè yú tàn* (血余炭, Crinis Carbonisatus, Carbonized Hair) ★

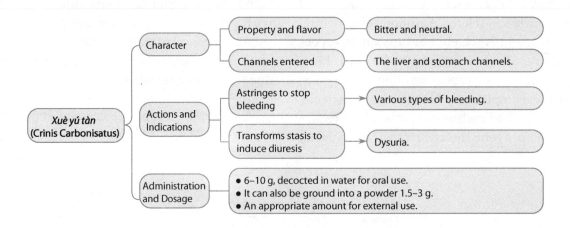

⑥ *Ǒu jié* (藕节, Nodus Nelumbinis Rhizomatis, Lotus Root Node)

Zōng lǔ tàn (Petiolus Trachycarpi), *xuè yú tàn* (Crinis Carbonisatus), *ǒu jié* (Nodus Nelumbinis Rhizomatis) and *zǐ zhū* (Folium Callicarpae Formosanae) have an astringent flavor, and can astringe to stop bleeding. They are used for various types of bleeding without stasis. *Xuè yú tàn* (Crinis Carbonisatus) and *ǒu jié* (Nodus Nelumbinis Rhizomatis) can not only astringe to stop bleeding, but can also transform stasis to stop bleeding. They are characterized by being able to stop bleeding without retaining blood stasis. These two medicinals can also be used for bleeding complicated by blood stasis. *Zōng lǔ tàn* (Petiolus Trachycarpi) has a pure and strong action, and is often used for metrorrhagia, metrostaxis, and excessive menstrual blood. *Xuè yú tàn* (Crinis Carbonisatus) is able to induce diuresis, and can be used to treat dysuria. *Zǐ zhū* (Folium Callicarpae Formosanae) is bitter and astringent in flavor, and cool in property. It can astringe and cool blood to stop bleeding. It is indicated for bleeding internally and externally, especially pulmonary and stomach bleeding. It can also clear heat and detoxify to treat scalds, burns, and ulcers due to heat toxins.

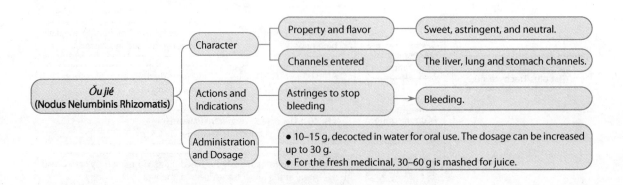

⑦ *Jì mù* (檵木, Flos Loropetali Chinensis, Chinese Loropetalum Flower)

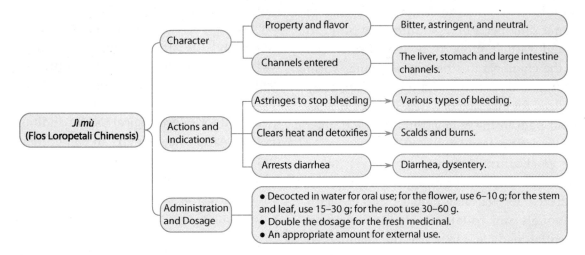

Section 4   Medicinals that Warm Channels to Stop Bleeding

Medicinals in this section are warm or hot in property, and can warm the internal organs, tonify the spleen yang, and consolidate the *chong* to govern and retain blood. They have the effect of warming the channels to stop bleeding, and are indicated for bleeding of a deficiency cold type due to failure of the spleen to govern blood and non-consolidation of the *chong*.

① *Ài yè* (艾叶, Folium Artemisiae Argyi, Argy Wormwood Leaf) ★ ★ ★

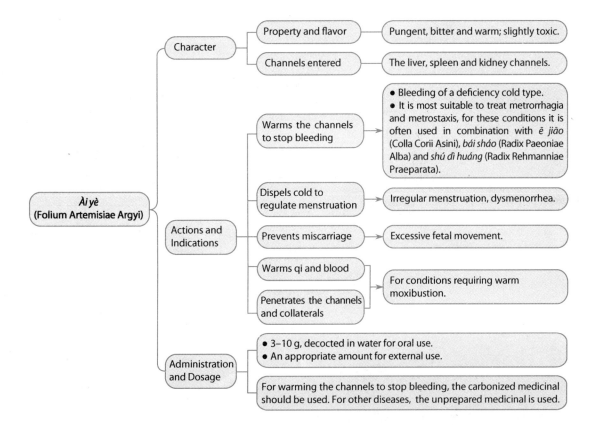

② *Páo jiāng* (炮姜, Rhizoma Zingiberis Praeparatum, Prepared Dried Ginger) ★

Ài yè (Folium Artemisiae Argyi) and *páo jiāng* (Rhizoma Zingiberis Praeparatum) are bitter in flavor and warm in property. Both medicinals can warm the channels to stop bleeding and warm the middle to dispel cold and relieve pain. They can be used for bleeding of a deficiency cold type, and cold pain in the epigastrium and abdomen caused by deficient cold in the middle *jiao*.

Ài yè (Folium Artemisiae Argyi) has a pungent and bitter flavor and a warm property. It is effective for warming qi and blood to warm the channels and collaterals. It is considered an essential medicinal to warm the channels to stop bleeding. It is especially suitable in treating deficient cold in the lower *jiao* (deficient cold in the uterus), manifesting as metrorrhagia, metrostaxis and profuse menstrual blood. *Xiān ài yè* (fresh Folium Artemisiae Argyi) can be used for bleeding due to blood heat if combined with medicinals for cooling blood and stopping bleeding. In addition, *ài yè* (Folium Artemisiae Argyi) is capable of warming the liver and kidney, dispelling cold to regulate menstruation, and preventing miscarriage. It is often used for deficiency cold in the lower *jiao* or pathogenic cold invasion of the uterus, manifesting as irregular menstruation, abdominal pain during menstrual bleeding, female infertility with uterine cold, leukorrhea with a thin discharge, vaginal bleeding during pregnancy, and excessive fetal movement. It is regarded as an essential medicinal for gynecological use. In addition, *ài yè* (Folium Artemisiae Argyi) can be lightly ground and made into a moxa stick for moxibustion, which can warm the qi and blood, and penetrate the channels and collaterals. It is considered a necessary medicinal of acupuncture and moxibustion.

Páo jiāng (Rhizoma Zingiberis Praeparatum) is bitter and astringent in flavor, warm in property. It is effective for warming the spleen to govern blood. It is indicated for deficient cold in the spleen and stomach, failure of the spleen to govern blood with bleeding (hematemesis, hemafecia), and cold pain in epigastrium and abdomen and diarrhea due to deficient cold in the middle *jiao*.

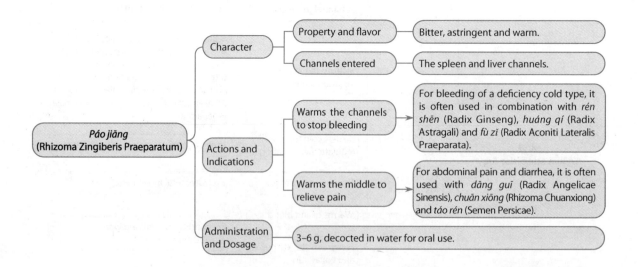

③ *Zào xīn tǔ* (灶心土, Terra Flava Usta, Furnace Soil)

Ài yè (Folium Artemisiae Argyi) and *zào xīn tǔ* (Terra Flava Usta) are pungent in flavor and warm in property. They can warm the channels to stop bleeding, and are used for bleeding of deficiency cold type.

Ài yè (Folium Artemisiae Argyi) has a pungent and bitter flavor and a warm property. It is effective for warming the qi and blood to warm the channels and collaterals. It is considered an essential medicinal to warm the channels to stop bleeding. It is especially suitable to treat deficiency cold in the lower *jiao* (deficiency cold in the uterus), manifesting as metrorrhagia, metrostaxis, and profuse menstrual blood. When combined with medicinals for cooling blood and stopping bleeding, *xiān ài yè* (fresh Folium Artemisiae Argyi) can be used for bleeding due to blood heat. In addition, *ài yè* (Folium Artemisiae Argyi) is capable of warming the liver and kidney, dispelling cold to regulate menstruation, and preventing miscarriage. It is often used for deficiency cold in the lower *jiao* or pathogenic cold invasion of the uterus, manifesting as irregular menstruation, abdominal pain during menstrual bleeding, female infertility with cold in the uterus, leukorrhea with thin discharge, vaginal bleeding during pregnancy, and excessive fetal movement. It is regarded as an essential medicinal in gynecology. In addition, *ài yè* (Folium Artemisiae Argyi) can be ground slightly and made into a moxa stick for moxibustion, which can warm the qi and blood, penetrate the channels and collaterals. It is considered a necessary medicinal of acupuncture and moxibustion.

Zào xīn tǔ (Terra Flava Usta) is pungent in flavor and warm in property. It has a local action in warming the middle to stop bleeding. It is indicated for deficiency cold in the spleen leading to failure of the spleen to govern blood, with manifestations such as hematemesis, hemafecia, metrorrhagia, and metrostaxis. In addition, it can warm the middle to relieve vomiting and diarrhea. It can also be used for vomiting due to stomach cold, vomiting during pregnancy, and chronic diarrhea due to spleen deficiency.

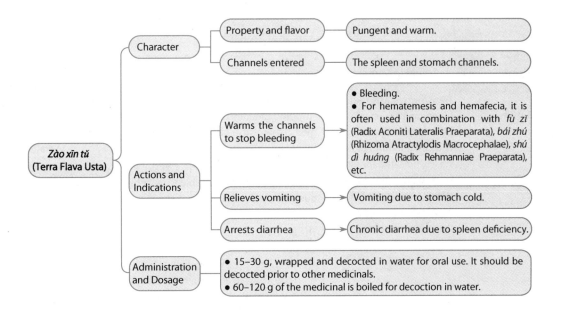

Actions of medicinals that stop bleeding are summarized in the following tables (Tables 18-1~18-4, see p.278~279):

Table 18-1: Summary of Medicinals that Cool Blood and Stop Bleeding:

Medicinal	Action in Common		Individual Character	
			Characteristic Actions	Other Actions
Dà jì (Herba seu Radix Cirsii Japonici)	Cools blood to stop bleeding, indicated for bleeding due to blood heat	Removes stasis, detoxifies and eliminates carbuncles	It has strong actions for removing stasis, detoxifing and eliminating carbuncles, it is often used for hematemesis, hemoptysis, metrorrhagia and metrostaxis	
Xiǎo jì (Herba Cirsii)			Induces diuresis, is effective for treating hematuria, or stranguria caused by hematuria	
Dì yú (Radix Sanguisorbae)			Detoxifies and treats infections on the surface of the body, an essential medicinal to treat scalds and burns	
Huái huā (Flos Sophorae)				Clears liver fire, reduces blood pressure
Bái máo gēn (Rhizoma Imperatae)		Especially suitable for blood heat in the lower jiao, manifesting as hemafecia, hemorrhoids with blood, dysentery with blood, metrorrhagia and metrostaxis	Clears heat to induce diuresis, especially used for hematuria, and stranguria caused by hematuria	Clears and purges heat accumulation in the lung and stomach
Zhù má gēn (Radix Boehmeriae)			Suitable to treat metrorrhagia, metrostaxis and profuse menstrual blood	Clears heat to prevent miscarriage, detoxifies
Cè bǎi yè (Cacumen Platycladi)			Astringes to stop bleeding, transforms phlegm to relieve cough, promotes generation of hair, blackens hair	
Yáng tí (Radix Rumicis Japonici)			Detoxifies to kill parasites, promotes defecation	

Table 18-2: Summary of Medicinals that Transform Stasis to Stop Bleeding:

Medicinal	Action in Common	Individual Character	
		Characteristic Actions	Other Actions
Sān qī (Radix et Rhizoma Notoginseng)	Transforms stasis to stop bleeding, characterized by stopping blood without retaining blood stasis, indicated for blood stasis obstruction in the interior leading to failure of blood to circulate in the blood vessels	It has a stronger action in transforming stasis and stopping bleeding, is regarded as an essential medicinal to stop bleeding. Extensively applied for bleeding, both internally and externally	Activates blood to relieve pain, an essential medicinal in traumatology
Qiàn cǎo (Radix et Rhizoma Rubiae)		Transforms stasis to stop bleeding, cools blood and stops bleeding, suitable to treat bleeding due to blood heat and blood stasis, especially bleeding due to blood heat with stasis	Activates blood and channels, an essential medicinal in gynecology
Pú huáng (Pollen Typhae)		The fresh medicinal has a cool property and a slippery action to transform stasis to stop bleeding. The parched medicinal has a warm property and can astringe to stop bleeding. It is suitable to treat bleeding from various causes, especially those of an excess type with stasis	Transforms blood stasis to relieve pain, induces diuresis to relieve stranguria
Huā ruǐ shí (Ophicalcitum)		Transforms stasis to stop bleeding	
Jiàng xiāng (Lignum Dalbergiae Odoriferae)			Regulates qi to relieve pain

Table 18-3: Summary of Medicinals that Astringe to Stop Bleeding:

Medicinal	Action in Common		Individual Character	
			Characteristic Actions	Other Actions
Bái jí (Rhizoma Bletillae)	Most medicinals are astringent in flavor. They can astringe to stop bleeding, and are suitable to treat bleeding without stasis		It has a sticky texture, a strong action in astringing to stop bleeding, and is often used for pulmonary and stomach bleeding.	Reduces swelling and promotes the generation of tissue
Xiān hè cǎo (Herba Agrimoniae)			With a neutral property, it is extensively used for various types of bleeding.	Arrests dysentery, prevents the recurrence of malaria, tonifies deficiency and strengthens the body, detoxifies and kills parasites
Zōng lǘ tàn (Petiolus Trachycarpi)			It has a pure and strong action, and is often used for metrorrhagia, metrostaxis and profuse menstrual bleeding.	
Xuè yú tàn (Crinis Carbonisatus)		Transforms stasis to stop bleeding, used for bleeding with stasis		Induces diuresis
Ǒu jié (Nodus Nelumbinis Rhizomatis)			Stops bleeding and transforms stasis if used unprepared, whereas when carbonized, it is used to astringe to stop bleeding	
Zǐ zhū (Folium Callicarpae Formosanae)			Cools blood and stops bleeding, is often used for pulmonary and stomach bleeding	Clears heat and detoxifies
Jì mù (Flos Loropetali Chinensis)				

Table 18-4: Summary of Medicinals that Warm Channels to Stop Bleeding:

Medicinal	Action in Common		Individual Character	
			Characteristic Actions	Other Actions
Ài yè (Folium Artemisiae Argyi)	Warms the channels to stop bleeding, indicated for bleeding of a deficiency cold type	Warms the middle and dispels cold to relieve pain	It is effective for warming qi and blood to warm the channels and collaterals, is regarded as an essential medicinal to warm the channels to stop bleeding. It is suitable for treating metrorrhagia, metrostaxis, and profuse menstrual blood due to deficient cold in the lower *jiao*. It can warm the liver and kidney, dispel cold to regulate the channels, and prevent miscarriage	
Páo jiāng (Rhizoma Zingiberis Praeparatum)		Warms the spleen to govern blood, indicated for hematemesis and hemafecia due to deficiency cold of the spleen qi failing to govern blood	It has a local action.	
Zào xīn tǔ (Terra Flava Usta)			Warms the middle to relieve vomiting and diarrhea	

Tables to test you herbal knowledge of the actions and indications of medicinals that stop bleeding are as follows (Tables 18-5~18-10, see p.280~282):

Table 18-5: Test your Herbal Knowledge of the Actions of Medicinals that Stop Bleeding (one):

Medicinal / Actions	Dà jì	Xiǎo jì	Dì yú	Huái huā	Cè bǎi yè	Bái máo gēn	Zhù má gēn	Yáng tí
Cools blood and stops bleeding								
Removes stasis, detoxifies and eliminates carbuncles								
Detoxifies to kill parasites								
Clears liver fire								
Transforms phlegm to relieve cough								
Clears heat to induce diuresis								
Prevents miscarriage								
Detoxifies								
Detoxifies to treat infections on the surface of the body								
Purges downwards								

Table 18-6: Test your Herbal Knowledge of the Actions of Medicinals that Stop Bleeding (two):

Medicinal / Actions	Sān qī	Qiàn cǎo	Pú huáng	Huā ruǐ shí	Jiàng xiāng	Páo jiāng	Ài yè	Zào xīn tǔ
Warms the channels to stop bleeding								
Activates blood to relieve pain								
Cools blood and stops bleeding								
Activates the channels								
Warms the middle to stop bleeding								
Regulates qi to relieve pain								
Transforms stasis to stop bleeding								
Warms the middle to relieve pain								
Dispels cold to regulate menstruation								
Prevents miscarriage								
Induces diuresis								
Relieves vomiting								
Relieves diarrhea								

Table 18-7: Test your Herbal Knowledge of the Actions of Medicinals that Stop Bleeding (three):

Medicinal / Actions	Bái jí	Xiān hè cǎo	Zǐ zhū	Zōng lǜ tàn	Xuè yú tàn	Ǒu jié	Cì wei pí
Clears heat and detoxifies							
Reduces swelling and promotes the generation of tissues							
Tonifies deficiency							
Transforms stasis to relieve pain							
Arrests dysentery							
Kills parasites							
Astringes to stop bleeding							
Induces diuresis							
Relieves seminal emission and reduces urine							
Removes stagnation							
Transforms stasis to stop bleeding							

Table 18-8: Test your Herbal Knowledge of the Indications of Medicinals that Stop Bleeding (one):

Medicinal / Indications	Dà jì	Xiăo jì	Dì yú	Huái huā	Cè băi yè	Bái máo gēn	Zhù má gēn	Yáng tí
Bleeding due to blood heat								
Stranguria due to heat, edema								
Scalds, eczema								
Flaring up of liver fire								
Cough due to lung heat								
Carbuncles and swellings due to heat toxin								
Vaginal bleeding during pregnancy, excessive fetal movement								
Scabies, tinea, favus								

Table 18-9: Test your Herbal Knowledge of the Indications of Medicinals that Stop Bleeding (two):

Medicinal / Indications	Sān qī	Qiàn căo	Pú huáng	Huā ruĭ shí	Jiàng xiāng	Páo jiāng	Ài yè	Zào xīn tŭ
Various types of bleeding, internally and externally								
Bi due to wind damp								
Chest blockage due to blood stasis								
Bleeding due to blood heat accompanied by stasis								
Amenorrhea due to blood stasis								
Injuries due to trauma								
Female infertility due to cold in the uterus								
Stranguria due to hematuria								
Bleeding due to blood stasis								
Bleeding of a deficiency cold type								
Eczema with itching								
Diarrhea due to deficient cold								
Dysmenorrhea due to deficiency cold								
Pain due to stagnation								
Vaginal bleeding due to pregnancy								
Excessive fetal movement								
Cough of a cold type								
Abdominal pain due to deficiency cold								
Vomiting due to deficiency cold								
Nausea due to deficiency cold								
Vomiting during pregnancy								
Chronic diarrhea due to deficiency cold								

Table 18-10: Test your Herbal Knowledge of the Indications of Medicinals that Stop Bleeding (three):

Indications \ Medicinal	Bái jí	Xiān hè căo	Zǐ zhū	Zōng lǚ tàn	Xuè yú tàn	Ǒu jié	Cì wei pí
Various types of bleeding							
Leukorrhagia							
Scalds and burns							
Various types of internal bleeding							
Diarrhea and dysentery							
Pulmonary and stomach bleeding							
Infant's abdominal distention due to malnutrition							
Carbuncles, ulcers							
Seminal emission, enuresis							
Stomachache, regurgitation							
Rhagades							
Anal fissure							
Internal injury due to overstrain							

Chapter 19
Medicinals that Invigorate Blood and Transform Stasis

Concept

Medicinals that have actions of promoting blood flow and removing blood stasis are called medicinals that invigorate blood and transform stasis. They are also called medicinals for invigorating blood and removing blood stasis, medicinals for activating blood, and medicinals for transforming stasis. Among such medicinals, the ones with stronger actions to activate blood are known as medicinals for breaking up blood stasis.

Character and Actions

Medicinals of this chapter are mostly pungent and bitter in flavor and warm in property. Some of the animal medicinals have a salty flavor. They enter the heart and liver channels. The pungent flavor can disperse and promote, while the bitter flavor is able to purge and dredge. Both pungent and bitter flavors enter the blood to promote blood flow and activate blood, so as to facilitate blood flow and transform stasis. Medicinals that invigorate blood and transform stasis will achieve therapeutic effects such as activating blood to relieve pain, activating blood to regulate menstruation, activating blood to reduce swelling, activating blood to treat trauma, activating blood to eliminate carbuncles, and breaking blood to remove blood stasis.

Indications

They are indicated for various types of blood stasis in internal medicine, surgery, gynecology, pediatrics, traumatology, etc. For example, they treat stabbing and fixed pain in the chest, abdomen and head; abdominal masses; stroke with hemiparalysis and numb limbs; chronic *bi* in the joints; injuries due to trauma, swelling pain due to stasis; ulcers; irregular menstruation, amenorrhea, dysmenorrhea, and postpartum abdominal pain.

Classification

According to their action characteristics and clinical applications medicinals that invigorate blood and transform stasis are divided into four categories: Medicinals that invigorate blood to relieve pain; medicinals that invigorate blood to regulate menstruation; medicinals that invigorate blood to treat trauma; and medicinals that break up blood stasis.

Combinations

When using medicinals that invigorate blood and transform stasis in clinical practice, doctors should chose medicinals with certain actions according to the syndrome present. They should also use the correct combination aiming at the specific cause of blood stasis, in order to treat both the root and branch. For blood stasis due to cold congealing, combine with medicinals for warming the interior to dispel cold, and warming and activating the channels and vessels. For heat burning the blood leading to a mix of stasis and heat, combine with medicinals for clearing heat and cooling blood, or purging fire and detoxifying. For disturbance in blood circulation due to phlegm damp obstruction, combine with medicinals that transform phlegm and remove damp. For wind damp obstruction in the channels and collaterals, combine with medicinals for expelling wind damp and activating the collaterals. For weakness due to protracted blood stasis or stasis resulting from deficiency, add medicinals that tonify. For abdominal masses due to blood stasis, add medicinals for softening hard masses and removing stasis. There is a close relationship between qi and blood. Therefore, when using medicinals for invigorating qi and transforming blood, always combine with medicinals for promoting qi circulation, so as to strengthen the therapeutic effect.

Precautions

Medicinals in this chapter are prone to consuming blood, therefore they are not recommended for women with excessive menstrual blood, or bleeding without blood stasis. They should be used cautiously or prohibited during pregnancy.

Section 1 Medicinals that Invigorate Blood to Relieve Pain

Medicinals in this section mostly have a pungent flavor. They enter the *xue* level as well as the qi level to invigorate blood and promote qi circulation, which both contribute to relieving pain. They are indicated for various types of pain caused by blood stasis and qi stagnation, such as headache, chest and hypochondriac pain, chest and abdominal pain, dysmenorrhea, postpartum abdominal pain, *bi,* and pain due to stasis resulting from injuries due to trauma. They are also used for other diseases caused by blood stasis.

① *Chuān xiōng* (川芎, Rhizoma Chuanxiong, Chuanxiong Root) ★★★

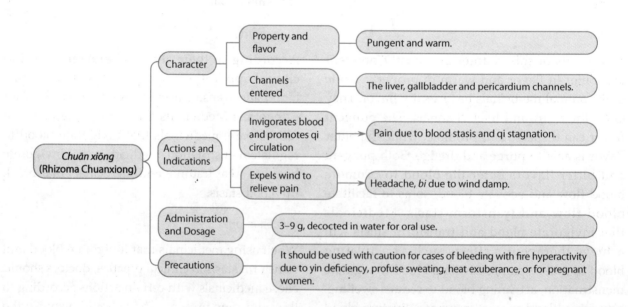

② *Yán hú suǒ* (延胡索, Rhizoma Corydalis, Yanhusuo) ★★★

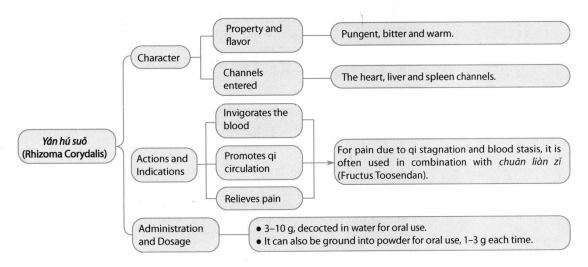

③ *Yù jīn* (郁金, Radix Curcumae, Turmeric Root Tuber) ★★★

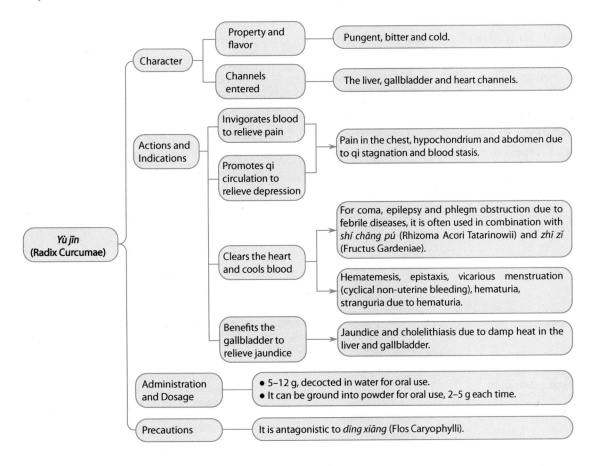

④ *Jiāng huáng* (姜黄, Rhizoma Curcumae Longae, Turmeric Root Tuber) ★★

Both *yù jīn* (Radix Curcumae) and *jiāng huáng* (Rhizoma Curcumae Longae) are pungent and bitter, and can invigorate blood and promote qi circulation to relieve pain. They are used in

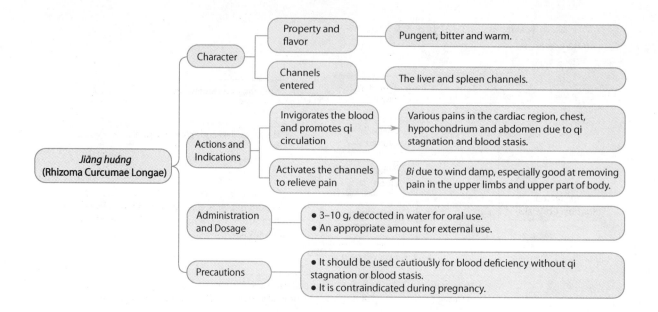

combination for mutual reinforcement to treat pain in the chest, hypochondrium, epigastrium and abdomen, amenorrhea, dysmenorrhea, irregular menstruation, postpartum abdominal pain and abdominal masses caused by qi stagnation and blood stasis, as well as injuries due to trauma. Their differences are as follows: *Yù jīn* (Radix Curcumae) is cold and appropriate for qi stagnation and blood stasis with heat manifestations. It can cool blood, clear the heart to relieve depression and benefit the gallbladder to relieve jaundice. It is used for coma, epilepsy and phlegm obstruction in febrile diseases;

bleeding due to adverse flow of qi and fire (manifesting as hematemesis, epistaxis and vicarious menstruation); jaundice of a damp heat type, and cholelithiasis. *Jiāng huáng* (Rhizoma Curcumae Longae) is warm in property, and is suitable for qi stagnation and blood stasis with cold congealing. It can also expel wind-cold damp, activate the channels to relieve pain, and is especially effective for relieving *bi* in the upper part of the body. It is used for *bi* due to wind-cold damp, and pain in the shoulders and arms.

⑤ *Rǔ xiāng* (乳香, Olibanum, Boswellin) ★★

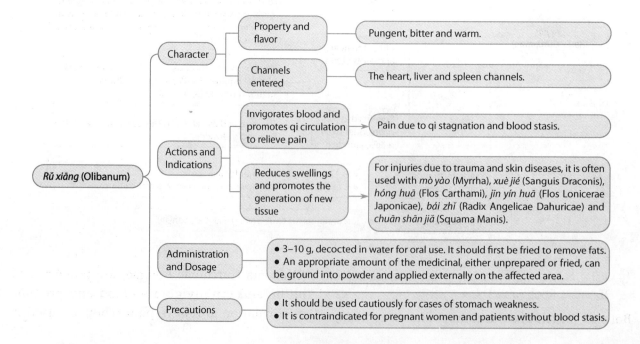

⑥ *Mò yào* (没药, Myrrha, Myrrh) ★

Rǔ xiāng (Olibanum) and *mò yào* (Myrrha) are pungent and bitter in flavor, and can invigorate blood to relieve pain, reduce swelling and promote the generation of new tissue. They have a pronounced pain-relieving action, and are the most commonly used medicinals for invigorating blood to relieve pain. They are used for various types of pain due to blood stasis and qi stagnation, manifesting as amenorrhea, dysmenorrhea, angina due to chest blockage, epigastric and abdominal pain, *bi* due to wind damp, injuries due to trauma, swelling and pain due to carbuncles, and abdominal pain due to intestinal abscesses. They are also used for skin diseases which have ruptured but have not healed for a long time. *Rǔ xiāng* (Olibanum) has a warm property, and can mainly promote qi circulation to stretch the sinews. *Mò yào* (Myrrha) has a neutral property and can mainly transform blood stasis, and therefore is often used for stomachache with severe blood stasis and qi stagnation.

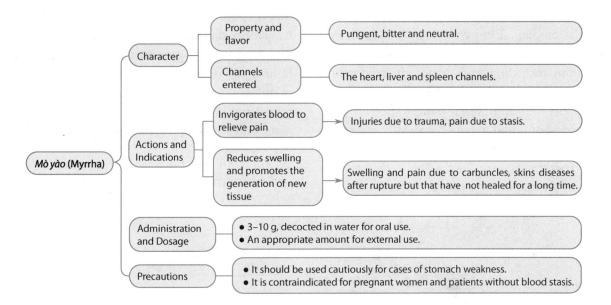

⑦ *Wǔ líng zhī* (五灵脂, Faeces Trogopterori, Trogopterus Dung) ★

Chuān xiōng (Rhizoma Chuanxiong), *yán hú suǒ* (Rhizoma Corydalis) and *wǔ líng zhī* (Faeces

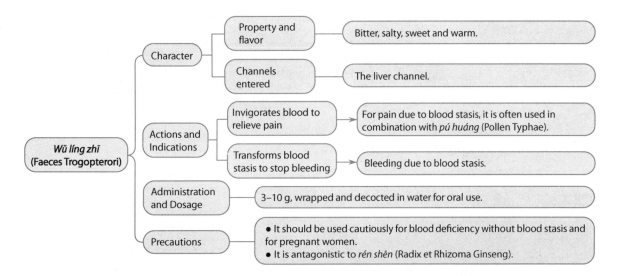

Trogopterori) can invigorate blood to relieve pain. They can be used for various types of pain due to blood stasis, such as amenorrhea, dysmenorrhea, postpartum abdominal pain due to blood stasis, chest and hypochondriac pain, epigastric and abdominal pain, and trauma. *Chuān xiōng* (Rhizoma Chuanxiong) and *yán hú suǒ* (Rhizoma Corydalis) are capable of invigorating qi as well as promoting qi circulation, and are suitable for pain due to both qi stagnation and blood stasis. *Chuān xiōng* (Rhizoma Chuanxiong) enters the liver, gallbladder and pericardium channels, and can regulate menstruation and relieve depression. Therefore it is considered an essential medicinal in gynecology. It is indicated for various diseases caused by blood stasis and qi stagnation, including amenorrhea, dysmenorrhea, irregular menstruation, postpartum abdominal pain, chest and abdominal pain, hypochondriac pain and abdominal masses, especially ones with cold manifestations. In addition, it has a lifting and dispersing nature, "*ascending to the head and activating the channels and collaterals*", and therefore

can expel wind to relieve pain. It is commonly used to treat headache and *bi* due to wind damp. It is regarded as an essential medicinal to treat headache. It is used for headache from wind cold, wind heat, wind damp, blood deficiency, or blood stasis. Physicians in ancient times believed that whenever there was a headache, *chuān xiōng* (Rhizoma Chuanxiong) was the medicinal to use. *Yán hú suǒ* (Rhizoma Corydalis) has an excellent action in relieving pain, and its focus is treating various types of pain all over the body. Clinically, it is widely used for pain in different regions of body caused by qi stagnation and blood stasis. *Wǔ líng zhī* (Faeces Trogopterori) can transform stasis to stop bleeding, and is used for bleeding resulting from blood stasis causing a failure of blood to travel inside the blood vessels, manifesting as metrorrhagia, metrostaxis, profuse menstrual blood, purplish menstrual blood with clots, and stabbing pain in the lower abdomen.

⑧ *Xià tiān wú* (夏天无, Rhizoma Corydalis Decumbentis, Decumbent Corydalis Rhizome)

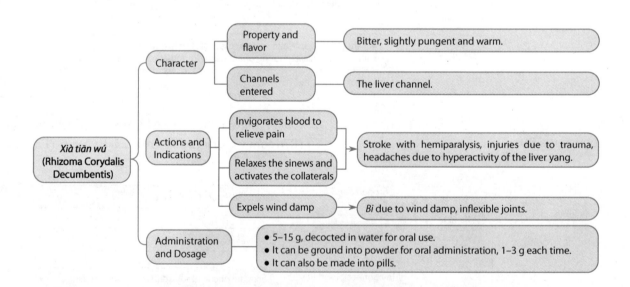

⑨ *Fēng xiāng zhī* (枫香脂, Resina Liquidambaris, Beautiful Sweetgum Resin)

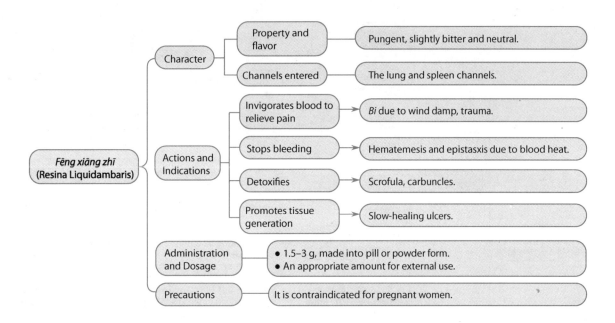

Section 2   Medicinals that Invigorate Blood to Regulate Menstruation

Medicinals in this section are often pungent and bitter in flavor. They mainly enter the *xue* level of the liver channel to invigorate blood in order to transform stasis, and are effective for activating blood to regulate menstruation. They are indicated for irregular menstruation, amenorrhea, dysmenorrhea, and postpartum abdominal pain due to blood stasis. They are also commonly used for pain due to blood stasis, including abdominal masses, injuries due to trauma, and suppurating infections on the surface of the body.

① *Dān shēn* (丹参, Radix et Rhizoma Salviae Miltiorrhizae, Danshen Root) ★★★

Chuān xiōng (Rhizoma Chuanxiong) and *dān shēn* (Radix et Rhizoma Salviae Miltiorrhizae) are commonly used medicinals for invigorating the blood. Both medicinals can invigorate blood to regulate menstruation and remove stasis to relieve pain. They can be used for blood stasis with symptoms such as amenorrhea, dysmenorrhea, irregular menstruation, postpartum abdominal pain, abdominal masses, and injuries due to trauma. The two medicinals can be used for various diseases

caused by blood stasis, and are considered essential gynecological medicinals to invigorate the blood in order to regulate menstruation. *Chuān xiōng* (Rhizoma Chuanxiong) is pungent and warm, and can invigorate blood and promote qi circulation. It is said to travel in the *xue* level as well as the qi level. It is most suitable to treat diseases induced by qi stagnation and blood stasis accompanied by cold congealing. In addition, it has a lifting and dispersing nature – it is said to *"ascend to the head and activate the channels and collaterals"*. Therefore it can expel wind to relieve pain. It is commonly used to treat headaches and *bi* due to wind damp, and it is regarded as an essential medicinal to treat headaches. It is used to treat various types of headache when combined properly with other medicinals. *Dān shēn* (Radix et Rhizoma Salviae Miltiorrhizae) is bitter and slightly cold, and can invigorate and cool the blood, and therefore is most suitable for blood stasis with heat. It can also cool blood to eliminate carbuncles and relieve vexation to tranquilize the mind. It is commonly used for suppurating infections on the surface of the body; heat *bi* due to wind damp with red swellings and painful sensations in the limbs and joints; epidemic febrile diseases with heat invading the heart blood, with manifestations such as high fever, vexation, insomnia, or indistinct maculae, or even coma, and delirium; and palpitations and

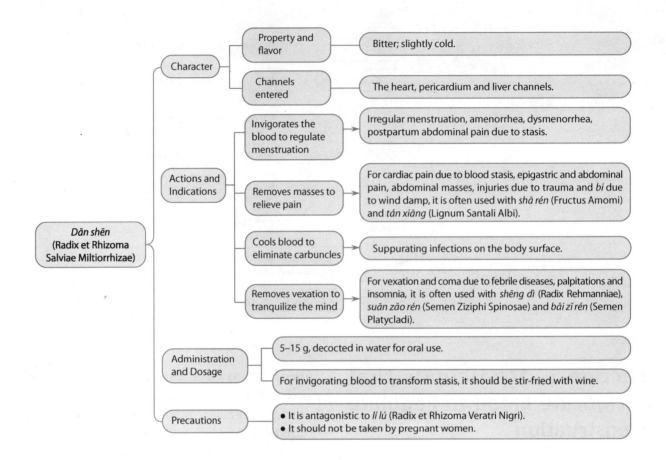

insomnia due to failure of the blood to nourish the heart resulting from stubborn diseases.

② *Hóng huā* (红花, Flos Carthami, Safflower) ★ ★ ★

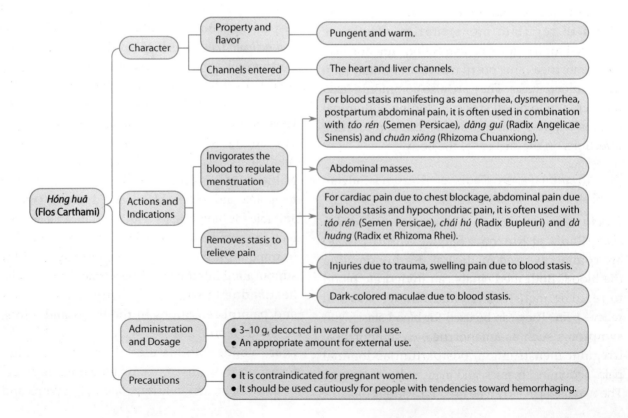

③ *Táo rén* (桃仁, Semen Persicae, Peach Seed)
★ ★ ★

Both *táo rén* (Semen Persicae) and *hóng huā* (Flos Carthami) can invigorate blood to remove stasis and regulate menstruation. They are always used in combination for mutual reinforcement to treat various types of blood stasis, such as amenorrhea, dysmenorrhea, irregular menstruation, postpartum abdominal pain, abdominal masses, stabbing pain in chest and abdomen, and injuries due to trauma. *Táo rén* (Semen Persicae) is pungent, sweet and neutral with a slight toxicity. It can invigorate the blood and eliminate internal carbuncles, and is commonly used for pulmonary and intestinal abscesses. It can also moisten the intestines to promote defecation, and relieve cough and asthma. It is used for constipation due to dry intestines, and cough with dyspnea.

Hóng huā (Flos Carthami) is pungent and warm, and enters the *xue* level and therefore has a strong action in invigorating blood to induce menstruation, and removing stasis to relieve pain. It can invigorate the blood if used in a small dosage and break up stasis if used in a large dosage. It is also used for dark-colored maculae due to stagnant blood accumulation. In addition, *fān hóng huā* (番红花, Stigma Croci, Saffron) has a similar but stronger action than *hóng huā* (Flos Carthami). It can also cool blood and detoxify and is used for blood stasis with heat retention, dark maculae and epidemic febrile diseases with heat invading the *ying* blood. *Xī hóng huā* (Stigma Croci) is rare and expensive, so it is not often used in the clinic, and when it is, it should be used in a smaller dosage.

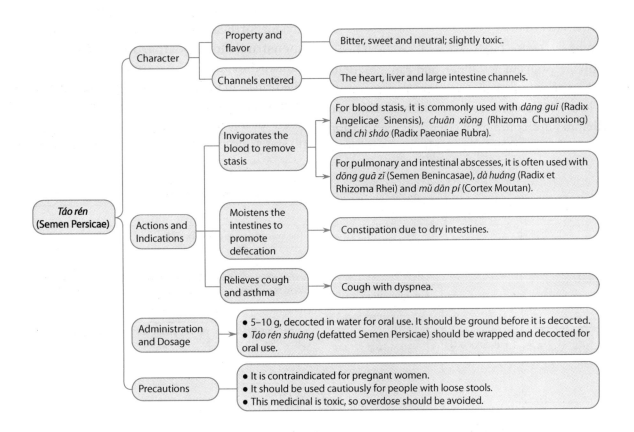

④ *Yì mǔ cǎo* (益母草, Herba Leonuri, Motherwort Herb) ★★★

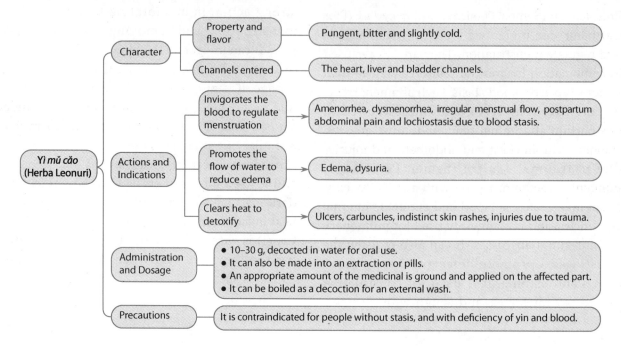

⑤ *Zé lán* (泽兰, Herba Lycopi, Hirsute Shiny Bugleweed Herb)

Yì mǔ cǎo (Herba Leonuri) and *zé lán* (Herba Lycopi) are pungent and bitter, and can invigorate blood to regulate menstruation and promote the flow of water to reduce edema. The two medicinals are commonly used in combination for mutual reinforcement to treat stagnant blood (in gynecology), manifesting as amenorrhea, dysmenorrhea, irregular menstruation, irregular menstrual flow, postpartum abdominal pain, and lochiostasis. They are considered effective medicinals in treating diseases during menstruation and pregnancy as well as post partum. They are also used for injuries due to trauma, swelling pain due to stasis, ulcers and carbuncles; edema and dysuria,

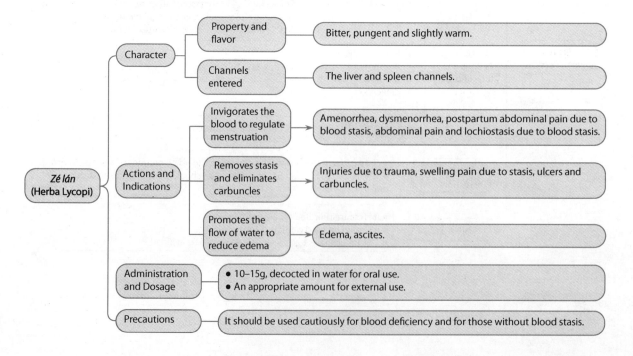

and edema from a mix of water with stasis. *Yì mǔ cǎo* (Herba Leonuri) has a slightly cold property, and is suitable to treat stasis with blood heat. It has a strong action in invigorating the blood to regulate menstruation. It is commonly used for edema from either acute or chronic nephritis. It can also clear heat to detoxify, and is often used for ulcers, carbuncles and indistinct skin rashes. It is also used for headaches due to liver heat, blood-shot eyes, swollen and painful eyes, and blurred vision due to deficiency in both the liver and kidney. *Zé lán* (Herba Lycopi) has a moderate action and can remove stasis without impairing the right qi. It is commonly used for puffiness and dysuria post partum. In addition, *chōng wèi zǐ* (Fructus Leonuri) is the dried fruit of Leonurus japonicus Houtt. It has similar actions to *yì mǔ cǎo* (Herba Leonuri) and can also cool the liver to promote eyesight.

⑥ *Niú xī* (牛膝, Radix Achyranthis Bidentatae, Twotoothed Achyranthes Root) ★ ★ ★

Both *huái niú xī* (Radix Achyranthis Bidentatae) and *chuān niú xī* (川牛膝, Radix Cyathulae, Yathula Root) are called *niú xī*. They are bitter, sweet, sour and neutral in character with a descending action, and enter the liver and kidney channels. They can invigorate blood to remove stasis, nourish the liver and kidney, strengthen sinews and bones, induce diuresis to relieve stranguria, guide the blood and fire downwards. Both medicinals are used for blood stasis manifesting as amenorrhea, dysmenorrhea, irregular menstruation, postpartum abdominal pain, lochiostasis and injuries due to trauma; aching of the waist and knees, flaccidity of the lower limbs due to liver and kidney deficiency, paralysis and flaccidity of feet and knees caused

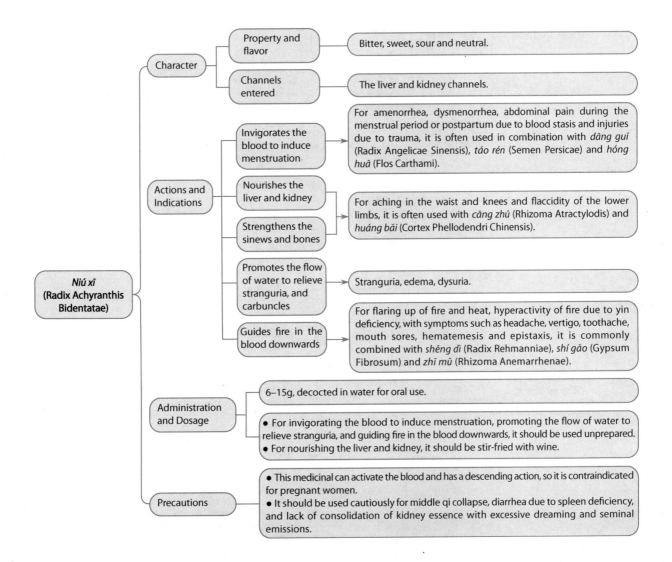

by damp heat; stranguria, edema and dysuria; headache and vertigo due to yang hyperactivity from yin deficiency; swollen and painful gums and mouth sores due to flaring up of deficient fire; and bleeding such as hematemesis and epistaxis resulting from the adverse flow of qi and fire. *Huái niú xī* (Radix Achyranthis Bidentatae) and *chuān niú xī* (Radix Cyathulae) can guide other medicinals to move downwards to treat diseases in the lower part of the body. There are differences between the two. *Huái niú xī* (Radix Achyranthis Bidentatae) is effective for nourishing the liver and kidney, strengthening the bones and sinews, and is commonly used for aching of the waist and knees and flaccidity of the lower limbs caused by deficiency of the liver and kidney. *Chuān niú xī* (Radix Cyathulae) is effective for invigorating the blood to remove stasis and activating the channels, and is often used for various diseases caused by blood stasis.

⑦ *Jī xuè téng* (鸡血藤, Caulis Spatholobi, Suberect Spatholobus Stem) ★ ★ ★

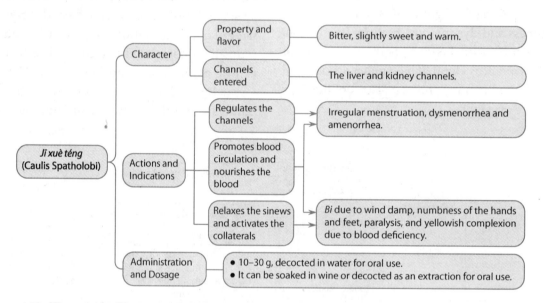

⑧ *Wáng bù liú xíng* (王不留行, Semen Vaccariae, Cowherb Seed)

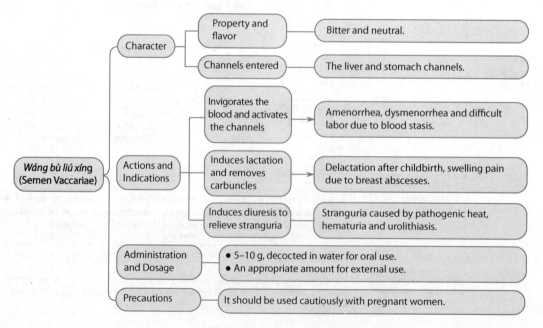

⑨ *Yuè jì huā* (月季花, Flos Rosae Chinensis, Chinese Rose Flower)

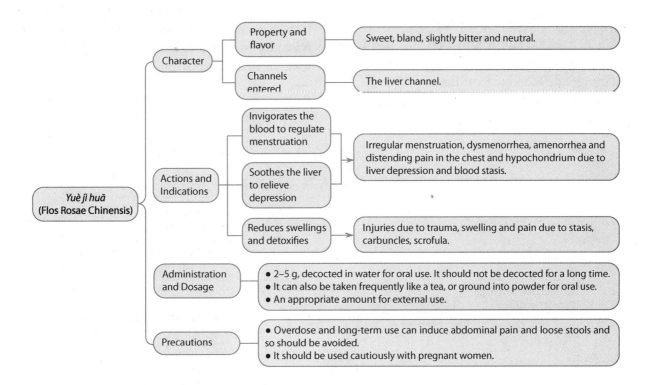

⑩ *Líng xiāo huā* (凌霄花, Flos Campsis, Trumpetcreeper Flower)

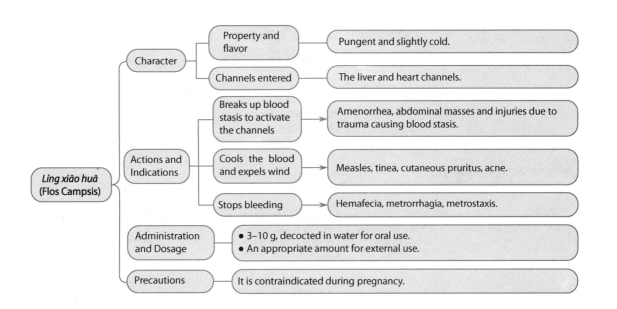

Section 3 Medicinals that Invigorate Blood to Treat Trauma

Medicinals whose principal effect is to invigorate blood to treat trauma and that are used for diseases of traumatology are called medicinals that invigorate blood to treat trauma.

Medicinals in this section are mostly pungent, bitter and salty, and enter the liver and kidney channels. They can invigorate blood, transform stasis, reduce swellings to relieve pain, mend fractures, stop bleeding, promote tissue regeneration, and heal wounds. They are indicated for injures due to trauma, swelling and pain due to blood stasis, bone fractures, and bleeding due to trauma. They are also used for other diseases caused by blood stasis.

①*Tŭ biē chóng* (土鳖虫, Eupolyphaga seu Steleophaga, Ground Beetle) ★★★

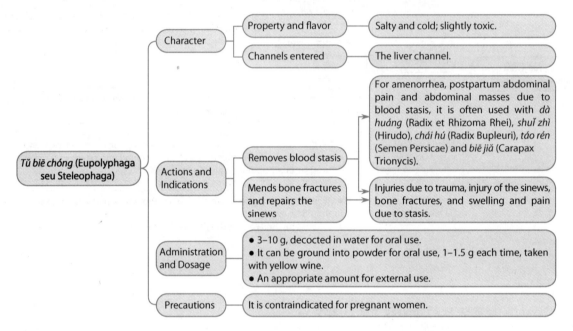

②*Mă qián zĭ* (马钱子, Semen Strychni, Nux Vomica) ★★★

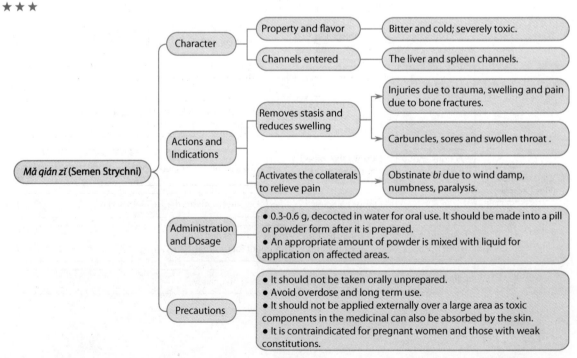

③ *Zì rán tóng* (自然铜, Pyritum, Pyrite) ★

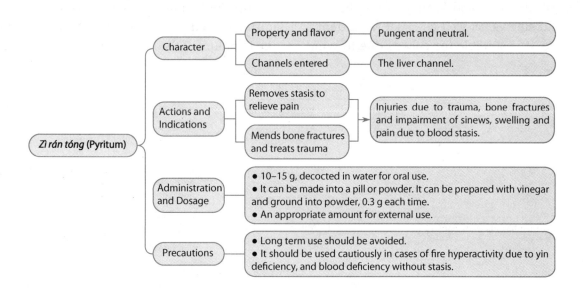

④ *Sū mù* (苏木, Lignum Sappan, Sappan Wood) ★

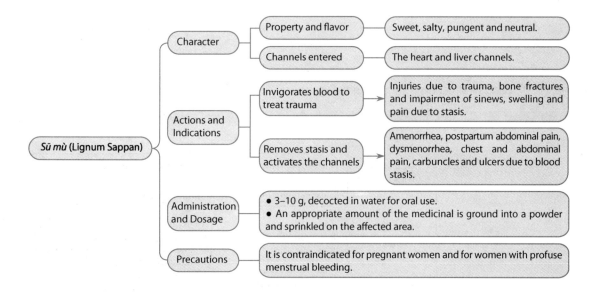

⑤ *Gǔ suì bǔ* (骨碎补, Rhizoma Drynariae, Drynaria Root) ★

Both *gǔ suì bǔ* (Rhizoma Drynariae) and *gǒu jǐ* (Rhizoma Cibotii) enter the liver and kidney channels, and can nourish the liver and kidney, and strengthen the bones and sinews. They are used in combination to treat waist pain, weak legs, and flaccidity due to deficiency of the liver and kidney. Their differences are as follows: *Gǔ suì bǔ* (Rhizoma Drynariae) is effective for invigorating the blood to treat trauma and is commonly used for injuries due to trauma, bone fractures and impairment of the sinews, and swelling and pain due to stasis. In addition, it is also used for tinnitus, deafness, toothache, and chronic diarrhea. *Gǒu jǐ* (Rhizoma Cibotii) is able to nourish the liver and kidney, strengthen the bones and sinews, as well as expel wind damp. Therefore, it is suitable for cold *bi* due to wind damp complicated by deficiency in the liver and kidney. It can also warm and nourish the kidney to stop the leaking of essence, and is used for enuresis, frequent urination and leukorrhagia due to failure of the kidney qi to consolidate.

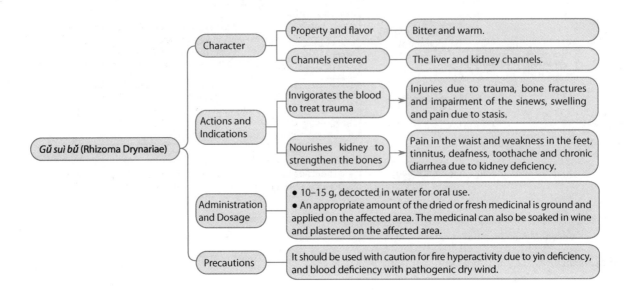

6 *Xuè jié* (血竭, Sanguis Draconis, Dragon's Blood) ★

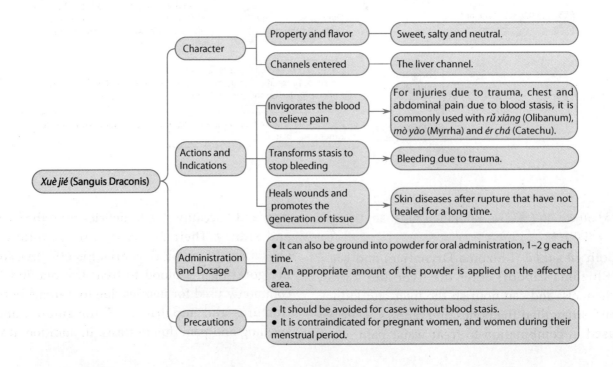

⑦ *Ér chá* (儿茶, Catechu, Cutch)

Xuè jié (Sanguis Draconis) and *ér chá* (Catechu) can invigorate blood to treat trauma, transform stasis to stop bleeding, promote the generation of tissue, and heal wounds. They are used in combination to treat injuries due to trauma, swelling and pain due to stasis, bleeding due to trauma; and skin diseases which have ruptured but that have not healed for a long time. Their differences are as follows: *Xuè jié* (Sanguis Draconis) is able to invigorate the blood to relieve pain, and is also used for stabbing pain in the chest and abdomen, amenorrhea, dysmenorrhea and postpartum abdominal pain due to blood stasis. *Ér chá* (Catechu) is used externally to remove dampness and heal wounds, and is used for damp ulcers with watery effusion, ulcerative gingivitis and mouth sores. In addition, when taken orally it can clear the lung to transform phlegm, and is used for cough due to lung heat.

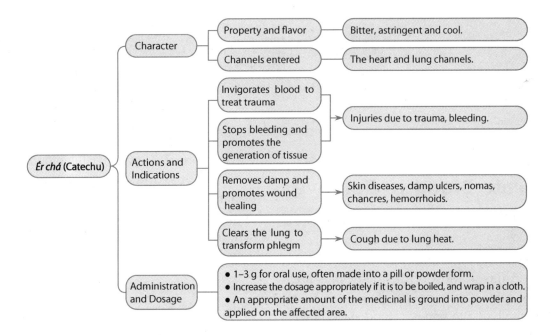

⑧ *Liú jì nú* (刘寄奴, Herba Artemisiae Anomalae, Diverse Wormwood Herb)

Zì rán tóng (Pyritum), *liú jì nú* (Herba Artemisiae Anomalae) and *sū mù* (Lignum Sappan) can invigorate the blood to treat trauma and remove stasis to relieve pain. They are commonly used for injuries due to trauma, impairment of the sinews and bone fractures, and are commonly used medicinals in traumatology and orthopedics. *Liú jì nú* (Herba Artemisiae Anomalae) and *sū mù* (Lignum Sappan) can invigorate the blood and activate the channels, and are used for amenorrhea, dysmenorrhea, and postpartum abdominal pain due to blood stasis.

Zì rán tóng (Pyritum) is effective for promoting the healing of bone fractures, and is regarded as an essential medicinal to mend bone fractures and treat the impairment of sinews. It can be used both internally and externally. *Liú jì nú* (Herba Artemisiae Anomalae) is able to stop bleeding, and promote digestion to remove food retention. It is often used for bleeding due to trauma, abdominal pain, and dysentery with bloody and purulent discharge due to food retention. *Sū mù* (Lignum Sappan) can invigorate the blood if used in a small dosage, and can remove blood stasis if used in a large dosage.

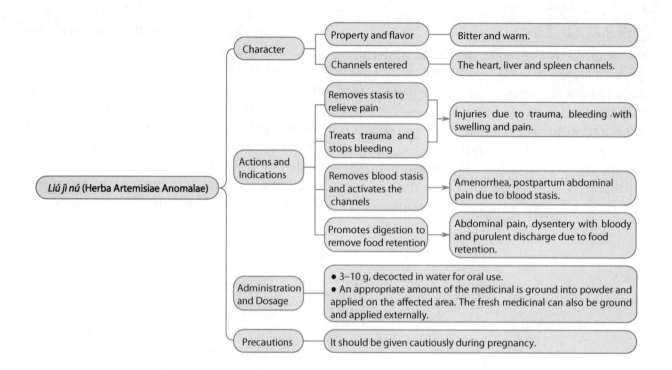

Section 4　Medicinals that Invigorate Blood to Remove Blood Stasis

Medicinals in this section are often pungent and bitter in flavor. Most of the medicinals are insects, and have a salty flavor. Medicinals that invigorate the blood to remove blood stasis enter the liver channel. They enter the blood and have drastic actions, and can remove blood stasis and masses. They are indicated for severe and chronic abdominal masses. They are also used for amenorrhea, swelling and pain due to stasis, and paralysis.

①*É zhú* (莪术, Rhizoma Curcumae, Blue Turmeric Rhizome) ★★★

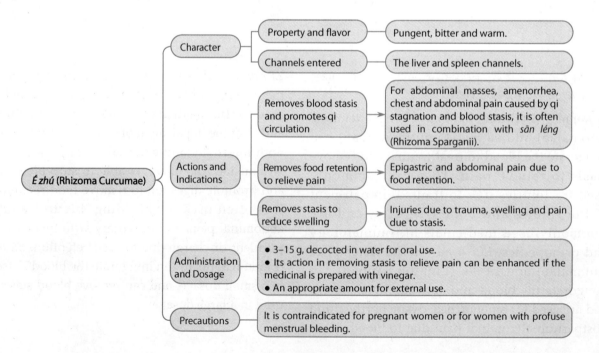

② *Sān léng* (三棱, Rhizoma Sparganii, Common Burreed Tuber) ★

Both *sān léng* (Rhizoma Sparganii) and *é zhú* (Rhizoma Curcumae) are pungent and bitter in flavor, and are commonly used for removing blood stasis and eliminating hard masses. They can remove blood stasis, promote qi circulation, and remove food retention so as to relieve pain. The two medicinals are used in combination for mutual reinforcement for qi stagnation and blood stasis with symptoms such as abdominal hard masses, amenorrhea, dysmenorrhea, chest and abdominal pain, injuries due to trauma, and swelling and pain due to stasis; and epigastric and abdominal distending pain due to food retention with qi stagnation. *Sān léng* (Rhizoma Sparganii) has a neutral property, which puts emphasis on its ability to remove blood stasis. *É zhú* (Rhizoma Curcumae) has a warm property and is effective for removing qi stagnation and food retention.

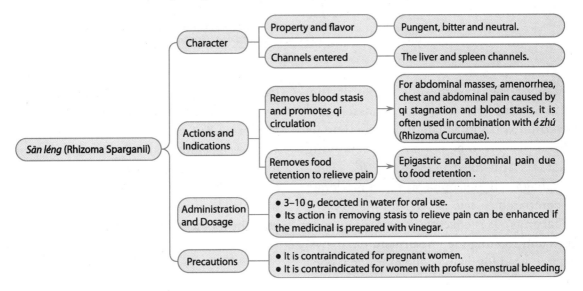

③ *Shuǐ zhì* (水蛭, Hirudo, Leech) ★★★

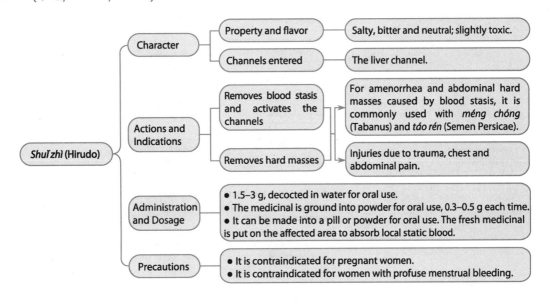

④ *Méng chóng* (虻虫, Tabanus, Gadfly)

Tǔ biē chóng (Eupolyphaga seu Steleophaga), *shuǐ zhì* (Hirudo) and *méng chóng* (Tabanus) are slightly toxic insect medicinals. They have drastic actions and can remove blood stasis and hard masses. They are used in combination for severe

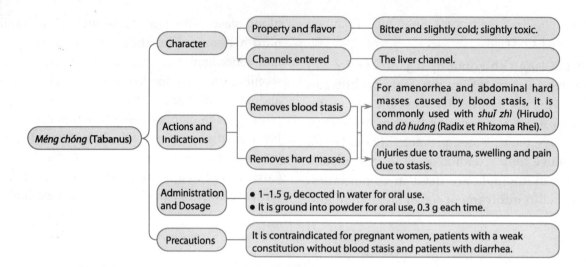

cases of blood stasis manifesting as postpartum abdominal pain, abdominal hard masses, and injuries due to trauma. The three medicinals have been proven to be effective in removing blood stasis and hard masses. *Tŭ biē chóng* (Eupolyphaga seu Steleophaga) has a moderate action compared to *shuĭ zhì* (Hirudo) and *méng chóng* (Tabanus). It is effective for mending bone fractures and treating the impairment of sinews, and is often used for injuries due to trauma, bone

fractures, impairment of the sinews, swelling and pain due to stasis. *Shuĭ zhì* (Hirudo) has a moderate but constant action compared with *méng chóng* (Tabanus). It is effective for removing hard masses. *Méng chóng* (Tabanus) has a drastic action. After taking *méng chóng* (Tabanus), patients can have diarrhea, but it will be relieved after the medicinal has finished acting.

⑤ *Bān máo* (斑蝥, Mylabris, Large Blister Beetle)

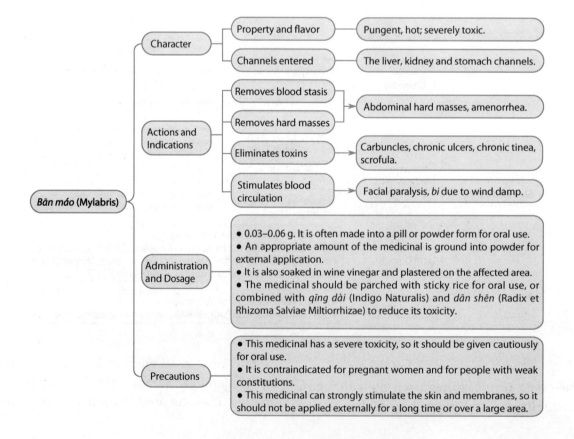

⑥ *Chuān shān jiǎ* (穿山甲, Squama Manitis, Pangolin Scales)

Both *chuān shān jiǎ* (Squama Manitis) and *wáng bù liú xíng* (Semen Vaccariae) can invigorate the blood, activate the channels, and induce lactation, they are considered essential medicinals to activate the channels to induce lactation. They are indicated for amenorrhea, dysmenorrhea, and postpartum abdominal pain due to blood stasis; delactation during the breast feeding period, and swelling pain due to mammary abscesses. The two medicinals are commonly used in combination for mutual reinforcement. *Chuān shān jiǎ* (Squama Manitis) migrates throughout the body and has a drastic action in invigorating blood to remove hard masses, reducing swelling and promoting the discharge of pus. It can be used for abdominal hard masses; *bi* due to wind damp, stroke with paralysis; carbuncles, ulcers, scrofula, and superficial nodules. *Wáng bù liú xíng* (Semen Vaccariae) is able to induce diuresis to relieve stranguria, and is often used for stranguria.

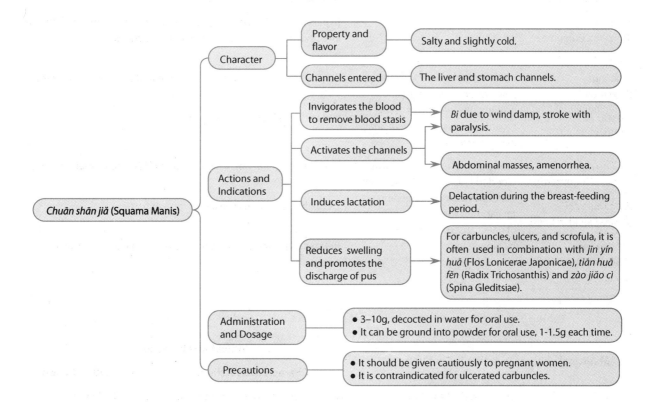

Actions and indications of medicinals that invigorate the blood and transform stasis are summarized in the following tables (Tables 19-1~19-4, see p.304~306):

Table 19-1: Summary of Medicinals that Invigorate the Blood to Relieve Pain:

Medicinal	Action in Common	Individual Character	
		Characteristic Actions	**Other Actions**
Chuān xiōng (Rhizoma Chuanxiong)	Invigorates the blood and promotes qi circulation to relieve pain, often indicated for various types of pain caused by qi stagnation and blood stasis	A medicinal with the action of invigorating blood as well as promoting qi circulation. It can regulate menstruation and remove depression, and is regarded as an essential medicinal in gynecology. It is suitable for various diseases induced by qi stagnation and blood stasis.	It is effective for dispelling wind to relieve pain, and is regarded as an essential medicinal to treat headache.
Yán hú suǒ (Rhizoma Corydalis)		It is effective for relieving pain, and is extensively indicated for pain all over the body caused by qi stagnation and blood stasis.	
Yù jīn (Radix Curcumae)		Cools blood, clears the heart to relieve depression, benefits the gallbladder to relieve jaundice	
Jiāng huáng (Rhizoma Curcumae Longae)		Expels wind cold and damp, promotes qi and blood circulation, is effective for relieving *bi* in the shoulders and arms.	
Rǔ xiāng (Olibanum)	Invigorates the blood to relieve pain, reduces swelling to promote generation of tissue, regarded as essential medicinals in traumatology	Emphasis on promoting qi circulation and stretching the sinews	
Mò yào (Myrrha)		It is effective for removing blood stasis	
Wǔ líng zhī (Faeces Trogopterori)	Invigorates the blood to relieve pain, indicated for various types of pain caused by blood stasis	Transforms stasis to stop bleeding	With a stronger action than *fēng xiāng zhī* (Resina Liquidambaris)
Fēng xiāng zhī (Resina Liquidambaris)			Detoxifies, promotes the generation of tissue
Xià tiān wú (Rhizoma Corydalis Decumbentis)			Relaxes the sinews and activates the collaterals, expels wind damp

Table 19-2: Summary of Medicinals that Invigorate the Blood to Regulate Menstruation:

Medicinal	Action in Common	Individual Character	
		Characteristic Actions	**Other Actions**
Dān shēn (Radix et Rhizoma Salviae Miltiorrhizae)	Invigorates the blood to regulate menstruation	Cools blood, suitable for blood heat with stasis. Effective for invigorating the blood to remove stasis and relieve pain, extensively used for various diseases caused by blood stasis	Eliminates carbuncles, relieves vexation to tranquilize the mind
Jī xuè téng (Caulis Spatholobi)		Nourishes blood, suitable for blood stasis and blood deficiency	Relaxes the sinews and activates the collaterals
Táo rén (Semen Persicae)	Invigorates the blood to remove stasis and activates the channels	Eliminates internal carbuncles, moistens the intestines to promote defecation, relieves cough and asthma	
Hóng huā (Flos Carthami)		It has a strong action on invigorating blood, activating channels and removing stasis to relieve pain. It is able to invigorate the blood if used in small dosages, and can remove blood stasis if used in large dosages	

Table 19-2: Summary of Medicinals that Invigorate the Blood to Regulate Menstruation:

continued

Medicinal	Action in Common	Individual Character	
		Characteristic Actions	**Other Actions**
Yì mǔ cǎo (Herba Leonuri)	Invigorates the blood to regulate menstruation	It has a strong action, regarded as an essential medicinal in gynecology	Clears heat and detoxifies
Zé lán (Herba Lycopi)		It has a moderate action, removes stasis without impairing the right qi	
Niú xī (Radix Achyranthis Bidentatae)	With a descending nature, both medicinals can invigorate the blood to remove stasis, nourish the liver and kidney, strengthen the bones and sinews, induce diuresis to relieve stranguria, guide blood (fire) and other medicinals downwards	It is effective for nourishing the liver and kidney, strengthening the bones and sinews	
chuān niú xī (Radix Cyathulae)		It is effective for invigorating the blood, removing stasis and activating the channels	
Wáng bù liú xíng (Semen Vaccariae)	Invigorates the blood and activates the channels	Induces lactation, eliminates carbuncles, induces diuresis to relieve stranguria	
Líng xiāo huā (Flos Campsis)		Cools blood and expels wind	
Yuè jì huā (Flos Rosae Chinensis)	Invigorates the blood to regulate menstruation, soothes the liver to relieve depression, reduces swelling and detoxifies		

Table 19-3: Summary of Medicinals that Invigorate the Blood to Treat Trauma:

Medicinal	Action in Common	Individual Character	
		Characteristic Actions	**Other Actions**
Tǔ biē chóng (Eupolyphaga seu Steleophaga)	Breaks up blood stasis, mends bone fractures and treats the impairment of sinews, it is regarded as an essential medicinal to treat bone fractures, impairment of sinews and abdominal masses		
Zì rán tóng (Pyritum)	Invigorates the blood to treat trauma, removes stasis to relieve pain		It is effective for promoting the healing of bone fractures, and is regarded as an essential medicinal to mend bone fractures and treat the impairment of sinews
Liú jì nú (Herba Artemisiae Anomalae)		Invigorates the blood and activates the channels	Stops bleeding, promotes digestion to remove food retention
Sū mù (Lignum Sappan)			Invigorates the blood if used in small dosages, breaks up blood stasis if used in large dosages
Mǎ qián zǐ (Semen Strychni)	Removes masses, reduces swelling, activates the channels to relieve pain		
Gǔ suì bǔ (Rhizoma Drynariae)	Invigorates the blood to treat trauma, nourishes the kidney to strengthen the bones		
Xuè jié (Sanguis Draconis)	Invigorates the blood to treat trauma, transforms stasis to stop bleeding, promotes the generation of tissue and wound healing	Invigorates the blood to relieve pain	
Ér chá (Catechu)		Removes damp and promotes wound healing	

Table 19-4: Summary of Medicinals that Break up Blood Stasis:

Medicinal	Action in Common	Individual Character	
		Characteristic Actions	**Other Actions**
É zhú (Rhizoma Curcumae)	Breaks up blood stasis, promotes qi circulation, removes food retention to relieve pain	It is effective for removing qi stagnation and food retention	
Sān léng (Rhizoma Sparganii)		It is effective for breaking up blood stasis	
Shuǐ zhì (Hirudo)	Slightly toxic, breaks up blood stasis to remove hard masses	It has a more moderate and lasting action than *méng chóng* (Tabanus)	
Méng chóng (Tabanus)		It has a drastic action, the patient can have diarrhea after taking the medicinal, but it will cease when the medicinal is discontinued.	
Bān máo (Mylabris)	It has a severe toxicity; it can break up blood stasis, and remove hard masses. It is effective for treating hepatic cancer. It removes toxic materials.		
Chuān shān jiǎ (Squama Manis)	It has a migrating nature, it can invigorate the blood to remove hard masses, activate the channels to induce lactation, reduce swelling and promote the discharge of pus. It is regarded as an essential medicinal to treat galactostasis postpartum.		

Tables to test your herbal knowledge of actions and indications of medicinals that invigorate the blood and transform stasis are as follows (Table 19-5~19-12):

Table 19-5: Test your Herbal Knowledge of the Actions of Medicinals that Invigorate the Blood to Relieve Pain:

Medicinal Actions	Chuān xiōng	Yán hú suǒ	Yù jīn	Jiāng huáng	Rǔ xiāng	Mò yào	Wǔ líng zhī
Invigorates the blood and promotes qi circulation							
Expels wind to relieve pain							
Invigorates the blood							
Promotes qi circulation							
Activates the channels to relieve pain							
Invigorates the blood and promotes qi circulation to relieve pain							
Clears the heart to relieve depression							
Transforms stasis to stop bleeding							
Cools blood							
Relieves pain							
Reduces swelling and promotes the regeneration of tissue							
Invigorates the blood to relieve pain							
Benefits the gallbladder to relieve jaundice							

Table 19-6: Test your Herbal Knowledge of the Actions of Medicinals that Invigorate the Blood to Regulate Menstruation:

Actions / Medicinal	Dān shēn	Hóng huā	Táo rén	Yì mǔ cǎo	Zé lán	Niú xī	Jī xuè téng	Wáng bù liú xíng	Yuè jì huā	Líng xiāo huā
Strengthens the bones and sinews										
Cools the blood and eliminates carbuncles										
Tranquilizes the mind										
Invigorates the blood and activates the channels										
Removes stasis to relieve pain										
Induces lactation										
Promotes the flow of water to reduce edema										
Nourishes the liver and kidney										
Invigorates the blood to regulate menstruation										
Promotes the flow of water to relieve stranguria										
Guides fire and blood downwards										
Nourishes the blood										
Relaxes the sinews and activates the collaterals										
Moistens the intestines to promote defecation										
Eliminates carbuncles										
Relieves depression										
Reduces swellings										
Cools the blood and expels wind										

Table 19-7: Test your Herbal Knowledge of the Actions of Medicinals that Invigorate the Blood to Treat Trauma:

Actions / Medicinal	Tǔ biē chóng	Zì rán tóng	Sū mù	Gǔ suì bǔ	Mǎ qián zǐ	Xuè jié	Ér chá	Liú jì nú
Nourishes the kidney to strengthen bones								
Cures bone fractures and impairment of the sinews								
Removes stasis to relieve pain								
Activates collaterals to relieve pain								
Invigorates the blood to treat trauma								
Removes stasis and activates channels								
Invigorates the blood to cure bone fractures								
Breaks up blood stasis								
Removes stasis to reduce swelling								
Cures bone fractures and treats trauma								
Stops bleeding, promotes regeneration of tissue and wound healing								
Activates channels								
Stops bleeding								

Table 19-8: Test your Herbal Knowledge of the Actions of Medicinals that Break up Blood Stasis:

Actions / Medicinal	É zhú	Sān léng	Shuǐ zhì	Méng chóng	Bān máo	Chuān shān jiǎ
Breaks up blood stasis						
Activates the channels						
Breaks up blood stasis, removes abdominal hard masses						
Eliminates toxic material						
Invigorates the blood to remove abdominal masses						
Removes food retention to relieve pain						
Induces lactation						
Reduces swelling and promotes the discharge of pus						

Table 19-9: Test your Herbal Knowledge of the Indications of Medicinals that Invigorate the Blood to Relieve Pain:

Indications / Medicinal	Chuān xiōng	Yán hú suǒ	Yù jīn	Jiāng huáng	Rǔ xiāng	Mò yào	Wǔ líng zhī
Various types of pain caused by blood stasis and qi stagnation							
Skin diseases							
Headaches							
Bi due to wind damp							
Injuries due to trauma							
Bleeding due to blood stasis							
Epilepsy and fainting due to phlegm obstruction							
Damp heat in the liver and gallbladder							
Bleeding due to blood heat							
Chest blockage due to blood stasis							
Toothache							
Hyperlipidemia							
Coma due to febrile diseases							
Scrofula, superficial nodules							

Table 19-10: Test your Herbal Knowledge of the Indications of Medicinals that Invigorate the Blood to Regulate Menstruation:

Medicinal / Indications	Dān shēn	Hóng huā	Fān hóng huā	Táo rén	Yì mǔ cǎo	Zé lán	Niú xī	Jī xuè téng	Wáng bù liú xíng	Yuè jì huā	Líng xiāo huā
Irregular menstruation											
Palpitations and insomnia due to stubborn diseases											
Postpartum abdominal pain due to blood stasis											
Chest blockage due to blood stasis											
Abdominal hard masses											
Pulmonary and intestinal abscesses											
Skin diseases											
Vexation and coma due to febrile diseases											
Amenorrhea and dysmenorrhea due to blood stasis											
Injuries due to trauma											
Dark maculae											
Constipation due to dry intestines											
Bi due to wind damp											
Edema, dysuria											
Stranguria											
Waist pain due to kidney deficiency											
Liver qi constraint											
Flaring up of fire and heat											
Galactostasis postpartum, breast abscesses											
Stroke with paralysis											
Aching in the waist and knees due to chronic bi											

Table 19-11: Test your Herbal Knowledge of the Indications of Medicinals that Invigorate the Blood to Treat Trauma:

Indications \ Medicinal	Tŭ biē chóng	Zì rán tóng	Sū mù	Gŭ suì bŭ	Mă qián zĭ	Xuè jié	Ér chá	Liú jì nú
Carbuncle, ulcers								
Bone fractures, impairment of the sinews								
Swelling and pain due to stasis								
Amenorrhea due to blood stasis								
Numbness, paralysis								
Abdominal hard masses due to blood stasis								
Cardiac and abdominal pain due to blood stasis								
Injuries due to trauma								
Waist pain and weak legs due to kidney deficiency								
Tinnitus and deafness due to kidney deficiency								
Abdominal pain caused by food retention								
Alopecia areata, vitiligo								
Stubborn bi due to wind damp								
Postpartum abdominal pain due to blood stasis								
Bleeding due to trauma								
Skin diseases with rupture failing to heal for a long time								
Chronic diarrhea and toothache due to kidney deficiency								
Dysentery with bloody and purulent discharge								
Cough due to lung heat								

Table 19-12: Test your Herbal Knowledge of the Indications of Medicinals that Break Up Blood Stasis:

Indications \ Medicinal	É zhú	Sān léng	Shuĭ zhì	Méng chóng	Bān máo	Chuān shān jiă
Stubborn tinea						
Amenorrhea due to blood stasis						
Cardiac and abdominal pain due to blood stasis						
Bleeding due to trauma						
Injuries due to trauma						
Carbuncles, chronic ulcers						
Abdominal hard masses due to blood stasis						
Bi due to wind damp						
Galactostasis postpartum						
Superficial nodules						
Abdominal pain due to food retention						

Chapter 20
Medicinals that Stop Cough, Calm Panting and Transform Phlegm

Concept

Medicinals that help to remove or dissolve phlegm and are used to treat phlegm syndrome are called medicinals that transform phlegm. Medicinals with the main actions of stopping or relieving cough and panting are called medicinals that stop cough and calm panting. Medicinals that transform phlegm always have the actions of stopping cough and calming panting, and medicinals for stopping cough and calming panting can often transform phlegm. Therefore these two kinds of medicinals are compiled in one chapter.

Indications

Medicinals for transforming phlegm are indicated for phlegm syndrome. Phlegm is both a pathological product and causative factor. It moves with qi activity and exists everywhere. Therefore, phlegm syndrome can cause different diseases, like cough with profuse phlegm due to phlegm obstruction in the lung; coma and epilepsy induced by phlegm obstruction in the heart orifice; numbness in the limbs and trunk, hemiparalysis and facial distortion due to phlegm retention in the channels and collaterals; scrofula and goiter due to mingling of phlegm with fire; and multiple abscesses due to phlegm retention in the muscles. Medicinals for stopping cough

and calming panting are used for cough and panting caused by either external invasion or internal injury.

Combinations

Medicinals for transforming phlegm or medicinals for stopping cough and calming panting are selected according to different symptoms and signs. In addition, cough and panting are always accompanied by phlegm, while profuse phlegm can often cause cough. Therefore, medicinals for transforming phlegm and medicinals for stopping cough and calming panting are commonly used together. In addition, combinations should be based on different causative factors of phlegm, cough and panting, so as to treat the root with consideration of the branch. For diseases caused by external invasion, combine with medicinals for dispersing external pathogens to relieve the exterior syndrome. For fire and heat syndrome, combine with medicinals for clearing heat and purging fire. For cold in the interior, add medicinals for warming the interior to dispel cold. For internal injury due to overstrain, add medicinals with the action of nourishing deficiency. For epilepsy, convulsion, vertigo and coma, combine with medicinals for calming the liver to extinguish wind, opening the orifices, and tranquilizing the mind. For superficial nodules, scrofula and goiter, add medicinals for softening hard masses and removing stasis. For multiple abscesses, add medicinals with the actions of warming yang and removing stagnation. Different medicinals with the action of transforming phlegm are selected according to different kinds of phlegm syndrome. Furthermore, treatment should be based on the pathogenesis of phlegm. "*Spleen is the source of phlegm*" and spleen deficiency leads to a failure of the body fluids to be transformed. These fluids then gather and form phlegm. Therefore, medicinals for invigorating phlegm to dry damp are often used in combination. Phlegm can easily stagnate qi activity, "*qi stagnation will lead to production of phlegm, while normal qi circulation can transform phlegm*", and therefore medicinals for regulating qi activity are always added to enhance the effect of transforming phlegm.

Precautions

Some medicinals for transforming phlegm are harsh and stimulating, so they are not suitable for syndromes of hemorrhagic tendencies, such as phlegm accompanied by blood. For cases of cough due to measles during the initial stage with external pathogens, medicinals for stopping cough should not be used alone. The principle of clearing lung heat should be used, so as not to retain pathogenic factors. Retention of pathogens can cause chronic panting and affect the smooth eruption of measles. Astringent medicinals and medicinals with a warm and dry nature also should be avoided.

Classification

According to their different characters, effects and indications, medicinals for stopping cough, calming panting, and transforming phlegm are classified into three categories: Medicinals that warm and transform cold phlegm, medicinals that clear heat and transform phlegm, and medicinals that stop cough and calm panting.

Section 1 Medicinals that Warm and Transform Cold Phlegm

Medicinals in this section usually have a pungent and bitter flavor, and a warm and dry property. They often enter the lung, spleen and liver channels to warm the lung and dispel cold, dry damp, and transform phlegm. They are indicated for cold phlegm and damp phlegm syndrome, manifesting as cough with panting, profuse white phlegm, a greasy tongue coating; vertigo, numbness, and multiple abscesses induced by cold and damp phlegm. Warm medicinals that transform cold phlegm are not suitable for heat phlegm or dry phlegm syndrome.

① *Bàn xià* (半夏, Rhizoma Pinelliae, Pinellia Tuber)
★★★

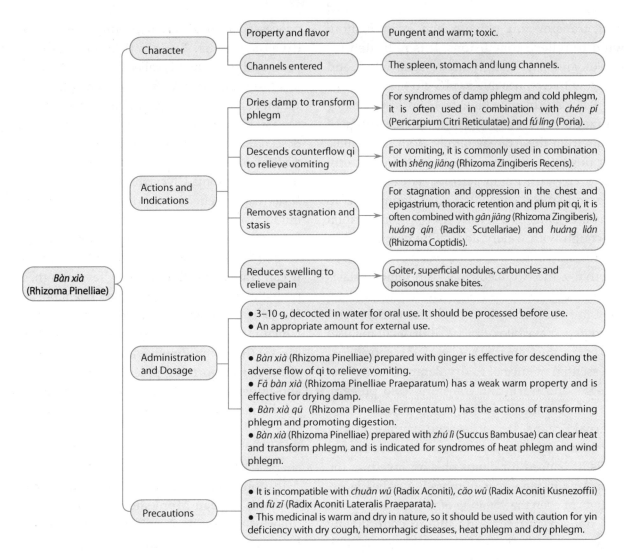

Bàn xià (Rhizoma Pinelliae)

- Character
  - Property and flavor → Pungent and warm; toxic.
  - Channels entered → The spleen, stomach and lung channels.
- Actions and Indications
  - Dries damp to transform phlegm → For syndromes of damp phlegm and cold phlegm, it is often used in combination with *chén pí* (Pericarpium Citri Reticulatae) and *fú líng* (Poria).
  - Descends counterflow qi to relieve vomiting → For vomiting, it is commonly used in combination with *shēng jiāng* (Rhizoma Zingiberis Recens).
  - Removes stagnation and stasis → For stagnation and oppression in the chest and epigastrium, thoracic retention and plum pit qi, it is often combined with *gān jiāng* (Rhizoma Zingiberis), *huáng qín* (Radix Scutellariae) and *huáng lián* (Rhizoma Coptidis).
  - Reduces swelling to relieve pain → Goiter, superficial nodules, carbuncles and poisonous snake bites.
- Administration and Dosage
  - 3–10 g, decocted in water for oral use. It should be processed before use.
  - An appropriate amount for external use.
  - *Bàn xià* (Rhizoma Pinelliae) prepared with ginger is effective for descending the adverse flow of qi to relieve vomiting.
  - *Fǎ bàn xià* (Rhizoma Pinelliae Praeparatum) has a weak warm property and is effective for drying damp.
  - *Bàn xià qū* (Rhizoma Pinelliae Fermentatum) has the actions of transforming phlegm and promoting digestion.
  - *Bàn xià* (Rhizoma Pinelliae) prepared with *zhú lì* (Succus Bambusae) can clear heat and transform phlegm, and is indicated for syndromes of heat phlegm and wind phlegm.
- Precautions
  - It is incompatible with *chuān wū* (Radix Aconiti), *cǎo wū* (Radix Aconiti Kusnezoffii) and *fù zǐ* (Radix Aconiti Lateralis Praeparata).
  - This medicinal is warm and dry in nature, so it should be used with caution for yin deficiency with dry cough, hemorrhagic diseases, heat phlegm and dry phlegm.

② *Tiān nán xīng* (天南星, Rhizoma Arisaematis, Jackinthepulpit Tuber) ★★

Addition: *Dǎn nán xīng* (胆南星, Arisaema cum Bile, Bile Arisaema) has the actions of clearing

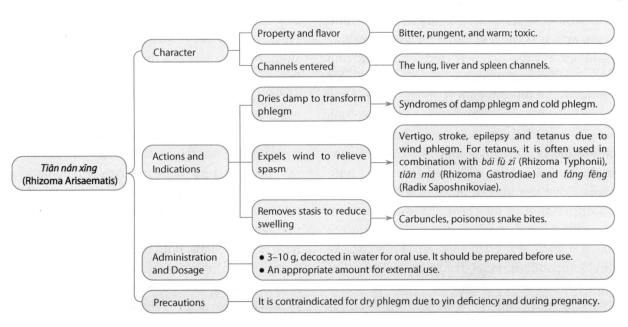

Tiān nán xīng (Rhizoma Arisaematis)

- Character
  - Property and flavor → Bitter, pungent, and warm; toxic.
  - Channels entered → The lung, liver and spleen channels.
- Actions and Indications
  - Dries damp to transform phlegm → Syndromes of damp phlegm and cold phlegm.
  - Expels wind to relieve spasm → Vertigo, stroke, epilepsy and tetanus due to wind phlegm. For tetanus, it is often used in combination with *bái fù zǐ* (Rhizoma Typhonii), *tiān má* (Rhizoma Gastrodiae) and *fáng fēng* (Radix Saposhnikoviae).
  - Removes stasis to reduce swelling → Carbuncles, poisonous snake bites.
- Administration and Dosage
  - 3–10 g, decocted in water for oral use. It should be prepared before use.
  - An appropriate amount for external use.
- Precautions → It is contraindicated for dry phlegm due to yin deficiency and during pregnancy.

heat, transforming phlegm, and extinguishing wind to relieve convulsions. It is indicated for stroke, epilepsy, vertigo due to head wind, and cough with dyspnea due to phlegm fire.

Bàn xià (Rhizoma Pinelliae) and *tiān nán xīng* (Rhizoma Arisaematis) are the dried tuber of plants from the Araceae family. Both medicinals are pungent in flavor, warm and dry in property and toxic with harsh actions. They enter the lung and spleen channels to dry damp so as to transform phlegm. They are used in combination for cough with watery and white expectoration due to damp phlegm and cold phlegm. When used externally, the two medicinals can remove stasis and reduce swellings so as to relieve pain, and are used to treat carbuncles, superficial nodules and poisonous snake bites. *Bàn xià* (Rhizoma Pinelliae) also enters the stomach channel, and is considered an essential medicinal to dry damp to transform phlegm, and warm and transform cold phlegm. It is effective for dissolving damp phlegm in the internal organs. It can descend counterflow qi to relieve vomiting, and remove stagnation and stasis. It is used for damp phlegm invading the clear yang in the upper, manifesting as headache, vertigo, or even the vomiting of phlegm and saliva, and nausea and vomiting due to counterflow stomach qi. When used in combination with other medicinals, it is an essential medicinal to relieve vomiting. It is used for vomiting caused by various factors such as stomach cold, stomach heat, stomach deficiency, phlegm-fluids, and pregnancy. It is most suitable for vomiting due to phlegm-fluids, stomach cold; epigastric and abdominal stagnation, thoracic accumulation due to mingling of phlegm with heat; and plum pit qi caused by phlegm congealing due to qi constraint. *Tiān nán xīng* (Rhizoma Arisaematis) has stronger actions and is more toxic than *bàn xià* (Rhizoma Pinelliae). It is commonly used for cough with dyspnea due to stubborn phlegm, and distension and oppression in the chest and diaphragm. It enters the liver channel, and can dispel wind to relieve spasms. It is often used for vertigo, stroke with hemiparalysis, facial distortion, epilepsy, and tetanus due to wind phlegm.

In addtion, *bàn xià* (Rhizoma Pinelliae) is processed into different products, which have diverse actions. *Bàn xià* (Rhizoma Pinelliae) processed with alum is called *qīng bàn xià*, which is less toxic, and effective for dissolving phlegm. *Bàn xià* prepared with ginger and alum is called *jiāng bàn xià*. It has even less toxicity and is effective for descending counterflow qi to relieve vomiting. *Bàn xià* (Rhizoma Pinelliae) prepared with alum, *gān cǎo* (Radix et Rhizoma Glycyrrhizae) and lime is called *fǎ bàn xià*. It is effective for drying damp and has a mildly warm property. *Bàn xià* (Rhizoma Pinelliae) fermented with flour and ginger juice is called *bàn xià qū* (半夏曲, Rhizoma Pinelliae Fermentatum). It can transform phlegm to relieve cough, and promote digestion to remove food retention. *Zhú lì bàn xià* is prepared with *zhú lì* (Succus Bambusae), which moderates the warm and dry property of *bàn xià* (Rhizoma Pinelliae), and strengthens the effect of transforming phlegm. It is able to clear and transform heat phlegm, and is indicated for syndromes of hot phlegm and wind phlegm.

③ *Yǔ bái fù* (禹白附, Rhizoma Typhonii, Giant Typhonium Tuber) ★

Addition: **Guān bái fù (关白附, Radix Aconiti Coreani, Korean Monkshood Root)** is the root tuber of the family *Aconitum coreanum* Rapaics, Ranunculaceae. *Bái fù zǐ*, as recorded in ancient herbal documents, actually refers to *guān bái fù* (Radix Aconiti Coreani). Both *yǔ bái fù* (Rhizoma Typhonii) and *guān bái fù* (Radix Aconiti Coreani) can dispel wind phlegm to relieve spasm. However, *yǔ bái fù* (Rhizoma Typhonii) has a slight toxicity, but can detoxify to remove stasis. It is now extensively used as the correct species of *bái fù zǐ*. *Guān bái fù* (Radix Aconiti Coreani) has a severe toxicity. It has a strong emphasis on dispelling cold and damp to relieve pain, and is indicated for migraines, headaches and *bi*.

Tiān nán xīng (Rhizoma Arisaematis) and *yǔ bái fù* (Rhizoma Typhonii) come from the dried tuber of plants from the family Araceae. They are pungent in flavor, warm in property, toxic, and have harsh actions. Both medicinals can dry damp to transform phlegm and expel wind to relieve spasms, and are capable of removing wind phlegm in the channels and collaterals. The two medicinals

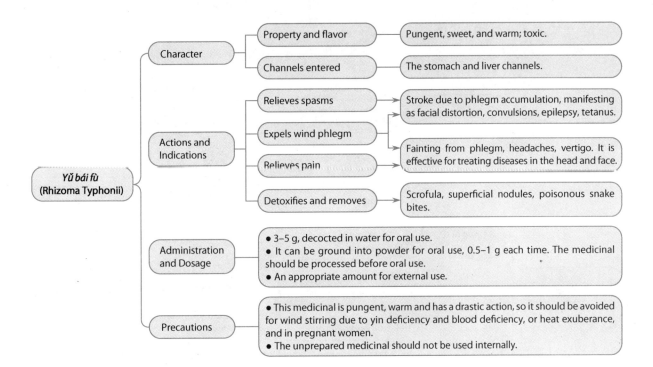

are used in combination to treat vertigo, facial distortion, epilepsy, and tetanus due to wind phlegm. They can also be used externally to remove toxic materials, and dispel stasis to reduce swelling. Therefore they are used for carbuncles, scrofula, superficial nodules, and poisonous snake bites. Their differences are as follows: *Tiān nán xīng* (Rhizoma Arisaematis) can dry damp to transform phlegm. It enters the lung channel to treat syndromes of cold phlegm and damp phlegm,

cough due to stubborn phlegm, and distension and distress in the chest and diaphragm. *Yǔ bái fù* (Rhizoma Typhonii) has an ascending nature. It guides other medicinals upwards to the head and face, and therefore is effective for treating various diseases on the head and face, such as fainting from phlegm, headaches, and migraines.

④ *Bái jiè zǐ* (白芥子, Semen Sinapis, White Mustard Seed) ★

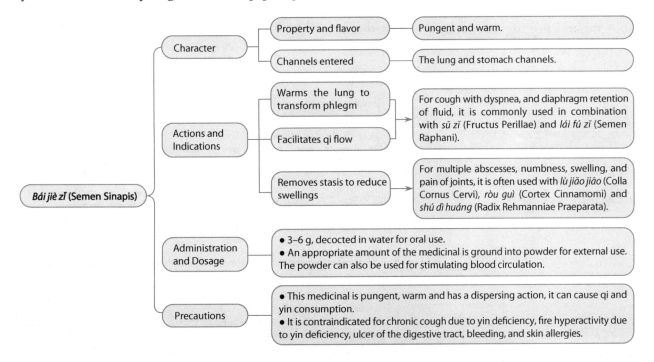

⑤ *Zào jiá* (皂荚, Fructus Gleditsiae, Chinese Honeylocust Fruit) ★

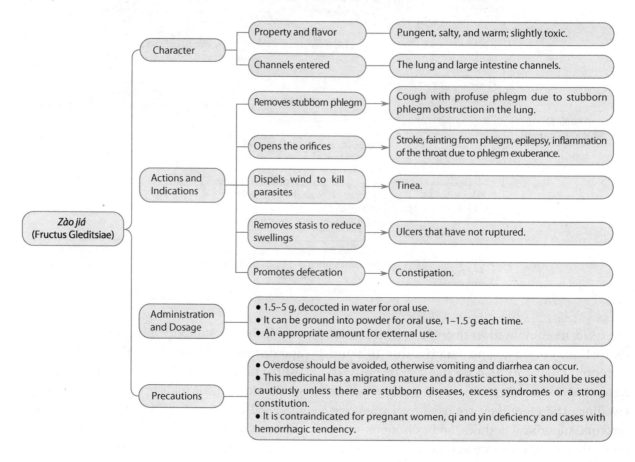

Zào jiá
(Fructus Gleditsiae)

- **Character**
  - Property and flavor — Pungent, salty, and warm; slightly toxic.
  - Channels entered — The lung and large intestine channels.

- **Actions and Indications**
  - Removes stubborn phlegm — Cough with profuse phlegm due to stubborn phlegm obstruction in the lung.
  - Opens the orifices — Stroke, fainting from phlegm, epilepsy, inflammation of the throat due to phlegm exuberance.
  - Dispels wind to kill parasites — Tinea.
  - Removes stasis to reduce swellings — Ulcers that have not ruptured.
  - Promotes defecation — Constipation.

- **Administration and Dosage**
  - 1.5–5 g, decocted in water for oral use.
  - It can be ground into powder for oral use, 1–1.5 g each time.
  - An appropriate amount for external use.

- **Precautions**
  - Overdose should be avoided, otherwise vomiting and diarrhea can occur.
  - This medicinal has a migrating nature and a drastic action, so it should be used cautiously unless there are stubborn diseases, excess syndromes or a strong constitution.
  - It is contraindicated for pregnant women, qi and yin deficiency and cases with hemorrhagic tendency.

⑥ *Xuán fù huā* (旋覆花, Flos Inulae, Intussusceer) ★

Bái jiè zǐ (Semen Sinapis), *xuán fù huā* (Flos Inulae) and *zào jiá* (Fructus Gleditsiae) can remove phlegm, and are used for cough with profuse phlegm. Their differences are as follows: *Bái jiè zǐ* (Semen Sinapis) is pungent and warm with a dispersing action. It can warm the lung to transform phlegm, and is indicated for cough

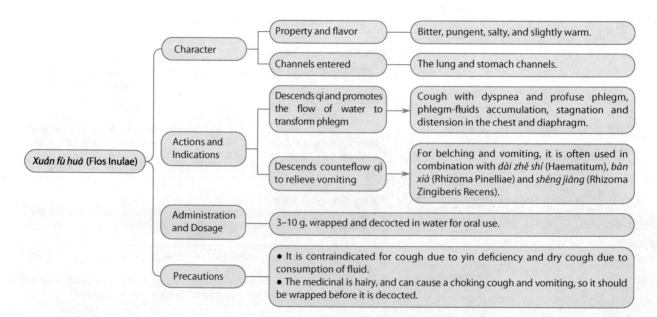

Xuán fù huā (Flos Inulae)

- **Character**
  - Property and flavor — Bitter, pungent, salty, and slightly warm.
  - Channels entered — The lung and stomach channels.

- **Actions and Indications**
  - Descends qi and promotes the flow of water to transform phlegm — Cough with dyspnea and profuse phlegm, phlegm-fluids accumulation, stagnation and distension in the chest and diaphragm.
  - Descends counteflow qi to relieve vomiting — For belching and vomiting, it is often used in combination with *dài zhě shí* (Haematitum), *bàn xià* (Rhizoma Pinelliae) and *shēng jiāng* (Rhizoma Zingiberis Recens).

- **Administration and Dosage** — 3–10 g, wrapped and decocted in water for oral use.

- **Precautions**
  - It is contraindicated for cough due to yin deficiency and dry cough due to consumption of fluid.
  - The medicinal is hairy, and can cause a choking cough and vomiting, so it should be wrapped before it is decocted.

with dyspnea due to cold phlegm, diaphragm fluid retention with cough and panting, and thoracic accumulation and hypochondriac pain. It can also facilitate qi activity and remove stasis, activate the collaterals and reduce swelling to relieve pain. It is often used for dorsal furuncles due to damp phlegm oozing in the body; pain in the body and joints, and numbness due to damp phlegm obstruction in the channels and collaterals. *"Phlegm in the hypochondrium and subcutaneous area can only be removed by bái jiè zǐ (Semen Sinapis)."* *Xuán fù huā* (Flos Inulae) can descend qi and promote the flow of water so as to transform phlegm, and is indicated for cough with profuse phlegm due to phlegm accumulation in the lung, phlegm-fluids accumulation with stagnation, and oppression in the chest and diaphragm. It is effective for descending counterflow qi to relieve vomiting and belching, therefore it is commonly used for belching, vomiting, stagnation in the epigastrium due to phlegm-turbidity obstruction in the middle and counterflow stomach qi. *Zào jiá* (Fructus Gleditsiae) is pungent, warm and toxic. It can eliminate stubborn phlegm, and is frequently used for cough with dyspnea, expectoration of thick phlegm, and difficulty lying flat in bed. In addition, it can open the orifices to induce resuscitation, and dispel wind to kill parasites. It is also used for stroke, fainting due to phlegm, epilepsy, inflammation of the throat, and tinea.

⑦ *Bái qián* (白前, Rhizoma et Radix Cynanchi Stauntonii, Cynanchum Root and Rhizome) ★

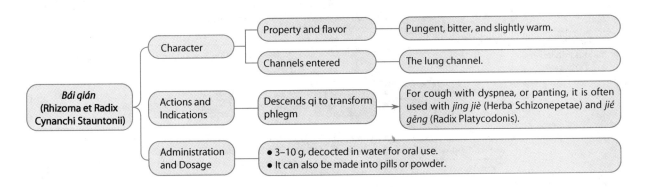

⑧ *Māo zhuǎ cǎo* (猫爪草, Radix Ranunculi Ternati, Catclaw Buttercup Root)

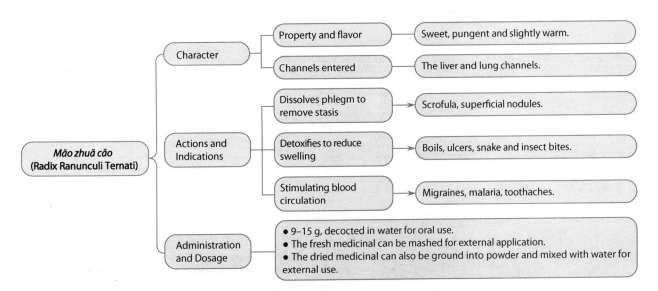

Section 2   Medicinals that Clear Heat and Transform Phlegm

Medicinals in this section are mostly cool or cold in property with the actions of clearing heat and transforming phlegm. Some of the medicinals have a moist texture, and can moisten dryness. Some have a salty flavor and can soften hard masses and remove stasis. Medicinals for clearing heat and transforming phlegm are indicated for syndromes of heat phlegm, such as cough with dyspnea, and yellow and thick expectoration.

For dry phlegm with manifestations such as thick sputum that is difficult to expectorate, dry lips and mouth, choose moist medicinals for transforming phlegm. For phlegm heat with epilepsy, stroke with convulsions and syncope, goiter, and scrofula due to phlegm fire, use medicinals for clearing heat and transforming phlegm. However, the two kinds of medicinals mentioned above are not suitable for cold phlegm or damp phlegm.

① *Chuān bèi mǔ* (川贝母, Bulbus Fritillariae Cirrhosae, Tendrilled Fritillaria Bulb) ★★★

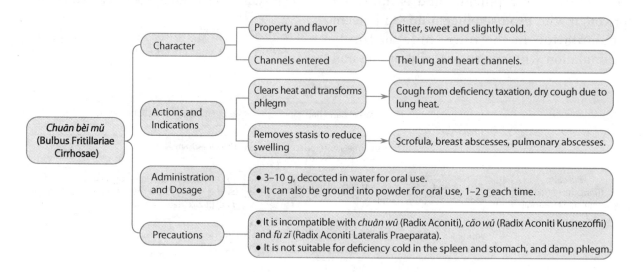

② *Zhè bèi mǔ* (浙贝母, Bulbus Fritillariae Thunbergii, Thunberg Fritillary Bulb) ★★★

When people refer to *bèi mǔ*, they are actually talking about two different types *chuān bèi mǔ*

(Bulbus Fritillariae Cirrhosae) and *zhè bèi mǔ* (Bulbus Fritillariae Thunbergii). Before the compilation of the *Compendium of the Materia Medica*, these two medicinals were written simply

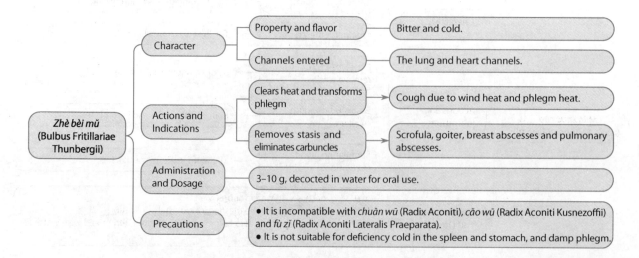

as *bèi mǔ* in herbal documents. *"Chuān bèi mǔ (Bulbus Fritillariae Cirrhosae) has a better therapeutic effect"* is initially recorded in *A Grand Collection of the Materia Medica (Běn Cǎo Huì Yán, 本草汇言)*. *Zhè bèi mǔ* (Bulbus Fritillariae Thunbergii) was first mentioned in *The Materia Medica of Rescuing (Xuān Qí Jiù Zhèng Lùn, 轩岐救正论)* of the *Qing* Dynasty. Both *chuān bèi mǔ* (Bulbus Fritillariae Cirrhosae) and *zhè bèi mǔ* (Bulbus Fritillariae Thunbergii) are bitter in flavor and cold in property. They enter the lung and heart channels to clear heat, transform phlegm, and remove stasis to reduce swelling. Both of these herbs can be used for cough due to phlegm heat or dry heat; scrofula, breast abscesses, and pulmonary abscesses. *Chuān bèi mǔ* (Bulbus Fritillariae Cirrhosae) is bitter and sweet in flavor, and slightly cold in property. It has a moist texture and therefore can moisten the lung to stop cough. It is most suitable for chronic cough due to internal injury, cough from over-strain due to yin deficiency, and dry cough with sticky phlegm. *Zhè bèi mǔ* (Bulbus Fritillariae Thunbergii) is bitter and cold with a stronger action in clearing heat, relieving depression, and removing stasis.

It is commonly used for cough due to wind heat invading the lung or phlegm heat retention in the lung, ulcers, breast abscesses, goiters, scrofula, and pulmonary abscesses.

③ *Guā lóu* (瓜蒌, Fructus Trichosanthis, Snakegourd Fruit) ★ ★ ★

In clinical practice, *guā lóu pí* (Pericarpium Trichosanthis), *guā lóu rén* (Semen Trichosanthis), *guā lóu shuāng* (defatted Semen Trichosanthis) and *quán guā lóu* (Fructus Trichosanthis) are all used. *Guā lóu pí* (Pericarpium Trichosanthis) can mainly clear the lung to transform phlegm, facilitate qi flow, and soothe the chest. *Guā lóu rén* (Semen Trichosanthis) has a moist texture and can moisten dryness, transform phlegm, and moisten the intestines to promote defecation. *Guā lóu shuāng* (defatted Semen Trichosanthis) has a similar but slower action than *guā lóu rén* (Semen Trichosanthis). *Quán guā lóu* (Fructus Trichosanthis) has the actions of clearing heat and moistening dryness to transform phlegm, soothing the chest to remove stasis, and moistening the intestines to promote defecation.

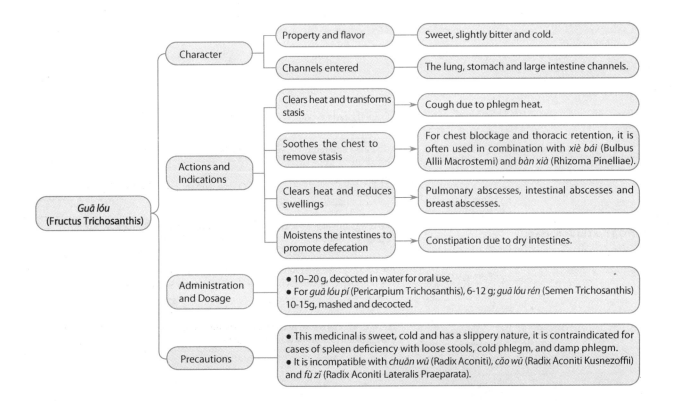

Guā lóu (Fructus Trichosanthis)	Character	Property and flavor	Sweet, slightly bitter and cold.
		Channels entered	The lung, stomach and large intestine channels.
	Actions and Indications	Clears heat and transforms stasis	Cough due to phlegm heat.
		Soothes the chest to remove stasis	For chest blockage and thoracic retention, it is often used in combination with *xiè bái* (Bulbus Allii Macrostemi) and *bàn xià* (Rhizoma Pinelliae).
		Clears heat and reduces swellings	Pulmonary abscesses, intestinal abscesses and breast abscesses.
		Moistens the intestines to promote defecation	Constipation due to dry intestines.
	Administration and Dosage		• 10–20 g, decocted in water for oral use. • For *guā lóu pí* (Pericarpium Trichosanthis), 6-12 g; *guā lóu rén* (Semen Trichosanthis) 10-15g, mashed and decocted.
	Precautions		• This medicinal is sweet, cold and has a slippery nature, it is contraindicated for cases of spleen deficiency with loose stools, cold phlegm, and damp phlegm. • It is incompatible with *chuān wū* (Radix Aconiti), *cǎo wū* (Radix Aconiti Kusnezoffii) and *fù zǐ* (Radix Aconiti Lateralis Praeparata).

④ *Zhú rú* (竹茹, Caulis Bambusae in Taenia, Bamboo Shavings) ★★

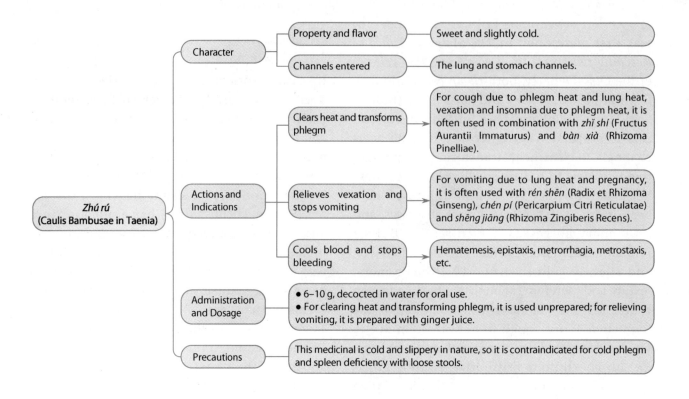

⑤ *Zhú lì* (竹沥, Succus Bambusae, Bamboo Juice) ★

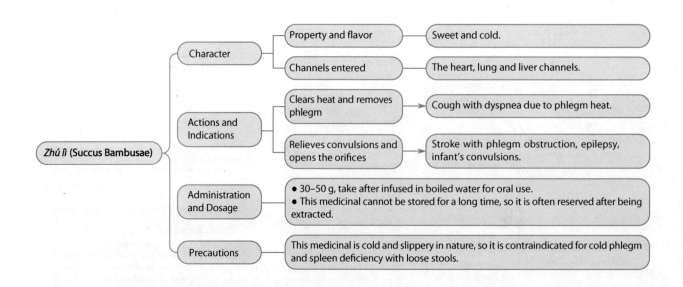

⑥ *Tiān zhú huáng* (天竺黄, Concretio Silicea Bambusae, Tabasheer)

Guā lóu (Fructus Trichosanthis), *zhú rú* (Caulis Bambusae in Taenia), *zhú lì* (Succus Bambusae) and *tiān zhú huáng* (Concretio Silicea Bambusae) are sweet in flavor, cold in property, and can clear heat and transform phlegm. They are used together to treat cough with yellow and sticky expectoration due to lung heat. *Guā lóu* (Fructus Trichosanthis) can moisten dryness to transform stasis, soothe the chest to remove stasis and moisten the intestines to promote defecation. It is used for dry cough without phlegm or with incomplete expectoration of scanty and sticky sputum, caused by dry heat impairing the lung; cardiac pain from chest blockage due to the binding of phlegm with qi, and inactivity of the chest yang. For such diseases, it is commonly used in combination with *xiè bái* (Bulbus Allii Macrostemi). It is considered an essential medicinal to treat chest blockage. For phlegm heat obstruction in the chest, manifesting as stagnation and oppression in the chest and diaphragm with pain upon palpation, it is often combined with *huáng lián* (Rhizoma Coptidis) and *bàn xià* (Rhizoma Pinelliae). It is also used for expectoration of purulent and bloody discharge due to pulmonary abscesses, abdominal pain due to intestinal abscesses, swelling and pain due to breast abscesses, as well as constipation

due to dry intestines. *Zhú rú* (Caulis Bambusae in Taenia) is effective for clearing heat and transforming phlegm to remove vexation and clearing the stomach to relieve vomiting. It is commonly used for chest oppression with profuse phlegm, vexation and insomnia due to gallbladder fire mingled with phlegm invading the lung and disturbing the heart; vomiting due to lung heat, and pregnancy. In addition, *zhú rú* (Caulis Bambusae in Taenia) can cool the blood and stop bleeding, and therefore is used for bleeding due to blood heat. *Zhú lì* (Succus Bambusae) has a slippery nature and a strong action in removing phlegm. It can clear heat to remove phlegm, and is most suitable for cough with dyspnea due to phlegm heat, incomplete expectoration of thick discharge, and stubborn phlegm. It is able to relieve convulsions and open the orifices, and is also used for stroke with phlegm obstruction, epilepsy, and convulsions in infants. *Tiān zhú huáng* (Concretio Silicea Bambusae) can clear heat and transform phlegm, and clear the heart to relieve convulsions. It has similar actions to *zhú lì* (Succus Bambusae) without the cold and slippery nature. It is commonly used for phlegm heat in the heart and liver channels, manifesting as infant's convulsions, stroke, epilepsy, and coma due to febrile diseases. It is also regarded as an essential medicinal to treat various infant's diseases caused by phlegm heat.

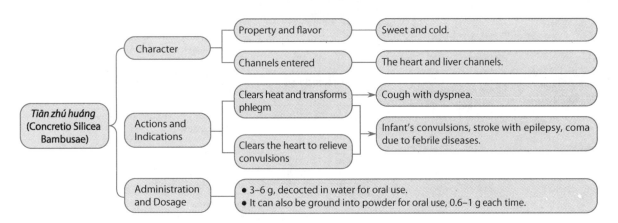

⑦ *Qián hú* (前胡, Radix Peucedani, Peucedanum Root) ★

Bái qián (Rhizoma et Radix Cynanchi Stauntonii)

and *qián hú* (Radix Peucedani) are pungent and bitter in character with a descending action. They can descend qi to transform phlegm, and are

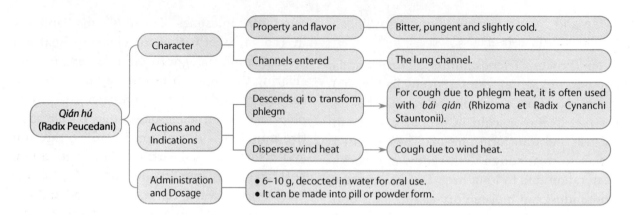

used for cough with excessive phlegm caused by counterflow qi due to phlegm accumulation. *Bái qián* (Rhizoma et Radix Cynanchi Stauntonii) has a slightly warm property. It can mainly warm and transform cold phlegm, and is used for cough with dyspnea due to cold phlegm. It can be used for cough of various kinds, and therefore is regarded as an essential medicinal in treating cough. *Qián hú* (Radix Peucedani) has a slightly cold property. It can clear heat and transform phlegm and is

indicated for cough with dyspnea due to phlegm heat. It is able to diffuse the lung and disperse wind heat. It is commonly used for cough with profuse phlegm, general fever, and headache caused by external invasion by wind heat and blocked lung qi. It is known as a medicinal with the action of diffusing and descending.

⑧ *Jié gěng* (桔梗, Radix Platycodonis, Platycodon Root) ★★★

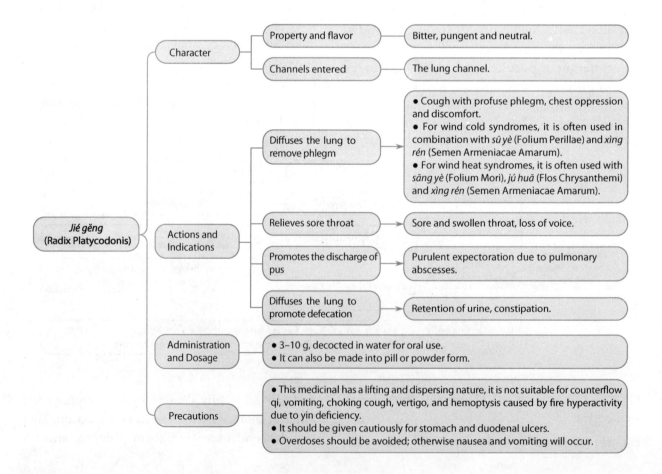

⑨ *Pàng dà hǎi* (胖大海, Semen Sterculiae Lychnophorae, Boat-fruited Sterculia Seed)

Both *jié gěng* (Radix Platycodonis) and *pàng dà hǎi* (Semen Sterculiae Lychnophorae) can diffuse the lung to transform stasis and relieve sore throat. They are used for sore and swollen throat and loss of voice. *Jié gěng* (Radix Platycodonis) is pungent and bitter in flavor, neutral in property, and has a strong action in diffusing the lung to remove phlegm. It can be used for sore throat and loss of voice caused by external pathogens invading the lung or heat toxin accumulation. It can also promote the discharge of pus, and guide other medicinals to move upwards. It is used in combination with other medicinals to treat cough with profuse phlegm of wind cold, wind heat, lung cold, or lung heat. It is also used for chest oppression and discomfort due to qi stagnation and phlegm obstruction; cough with chest pain and expectoration of foul and fishy sputum due to pulmonary abscesses. It has the effect of guiding other medicinals to move upward to treat diseases in the chest and above the diaphragm. In addition, it can diffuse lung qi to induce urination and defecation, and is used for the retention of urine and constipation. *Pàng dà hǎi* (Semen Sterculiae Lychnophorae) can mainly clear the lung to transform stasis and relieve sore throat. It is commonly used for hoarseness, sore throat, and cough due to lung heat. It can moisten the intestines to promote defecation, and therefore is used for constipation, headache, and blood-shot eyes due to dry heat.

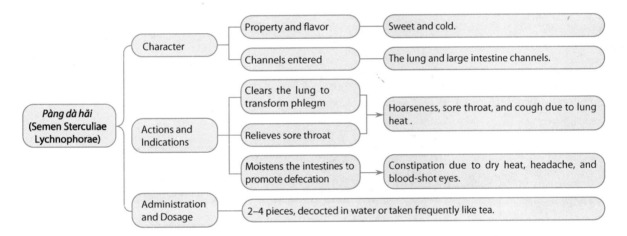

⑩ *Hǎi zǎo* (海藻, Sargassum, Seaweed) ★

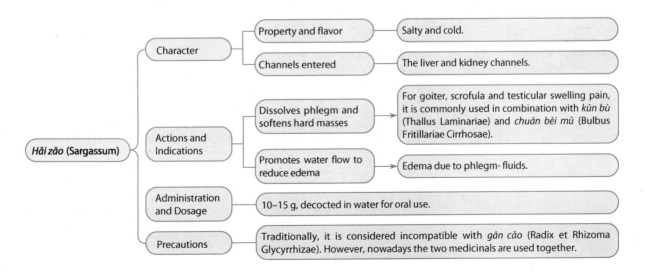

⑪ *Kūn bù* (昆布, Thallus Laminariae, Kelp) ★

Both *hǎi zǎo* (Sargassum) and *kūn bù* (Thallus Laminariae) have a salty flavor and cold property. Both medicinals can dissolve phlegm and soften hard masses, and promote the flow of water to

reduce edema. They are used in combination for mutual reinforcement to treat goiters, scrofula, testicular swelling pain, edema, and beriberi with swelling. They are essential medicinals to treat goiter and scrofula.

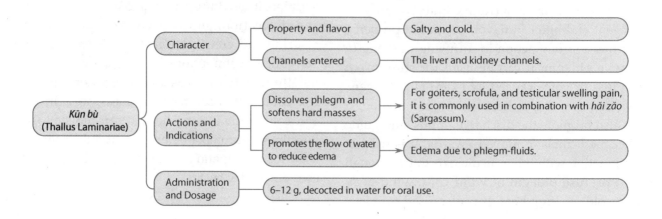

⑫ *Huáng yào zǐ* (黄药子, Rhizoma Dioscoreae Bulbiferae, Airpotato Yam) ★

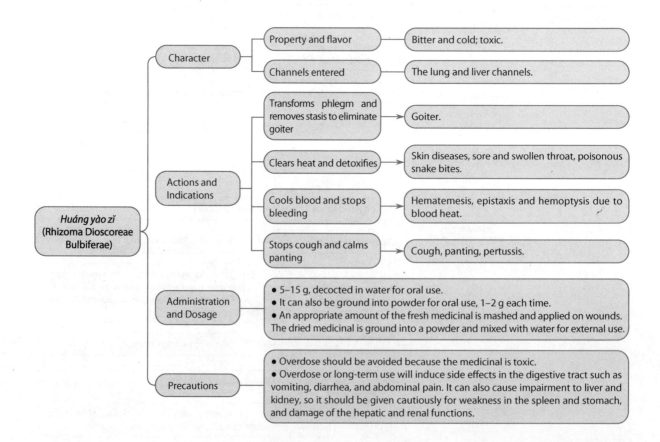

⑬ *Hǎi gé qiào* (海蛤壳, Concha Meretricis seu Cyclinae, Clam Shell) ★

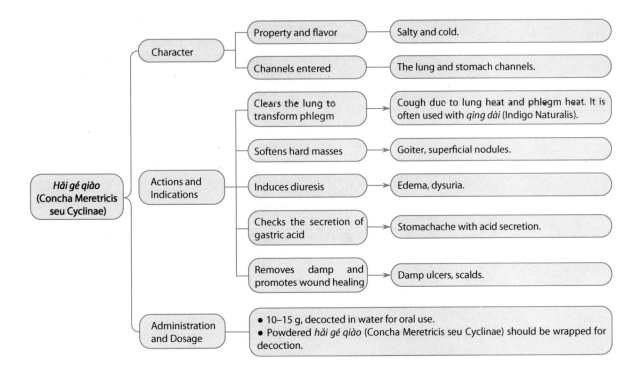

⑭ *Hǎi fú shí* (海浮石, Pumex, Pumice)

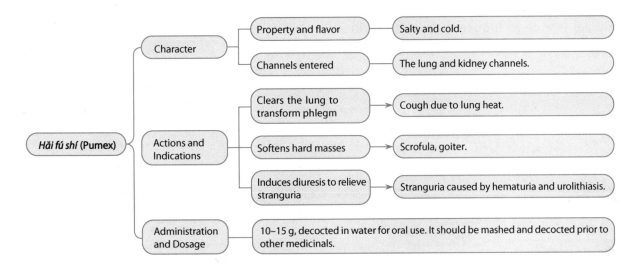

⑮ *Wǎ léng zǐ* (瓦楞子, Concha Arcae, Arc Shell)

Hǎi gé qiào (Concha Meretricis seu Cyclinae), *hǎi fú shí* (Pumex) and *wǎ léng zǐ* (Concha Arcae) are salty in flavor. They can dissolve phlegm, soften hardness, and remove stasis. They are used in combination to treat goiter, scrofula, and superficial nodules caused by the binding of accumulated phlegm and fire. *Hǎi gé qiào* (Concha Meretricis seu Cyclinae) and *hǎi fú shí* (Pumex) can clear the lung to transform phlegm, and are

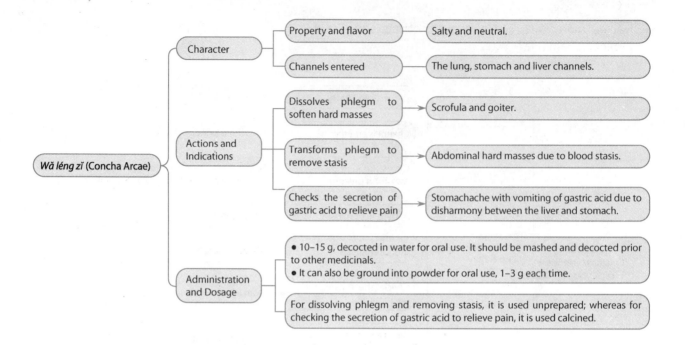

used for cough with dyspnea and expectoration of yellow and thick sputum caused by lung heat and phlegm fire. *Hǎi gé qiào* (Concha Meretricis seu Cyclinae) and *wǎ léng zǐ* (Concha Arcae) can check the secretion of gastric acid to relieve pain, and are used for stomachache with vomiting of gastric acid. *Hǎi gé qiào* (Concha Meretricis seu Cyclinae) is able to induce diuresis to reduce edema, and is used for edema and dysuria. *Hǎi*

fú shí (Pumex) can induce diuresis to relieve and treat stranguria caused by hematuria and urolithiasis. *Wǎ léng zǐ* (Concha Arcae) is capable of transforming and removing stasis, and is used for abdominal masses due to blood stasis and enlargement of the spleen and liver.

⑯ *Méng shí* (礞石, Chlorite-schist, Phlopopitum)

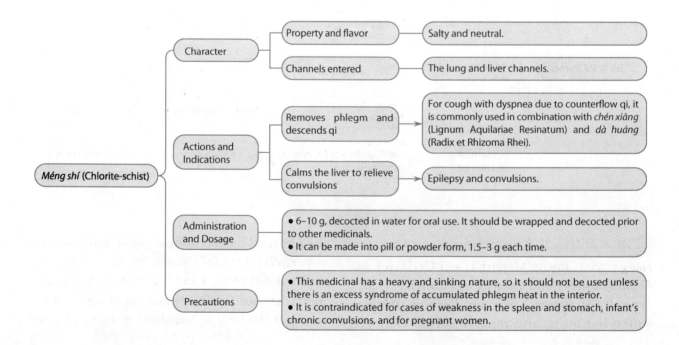

Section 3 Medicinals that Stop Cough and Calm Panting

Medicinals in this section enter the lung channel, and are pungent, bitter or sweet in flavor, and warm or cold in property. They have the actions of diffusing the lung, clearing the lung, moistening the lung, descending the lung qi, and astringing the lung in accordance with their characters. Some of them may have the principal effect of stopping cough, while some can mainly calm panting, and some may have the effect of both stopping cough and calming panting.

Medicinals of this kind are indicated for cough and panting. Cough and panting are caused by either external invasion or internal injury with manifestations of cold, heat, deficiency or excess. Medicinals for stopping cough and calming panting should be selected and properly combined with other medicinals according to the different syndromes present.

① *Kǔ xìng rén* (苦杏仁, Semen Armeniacae Amarum, Bitter Apricot Seed) ★ ★ ★

Addition: ***Tián xìng rén* (甜杏仁, Semen Armeniacae Dulce, Sweet Almond)** is sweet in flavor and neutral in property. It has a similar but mild action to *kǔ xìng rén* (Semen Armeniacae

Amarum). It can mainly moisten the lung to relieve cough. It is indicated for deficiency taxation cough and constipation due to fluid consumption.

Kǔ xìng rén (Semen Armeniacae Amarum) and *táo rén* (Semen Persicae) are bitter and moist, and can stop cough, calm panting and moisten the intestines to promote defecation. They are used for cough with dyspnea due to counterflow of lung qi; and constipation due to dry intestines. *Kǔ xìng rén* (Semen Armeniacae Amarum) is slightly warm and has a strong action in stopping cough and calming panting. It can be used for various types of cough caused by wind cold, wind heat, lung cold, lung heat, or dry heat. It is therefore regarded as an essential medicinal to stop cough and calm panting. In addition, it can diffuse and descend the lung qi, and is used for damp warmth in the initial stage with pathogens in the qi level and summer-heat warmth with damp. *Táo rén* (Semen Persicae) is neutral in property, and is effective for invigorating blood to remove stasis and activating the channels. It is indicated for irregular menstruation, amenorrhea, dysmenorrhea, postpartum abdominal pain, cardiac and abdominal pain, abdominal masses, injuries due to trauma, swelling and pain due to blood stasis; abdominal pain due to intestinal abscesses, and expectoration of purulent sputum

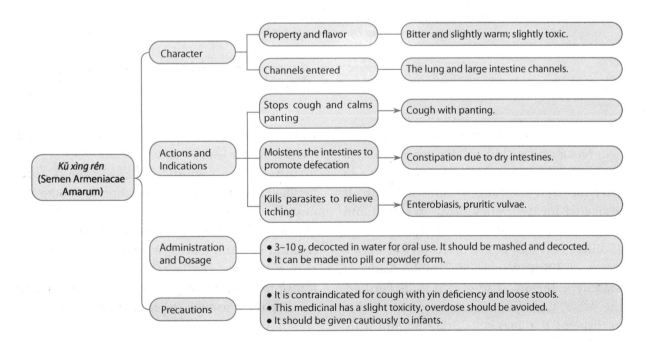

Kǔ xìng rén (Semen Armeniacae Amarum)	Character	Property and flavor	Bitter and slightly warm; slightly toxic.
		Channels entered	The lung and large intestine channels.
	Actions and Indications	Stops cough and calms panting	Cough with panting.
		Moistens the intestines to promote defecation	Constipation due to dry intestines.
		Kills parasites to relieve itching	Enterobiasis, pruritic vulvae.
	Administration and Dosage	• 3–10 g, decocted in water for oral use. It should be mashed and decocted. • It can be made into pill or powder form.	
	Precautions	• It is contraindicated for cough with yin deficiency and loose stools. • This medicinal has a slight toxicity, overdose should be avoided. • It should be given cautiously to infants.	

due to pulmonary abscesses. It is a commonly used medicinal to invigorate blood and transform stasis.

② *Zǐ sū zǐ* (紫苏子, Fructus Perillae, Perilla Fruit) ★ ★

Both *kǔ xìng rén* (Semen Armeniacae Amarum) and *zǐ sū zǐ* (Fructus Perillae) are warm in property and have a moist texture. They enter the lung and intestine, and can descend qi to stop cough and calm panting, and moisten the intestines to promote defecation. They are used for cough with dyspnea due to counterflow lung qi; constipation due to dry intestines, especially the kind that is complicated by counterflow lung qi. *Kǔ xìng rén* (Semen Armeniacae Amarum) is bitter in flavor, slightly warm in property, and

has a slight toxicity. It is able to descend the lung qi and diffuse the lung to stop cough and calm panting. It has a strong action in stopping cough and calming panting, and therefore is an essential medicinal for this. In addition, it is used for damp warmth in the initial stage with pathogens in the qi level and summer-heat warmth with damp, manifesting as fever after noon, chest oppression, no appetite, headache, and heaviness. *Zǐ sū zǐ* (Fructus Perillae) is pungent in flavor and warm in property. It can descend qi to transform phlegm, stop cough and calm panting. It is indicated for cough with dyspnea, profuse phlegm, stagnation, and oppression in the chest and diaphragm, and even difficulty lying down in bed.

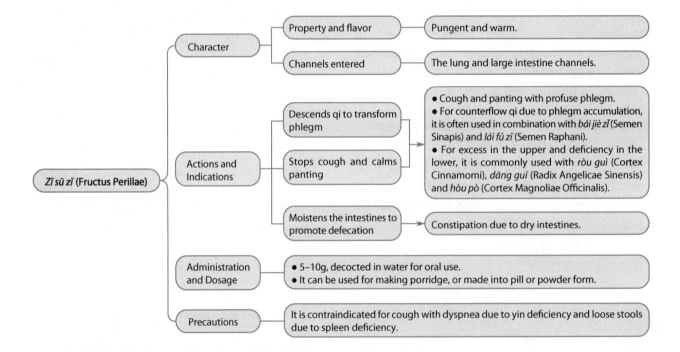

In addition, *tián xìng rén* (Semen Armeniacae Dulce) has a similar but milder action than *kǔ xìng rén* (Semen Armeniacae Amarum). It can mainly moisten the lung to relieve cough. It is indicated for deficiency taxation cough and constipation due to fluid consumption. *Zǐ sū yè* (Folium Perillae) is the dried leaf of *Perilla frutescens* (L.) Britt. Var. *acuta* (Thunb.) Kudo. of the family Labiatae. *Zǐ sū gěng* (Caulis Perillae) is the dried stem from the same plant, and *zǐ sū zǐ* (Fructus Perillae) is its dried mature fruit,

while *zǐ sū* (Folium et Caulis Perillae) is the dried stem with the leaf. *Zǐ sū yè* (Folium Perillae) can mainly disperse wind cold; *zǐ sū gěng* (Caulis Perillae) can promote qi circulation to soothe the middle and prevent miscarriage; *zǐ sū* (Folium et Caulis Perillae) has the effect of both *zǐ sū yè* (Folium Perillae) and *zǐ sū gěng* (Caulis Perillae); *zǐ sū zǐ* (Fructus Perillae) is able to descend qi to transform phlegm, stop cough, calm panting and moisten the intestines to promote defecation.

③ *Băi bù* (百部, Radix Stemonae, Stemona Root)
★ ★ ★

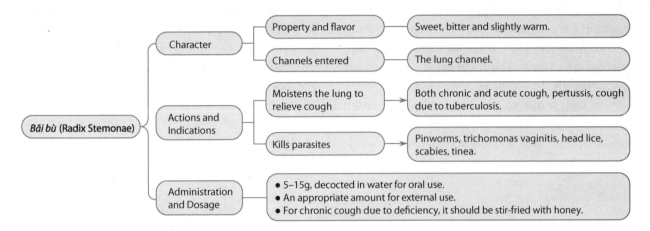

④ *Zĭ wăn* (紫菀, Radix et Rhizoma Asteris, Tatarian Aster Root) ★ ★

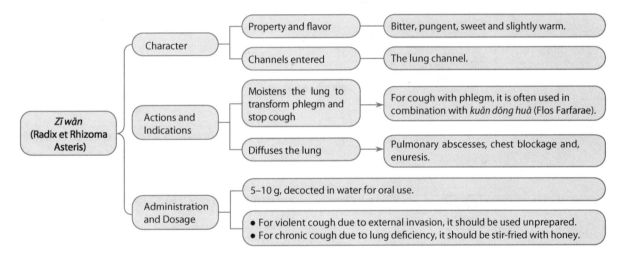

⑤ *Kuăn dōng huā* (款冬花, Flos Farfarae, Common Coltsfoot Flower) ★ ★

Băi bù (Radix Stemonae), *zĭ wăn* (Radix et Rhizoma Asteris) and *kuăn dōng huā* (Flos

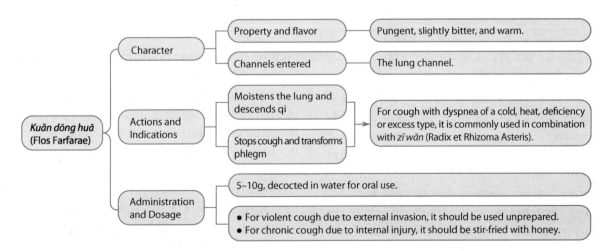

Farfarae) are slightly warm in property, and are moist and effective for moistening the lung and descending qi to relieve cough. They can be combined for coughs that are acute, chronic, from external invasion, from internal injury, cold, hot, deficient or excess. They are most suitable for chronic cough due to lung deficiency, deficiency taxation cough due to yin deficiency, and cough due to lung cold. The three medicinals are often used in combination to enhance their therapeutic effects. *Băi bù* (Radix Stemonae) and *kuăn dōng huā*

(Flos Farfarae) are effective for stopping cough. *Kuăn dōng huā* (Flos Farfarae) and *zǐ wăn* (Radix et Rhizoma Asteris) are able to transform phlegm as well as to stop cough. In addition, *băi bù* (Radix Stemonae) is capable of killing parasites, and is used for trichomonas vaginalis, enterobiasis, head lice, body lice, scabies, and tinea.

⑥ *Mă dōu líng* (马兜铃, Fructus Aristolochiae, Dutohmanspipe Fruit) ★★

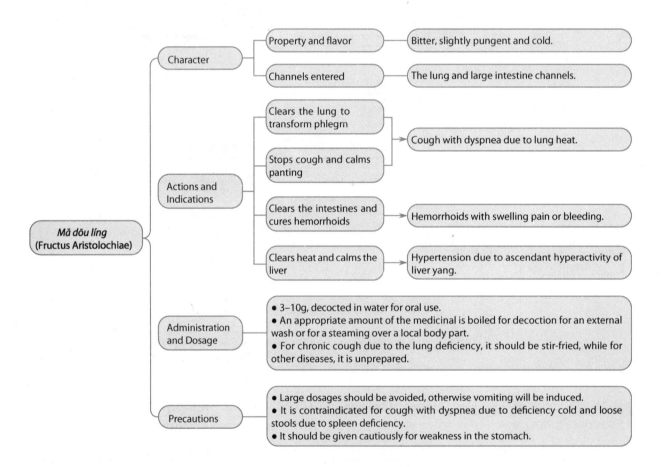

⑦ *Pí pá yè* (枇杷叶, Folium Eriobotryae, Loquat Leaf) ★★

Mă dōu líng (Fructus Aristolochiae) and *pí pá yè* (Folium Eriobotryae) are bitter in flavor and cold in property. They can clear the lung to transform phlegm, stop cough, and calm panting. They are indicated for cough with expectoration of yellow and sticky sputum due to lung heat. *Mă dōu líng* (Fructus Aristolochiae) can clear the lung to transform phlegm, stop cough and calm

panting in the upper body; clear intestines to cure hemorrhoids in the lower body, and is used for hemorrhoids with swelling pain or bleeding due to heat in the intestines. In addition, *mă dōu líng* (Fructus Aristolochiae) can clear heat and calm the liver to reduce blood pressure, and therefore is used for hypertension caused by ascendant hyperactivity of liver yang. *Pí pá yè* (Folium Eriobotryae) enters the lung channel to clear lung heat, and descend lung qi so as to transform

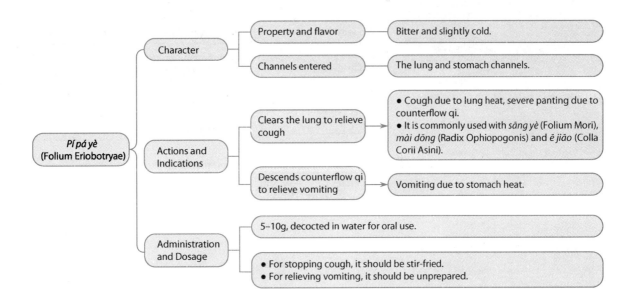

phlegm and stop cough. It is used for cough due to pathogenic wind, heat, dryness, or fire. It enters the stomach channel to clear stomach heat and descend stomach qi to relieve vomiting and belching. It is commonly used for vomiting, hiccups, and belching due to stomach heat.

⑧ *Sāng bái pí* (桑白皮, Cortex Mori, White Mulberry Root-bark) ★ ★ ★

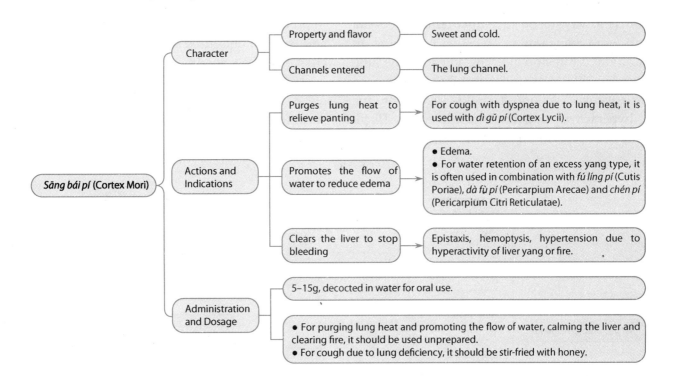

⑨ *Tíng lì zǐ* (葶苈子, Semen Lepidii, Pepperweed Seed) ★ ★ ★

Both *sāng bái pí* (Cortex Mori) and *tíng lì zǐ* (Semen Lepidii) are cold in property. They enter the lung channel, and can purge the lung to relieve panting and promote the flow of water to reduce edema. The two medicinals are used for cough with panting of an excess type; and edema and

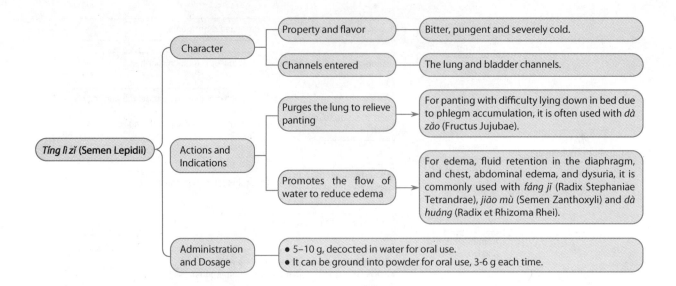

dysuria of an excess type. *Sāng bái pí* (Cortex Mori) is sweet in flavor and cold in property. It has an emphasis on purging fire in the lung as well as removing water to calm panting. It is indicated for cough with expectoration of yellow and thick sputum due to lung heat. It has a moderate action in promoting the flow of water to reduce edema, and is always used for subcutaneous edema and wind edema of an excessive yang type. In addition, it can stop bleeding and clear the lung to reduce blood pressure, and therefore is used for epistaxis, hemoptysis and hypertension due to hyperactivity of liver yang or liver fire. *Tíng lì zǐ* (Semen Lepidii) is pungent and bitter in flavor,

and severely cold in property. It specializes in removing water retention in the lung to calm panting and in stopping cough. It can also loosen the bowels, and is indicated for cough and panting with difficulty lying down in bed due to phlegm accumulation, and dysuria and defecation of an excess type. It has a strong action in promoting the flow of water to reduce edema, and is commonly used for fluid retention in the chest and hypochondria, and ascites.

⑩ *Bái guǒ* (白果, Semen Ginkgo, Ginkgo Nut) ★ ★

Addition: **Yín xìng yè (银杏叶, Folium Ginkgo, Ginkgo Leaf)** can astringe the lung to calm

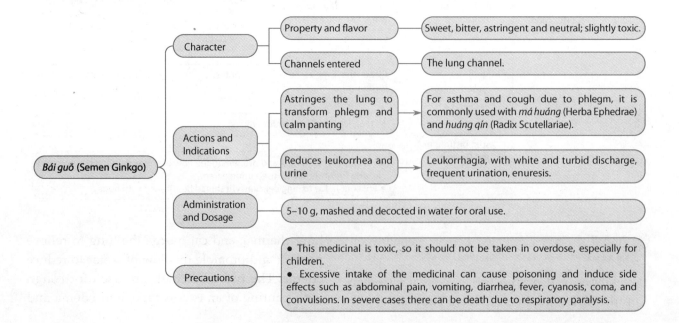

panting and activate the blood to relieve pain. It is indicated for hyperlipidemia, hypertension, coronary artery disease, angina and cerebral artery spasm.

⑪ *Ăi dì chá* (矮地茶, Herba Ardisiae Japonicae, Japanese Ardisia)

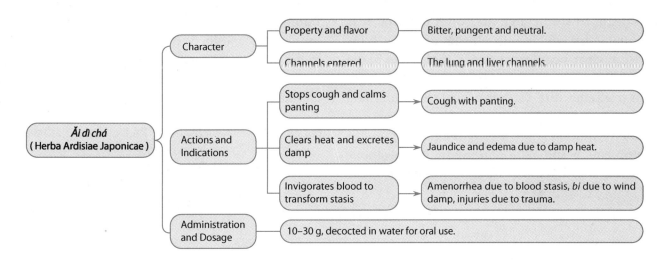

⑫ *Yáng jīn huā* (洋金花, Flos Daturae, Datura Flower)

Bái guŏ (Semen Ginkgo), *ăi dì chá* (Herba Ardisiae Japonicae) and *yáng jīn huā* (Flos Daturae) can stop cough and calm panting, and are therefore, used for cough and panting. *Bái guŏ* (Semen

Ginkgo) is astringent in flavor and is effective for astringing the lung to transform phlegm and calm panting. It is used for asthma and cough due to phlegm with lung cold, lung heat or deficiency in both the liver and kidney. Meanwhile, it can

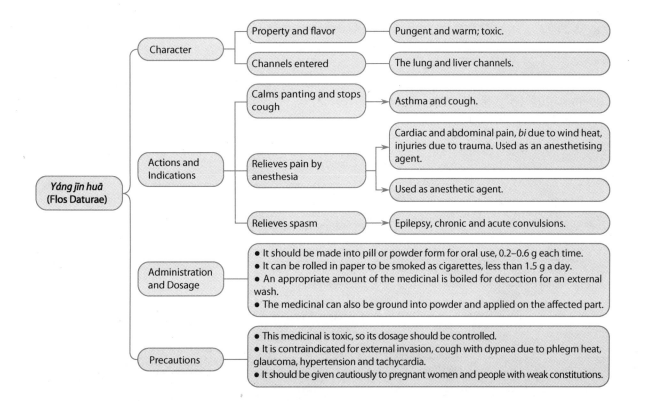

reduce leukorrhea and urine, and therefore is used for leukorrhagia with white and turbid discharge, enuresis and frequent urination. *Ăi dì chá* (Herba Ardisiae Japonicae) has a neutral and cool property, and a strong action in removing phlegm to stop cough and calm panting. It is suitable for cough with phlegm of a heat type. It can clear heat, expel damp, invigorate blood and transform stasis, and is used for jaundice and edema due to damp heat; amenorrhea, dysmenorrhea, *bi* due to wind damp, and injuries due to trauma. *Yáng jīn huā* (Flos Daturae) can stop cough and calm panting by its anesthetic action. It is used for cough in the adult or the elderly without phlegm or scanty phlegm which cannot be cured by other medicinals. It is effective for relieving pain by its anesthetic action, and is used for *bi* due to wind damp, cardiac and abdominal pain, injuries due to trauma, and swelling and pain due to stasis. It is an essential anesthetic medicinal for surgery and in the practice of Chinese medicine. In addition, it can relieve spasms, and is used for epilepsy and chronic convulsions in infants.

⑬ *Huà shān shēn* (华山参, Radix Physochlainae, Funnelid Physochlaina Root)

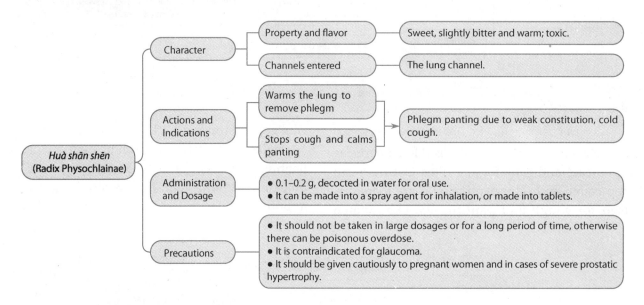

⑭ *Luó hàn guǒ* (罗汉果, Fructus Momordicae, Grosvenor Momordica Fruit)

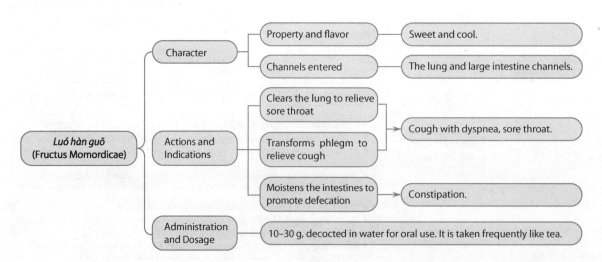

⑮ *Mǎn shān hóng* (满山红, Folium Rhododendri Daurici, Dahurian Rhododendron Leaf)

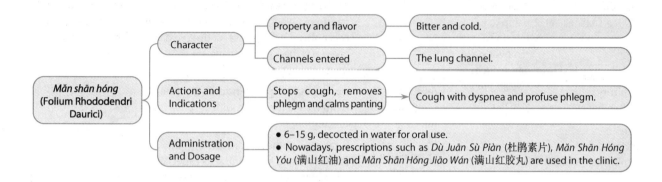

⑯ *Hú tuí zǐ yè* (胡颓子叶, Folium Elaegni Pungentis, Thorny Elaeagnus Leaf)

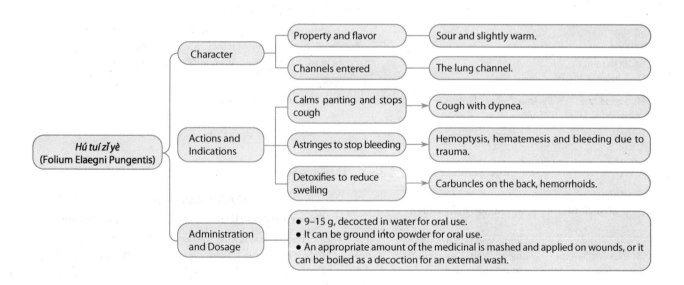

Actions of medicinals that transform phlegm, stop cough and calm panting are summarized in the following tables (Tables 20-1~20-3, see p.336~338):

Table 20-1: Summary of Medicinals that Warm and Transform Cold Phlegm:

Medicinal	Action in Common		Individual Character	
			Characteristic Actions	Other Actions
Bàn xià (Rhizoma Pinelliae)	Toxic, dries damp to transform stasis, removes stasis and reduces swelling to relieve pain		An essential medicinal to dry damp to transform phlegm, and warm and transform cold phlegm. It is effective for treating damp phlegm in the internal organs.	Descends counterflow qi to relieve vomiting, removes stagnation and stasis
Tiān nán xīng (Rhizoma Arisaematis)		Dispels wind to relieve spasm, is effective for removing wind phlegm in the channels and collaterals	With a stronger nature and harsher toxicity than *bàn xià* (Rhizoma Pinelliae), it is often used for cough with dyspnea due to stubborn phlegm.	
Yŭ bái fù (Rhizoma Typhonii)			It can guide other medicinals upwards to the face and head, and so is especially good at treating various diseases on the head and face.	
Bái jiè zĭ (Semen Sinapis)	Removes phlegm		It is effective for warming the lung to transform phlegm, facilitating qi flow to remove stasis, activating the channels and reducing swelling to relieve pain. It specializes in treating phlegm in the hypochondria and subcutaneous regions.	
Zào jiá (Fructus Gleditsiae)			Slightly toxic. It is effective for removing stubborn phlegm, and is often used for stubborn phlegm obstruction in the lung.	Opens the orifices, dispels wind to kill parasites
Xuán fù huā (Flos Inulae)	Descends qi to transform phlegm		It enters the lung channel to descend qi and promote the flow of water to transform phlegm, and enters the stomach channel to descend counterflow qi to relieve vomiting and belching.	
Bái qián (Rhizoma et Radix Cynanchi Stauntonii)			It is slightly warm in property but not dry, therefore it can be used for cough from external factors, internal injuries, of a chronic or acute kind. It is regarded as an important medicinal to treat lung diseases.	
Māo zhuă căo (Radix Ranunculi Ternati)	Transforms phlegm and removes stasis, detoxifies to reduce swelling			

Table 20-2: Summary of Medicinals that Clear Heat and Transform Phlegm:

Medicinal	Action in Common	Individual Character	
		Characteristic Actions	Other Actions
Chuān bèi mŭ (Bulbus Fritillariae Cirrhosae)	Clears heat and transforms phlegm, removes stasis to reduce swelling	It has a sticky nature, and is effective for moistening the lung to relieve cough. It is suitable for chronic cough due to internal injuries, deficiency taxation cough due to yin deficiency, and dry cough with sticky phlegm.	
Zhè bèi mŭ (Bulbus Fritillariae Thunbergii)		With a strong action in clearing heat, relieving depression and remove stasis, it is often used for cough due to wind heat and phlegm heat, carbuncles, goiters and scrofula.	
Guā lóu (Fructus Trichosanthis)	Clears heat and transforms phlegm	Moistens dryness to transform phlegm, soothes the chest to remove stasis, moistens the intestines to promote defecation. It is an essential medicinal to treat chest blockage.	
Zhú rú (Caulis Bambusae in Taenia)		It is effective for clearing heat and transforming phlegm to relieve vexation, clearing the stomach to relieve vomiting, cooling the blood, and stopping bleeding.	

Table 20-2: Summary of Medicinals that Clear Heat and Transform Phlegm:

continued

Medicinal	Action in Common	Individual Character	
		Characteristic Actions	Other Actions
Zhú lì (Succus Bambusae)	Clears heat and transforms phlegm	It has a slippery action, and is effective for clearing heat to remove phlegm. It is suitable for cough with difficult expectoration of thick sputum due to heat.	Relieves convulsions and opens the orifices
Tian zhú huáng (Concretio Silicea Bambusae)		Clears heat and transforms phlegm. It has a similar action to zhú lì (Succus Bambusae) in clearing the heart and relieving convulsions but without the disadvantage of cold and slippery action.	
Jié gěng (Radix Platycodonis)	Diffuses the lung to transform phlegm, relieves sore throat	It has a strong action in diffusing the lung to remove phlegm	Promotes the discharge of pus, guides other medicinals upwards
Pàng dà hǎi (Semen Sterculiae Lychnophorae)		It has a particular emphasis on clearing the lung to transform phlegm, relieving sore throat	Moistens the intestines to promote defecation
Hǎi zǎo (Sargassum)	Dissolves phlegm and softens hard masses, promotes the flow of water to reduce edema. They are regarded as essential medicinals to treat goiter and scrofula.		
Kūn bù (Thallus Laminariae)			
Hǎi fú shí (Pumex)	Dissolves phlegm, softens hard masses, removes stasis	Clears the lung to transform phlegm	Induces diuresis to relieve stranguria
Hǎi gé qiào (Concha Meretricis seu Cyclinae)			Checks the secretion of gastric acid to relieve pain: Induces diuresis to reduce edema
Wǎ léng zǐ (Concha Arcae)			Transforms and removes stasis
Qián hú (Radix Peucedani)	Descends qi to transform phlegm, disperses wind heat		
Méng shí (Chlorite-schist)	With a heavy and sinking nature, it can remove phlegm and descend qi, and calm the liver to relieve convulsions		
Huáng yào zǐ (Rhizoma Dioscoreae Bulbiferae)	Transforms phlegm, removes stasis to eliminate goiter, clears heat and detoxifies		

Table 20-3: Summary of Medicinals that Stop Cough and Calm Panting:

Medicinal	Action in Common	Individual Character	
		Characteristic Actions	Other Actions
Kǔ xìng rén (Semen Armeniacae Amarum)	Descends qi to stop cough and calm panting, moistens the intestines to promote defecation	It has a slight toxicity, and can descend lung qi as well as diffuse the lung to stop cough and calm panting. It is used for various coughs in the correct combinations.	
Zǐ sū zǐ (Fructus Perillae)		It has a particular emphasis on descending qi to transform phlegm, stopping cough and calming panting	
Bǎi bù (Radix Stemonae)	Warms and moistens, it is effective for moistening the lung and descending qi to relieve cough. It is combined with other medicinals for cough from external pathogens, internal injuries, cold, heat, deficiency, or excess, and chronic or acute.	It is effective for relieving cough	Kills parasites and lice
Kuǎn dōng huā (Flos Farfarae)			Transforms phlegm
Zǐ wǎn (Radix et Rhizoma Asteris)			

Table 20-3: Summary of Medicinals that Stop Cough and Calm Panting:

continued

Medicinal	Action in Common	Individual Character	
		Characteristic Actions	Other Actions
Mǎ dōu líng (Fructus Aristolochiae)	Clears the lung to transform phlegm, stops cough and calms phlegm	Clears the intestines and cures hemorrhoids, clears heat and calms the liver to reduce blood pressure	
Pí pá yè (Folium Eriobotryae)		It enters the lung channel to clear lung heat and descend lung qi to transform phlegm and stop cough, it enters the stomach channel to clear stomach heat and descend stomach qi to relieve vomiting and belching.	
Sāng bái pí (Cortex Mori)	Purges the lung to calm panting, promotes the flow of water to reduce edema	It has an emphasis on purging lung fire and water retention to calm panting, indicated for cough due to lung heat. It has a moderate action in promoting the flow of water to reduce edema.	
Tíng lì zǐ (Semen Lepidii)		It is specialized in purging fluid retention in the lung to calm panting and stop cough, and promote defecation. It is indicated for cough with dyspnea and difficulty in lying down in bed, difficulty with urination and defecation due to phlegm accumulation of an excess type. It has a strong action in promoting the flow of water to reduce edema.	
Bái guǒ (Semen Ginkgo)	Stops cough and calms panting	It has a particular emphasis on astringing the lung to transform phlegm and calm panting	Astringes to reduce leukorrhea and urine
Ǎi dì chá (Herba Ardisiae Japonicae)		It has a strong action in eliminating phlegm, stopping cough and calming panting	Clears heat and excretes damp, invigorates blood and transforms stasis
Yáng jīn huā (Flos Daturae)		Stops cough and calms panting, with an anesthetic action. It is effective for relieving pain by its anesthetic action, and is regarded as an essential medicinal in Chinese medicine	Relieves spasm
Huà shān shēn (Radix Physochlainae)		Warms the lung to remove phlegm	
Mǎn shān hóng (Folium Rhododendri Daurici)		Removes phlegm to stop cough	
Hú tuí zǐ yè (Folium Elaegni Pungentis)		Stops bleeding, detoxifies	
Luó hàn guǒ (Fructus Momordicae)	It has a particular emphasis on clearing the lung to relieve sore throat, transforming phlegm and stopping cough, and moistening the intestines to promote defecation		

Tables to test your herbal knowledge of actions and indications of medicinals that stop cough, calm panting and transform phlegm are as follows (Tables 20-4~20-11, see p.339~342)

Table 20-4: Test your Herbal Knowledge of the Actions of Medicinals that Transform Phlegm (one):

Actions \ Medicinal	Bàn xià	Tiān nán xīng	Dǎn nán xīng	Yǔ bái fù	Bái jiè zǐ	Zào jiá	Zào jiǎo cì	Xuán fù huā
Extinguishes wind to relieve convulsions								
Descends counterflow qi to relieve vomiting								
Removes stagnation and stasis								
Reduces swelling to relieve pain when used externally								
Facilitates qi to remove stasis								
Clears heat and transforms phlegm								
Dries damp to transform phlegm								
Removes wind phlegm								
Relieves pain								
Reduces swelling and promotes the discharge of pus								
Warms the lung to transform phlegm								
Expels wind to relieve spasm								
Eliminates stubborn phlegm								
Removes phlegm to open the orifices								
Dispels wind to kill parasites								
Detoxifies to remove stasis								
Descends qi to transform phlegm								

Table 20-5: Test your Herbal Knowledge of the Actions of Medicinals that Transform Phlegm (two):

Actions \ Medicinal	Bái qián	Qián hú	Jié gěng	Chuān bèi mǔ	Zhè bèi mǔ	Guā lóu	Zhú rú	Zhú lì	Tiān zhú huáng
Moistens the lung to relieve cough									
Disperses wind heat									
Diffuses the lung to remove phlegm									
Moistens the intestines to promote defecation									
Promotes the discharge of pus									
Clears heat and transforms phlegm									
Descends qi to transform phlegm									
Removes stasis to reduce swelling									
Relieves depression to remove stasis									
Clears the heart to relieve convulsions									
Relieves sore throat									
Removes dysphoria and relieves vomiting									
Clears heat and removes phlegm									
Relieves convulsions and opens the orifices									
Soothes the chest to remove stasis									

Table 20-6: Test your Herbal Knowledge of the Actions of Medicinals that Transform Phlegm (three):

Actions / Medicinal	Hǎi zǎo	Kūn bù	Huáng yào zǐ	Hǎi gé qiào	Hǎi fú shí	Wǎ léng zǐ	Méng shí	Pàng dà hǎi
Removes phlegm and descends qi								
Promotes the flow of water to reduce edema								
Clears heat and detoxifies								
Moistens the intestines to promote defecation								
Softens hard masses and removes stasis								
Transforms and removes stasis								
Dissolves phlegm to soften hard masses								
Calms the liver to relieve convulsions								
Relieves sore throat								
Clears the lung to transform phlegm								

Table 20-7: Test your Herbal Knowledge of the Actions of Medicinals that Stop Cough and Calm Panting:

Actions / Medicinals	Kǔ xìng rén	Zǐ sū zǐ	Bǎi bù	Zǐ wǎn	Kuǎn dōng huā	Mǎ dōu líng	Pí pá yè	Sāng bái pí	Tíng lì zǐ	Bái guǒ	Ǎi dì chá	Yáng jīn huā
Stops cough and calms panting												
Descends counterflow qi to relieve vomiting												
Descends qi to transform phlegm												
Moistens the lung to stop cough												
Stops leukorrhea												
Moistens the lung to transform phlegm and stop cough												
Clears the lung to transform phlegm												
Moistens the intestines to promote defecation												
Purges the lung to calm panting												
Promotes the flow of water to reduce edema												
Astringes the lung to calm panting												
Kills parasites												
Reduces urine												
Clears heat and excretes damp												
Invigorates blood to transform stasis												
Relieves pain and spasm												

Table 20-8: Test your Herbal Knowledge of the Indications of Medicinals that Transform Phlegm (one):

Medicinal / Indications	Bàn xià	Tiān nán xīng	Dǎn nán xīng	Yǔ bái fù	Bái jiè zǐ	Zào jiá	Xuán fù huā	Bái qián	Qián hú
Poisonous snake bites									
Vomiting due to counterflow stomach qi									
Stagnation and oppression in the chest and diaphragm									
Thoracic retention of phlegm heat									
Plum pit qi									
Phlegm obstruction in the channels, collaterals and joints									
Carbuncles									
Damp phlegm, cold phlegm									
Wind phlegm syndromes									
Heat phlegm syndromes									
Cough with dyspnea due to cold phlegm, fluid retention in diaphragm									
Syncope due to phlegm exuberance									
Goiter, superficial nodules									
Stubborn phlegm obstruction in the lung with cough, dyspnea and profuse phlegm									
Dorsal furuncles									
External invasion of wind cold with cough and phlegm									

Table 20-9: Test your Herbal Knowledge of the Indications of Medicinals that Transform Phlegm (two):

Medicinal / Indications	Jié gěng	Chuān bèi mǔ	Zhè bèi mǔ	Guā lóu	Zhú rú	Zhú lì	Tiān zhú huáng	Hǎi zǎo	Kūn bù
Cough with profuse phlegm, chest oppression and discomfort									
Sore and swollen throat, aphonia									
Intestinal abscesses									
Deficiency taxation cough									
Dry cough due to lung heat									
Scrofula									
Goiter and scrofula									
Chest blockage, thoracic retention									
Breast abscesses									
Expectoration of purulent sputum due to pulmonary abscesses									
Constipation due to dry intestines									
Testicular swelling and pain									
Stroke due to phlegm obstruction									
Epilepsy and convulsions									
Cough with dyspnea due to phlegm heat									
Vomiting due to stomach heat									
Edema, swelling due to beriberi									

Table 20-10: Test your Herbal Knowledge of the Indications of Medicinals that Transform Phlegm (three):

Medicinal Indications	Huáng yào zǐ	Hǎi gé qiào	Hǎi fú shí	Wǎ léng zǐ	Méng shí	Pàng dà hǎi
Goiter						
Hemoptysis due to phlegm fire						
Sore and swollen throat						
Cough with hoarseness due to lung heat						
Cough and panting due to lung heat						
Skin diseases						
Scrofula						
Abdominal masses due to blood stasis						
Stomachache with vomiting of gastric acid						
Stubborn phlegm						
Headache, blood-shot eyes						
Poisonous snake bites						
Constipation due to dry heat						
Epilepsy and convulsions due to fright						

Table 20-11: Test your Herbal Knowledge of the Indications of Medicinals that Stop Cough and Calm Panting:

Medicinals Indications	Kǔ xìng rén	Zǐ sū zǐ	Bǎi bù	Zǐ wǎn	Kuǎn dōng huā	Mǎ dōu líng	Pí pá yè	Sāng bái pí	Tíng lì zǐ	Bái guǒ
Trichomonas vaginalis										
Constipation due to dry intestines										
Counterflow qi due to phlegm accumulation										
Hemorrhoids with swelling pain										
Cough due to tuberculosis										
Enterobiasis										
Cough with dyspnea										
Head and body lice										
Scabies and tinea										
Cough with dyspnea due to lung heat										
Pertussis										
Vomiting due to stomach heat										
Frequent urination										
Epistaxis, hemoptysis										
Diaphragm fluid retention										
Chest and abdominal edema										
Heart failure due to pneumocardial disease										
Leukorrhagia with whitish and turbid discharge										
Edema										
Enuresis										
Asthma and cough due to phlegm										

Chapter 21
Medicinals that Calm the Mind

Concept

Medicinals whose principal effect is to calm the mind and treat mental disorders are referred to as medicinals that calm the mind.

Character and Actions

The heart stores the mind, while the liver stores the soul. Therefore, mental changes are closely related to functional activity of the heart and liver. Medicinals of this kind enter the heart and liver channels, and have the primary actions of tranquilizing the mind and nourishing the heart.

Indications

Medicinals that calm the mind are indicated for palpitations, and insomnia with frequent dreams. They are subsidiary medicinals for convulsions and epilepsy.

Combinations

When using medicinals that calm the mind, they should be properly chosen according to the various causative factors that are seen in the patient. For restlessness of an excess type, select heavy medicinals for calming the mind. For cases caused by fire heat, combine with medicinals for clearing and purging heart fire, soothing the liver to relieve depression, clearing the liver and purging fire. For cases caused by phlegm, add medicinals for eliminating phlegm and opening

the orifices. For cases induced by blood stasis, combine with medicinals for invigorating blood and transforming blood stasis. For liver yang hyperactivity, combine with medicinals for calming the liver to subdue yang. For epilepsy and convulsions, medicinals for transforming phlegm to open orifices or calming the liver to extinguish wind should be mainly used, with medicinals for calming the mind added secondarily. For restlessness of a deficient type, select medicinals for nourishing the heart to calm the mind. For cases due to blood and yin deficiency, medicinals that calm the mind should be combined with medicinals for enriching blood and nourishing yin. For deficiency in both the heart and spleen, combine with medicinals for tonifying the heart and spleen. For failure of the heart to communicate with the kidney, add medicinals for nourishing yin to descend fire and communicate the heart with the kidney.

Precautions

Medicinals of this kind usually treat signs and symptoms, especially the minerals for calming the mind and toxic medicinals. They should not be used for a long time, and should be discontinued if the pathological conditions improve. If mineral medicinals are made into a pill or powder form, they should be combined with medicinals for nourishing the stomach and invigorating the spleen so as not to impair the stomach and consume qi.

Classification

According to their clinical application, medicinals for calming the mind are classified into two categories: Heavy medicinals that calm the mind, and medicinals that nourish the heart to calm the mind.

Section 1   Heavy Medicinals that Calm the Mind

Medicinals of this section are mostly minerals and stones, which have a heavy texture and descending action. Heavy medicinals have the actions of tranquilizing the heart and calming the mind, relieving convulsions, and calming the liver to subdue yang. They are used for restlessness, palpitations, and insomnia of an excess type induced by heart fire exuberance, phlegm fire disturbing the heart, induced by fright and liver depression transforming into fire.

① *Zhū shā* (朱砂, Cinnabaris, Cinnabar) ★ ★ ★

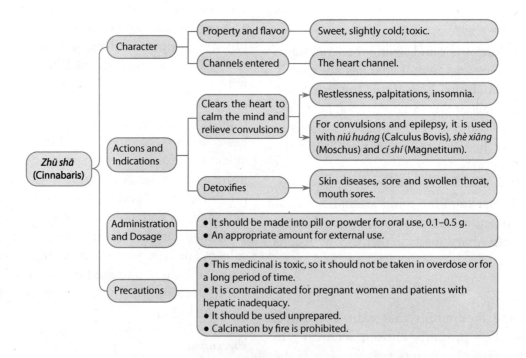

② *Cí shí* (磁石, Magnetitum, Magnetite) ★★★

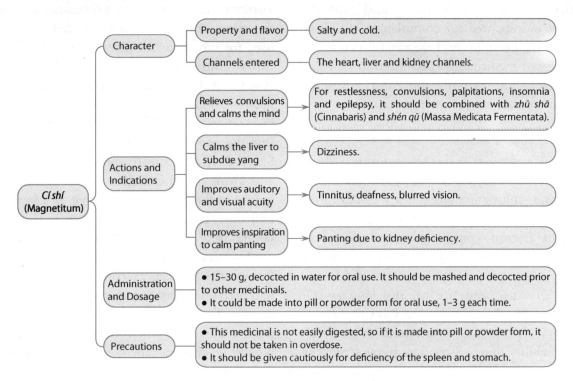

Cí shí (Magnetitum)

- **Character**
  - **Property and flavor** → Salty and cold.
  - **Channels entered** → The heart, liver and kidney channels.
- **Actions and Indications**
  - **Relieves convulsions and calms the mind** → For restlessness, convulsions, palpitations, insomnia and epilepsy, it should be combined with *zhū shā* (Cinnabaris) and *shén qū* (Massa Medicata Fermentata).
  - **Calms the liver to subdue yang** → Dizziness.
  - **Improves auditory and visual acuity** → Tinnitus, deafness, blurred vision.
  - **Improves inspiration to calm panting** → Panting due to kidney deficiency.
- **Administration and Dosage**
  - 15–30 g, decocted in water for oral use. It should be mashed and decocted prior to other medicinals.
  - It could be made into pill or powder form for oral use, 1–3 g each time.
- **Precautions**
  - This medicinal is not easily digested, so if it is made into pill or powder form, it should not be taken in overdose.
  - It should be given cautiously for deficiency of the spleen and stomach.

③ *Lóng gǔ* (龙骨, Os Draconis, Dragon Bones) ★★★

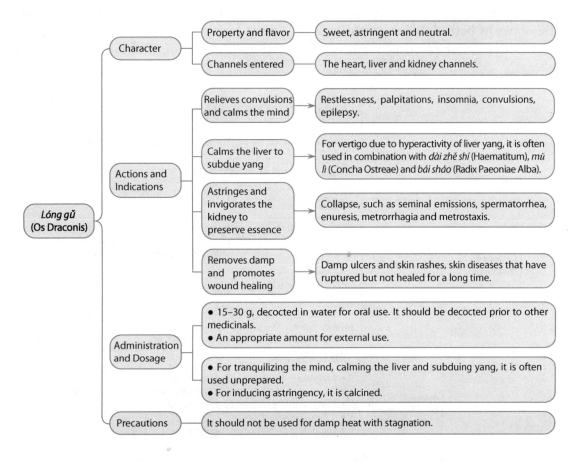

Lóng gǔ (Os Draconis)

- **Character**
  - **Property and flavor** → Sweet, astringent and neutral.
  - **Channels entered** → The heart, liver and kidney channels.
- **Actions and Indications**
  - **Relieves convulsions and calms the mind** → Restlessness, palpitations, insomnia, convulsions, epilepsy.
  - **Calms the liver to subdue yang** → For vertigo due to hyperactivity of liver yang, it is often used in combination with *dài zhě shí* (Haematitum), *mǔ lì* (Concha Ostreae) and *bái sháo* (Radix Paeoniae Alba).
  - **Astringes and invigorates the kidney to preserve essence** → Collapse, such as seminal emissions, spermatorrhea, enuresis, metrorrhagia and metrostaxis.
  - **Removes damp and promotes wound healing** → Damp ulcers and skin rashes, skin diseases that have ruptured but not healed for a long time.
- **Administration and Dosage**
  - 15–30 g, decocted in water for oral use. It should be decocted prior to other medicinals.
  - An appropriate amount for external use.
  - For tranquilizing the mind, calming the liver and subduing yang, it is often used unprepared.
  - For inducing astringency, it is calcined.
- **Precautions** → It should not be used for damp heat with stagnation.

Addition: *Lóng chǐ* (龙齿, **Dens Draconis, Dragon Teeth**) can relieve convulsions and calm the mind. It is indicated for convulsions, epilepsy, palpitations, insomnia and frequent dreams. The unprocessed medicinal is specialized in relieving convulsions and calming the mind, while the calcined one also has an astringent nature.

④ *Hǔ pò* (琥珀, Succinum, Amber) ★★

Zhū shā (Cinnabaris), *cí shí* (Magnetitum), *lóng gǔ* (Fossilia Ossis Mastodi) and *hǔ pò* (Succinum) are heavy and sinking in nature. They can calm the mind, and are used for restlessness, insomnia, frequent dreams, convulsions, epilepsy of an excess type due to excessive fire in the interior, yang qi upwardly disturbing the mind, and fright. *Cí shí* (Magnetitum), and *lóng gǔ* (Os Draconis) are able to calm the liver to subdue yang, and therefore are often used for dizziness and irritability due to ascendant hyperactivity of liver yang. *Zhū shā* (Cinnabaris) is sweet, cold and toxic. It enters the heart channel, and is able to calm and clear the heart to tranquilize the mind. It is considered an essential medicinal to calm the mind. It is often combined with other medicinals for restlessness of both deficiency and excess types. It is suitable for treating restlessness,

trembling with fear, palpitations, vexation and insomnia due to heart fire exuberance disturbing the mind. It can clear heat and detoxify, and is used for subcutaneous diseases, sore and swollen throat, and mouth sores. *Cí shí* (Magnetitum) is salty in flavor and cold in property. It can improve auditory and visual acuity, and induce inspiration to relieve panting. It is often used for tinnitus and deafness due to kidney deficiency; blurred vision due to deficiency in the liver and kidney; and deficiency panting due to the failure of the kidney to conserve qi. *Lóng gǔ* (Os Draconis) is sweet and astringent in flavor, and neutral in property. It is effective for astringing to treat seminal emission, spermatorrhea, enuresis, frequent urination, metrorrhagia, metrostaxis, leukorrhagia, spontaneous sweating, and night sweats. *Duàn lóng gǔ* (calcined Os Draconis), used externally, can remove damp, promote wound healing and the generation of tissue, and therefore is used for damp ulcers and skin rashes with itching, skin diseases that have ruptured but have not healed. *Hǔ pò* (Succinum) is sweet and neutral. It can invigorate blood to transform stasis and induce diuresis to relieve stranguria. It is used for amenorrhea, dysmenorrhea, postpartum abdominal pain, stabbing pain in the heart

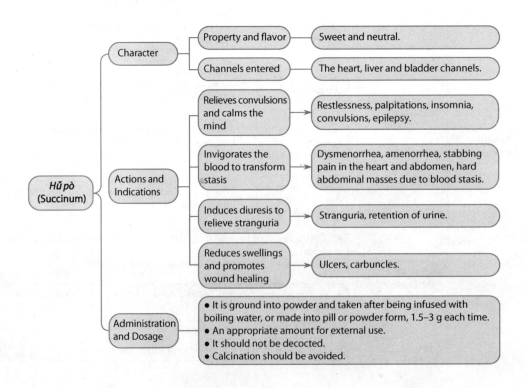

and abdomen, abdominal masses and injuries due to trauma due to blood stasis; stranguria, the retention of urine, and dysuria. It can also transform stasis to stop bleeding, and therefore is suitable for stranguria caused by hematuria. In addition, *hǔ pò* (Succinum) used externally can stop bleeding, promote the generation of tissues and wound healing. It is used for bleeding due to trauma and skin diseases that have not healed for a long time.

Section 2 Medicinals that Nourish the Heart to Calm the Mind

Medicinals in this section are mostly seeds and kernals, which are sweet, moist and nutritious. Therefore, they have the actions of nourishing the heart and liver, enriching yin and blood, and restoring communication between the heart and kidney. They are indicated for palpitations, vexation, insomnia, amnesia, frequent dreams, seminal emission and night sweats due to deficiency of yin and blood, deficiency of the heart and spleen and failure of the heart to communicate with the kidney.

① *Suān zǎo rén* (酸枣仁, Semen Ziziphi Spinosae, Spine Date Seed) ★★★

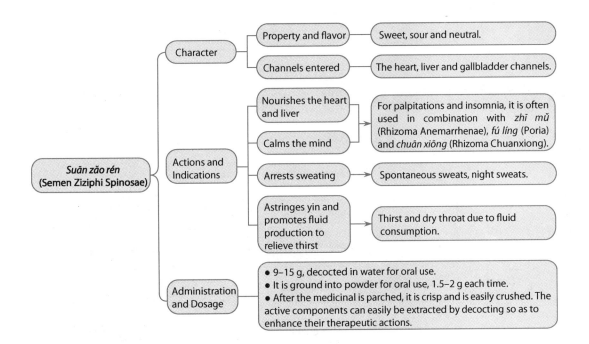

② *Băi zĭ rén* (柏子仁, Semen Platycladi, Arborvitae seed) ★★

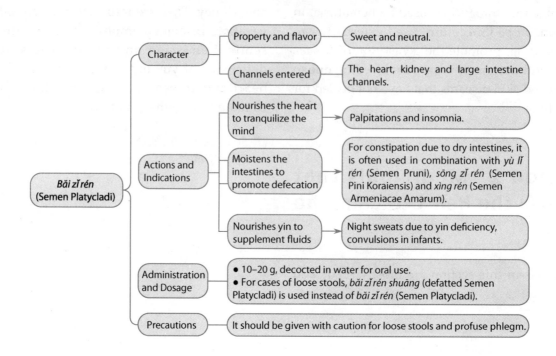

③ *Líng zhī* (灵芝, Ganoderma, Glossy Ganoderma)

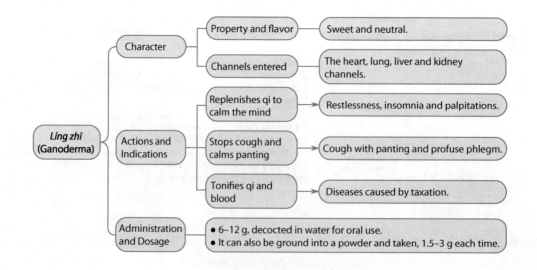

④ *Xié cǎo* (缬草, Rhizoma et Radix Valerianae Pseudoofficinalis, Chinese Common Valeriana Rhizome)

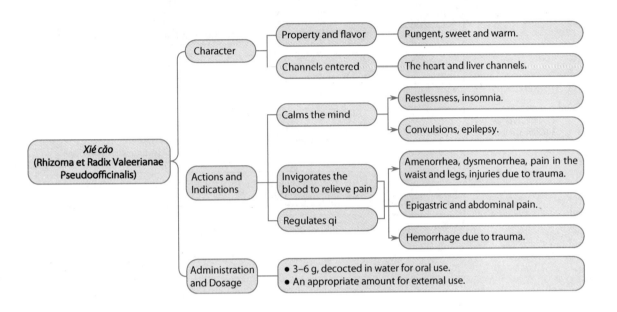

⑤ *Shǒu wū téng* (首乌藤, Caulis Polygoni Multiflori, Tuber Fleeceflower Stem) ★

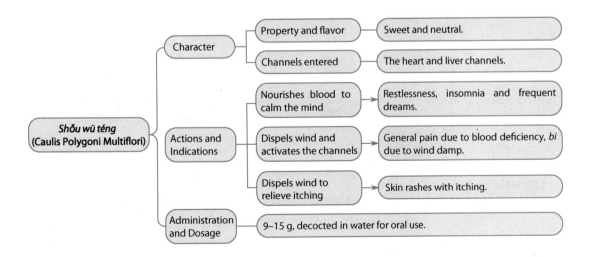

⑥ *Hé huān pí* (合欢皮, Cortex Albiziae, Silktree Albizia Bark) ★

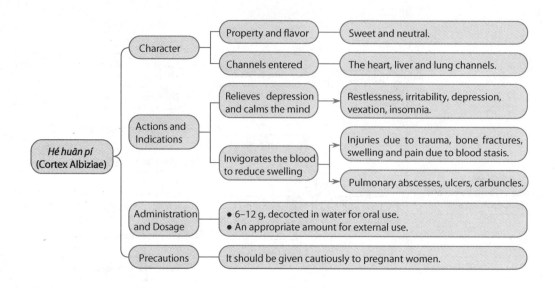

⑦ *Yuǎn zhì* (远志, Radix Polygalae, Thinleaf Milkwort Root) ★★

Suān zǎo rén (Semen Ziziphi Spinosae), *bǎi zǐ rén* (Semen Platycladi), *shǒu wū téng* (Caulis Polygoni Multiflori), *hé huān pí* (Cortex Albiziae) and *yuǎn zhì* (Radix Polygalae) are used for deficiency syndromes including palpitations, insomnia, frequent dreams and amnesia due to yin and blood deficiency, and both heart and spleen deficiency. *Suān zǎo rén* (Semen Ziziphi Spinosae), *bǎi zǐ rén* (Semen Platycladi) and *shǒu wū téng* (Caulis Polygoni Multiflori) have the actions of nourishing the heart to calm the mind. *Suān zǎo rén* (Semen Ziziphi Spinosae) is sweet, sour and neutral in character. It is effective for nourishing heart yin and heart and

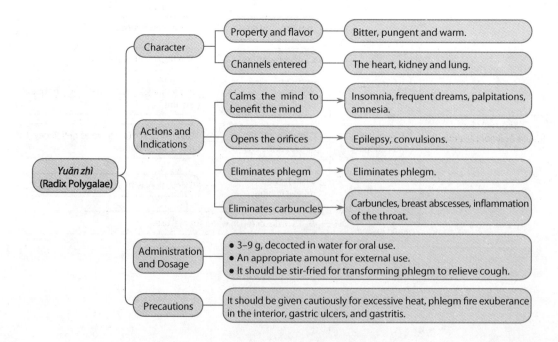

liver blood to calm and tranquilize the mind. They are essential medicinals for nourishing the heart to calm the mind. They are indicated for palpitations, insomnia, frequent dreams and amnesia due to yin and blood deficiency in the heart and liver. They can astringe to stop sweats, and promote fluid production to relieve thirst. They are indicated for spontaneous sweats due to deficiency, night sweats; thirst and dry throat due to fluid deficiency. *Bǎi zǐ rén* (Semen Platycladi) is moist; hence it can moisten the intestines to promote defecation. It is used for constipation due to intestinal dryness. *Shǒu wū téng* (Caulis Polygoni Multiflori) can expel wind and activate the collaterals and is used for general pain due to blood deficiency, *bi* due to wind damp and skin rashes with itching. *Hé huān pí* (Cortex Albiziae) is effective for relieving depression and calming the mind, and is considered an essential medicinal to calm the mind. It is indicated for vexation, insomnia, and restlessness due to emotional

disturbance. It can invigorate the blood to reduce swellings, and is used for bone fractures, swelling and pain due to stasis, pulmonary abscesses, ulcers, and carbuncles. *Yuǎn zhì* (Radix Polygalae) is bitter, pungent and warm, and is effective for re-establishing communication between the heart and kidney to calm the heart and tranquilize the mind, and benefit memory. It is indicated for restlessness, palpitations, insomnia and amnesia due to a failure of the heart to communicate with the kidney. It can remove phlegm to open the orifices, and eliminate carbuncles. It is used for mental disturbance, staring spells, epilepsy, spasms and convulsions due to phlegm due to failure of the heart to communicate with the kidney; cough with profuse phlegm due to cold phlegm; carbuncles, breast abscesses with swelling pain, and inflammation of the throat.

Actions of medicinals that calm the mind are summarized in the following table (Table 21-1):

Table 21-1: Summary of Medicinals that Calm the Mind:

Medicinal	Action in Common		Individual Character	
			Characteristic Actions	Other Actions
Zhū shā (Cinnabaris)	Medicinals for calming the mind with heavy and sinking natures, indicated for restlessness of an excessive type		Toxic. Tranquilizes and clears the heart to calm the mind, an essential medicinal to tranquilize the heart to calm the mind. It is suitable for restlessness, palpitations, vexation and insomnia due to heart fire exuberance disturbing the mind	Clears heat and detoxifies
Cí shí (Magnetitum)		Calms the liver to subdue yang		Improves auditory and visual acuity, induces inspiration to relieve panting
Lóng gǔ (Os Draconis)				It is effective for astringing and invigorating the kidney to preserve essence. Removes damp, promotes wound healing and the generation of tissue when used externally.
Hǔ pò (Succinum)				Invigorates blood to transform stasis, induces diuresis to relieve stranguria

Table 21-1: Summary of Medicinals that Calm the Mind:

continued

Medicinal	Action in Common		Individual Character	
			Characteristic Actions	Other Actions
Suān zǎo rén (Semen Ziziphi Spinosae)	Medicinals for nourishing the heart to calm the mind, indicated for restlessness of a deficient type	Nourishes the heart to calm the mind	Nourishes the heart yin, enriches blood in the heart and liver to calm the mind. It has a strong effect on nourishing the heart to calm the mind.	Astringes to stop sweating, promotes fluid production to relieve thirst
Bǎi zǐ rén (Semen Platycladi)				Moistens the intestines to promote defecation
Líng zhī (Ganoderma)				Replenishes qi and nourishes blood to relieve cough and calm panting
Shǒu wū téng (Caulis Polygoni Multiflori)				Expels wind and activates the collaterals
Xié cǎo (Rhizoma et Radix Valerianae Pseudoofficinalis)				Regulates qi and invigorates blood to relieve pain
Hé huān pí (Cortex Albiziae)			It is effective for relieving depression to calm the mind, is regarded as an essential medicinal to benefit the heart to calm the mind. It is indicated for vexation, insomnia and restlessness due to emotional disturbance.	Invigorates blood to reduce swelling
Yuǎn zhì (Radix Polygalae)			It is effective for reestablishing communication between the heart and kidney to calm the mind and improve memory. It is indicated for restlessness, palpitations, insomnia and amnesia due to a failure of the heart to communicate with the kidney.	Eliminates phlegm to open the orifices, eliminates carbuncles

Tables to test your herbal knowledge of actions and indications of medicinals that calm the mind are as follows (Tables 21-2~21-3):

Table 21-2: Test your Herbal Knowledge of the Actions of Medicinals that Calm the Mind:

Actions \ Medicinal	Zhū shā	Cí shí	Lóng gǔ	Hǔ pò	Suān zǎo rén	Bǎi zǐ rén	Yuǎn zhì	Hé huān pí	Shǒu wū téng
Astringes and invigorates the kidney to preserve essence									
Clears heat and detoxifies									
Calms the mind									
Calms the liver to subdue yang									
Nourishes the heart to calm the mind									
Induces inspiration to relieve panting									
Invigorates the blood to transform stasis									
Induces diuresis to relieve stranguria									
Nourishes the heart yin, enriches the liver blood									

Table 21-2: Test your Herbal Knowledge of the Actions of Medicinals that Calm the Mind:

continued

Actions / Medicinal	Zhū shā	Cí shí	Lóng gǔ	Hǔ pò	Suān zǎo rén	Bǎi zǐ rén	Yuǎn zhì	Hé huān pí	Shǒu wū téng
Stops sweating									
Improves auditory and visual acuity									
Invigorates the blood to reduce swelling									
Reestablishes communication between the heart and kidney to calm the mind									
Removes phlegm to open the orifices									
Eliminates carbuncles									
Relieves depression to calm the mind									
Moistens the intestines to promote defecation									
Expels wind and activates the collaterals									

Table 21-3: Test your Herbal Knowledge of the Indications of Medicinals that Calm the Mind:

Actions / Medicinal	Zhū shā	Cí shí	Lóng gǔ	Hǔ pò	Suān zǎo rén	Bǎi zǐ rén	Yuǎn zhì	Hé huān pí	Shǒu wū téng
Palpitations, insomnia									
Convulsions, epilepsy									
Blurred vision									
Sore and swollen throat									
Mouth sores									
Vertigo due to liver yang									
Skin diseases									
Tinnitus and deafness									
Retention of urine									
Prolapse									
Swollen and painful breasts									
Skin diseases that have ruptured but not healed for a long time									
Blood stasis									
Stranguria									
Panting due to kidney deficiency									
Bi due to wind damp									
General pain due to blood deficiency									
Constipation due to dry intestines									
Vexation and insomnia due to emotional disturbance									
Damp ulcers, skin rashes with itching									
Carbuncles									
Cough with profuse phlegm									
Epilepsy and madness due to phlegm obstruction in the heart orifice									
Profuse sweating due to deficiency									
Trauma and bone fractures									

Chapter 22
Medicinals that Calm the Liver and Extinguish Wind

Concept

Medicinals that have the main actions of calming the liver to subdue yang or extinguishing wind to relieve convulsions, and are indicated for ascendant hyperactivity of liver yang and internal stirring of liver wind, are referred to as medicinals that calm the liver and extinguish wind.

Character and Actions

Medicinals in this chapter all enter the liver channel. They are mostly shells, insects and minerals. They have the actions of calming the liver to subdue yang, and extinguishing wind to relieve convulsions.

Indications

Medicinals for calming the liver and extinguishing wind, indicated for diseases caused by ascendant hyperactivity of liver yang and internal stirring of liver wind.

Combinations

When using such medicinals, doctors should combine them with other medicinals that address the causative factors of disease and different manifesting complications. For instance, for diseases caused by yang activity due to yin deficiency, medicinals for nourishing the kidney yin should also be used, so as to nourish yin to restrain yang. For flaring up of liver fire, add medicinals for clearing and purging the liver. For cases complicated by restlessness, insomnia and frequent dreams, combine with medicinals for calming the mind. For internal stirring of liver wind due to liver yang transforming into wind, use medicinals for extinguishing wind to relieve convulsions as well as those that calm the liver to subdue yang. For liver wind stirring in the interior, combine with medicinals for clearing and purging fire and detoxifying. For liver wind stirring in the interior due to yin and blood deficiency, combine with medicinals that nourish yin and blood. For chronic convulsions due to spleen deficiency, add medicinals for replenishing qi and invigorating the spleen. For cases of coma due to the obstruction of the heart orifices, combine with medicinals that open the orifices. For cases complicated by phlegm, add medicinals for removing phlegm.

Precautions

Medicinals for calming the liver and extinguishing wind should be used according to their cold or warm natures. For chronic convulsions due to spleen deficiency, medicinals with a cold or cool property should not be used. For yin and blood deficiency, medicinals with a warm and dry property should be avoided.

Classification

Medicinals of this kind are classified into two categories: Medicinals that suppress liver yang and medicinals that extinguish wind to relieve convulsions.

Section 1 Medicinals that Suppress the Liver Yang

Medicinals in this section are mostly shells and minerals, which have the actions of suppressing liver yang or calming the liver to subdue yang. They are indicated for dizziness, headache and tinnitus due to ascendant hyperactivity of liver yang; flushing, oral bitterness, blood-shot, swollen and painful eyes, irritability, headache and dizziness due to flaring up of liver fire.

① *Shí jué míng* (石决明, Concha Haliotidis, Sea-ear Shell) ★ ★ ★

Both *shí jué míng* (Concha Haliotidis) and *cǎo jué míng* (Semen Cassiae) are cold in property, and can clear the liver to improve visual acuity. They are used for blood-shot, swollen and painful eyes, and nebulae due to flaring up of liver fire or wind heat invading the upper; dim eyesight, night blindness, and blurred vision due to yin and blood deficiency. The two medicinals are effective to improve visual acuity. *Shí jué míng* (Concha Haliotidis) is salty in flavor and cold in property. It has a strong action in calming the liver to subdue yang, and is often used for headache, dizziness, and irritability due to ascendant activity of liver yang. *Cǎo jué míng* (Semen Cassiae) (or *jué míng zǐ*) is the seed, and has a moist texture. It can moisten the intestines to promote defecation and is commonly used for constipation due to dry intestines caused by fluid

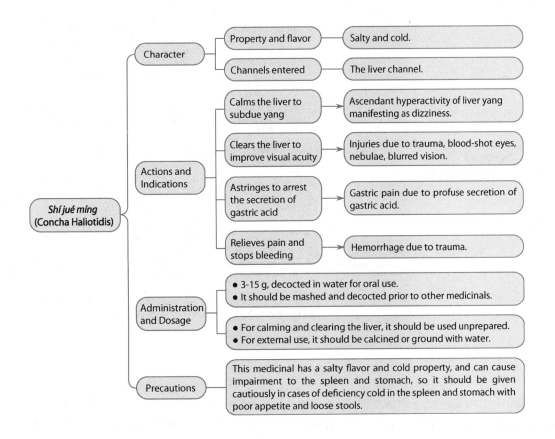

consumption resulting from internal heat.

② *Zhēn zhū mǔ* (珍珠母, Concha Margaritiferae Usta, Nacre) ★★

Both *shí jué míng* (Concha Haliotidis) and *zhēn zhū mǔ* (Concha Margaritiferae Usta) are salty in flavor and cold in property. They enter the liver channel to calm the liver to subdue yang and clear the liver to improve visual acuity. The two medicinals can be used in combination for dizziness, vexation and irritability due to ascendant hyperactivity of liver yang; blood-shot, swollen and painful eyes and nebulae due to flaring up of liver fire or wind heat invading upwards; dim eyesight, blurred vision, and night-blindness and twilight blindness due to liver blood deficiency. It is suitable for blood-shot, swollen and painful eyes due to flaring up of liver fire. *Shí jué míng* (Concha Haliotidis)

has a stronger action in calming and cooling the liver, and is efficient in treating eye diseases. In addition, *duàn shí jué míng* (calcined Concha Haliotidis) has the actions of astringing, checking the secretion of gastric acid, relieving pain and stopping bleeding. It can be used for gastric pain due to profuse secretion of gastric acid. It is ground into powder for external application to treat bleeding due to trauma. *Zhēn zhū mǔ* (Concha Margaritiferae Usta) has a more moderate action than *shí jué míng* (Concha Haliotidis). It can calm the mind to relieve convulsions, and is used for palpitations, insomnia, and restlessness. When it is calcined and ground into powder for external use, it can dry damp and promote wound healing, and is used for damp ulcers with itching, and non-healing ulcers.

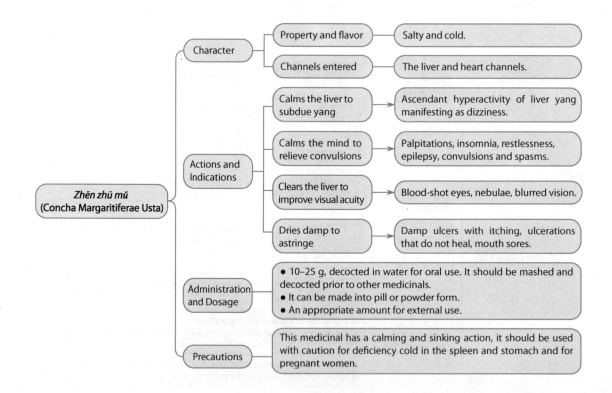

③ *Mǔ lì* (牡蛎, Concha Ostreae, Oyster Shell) ★★★

Both *lóng gǔ* (Os Draconis) and *mǔ lì* (Concha Ostreae) enter the liver and kidney channels. When used unprepared, they can calm the

liver to subdue yang and calm the mind. When calcined, they have the actions of astringing and invigorating the kidney to preserve essence. The two medicinals are used in combination

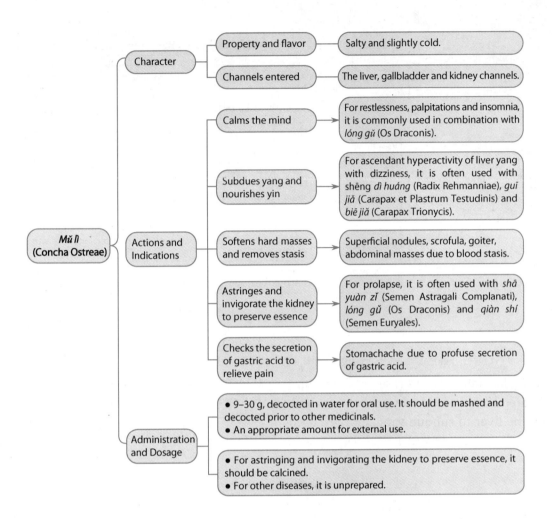

for dizziness, vexation, and irritability due to ascendant hyperactivity of liver yang; restlessness, palpitations, insomnia, amnesia, frequent dreams, convulsions and epilepsy due to mental disorders; seminal emission, spermatorrhea, enuresis, frequent urination, metrorrhagia, metrostaxis, leukorrhagia, spontaneous sweating, and night sweating due to deficiency. *Lóng gǔ* (Os Draconis) is sweet, astringent and neutral. It enters the heart channel and therefore has a strong action in calming the mind, and astringing and invigorating the kidney to preserve essence. It is often used for restlessness and prolapse from deficiency. *Duàn lóng gǔ* (calcined Os Draconis) can remove damp, promote wound healing and the generation of tissue when used externally, and is used for damp ulcers, skin rashes with itching, and skin diseases

that have ruptured but not healed. *Mǔ lì* (Concha Ostreae) is salty and slightly cold in character. It is effective for nourishing yin to subdue yang, softening hard masses and removing stasis. It is commonly used for convulsions of the limbs due to internal stirring of deficient fire caused by yin consumption, resulting from febrile diseases; goiter, scrofula, and superficial nodules due to binding of phlegm with fire; and abdominal masses due to qi stagnation and blood stasis. It has recently been used for splenohepatomegalia. In addition, *duàn mǔ lì* (calcined Concha Ostreae) has the effect of checking the secretion of gastric acid to relieve pain, and is used for stomachache due to profuse secretion of gastric acid.

④ *Zǐ bèi chǐ* (紫贝齿, Concha Cypraeae Violacae, Arabic Cowry Shell)

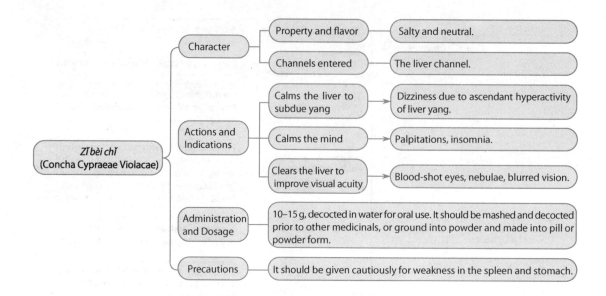

⑤ *Dài zhě shí* (代赭石, Haematitum, Hematite) ★ ★ ★
Dài zhě shí (Haematitum) and *cí shí* (Magnetitum) are iron ore. They are cold in property, which can calm the liver to subdue yang, and are used for dizziness, vexation and irritability due to ascendant activity of liver yang. *Dài zhě shí* (Haematitum) is bitter in flavor, and is effective for descending counterflow qi, cooling blood and arresting bleeding. It is used for vomiting, hiccups, and belching due to counterflow

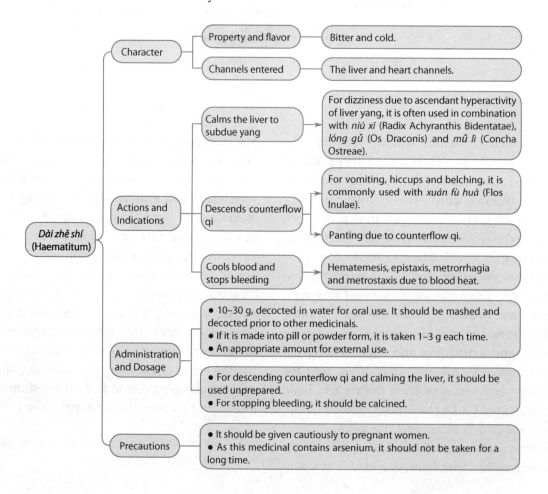

stomach qi; panting due to counterflow qi caused by deficiency in both the lung and kidney; hematemesis, epistaxis, metrorrhagia and metrostaxis due to blood heat. *Cí shí* (Magnetitum) is pungent and salty in flavor. It is effective for calming the mind, and is used for restlessness, palpitations, insomnia, convulsions and epilepsy caused by yang hyperactivity due to yin deficiency disturbing the mind or fright. It can improve auditory and visual acuity, induce inspiration to calm panting, and is used for tinnitus and deafness due to kidney deficiency; and deficiency panting due to failure of the kidney to preserve qi.

⑥ *Cì jí lí* (刺蒺藜, Fructus Tribuli, Caltrop Fruit) ★ ★

Both *dài zhě shí* (Haematitum) and *cì jí lí* (Fructus Tribuli) can calm liver yang, and are used for headache, dizziness, vexation, and irritability due to ascendant hyperactivity of liver yang. *Dài zhě shí* (Haematitum) is bitter, cold and heavy

in nature, and therefore has a stronger action in calming the liver to subdue yang. It is effective for descending counterflow qi, which is an essential medicinal to descend counterflow qi. It is able to cool blood and stop bleeding, and is commonly used in combination with *xuán fù huā* (Flos Inulae) for vomiting, hiccups, and belching due to counterflow stomach qi; panting due to counterflow qi; hematemesis, epistaxis, metrorrhagia and metrostaxis due to blood heat. *Cì jí lí* (Fructus Tribuli) can suppress liver yang, calm the liver to relieve depression, dispel wind to improve visual acuity, and dispel wind to relieve itching. It is also used for chest and hypochondriac distending pain, galactostasis, breast distending pain due to liver constraint with qi stagnation; blood-shot, swollen and painful eyes, excessive tearing and nebulae due to wind heat invading upwards; measles with itching, and vitiligo.

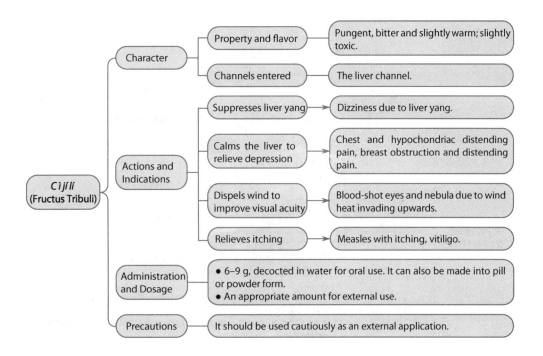

⑦ *Luó bù má* (罗布麻, Folium Apocyni Veneti, Dogbane Leaf)

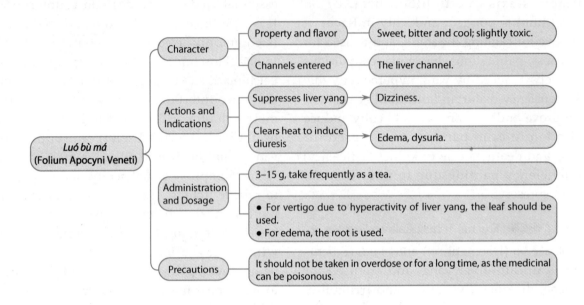

⑧ *Shēng tiě luò* (生铁落, Frusta Ferri, Pulvis Ferri)

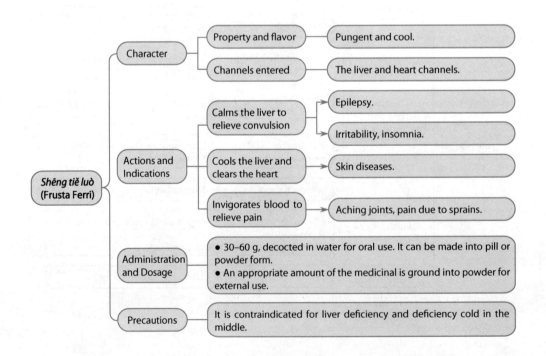

Section 2 Medicinals that Extinguish Wind to Relieve Convulsions

Medicinals in this section enter the liver channel and have the main actions of extinguishing liver wind and relieving spasms and convulsions. They are indicated for vertigo, susceptibility to falls, stiff neck, trembling, and spasms of the limbs due to extreme heat stirring wind caused by epidemic febrile diseases, liver yang transforming into wind, blood deficiency leading to wind; epilepsy, convulsions, and spasms due to wind yang accompanied by phlegm, phlegm heat disturbing upwards; tetanus with spasms, convulsions, and opisthotonus (hyperextension and spasticity in the head, neck and spinal column) due to wind toxin leading to internal wind.

① *Líng yáng jiǎo* (羚羊角, Cornu Saigae Tataricae, Antelope Horn) ★★★

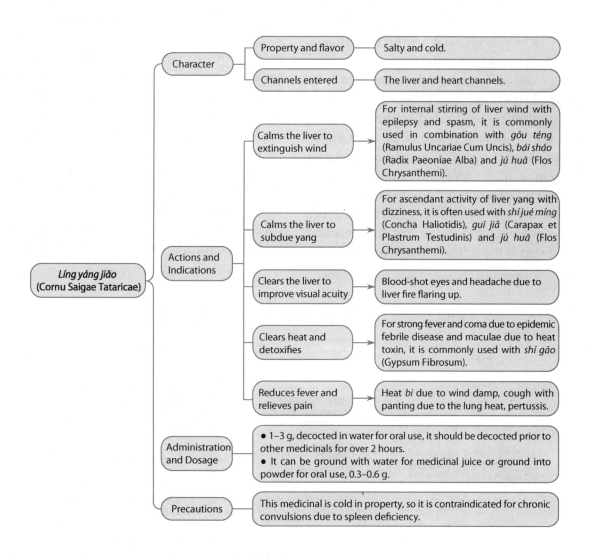

Líng yáng jiǎo
(Cornu Saigae Tataricae)

- **Character**
  - **Property and flavor**: Salty and cold.
  - **Channels entered**: The liver and heart channels.

- **Actions and Indications**
  - **Calms the liver to extinguish wind**: For internal stirring of liver wind with epilepsy and spasm, it is commonly used in combination with *gōu téng* (Ramulus Uncariae Cum Uncis), *bái sháo* (Radix Paeoniae Alba) and *jú huā* (Flos Chrysanthemi).
  - **Calms the liver to subdue yang**: For ascendant activity of liver yang with dizziness, it is often used with *shí jué míng* (Concha Haliotidis), *guī jiǎ* (Carapax et Plastrum Testudinis) and *jú huā* (Flos Chrysanthemi).
  - **Clears the liver to improve visual acuity**: Blood-shot eyes and headache due to liver fire flaring up.
  - **Clears heat and detoxifies**: For strong fever and coma due to epidemic febrile disease and maculae due to heat toxin, it is commonly used with *shí gāo* (Gypsum Fibrosum).
  - **Reduces fever and relieves pain**: Heat *bi* due to wind damp, cough with panting due to the lung heat, pertussis.

- **Administration and Dosage**
  - 1–3 g, decocted in water for oral use, it should be decocted prior to other medicinals for over 2 hours.
  - It can be ground with water for medicinal juice or ground into powder for oral use, 0.3–0.6 g.

- **Precautions**: This medicinal is cold in property, so it is contraindicated for chronic convulsions due to spleen deficiency.

② *Niú huáng* (牛黄, Calculus Bovis, Cow-bezoar) ★ ★ ★

Líng yáng jiǎo (Cornu Saigae Tataricae) and *niú huáng* (Calculus Bovis) are commonly used precious medicinals. They are cold in property and enter the heart and liver channels to cool the liver to extinguish wind to relieve convulsions, clear heat, and detoxify. Both medicinals are used for chronic and acute convulsions in infants, strong fevers, coma, convulsions, and spasms due to extreme heat generating wind during epidemic febrile diseases. *Líng yáng jiǎo* (Cornu Saigae Tataricae) is also used for maculae due to heat toxins. In addition, it is effective for calming the liver to subdue yang and clearing the liver to improve visual acuity. It is always used for dizziness, vertigo, vexation, and irritability caused by ascendant activity of liver yang; headaches, vertigo, blood-shot swollen and painful eyes, photophobia and excessive tearing due to liver fire flaring up. *Niú huáng* (Calculus Bovis) is often used for swollen and sore throat, mouth sores, swollen and painful gums, carbuncles and furuncles due to heat toxin accumulation and retention. In addition, it is effective for clearing the heart and transforming phlegm to open the orifices, and is used for heat attacking the pericardium due to epidemic febrile diseases; high fever, coma, lockjaw and wheezing phlegm due to phlegm heat obstruction in the heart orifice.

Niú huáng (Calculus Bovis) and *xióng dǎn* (熊胆, Ursi Fel, Bear Gall) are from animal bile. They are bitter in flavor, and cool in property. They enter the liver and heart channels and have the actions of clearing heat, detoxifying, cooling the liver and extinguishing wind, and relieving convulsions. The two medicinals are used for skin diseases, swollen and sore throat due to heat toxins; convulsions, epilepsy and spasms due to extreme heat generating wind. *Niú huáng* (Calculus Bovis) is the gall stone of cattle, or bile extraction from cattle and pigs. It is also used for mouth sores, and infant's carbuncles. It is effective for transforming phlegm to open the orifices and is often used for stroke, convulsions, and epilepsy caused by heat attacking the pericardium during epidemic febrile diseases, and the resulting coma, delirium, high fever, vexation, and lockjaw due to phlegm heat obstruction in the heart orifices. *Xióng dǎn* (Ursi Fel) is from the dried bile from *Ursus arctos* L. or *Selenarctos thibetanus* G.Cuvier. It can clear heat and detoxify to treat hemorrhoids with swelling and pain. It can also clear the liver

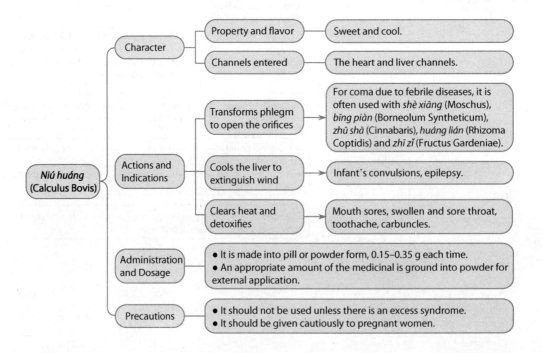

to improve visual acuity, and is used to treat blood-shot, swollen and painful eyes and nebulae due to liver heat while used both internally and externally.

③ *Zhēn zhū* (珍珠, Margarita, Pearl)

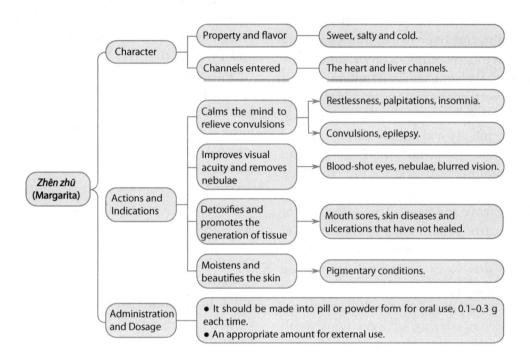

④ *Gōu téng* (钩藤, Ramulus Uncariae Cum Uncis, Gambir Plant) ★ ★ ★

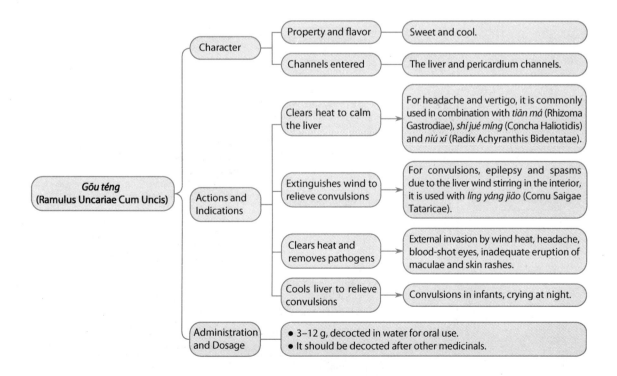

⑤ *Tiān má* (天麻, Rhizoma Gastrodiae, Tall Gastrodis Tuber) ★ ★ ★

Líng yáng jiǎo (Cornu Saigae Tataricae), *gōu téng* (Ramulus Uncariae Cum Uncis) and *tiān má* (Rhizoma Gastrodiae) enter the liver channel. They can calm the liver to subdue yang and extinguish wind to relieve convulsions. The three medicinals are used in combination for headaches, vertigo, vexation, and irritability due to ascendant hyperactivity of liver yang; convulsions, epilepsy and spasms due to internal stirring of liver wind. *Líng yáng jiǎo* (Cornu Saigae Tataricae) is salty and cold in character. It enters the heart channel and has a strong action in clearing the heart. It is effective for clearing liver fire to extinguish liver wind and calm liver yang. It is suitable for high fever and convulsions due to extreme heat generating wind and yang hyperactivity resulting from liver heat. It is considered an essential medicinal to treat internal stirring of liver wind with convulsions, epilepsy and spasms. *Líng yáng jiǎo* (Cornu Saigae Tataricae) is effective for clearing the liver to improve visual acuity, clearing heat, and detoxifying. It is used for headaches, vertigo, blood-shot, swollen and painful eyes, photophobia, and excessive tearing due to flaring up of liver fire; strong fevers, and coma due to epidemic febrile diseases; and maculae due to heat toxin. *Gōu téng* (Ramulus Uncariae Cum Uncis) is sweet and slightly cold. It can clear heat but is inferior to *líng yáng jiǎo* (Cornu Saigae Tataricae) in clearing heat, extinguishing wind, and calming the liver. It is indicated for acute convulsions in infants, constant strong fevers, and spasms of the hands and feet due to extreme heat generating wind. It is a commonly used medicinal to treat convulsions, epilepsy and spasms due to internal stirring of liver wind. It is also used for headache and vertigo due to liver fire invading upwards. *Tiān má* (Rhizoma Gastrodiae) is sweet and neutral; hence it has a moderate action. It is combined with other medicinals for convulsions and spasms of cold, heat, deficiency or excess types due to internal stirring of liver wind. It is considered an efficient medicinal to treat internal wind. In addition *tiān má* (Rhizoma Gastrodiae) is also used for vertigo and headache due to ascendant hyperactivity of liver yang, wind phlegm disturbing upwards, blood deficiency, and liver hyperactivity or wind syndrome of the head. In addition, *tiān má* (Rhizoma Gastrodiae) can expel wind and activate the collaterals. It is used for wind invading the channels and

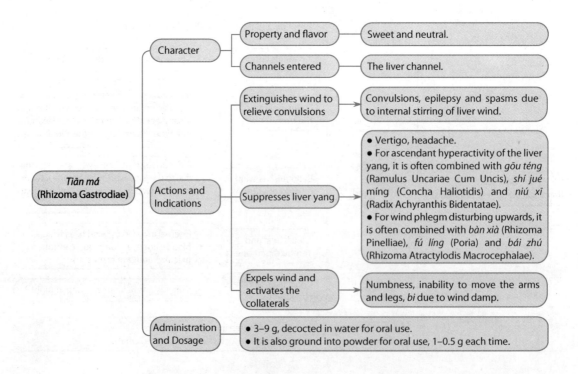

collaterals manifesting as numbness, *bi* due to wind damp, and inflexible joints.

⑥ *Dì lóng* (地龙, Pheretima, Earthworm) ★★

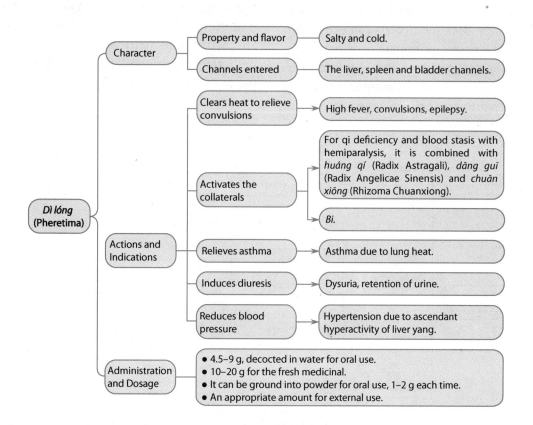

⑦ *Quán xiē* (全蝎, Scorpio, Scorpion) ★★

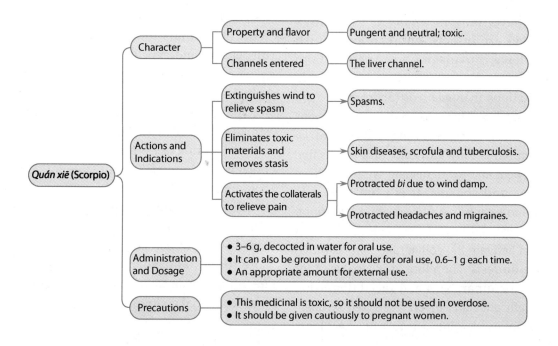

⑧ *Wú gōng* (蜈蚣, Scolopendra, Centipede) ★★

Quán xiē (Scorpio) and *wú gōng* (Scolopendra) are insects. They are pungent and toxic, and enter the liver channel. Both medicinals can extinguish wind to relieve spasms, eliminate toxic materials, remove stasis and activate the collaterals to relieve pain. They are essential medicinals to treat spasm. The two medicinals are used for spasm due to various causes such as acute convulsions, chronic stubborn *bi* due to wind damp, spasms of sinews and vessels or even deformity of joints; and stubborn migraines and headaches. *Quán xiē* (Scorpio) is neutral in property and has a moderate action; while *wú gōng* (Scolopendra) is warm in property and has a drastic action.

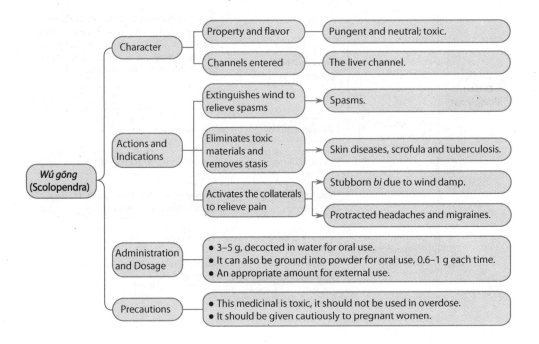

⑨ *Jiāng cán* (僵蚕, Bombyx Batryticatus, Stiff Silkworm) ★★

Dì lóng (Pheretima) and *jiāng cán* (Bombyx Batryticatus) are insects, and can extinguish wind to relieve convulsions and spasms. Both medicinals are without toxicity and have more moderate actions than *quán xiē* (Scorpio) and *wú gōng* (Scolopendra). They are used for convulsions and spasms due to internal stirring of liver wind. *Dì lóng* (Pheretima) is salty and cold, and is effective for clearing heat and extinguishing wind to relieve convulsions and spasms. It is used for acute convulsions in infants, high fever, comas, delirium, and spasms caused by extreme heat generating wind. It can activate the collaterals, calm panting, and induce diuresis. Therefore, it is also used for stroke with hemiparalysis and facial distortion due to qi deficiency and blood stasis; red swollen, painful and inflexible joints due to *bi* of a heat kind; asthma due to lung heat; and dysuria and retention of urine due to heat retention in the bladder. It is also used for cold *bi* due to wind damp if combined with medicinals for warming the channels to dispel cold and expelling wind to remove damp. *Jiāng cán* (Bombyx Batryticatus) is pungent and salty in flavor, and neutral in property. It is used for spasms due to acute and chronic convulsions, stroke with facial distortion and tetanus induced by internal stirring of liver wind. It can also transform phlegm, and therefore is suitable for convulsions and epilepsy with phlegm heat. It can dispel wind to relieve pain and itching, transform phlegm and detoxify to remove stasis. It is used for headache, blood-shot, swollen and painful eyes, swollen and sore throat, and hoarseness due to wind heat invading upwards; measles with itching; scrofula, and superficial nodules.

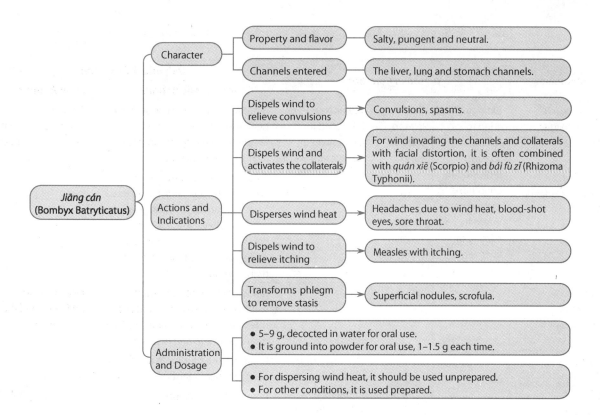

Actions of medicinals that calm the liver and extinguish wind are summarized in the following table (Table 22-1):

Table 22-1: Summary of Medicinals that Calm the Liver and Extinguish Wind:

Medicinal	Action in Common		Individual Character	
			Characteristic Actions	Other Actions
Shí jué míng (Concha Haliotidis)	Suppresses liver yang	Clears the liver to improve visual acuity	It has a strong action, it is an essential medicinal to calm and cool the liver. It is efficient for treating eye disease.	Astringes to check the secretion of gastric acid, relieves pain and stops bleeding when the medicinal is calcined.
Zhēn zhū mǔ (Concha Margaritiferae Usta)			Calms the mind to relieve convulsions. Dries damp and promotes wound healing when calcined.	
Mǔ lì (Concha Ostreae)	Suppresses liver yang, indicated for diseases caused by ascendant activity of liver yang		It is effective for nourishing yin to subdue yang, calming the mind, softening hard masses and removing stasis. It can restrain the secretion of gastric acid to relieve pain, when calcined.	
Dài zhě shí (Haematitum)			Descends counterflow qi, cools blood and stops bleeding	
Cì jí lí (Fructus Tribuli)			Soothes the liver to relieve depression, dispels wind to improve visual acuity, dispels wind to relieve itching	
Zǐ bèi chǐ (Concha Cypraeae Violacae)		Relieves convulsions to calm the mind	Clears the liver to improve visual acuity	
Shēng tiě luò (Frusta Ferri)			Reduces swellings to relieve pain	
Luó bù má (Folium Apocyni Veneti)			Clears heat to induce diuresis	

Table 22-1: Summary of Medicinals that Calm the Liver and Extinguish Wind:

continued

Medicinal	Action in Common			Individual Character	
				Characteristic Actions	Other Actions
Líng yáng jiǎo (Cornu Saigae Tataricae)	Extinguishes wind to relieve spasms, indicated for conditions caused by internal stirring of liver wind	Calms the liver to subdue yang	Clears heat, indicated for extreme heat generating wind	It has a strong action in clearing heat and is regarded as an essential medicinal to calm the liver to extinguish wind.	Clears the liver to improve visual acuity, clears heat and detoxifies
Gōu téng (Ramulus Uncariae Cum Uncis)				Clears heat and calms the liver. It is inferior to *líng yáng jiǎo* (Cornu Saigae Tataricae) in extinguishing wind to relieve spasms. It is commonly used for convulsions and spasms due to internal stirring of liver wind.	
Tiān má (Rhizoma Gastrodiae)				It has a moderate action. It is suitable for convulsions and spasms due to all causes. It is effective for treating vertigo and headache.	Dispels wind and activates the collaterals
Quán xiē (Scorpio)			It is toxic and migrating. Eliminates toxic materials and removes stasis, activates collaterals to relieve pain	It has a more moderate action than *wú gōng* (Scolopendra).	
Wú gōng (Scolopendra)				It has a drastic action.	
Niú huáng (Calculus Bovis)			Clears heat, indicated for extreme heat generating wind	Clears heat and detoxifies, transforms phlegm to open the orifices	
Dì lóng (Pheretima)				Activates the collaterals, calms panting, induces diuresis	
Jiāng cán (Bombyx Batryticatus)				Transforms phlegm. It is suitable for convulsions and epilepsy of a phlegm heat type.	Dispels wind to relieve pain and itching, transforms phlegm, detoxifies and removes stasis
Zhēn zhū (Margarita)				Calms the mind to relieve convulsions, improves visual acuity, removes nebula, sterilizes and promotes the generation of tissue	

Tables to test your herbal knowledge of the actions and indications of medicinals that calm the liver and extinguish wind are as follows (Tables 22-2~22-3):

Table 22-2: Test your Herbal Knowledge of the Actions of Medicinals that Calm the Liver and Extinguish Wind:

Medicinal / Actions	*Shí jué míng*	*Zhēn zhū mǔ*	*Mǔ lì*	*Dài zhě shí*	*Cì jí lí*	*Luó bù má*	*Líng yáng jiǎo*	*Niú huáng*	*Gōu téng*	*Tiān má*	*Dì lóng*	*Quán xiē*	*Wú gōng*	*Jiāng cán*
Calms the liver to subdue yang														
Clears the liver to promote visual acuity														

Table 22-2: Test your Herbal Knowledge of the Actions of Medicinals that Calm the Liver and Extinguish Wind:
continued

Medicinal / Actions	Shí jué míng	Zhēn zhū mǔ	Mǔ lì	Dài zhě shí	Cì jí lí	Luó bù má	Líng yáng jiǎo	Niú huáng	Gōu téng	Tiān má	Dì lóng	Quán xiē	Wú gōng	Jiāng cán
Dispels wind to improve visual acuity														
Astringes and invigorates the kidney to preserve essence														
Softens hard masses and removes stasis														
Calms the liver to extinguish wind														
Descends counterflow qi via its heavy texture														
Cools blood and stops bleeding														
Calms the heart to tranquilize the mind														
Suppresses liver yang														
Clears heat to induce diuresis														
Calms the liver														
Calms the liver to relieve convulsions														
Induces diuresis														
Extinguishes wind to relieve spasms														
Transforms phlegm to open the orifices														
Transforms phlegm to remove stasis														
Dispels wind and activates the collaterals														
Activates collaterals														
Calms panting														
Clears heat and detoxifies														
Eliminates toxic materials and removes stasis														
Activates the collaterals to relieve pain														
Dispels wind to relieve pain														
Clears heat to calm the liver														

Table 22-3: Test your Herbal Knowledge of the Indications of Medicinals that Calm the Liver and Extinguish Wind:

Medicinal / Actions	Shí jué míng	Zhēn zhū mǔ	Mǔ lì	Dài zhě shí	Cì jí lí	Luó bù má	Líng yáng jiǎo	Niú huáng	Gōu téng	Tiān má	Dì lóng	Quán xiē	Wú gōng	Jiāng cán
Blurred vision														
Blood-shot, swollen and painful eyes due to liver heat														
Nebula														
Ascendant hyperactivity of liver yang														
Palpitations, insomnia, restlessness														
Distending pain in the chest and hypochondrium														
Abdominal masses due to blood stasis														
Prolapse														
Cough with dyspnea due to lung heat														
Vomiting, hiccups														
Belching														
Panting due to counterflow qi														
Bleeding due to blood heat														
Scrofula, superficial nodules														
Breast abscesses with distending pain														
Edema, dysuria														
Convulsion and spasms due to internal stirring of liver wind														
Coma and convulsions due to febrile diseases														
Headache due to pathogenic wind heat														
Stomachache due to the profuse secretion of gastric acid														
Swollen and sore throat														
Carbuncles, furuncles														
Infant's night crying														
Skin diseases														
Headaches due to liver fire														
Stubborn headaches and migraines														
Maculae due to heat toxin														
Blood-shot, swollen and painful eyes due to wind heat														
Measles with itching														
Bi due to wind damp														

Chapter 23
Medicinals that Open the Orifices

Concept

Medicinals that are pungent, fragrant, and piercing, and whose principal effect is to open the orifices to arouse the spirit, and are used to treat coma from blockage patterns, are called medicinals that open the orifices.

Character and Actions

Medicinals of this kind are pungent, aromatic and penetrating. They enter the heart channel and have the action of opening the orifices to arouse the spirit.

Indications

Medicinals that open the orifices are indicated for sudden syncope and spasms due to coma, delirium, convulsions, epilepsy and stroke induced by heat invading the pericardium, and phlegm-turbidity attacking the clear orifices during febrile diseases.

Combinations

Both deficiency syndrome and excess syndrome can result in coma. The deficient types are referred to as desertion syndromes, while the excessive types are called blockage patterns. For desertion syndrome, the principles of tonifying the deficiency and rescuing desertion are applied. For blockage patterns, the principle of opening the orifices to arouse the spirit is used. The blockage type patterns can be treated by medicinals introduced in this chapter. Blockage patterns are divided into cold types and heat types. For cold type blockage patterns manifesting with cyanotic complexion, general coldness, a whitish tongue coating and a slow pulse, the principle of warming the interior and opening the orifices is used, and medicinals that are pungent and warm for opening the orifices are given, in combination with medicinals with the actions of warming the interior to dispel cold. For hot type blockage patterns manifesting with flushing, general fever, a yellowish tongue coat and a rapid pulse, the principles of cooling and opening the orifices should be used, and medicinals that are pungent and cool for opening the orifices are chosen in combination with medicinals for clearing heat, purging fire and detoxifying. For coma due to blockage patterns accompanied by convulsions and spasms, combine with medicinals that have the actions of calming the liver to extinguish wind and relieve spasms. For cases with vexation, add medicinals for calming the mind to relieve convulsions. For phlegm-turbidity accumulation, combine with medicinals for transforming damp and eliminating phlegm.

Precautions

Medicinals in this chapter are pungent and aromatic in flavor, and are penetrating. They

371

are often used for emergent cases or treating the branch of a pattern, and can consume the right qi, so they are recommended for short term use. The active components in such medicinals are easily volatized; therefore they should not be decocted, and should be made into pill or powder form for oral use.

① *Shè xiāng* (麝香, Moschus, Musk) ★ ★ ★

Shè xiāng (Moschus) and *niú huáng* (Calculus Bovis) are precious medicinals for opening the orifices to arouse the spirit. They are used in combination for blockage patterns of a heat type, manifesting as coma, lockjaw, clenched fists, unconsciousness, flushing, general fever, a yellow tongue coating, and a rapid pulse. *Shè xiāng* (Moschus) is pungent in flavor and warm in property. It has a strong aroma and can be penetrating. It has a drastic action in opening the orifices to arouse the spirit and is regarded as an essential medicinal to arouse the spirit and restore the mind. It is used for coma due to blockage patterns of both cold and heat types. At the same time, it can invigorate the blood and activate the channels, reduce swelling to relieve pain, and induce labor. It is used for skin diseases, sore and swollen throats; amenorrhea due to blood stasis, abdominal pain, violent pain in the chest and abdomen, headaches, injuries due to trauma, cold *bi* due to wind damp; abnormal or difficult childbirth, fetal death, and retention of the lochia. *Niú huáng* (Calculus Bovis) is bitter and cool, and can clear heat and transform phlegm. It is suitable for coma due to blockage patterns caused by phlegm heat invading the heart orifice. It can also extinguish wind to relieve spasms, clear heat and detoxify, and therefore is used for convulsions in infants with strong fever, coma and spasms due to extreme heat generating wind caused by epidemic febrile diseases; sore and swollen throat, mouth sores, and carbuncles and furuncles due to heat toxin accumulation.

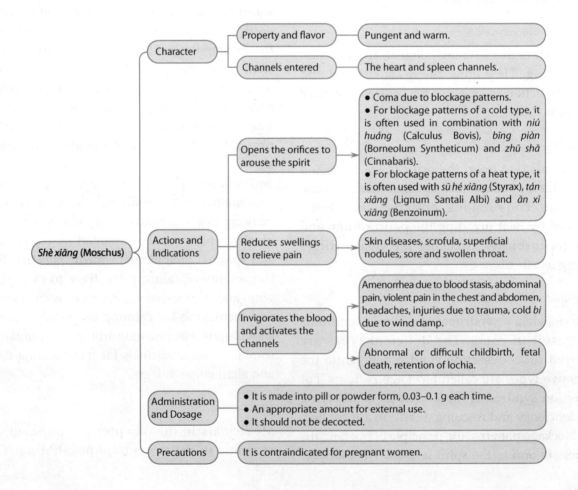

② *Bīng piàn* (冰片, Borneolum Syntheticum, Borneol) ★★

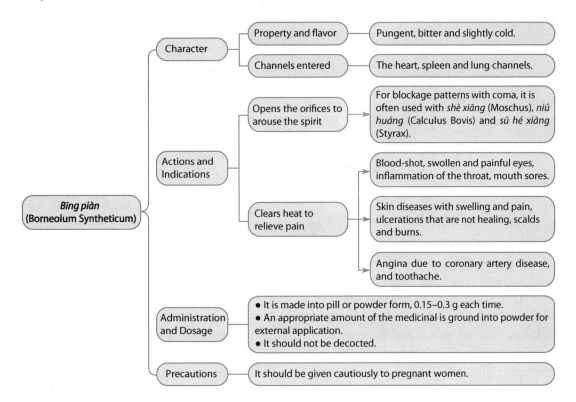

③ *Sū hé xiāng* (苏合香, Styrax, Storax) ★

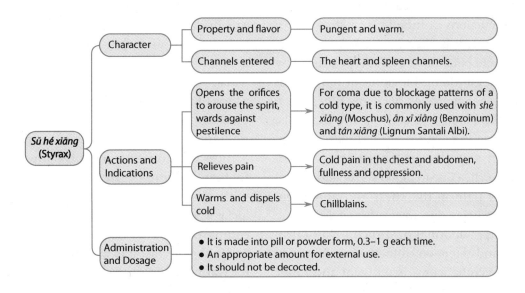

④ *Shí chāng pú* (石菖蒲, Rhizoma Acori Tatarinowii, Grassleaf Sweetflag Rhizome) ★★★

Shè xiāng (Moschus), *bīng piàn* (Borneolum Syntheticum), *sū hé xiāng* (Styrax) and *shí chāng pú* (Rhizoma Acori Tatarinowii) are pungent, aromatic and penetrating. They can open the orifices to arouse the spirit, and are used for coma due to blockage patterns. In addition, *shè xiāng* (Moschus), *bīng piàn* (Borneolum Syntheticum) and *sū hé xiāng* (Styrax) are commonly used for

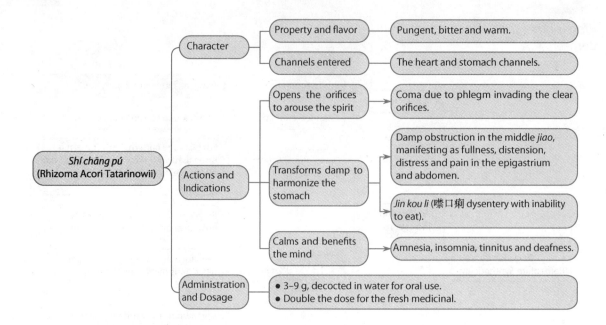

coronary artery disease and angina. *Shè xiāng* (Moschus) is pungent in flavor and warm in property. It has a strong aroma and is penetrating. It has a drastic action in opening the orifices to arouse the spirit and is regarded as an essential medicinal to arouse the spirit and restore the mind. It is suitable for coma due to blockage patterns of a heat type induced by heat invading the pericardium, phlegm heat invading the heart orifices, convulsions in infants, and stroke with phlegm syncope. It is effective for treating coma due to blockage patterns of a cold type caused by cold and phlegm damp blocking qi movement and invading the mind. At the same time, it can invigorate the blood and activate the channels, reduce swelling to relieve pain, and induce labor. It is used for skin diseases, sore and swollen throat; amenorrhea due to blood stasis, abdominal pain, violent pain in the chest and abdomen, headaches, injuries due to trauma, cold *bi* due to wind damp; abnormal or difficult childbirth, fetal death, and retention of the lochia. *Bīng piàn* (Borneolum Syntheticum) is pungent and bitter in flavor, and slightly cold in property. It has a similar but slower action than *shè xiāng* (Moschus) in opening the orifices to arouse the spirit. They are used in combination for mutual reinforcement to treat coma due to blockage patterns. However, *bīng piàn* (Borneolum Syntheticum) is suitable for blockage patterns of a heat type, manifesting

as coma, phlegm heat obstruction in the interior, syncope due to summer heat, and convulsions in infants. It is also used for blockage patterns of a cold type, if it is combined with medicinals for warming the interior to dispel cold or warm medicinals with the action of opening the orifices. In addition, it can clear heat to relieve pain, and is commonly used for blood-shot, swollen and painful eyes, mouth sores, earaches with pus discharge, skin diseases that have swelling, pain, and rupture, but have not healed, scalds, and burns. *Sū hé xiāng* (Styrax) is pungent, warm and aromatic. It has similar but inferior actions to *shè xiāng* (Moschus). It is indicated for blockage patterns of a cold type caused by cold phlegm and foul turbidity invading the clear orifices including stroke, invasion by pestilent factors, qi constraint, and phlegm syncope, with manifestations such as sudden syncope, lockjaw, clenched fists, unconsciousness, cyanotic complexion, a cold body, a whitish tongue coat, and a slow pulse. It is a representative medicinal for warming and opening the orifices. In addition, it has a good action in warming and activating the channels to relieve pain, and therefore is used for fullness, distress, and cold pain in the chest and abdomen caused by cold congealing phlegm-turbidity, qi stagnation, and blood stasis. *Shí chāng pú* (Rhizoma Acori Tatarinowii) is pungent, bitter, dry and warm in nature. It has a slow action in opening the orifices, but is effective for transforming damp, removing phlegm and driving away pestilent factors so as to open the orifices, and calm and benefit the mind. It is indicated for coma, epilepsy and dementia due to phlegm, damp and foul turbidity invading the clear orifices, as well as dizziness, drowsiness, amnesia, tinnitus and deafness. Meanwhile, it is effective for transforming damp to harmonize the stomach, and is used for epigastric and abdominal fullness and masses with distention, pain and distress; and *jin kou li* (dysentery with inability to eat) due to damp turbidity and heat toxin accumulating in the intestines.

Both *shí chāng pú* (Rhizoma Acori Tatarinowii) and *yuǎn zhì* (Radix Polygalae) can transform phlegm to open the orifices, calm the heart, and tranquilize the mind. They are used for coma, epilepsy and dementia due to phlegm, damp and foul turbidity invading the clear orifices; restlessness, amnesia, and insomnia due to phlegm-turbidity disturbing the interior. The two medicinals are commonly used in combination for mutual reinforcement. *Shí chāng pú* (Rhizoma Acori Tatarinowii) is aromatic, and has a particular emphasis on transforming damp to harmonize the stomach. It is often used for epigastric and abdominal fullness and masses with distention, pain and distress; and *jin kou li* (dysentery with inability to eat) due to damp turbidity and heat toxin accumulating in the intestines. *Yuǎn zhì* (Radix Polygalae) is effective for restoring communication between the heart and kidney in order to calm the heart and tranquilize the mind. It is indicated for restlessness, palpitations, amnesia, insomnia, and frequent dreams due to failure of the heart to communicate with the kidney. It can mainly transform phlegm and relieve cough, and therefore is used for cough with profuse phlegm that is not easy to expectorate. It can also eliminate carbuncles, and is used for carbuncles with swelling and pain, and breast swellings with pain.

Actions of medicinals that open the orifices are summarized in the following table (Table 23-1):

Table 23-1: Summary of Medicinals that Open the Orifices:

Medicinal	Action in Common	Individual Character	
		Characteristic Actions	Other Actions
Shè xiāng (Moschus)	Opens the orifices to arouse the spirit	Pungent and warm with a strong aroma, it has a drastic penetrating action. It has a strong action in opening the orifices to arouse the spirit, and is regarded as an essential medicinal for this. It is suitable for coma due to blockage patterns of both cold and heat types.	Invigorates the blood, activates the channels, reduces swellings to relieve pain, induces labor
Bīng piàn (Borneolum Syntheticum)		It is pungent and bitter in flavor, and slightly cold in property. It has similar but slower action than *shè xiāng* (Moschus) in opening the orifices to arouse the spirit. It is suitable for coma due to blockage patterns of a heat type.	Clears heat to relieve pain
Sū hé xiāng (Styrax)		It is pungent, warm and aromatic. It has a similar but inferior action to *shè xiāng* (Moschus) in opening the orifices to arouse the spirit. It is a representative medicinal for warming and opening the orifices, and is indicated for coma due to blockage patterns of a cold type.	Warms the interior to relieve pain
Shí chāng pú (Rhizoma Acori Tatarinowii)		It is pungent, bitter, dry and warm in nature. It has a slow action in opening the orifices, but is effective for transforming damp, removing phlegm and driving away pestilent factors to open the orifices, calming and benefitting the mind. It is indicated for coma, epilepsy and dementia due to phlegm, damp and foul turbidity invading the clear orifices, as well as dizziness, drowsiness, amnesia, tinnitus and deafness.	Transforms damp to harmonize the stomach

Tables to test your herbal knowledge of the actions and indications of medicinals that open the orifices are as follows (Tables 23-2 and 23-3):

Table 23-2: Test your Herbal Knowledge of the Actions of Medicinals that Open the Orifices:

Actions \ Medicinal	Shè xiāng	Bīng piàn	Sū hé xiāng	Shí chāng pú	Chán sū	Zhāng nǎo
Detoxifies						
Invigorates the blood and activates the channels						
Warms the channels to relieve pain						
Induces labor						
Clears heat to relieve pain						
Wards off pestilence to relieve pain						
Calms the heart and tranquilizes the mind						
Transforms damp to harmonize the stomach						
Opens the orifices to arouse the spirit						
Removes damp and kills parasites						
Relieves pain						

Table 23-3: Test your Herbal Knowledge of the Indications of Medicinals that Open the Orifices:

Indications \ Medicinal	Shè xiāng	Bīng piàn	Sū hé xiāng	Shí chāng pú	Chán sū	Zhāng nǎo
Blood-shot, swollen and painful eyes						
Skin diseases with swelling and pain						
Sore and swollen throat						
Coma due to blockage patterns of a heat type						
Violent pain in the chest and abdomen						
Injuries due to trauma						
Bi due to wind damp						
Abnormal or difficult childbirth, fetal death, retention of lochia						
Coma due to blockage patterns						
Skin diseases that have ruptured but are not healing						
Amenorrhea due to blood stasis						
Toothache						
Chest and abdominal fullness, distress, and cold pain						
Coma due to phlegm-damp invading the clear orifices						
Epigastric and abdominal distending pain due to damp obstruction in the middle jiao						
Abdominal pain, vomiting and diarrhea due to summer-heat gastric disturbance						
Stubborn ulcers, carbuncles, furuncles, and boils						
Coma due to blockage pattern of a cold type						
Swelling from cancer						
Scabies, tinea, damp ulcers and pruritus						

Chapter 24
Medicinals that Tonify Deficiency

Concept

Medicinals whose principal effect is to tonify deficiency, support weakness, and correct pathological tendencies in the body from deficiency and debilitation of qi, blood, yin and yang are referred to as medicinals that tonify deficiency.

Character

Medicinals of this kind can strengthen the right qi and supplement the essence. The sweet flavor is able to tonify, so such medicinals mostly have a sweet flavor. The characters and actions of the different kinds of medicinals that tonify deficiency vary greatly. They are discussed later in this chapter.

Actions and Indications

Medicinals that tonify deficiency are indicated for low spirits, lassitude, a whitish or yellowish complexion, palpitations, shortness of breath, and a weak pulse due to consumption of essence and deficiency of the right qi. The medicinals that treat qi deficiency, yang deficiency, blood deficiency, or yin deficiency syndrome, can correspondingly replenish yin, supplement yang, nourish yin and enrich yang.

Combinations

When using medicinals that tonify deficiency, corresponding individual medicinals should be chosen according to the different syndromes of qi deficiency, yang deficiency, blood deficiency or yin deficiency. Generally speaking, medicinals for replenishing qi should be selected for qi deficiency syndrome; medicinals for supplementing yang should be selected for yang deficiency; medicinals for enriching blood should be selected for blood deficiency; and medicinals for nourishing yin should be selected for yin deficiency. Moreover, qi, blood, yin and yang within the human body interact with each other both physically and pathologically. Clinically, simple deficiency syndromes are not commonly seen. Therefore, it is necessary to combine medicinals that tonify different types of deficiencies. For instance, for cases of qi deficiency developing into yang deficiency, medicinals for replenishing qi and supplementing yang should be used simultaneously, because yang deficiency always causes qi deficiency. Blood generates from qi, and qi deficiency will lead to blood deficiency. Blood stores qi, so blood deficiency can cause qi deficiency. Therefore medicinals for replenishing qi and enriching blood are often used together. Qi belongs to yang, while fluid belongs to yin. Qi can promote generation of fluids, and fluids can carry qi. The deficiency of qi affects the production of fluids and leads to deficiency of fluids. Consumption of fluids will also cause qi collapse with fluid depletion. Yin is easily consumed during febrile diseases. Strong fire can consume qi. Therefore medicinals for replenishing qi and nourishing yin are often used together. Fluids and blood share the same origin. Fluids are an important component of blood. Blood belongs to yin, so blood deficiency will result in yin deficiency, while consumption of yin fluids will in turn lead to blood dryness and fluid consumption. Blood deficiency and yin consumption often appear together during the course of a disease. Yin and yang are interdependent. Yin cannot exist alone without yang, and vice versa. If both yin and yang are impaired to a certain extent, conditions of yin consumption involving yang or yang consumption involving yin will occur, which finally lead to both yin and yang deficiency. For such cases, medicinals for nourishing yin and supplementing yang are used simultaneously.

In addition, medicinals for tonifying deficiency are used with medicinals of other kinds to strengthen the right qi to expel pathogens. They can also be combined with medicinals that easily damage the right qi, so as to protect the right qi and anticipate any possible deficiency.

Precautions

1. Avoid tonification by mistake. For excess syndromes without deficiency, the application of medicinals that tonify deficiency will cause an exacerbation of the pathological condition. Improper use of tonic medicinals can damage the relative balance between yin and yang, which will lead to new pathological changes.

2. Avoid improper tonification. Blind use of medicinals that tonify deficiency can, not only fail to achieve expected therapeutic actions, but lead to unwanted side effects. For example, if medicinals for supplementing yang are used for a syndrome of yin deficiency with heat, they will help the heat to consume yin. If medicinals for nourishing yin are mistakenly used for syndromes of yang deficiency with cold, they will help cold to impair yang.

3. The relation between strengthening the right qi and eliminating pathogens should be understood correctly. Therefore, medicinals for tonifying deficiency should be avoided if they will influence the effect of eliminating pathogens.

4. Medicinals for tonifying deficiency should be used in such a way so as not to cause stagnation. Some medicinals for tonifying deficiency are greasy and are not easily digested. Overdose or use of medicinals that tonify deficiency in patients with dysfunction of the spleen's ability to transport and transform may lead to a functional disturbance of the spleen and stomach. Therefore, they should be used properly with medicinals for invigorating the spleen to digest food. At the same time, replenishing qi should be assisted with promoting qi circulation, removing damp, or transforming phlegm. Enriching blood should be assisted with promoting blood circulation. In addition, medicinals that tonify deficiency should be simmered over a low fire to ensure their therapeutic effects. Deficiency syndromes always have a long course of disease. Therefore, medicinals can be prepared as honey pills, extractions, and liquids for convenient administration and to enhance their therapeutic effects.

Classification

According to their characters, actions and indications, medicinals for tonifying deficiency are divided into four categories: Medicinals that replenish qi, medicinals that supplement yang, medicinals that enrich blood, and medicinals that nourish yin.

Section 1   Medicinals that Replenish Qi

Medicinals in this section have the effect of replenishing qi to rectify pathological conditions of qi deficiency. Replenishing qi includes replenishing spleen qi, lung qi, heart qi and original qi. They are indicated for spleen qi deficiency, manifesting as poor appetite, deficiency distension in the epigastrium and abdomen, loose stools, lassitude, low spirit, a yellowish complexion, emaciation, and puffiness or even prolapse of the internal organs, and failure of the spleen to govern blood; lung qi deficiency, with manifestations such as shortness of breath worsening with movement, forceless cough, low voice, or even dyspnea, lassitude, low spirits, and sweating due to deficiency; heart qi deficiency manifesting as palpitations, chest oppression, shortness of breath worsening with activity; original qi deficiency, manifesting as qi deficiency in some *zang* organs in mild cases, and shortness of breath, and a faint, weak and indistinct pulse in severe cases.

Medicinals that replenish qi are mostly sweet in flavor, and warm or neutral in property. Some of them have actions of clearing fire or drying damp, and therefore have a bitter flavor. Types that can clear fire have a cold property. Most of the medicinals can replenish qi in the spleen and lung, and enter the spleen and lung channels. A few of them are able to replenish the heart qi, and therefore also enter the heart channel.

① *Rén shēn* (人参, Radix et Rhizoma Ginseng, Ginseng) ★★★

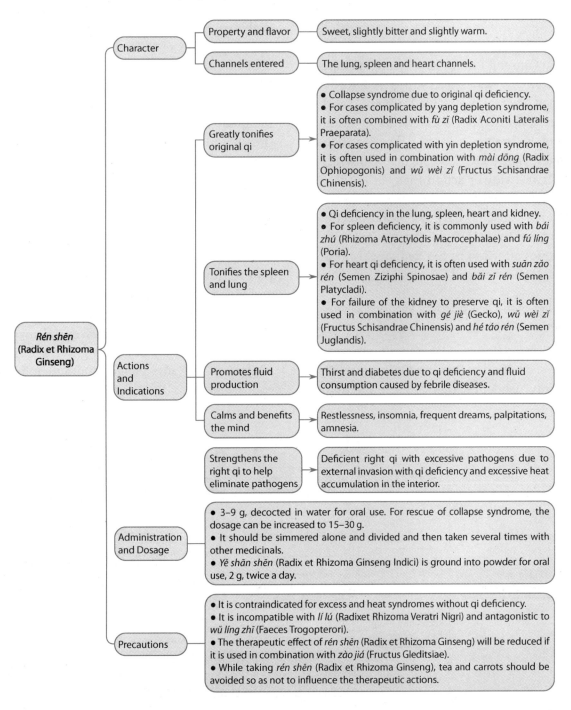

Rén shēn (Radix et Rhizoma Ginseng)

- **Character**
  - **Property and flavor** — Sweet, slightly bitter and slightly warm.
  - **Channels entered** — The lung, spleen and heart channels.

- **Actions and Indications**
  - **Greatly tonifies original qi**
    - Collapse syndrome due to original qi deficiency.
    - For cases complicated by yang depletion syndrome, it is often combined with *fù zǐ* (Radix Aconiti Lateralis Praeparata).
    - For cases complicated with yin depletion syndrome, it is often used in combination with *mài dōng* (Radix Ophiopogonis) and *wǔ wèi zǐ* (Fructus Schisandrae Chinensis).
  - **Tonifies the spleen and lung**
    - Qi deficiency in the lung, spleen, heart and kidney.
    - For spleen deficiency, it is commonly used with *bái zhú* (Rhizoma Atractylodis Macrocephalae) and *fú líng* (Poria).
    - For heart qi deficiency, it is often used with *suān zǎo rén* (Semen Ziziphi Spinosae) and *bǎi zǐ rén* (Semen Platycladi).
    - For failure of the kidney to preserve qi, it is often used in combination with *gé jiè* (Gecko), *wǔ wèi zǐ* (Fructus Schisandrae Chinensis) and *hé táo rén* (Semen Juglandis).
  - **Promotes fluid production** — Thirst and diabetes due to qi deficiency and fluid consumption caused by febrile diseases.
  - **Calms and benefits the mind** — Restlessness, insomnia, frequent dreams, palpitations, amnesia.
  - **Strengthens the right qi to help eliminate pathogens** — Deficient right qi with excessive pathogens due to external invasion with qi deficiency and excessive heat accumulation in the interior.

- **Administration and Dosage**
  - 3–9 g, decocted in water for oral use. For rescue of collapse syndrome, the dosage can be increased to 15–30 g.
  - It should be simmered alone and divided and then taken several times with other medicinals.
  - *Yě shān shēn* (Radix et Rhizoma Ginseng Indici) is ground into powder for oral use, 2 g, twice a day.

- **Precautions**
  - It is contraindicated for excess and heat syndromes without qi deficiency.
  - It is incompatible with *lí lú* (Radixet Rhizoma Veratri Nigri) and antagonistic to *wǔ líng zhī* (Faeces Trogopterori).
  - The therapeutic effect of *rén shēn* (Radix et Rhizoma Ginseng) will be reduced if it is used in combination with *zào jiá* (Fructus Gleditsiae).
  - While taking *rén shēn* (Radix et Rhizoma Ginseng), tea and carrots should be avoided so as not to influence the therapeutic actions.

Yě shān shēn (野山参, Radix et Rhizoma Ginseng Indici, Wild Ginseng) has a strong action for tonifying deficiency, however, it is rare and expensive, and therefore is not often used in the clinic. *Rén shēn* (Radix et Rhizoma Ginseng) is inferior to *yě shān shēn* (Radix et Rhizoma Ginseng Indici) in tonifying deficiency, but is commonly used in the clinic, because it is produced more abundantly, and is less expensive. *Gāo lì shēn* (高丽参, Korean Ginseng) has a stronger action than *hóng shēn* (红参, Radix et Rhizoma Ginseng Rubra, Red Ginseng). *Shēng shài shēn* (生晒参, Sun-dried Ginseng) and *hóng shēn* (Radix et Rhizoma Ginseng Rubra) have strong therapeutic effects. *Shēng shài shēn* (sun-dried Radix et Rhizoma Ginseng) is suitable for both qi and yin deficiency, while *hóng shēn* (Radix et Rhizoma Ginseng Rubra) is suitable for qi and yang deficiency. *Táng shēn* (糖参, Sugared Ginseng) has a similar but slower action than *shēng shài shēn* (Sun-dried Ginseng). Rootlets of *rén shēn* (Radix et Rhizoma Ginseng) have the weakest action. It is suitable for those with deficiency syndrome but who cannot afford to be tonified quickly. It is the cheapest type among all Ginsengs.

② *Xī yáng shēn* (西洋参, Radix Panacis Quinquefolii, American Ginseng) ★★

Both *rén shēn* (Radix et Rhizoma Ginseng) and *xī yáng shēn* (Radix Panacis Quinquefolii) are commonly used precious Chinese medicinals.

They are from the root of perennial plants, of the family Araliceae. Both medicinals can tonify original qi, replenish spleen and lung qi, and promote fluid production to relieve thirst. They are used for shortness of breath, low spirits, and a thready and powerless pulse due to qi deficiency with collapse syndrome; lassitude and poor appetite due to deficiency of spleen qi; cough, shortness of breath, dyspnea, indolence of speech, a low voice, and a weak pulse due to lung qi deficiency; vexation, lassitude, thirst and diabetes due to heat consuming qi and fluids. *Rén shēn* (Radix et Rhizoma Ginseng) is from the root of *Panax ginseng* C.A. Mey., of the family Campanulaceae. It is sweet and slightly bitter in flavor, and slightly warm in property. It is effective for greatly tonifying original qi, and tonifying the spleen and lung. It has a strong action in replenishing qi to rescue collapse syndrome even when used alone. It is indicated for collapse syndrome due to qi deficiency with deficiency of spleen and lung qi. At the same time, it can replenish qi in the heart and kidney, and calm and benefit the mind. Therefore it is used for palpitations, insomnia and amnesia due to qi and blood deficiency. *Rén shēn* (Radix et Rhizoma Ginseng) is the first choice for internal injury due to overstrain, and an essential medicinal to tonify deficiency and strengthen the right qi. *Xī yáng shēn* (Radix Panacis Quinquefolii) is the root from *Panax Puinquefolium* L., of the family

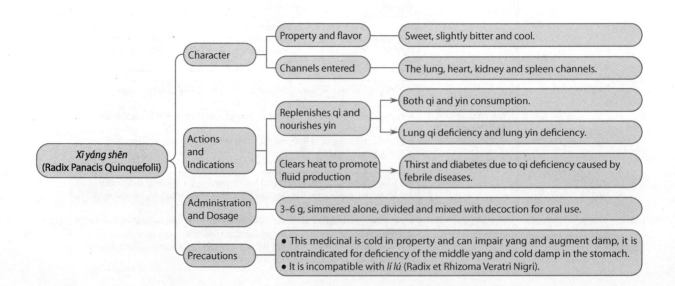

Campanulaceae. It is bitter and slightly sweet in flavor, and cold in property. It is inferior to *rén shēn* (Radix et Rhizoma Ginseng) in replenishing qi, but is effective for nourishing yin and clearing fire to promote fluid production. It is suitable for

qi and yin depletion due to febrile diseases, and both qi and yin deficiency in the spleen and lung.

③ *Dǎng shēn* (党参, Radix Codonopsis, Tangshen Root) ★★★

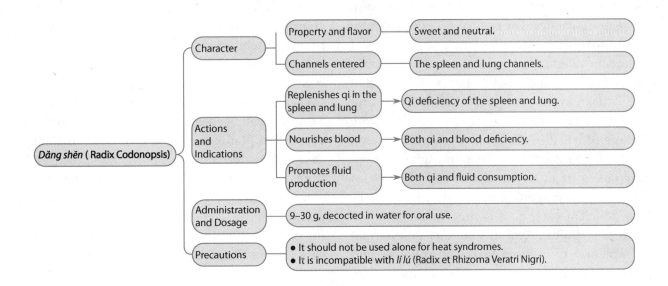

④ *Tài zǐ shēn* (太子参, Radix Pseudostellariae, Heterophylly Falsesatarwort Root) ★

Rén shēn (Radix et Rhizoma Ginseng), *dǎng shēn* (Radix Codonopsis) and *tài zǐ shēn* (Radix Pseudostellariae) are sweet in flavor, and enter the spleen and lung channels. They can tonify the spleen and stomach, and promote fluid production to relieve thirst. The two medicinals are used in combination for lassitude, poor appetite and loose stools due to deficiency of

spleen qi; cough, shortness of breath, dyspnea, indolence of speech, a low voice, spontaneous sweating, and a weak pulse due to lung qi deficiency; shortness of breath and thirst due to both qi and fluid consumption. *Rén shēn* (Radix et Rhizoma Ginseng) is sweet and slightly bitter in flavor, and slightly warm in property. It also enters the heart channel and therefore has the strongest action in tonifying. It is effective for greatly tonifying original qi, and is regarded as

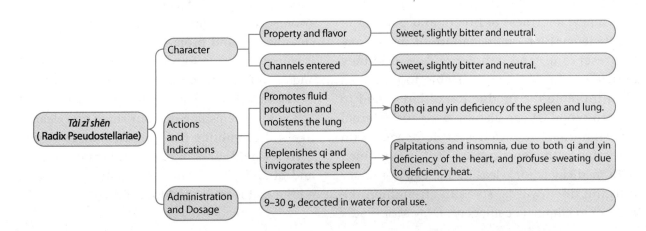

an essential medicinal to tonify deficiency and strengthen the right qi. It is the first choice for internal injury due to overstrain, and is used for deficiency of qi, blood and fluids. In the modern clinic, it is mainly used for emergency cases of collapse syndrome due to qi deficiency and critical cases of chronic diseases due to right qi deficiency. For critical cases of collapse syndrome due to extreme deficiency of original qi, manifesting as shortness of breath, low spirit, and a faint and indistinct pulse, no matter what the causes are (severe blood loss, vomiting, diarrhea, chronic or acute disease), a large dosage of *rén shēn* (Radix et Rhizoma Ginseng) of 15-30 g is used alone in a strong decoction. For cases of collapse syndrome due to qi deficiency accompanied by sweating, cold limbs and deficient yang qi, it is used in combination with *fù zǐ* (Radix Aconiti Lateralis Praeparata) to replenish qi in order to rescue collapse, and restore depleted yang to induce resuscitation. For collapse syndrome due to qi deficiency complicated by qi and yin consumption, with manifestations such as sweating, a warm body, thirst and a preference for cold drinks, it should be combined with *mài dōng* (Radix Ophiopogonis) and *wǔ wèi zǐ* (Fructus Schisandrae Chinensis) to replenish qi, nourish yin, arrest sweating, and rescue collapse. In addition, *rén shēn* (Radix et Rhizoma Ginseng) can replenish qi in the heart and kidney, and calm and benefit the mind. It is used for palpitations, chest oppression, shortness of breath, and a weak pulse due to heart qi deficiency; insomnia, frequent dreams, and amnesia due to qi and blood deficiency, or yin and blood deficiency due to both heart and kidney deficiency; shortness of breath and panting of a deficiency type due to failure of the kidney to preserve qi, and impotence due to kidney deficiency. In addition, it is able to replenish qi to promote the production of blood and to govern blood. It can also be used for external invasion due to deficiency or deficiency with excessive pathogenic factors, if it is combined with medicinals for releasing the exterior or for purging downwards, so as to strengthen the right qi to eliminate pathogens. *Dǎng shēn* (Radix

Codonopsis) is sweet in flavor and neutral in property. It has similar but weaker action than *rén shēn* (Radix et Rhizoma Ginseng) in tonifying qi of the spleen and lung, and promoting fluid production. It is an effective medicinal to tonify the middle and replenish qi and can also nourish blood. It is often used for a yellowish complexion, dizziness, and palpitations caused by qi deficiency of the spleen and stomach, deficiency of the middle qi, lung qi deficiency, or both qi and fluid consumption; as well as external invasion due to deficiency, or deficiency with excessive pathogens. It is commonly used instead of *rén shēn* (Radix et Rhizoma Ginseng) for mild cases of qi deficiency in both the spleen and lung. However, *dǎng shēn* (Radix Codonopsis) cannot tonify original qi and replenish qi to rescue collapse, and therefore should not be used for collapse due to original qi depletion. *Tài zǐ shēn* (Radix Pseudostellariae) has a neutral but a slightly cool property. It has a weaker action than *dǎng shēn* (Radix Codonopsis) in tonifying qi of the spleen and lung. It is a medicinal with the ability to both tonify and clear. It can nourish yin and moisten the lung, and is commonly used for both qi and fluid consumption, and qi and yin deficiency after a treatment which was not suitable for warm tonification.

Xī yáng shēn (Radix Panacis Quinquefolii) and *tài zǐ shēn* (Radix Pseudostellariae) can tonify both qi and yin. They are able to tonify qi and yin of both the spleen and lung, and promote fluid production to relieve thirst. The two medicinals are used for diseases caused by both qi and fluid consumption, and qi and yin deficiency. *Xī yáng shēn* (Radix Panacis Quinquefolii) has strong actions in replenishing qi, nourishing yin, clearing fire and promoting fluid production. It is commonly used for qi and fluid consumption, and qi and yin consumption with fire exuberance. *Tài zǐ shēn* (Radix Pseudostellariae) has a weak action in replenishing qi, nourishing yin, clearing fire and promoting fluid production. It is often used for mild cases of qi and fluid consumption, and qi and yin consumption with little fire. In addition, it is often used for children.

⑤ *Huáng qí* (黄芪, Radix Astragali, Astragalus Root)
★ ★ ★

Both *rén shēn* (Radix et Rhizoma Ginseng) and *huáng qí* (Radix Astragali) are sweet in flavor and slightly warm in property. They can replenish qi in the spleen and lung, enrich blood, govern blood, and promote fluid production to relieve thirst. Both medicinals are used for lassitude, poor appetite, and loose stools due to spleen qi deficiency and deficiency of middle qi; shortness of breath, dyspnea, indolence of speech, a low voice, spontaneous sweating and a weak pulse due to lung qi deficiency; a pale or yellowish complexion, lassitude, dizziness, and palpitations due to qi and blood deficiency; hemafecia, metrorrhagia and metrostaxis due to failure of the deficient qi to control blood; shortness of breath, thirst and diabetes due to both qi and fluid consumption. *Rén shēn* (Radix et Rhizoma Ginseng) has a strong action, and is effective for greatly tonifying original qi, and replenishing qi to treat collapse. It is used for collapse due to qi deficiency, manifesting as an indistinct and faint pulse. It can calm and benefit the mind, replenish qi, and invigorate yang. It is also used for palpitations, insomnia and amnesia due to qi and blood deficiency; and impotence due to kidney deficiency. It is an essential medicinal for tonifying deficiency and strengthening the right qi. It is considered the first choice for internal injury due to overstrain. *Huáng qí* (Radix Astragali) is inferior to *rén shēn* (Radix et Rhizoma Ginseng) in replenishing qi. However, it has a good effect in lifting yang. It is considered

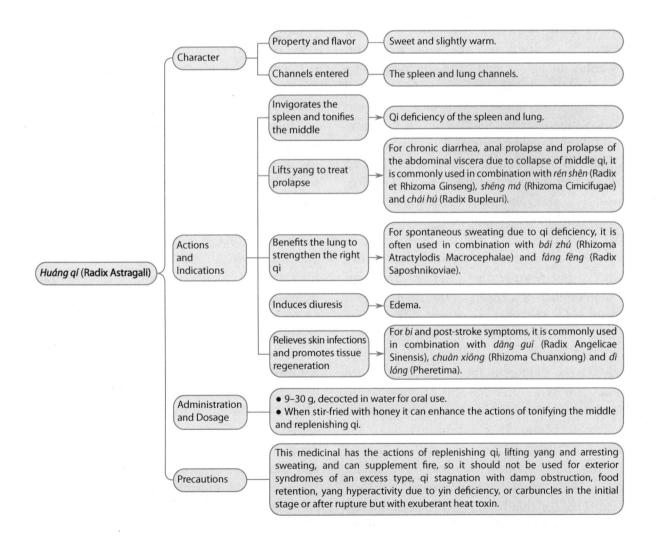

an essential medicinal to replenish qi and lift yang, which is suitable for chronic diarrhea, prolapse of the internal organs including anal, uterine and stomach prolapse, due to middle qi collapse from spleen deficiency. It can benefit the lung to strengthen the right qi, induce diuresis to reduce swellings, clear skin infections, promote tissue regeneration, and replenish qi to remove stagnation. It is commonly used for spontaneous sweating due to qi deficiency. It is also an essential medicinal to treat edema due to qi deficiency, and is used for swelling and decreased urine production due to failure of the deficient spleen to transport damp; skin diseases that are not rupturing, or that have ruptured but have not healed for a long time, caused by qi and blood deficiency; and *bi*, numbness and stroke with hemiparalysis due to malnutrition of the sinews and vessels caused by qi stagnation and blood stasis.

Both *huáng qí* (Radix Astragali) and *dǎng shēn* (Radix Codonopsis) are sweet in flavor. They enter the spleen and lung channels. They can replenish qi of the spleen and lung, and can promote fluid and blood production. Both medicinals are essential medicinals for tonifying the middle and replenishing qi. They are used for lassitude, poor appetite and loose stools caused by deficiency of the middle qi and spleen qi deficiency; cough, shortness of breath, dyspnea, indolence of speech, a low voice, spontaneous sweating, and a weak pulse due to lung qi deficiency; a pale or yellowish complexion, lassitude, dizziness, and palpitations due to qi and blood deficiency. *Huáng qí* (Radix Astragali) is effective for replenishing qi and lifting yang, and is an essential medicinal to treat prolapse due to qi deficiency. It is able to benefit the lung to strengthen the right qi, induce diuresis to reduce edema, clear skin infections and promote tissue regeneration, replenish qi to remove stagnation, and govern blood. It is commonly used for spontaneous sweating due to qi deficiency; edema and urine retention due to failure of the deficient spleen to transport damp; skin diseases that have not ruptured, or that have ruptured but are not healing, caused by qi and blood deficiency; *bi*,

numbness and stroke with hemiparalysis due to malnutrition of sinews and vessels caused by qi stagnation and blood stasis; blood loss due to a deficient spleen failing to govern blood. However, *dǎng shēn* (Radix Codonopsis) specializes in replenishing the qi of the spleen and lung as well as nourishing blood.

⑥ *Bái zhú* (白术, Rhizoma Atractylodis Macrocephalae, Atractylodes Rhizome) ★ ★ ★

Both *bái zhú* (Rhizoma Atractylodis Macrocephalae) and *cāng zhú* (Rhizoma Atractylodis) are referred to as *zhú* in *Shennong's Herbal Classic*, and they were treated as one medicinal at that time. Until the *Part Record of Famous Physicians*, there were records on *chì zhú*, which is also called *cāng zhú* (Rhizoma Atractylodis) nowadays. The name *cāng zhú* (Rhizoma Atractylodis) was initially mentioned in the *Classified Materia Medica from Historical Classics for Emergency*. *Bái zhú* (Rhizoma Atractylodis Macrocephalae) and *cāng zhú* (Rhizoma Atractylodis) are bitter in flavor and warm in property. They enter the spleen and stomach channels and have the actions of drying damp and invigorating the spleen. Both the medicinals are used for loose stools, edema, leukorrhagia and phlegm-fluids due to damp exuberance in the spleen. They are often used in combination for mutual reinforcement for damp exuberance in the spleen. *Bái zhú* (Rhizoma Atractylodis Macrocephalae) has a sweet flavor. It is effective for replenishing qi and invigorating the spleen, and therefore is used for damp obstruction in the spleen of a deficiency kind. It can also induce diuresis, strengthen the right qi to arrest sweating, and prevent miscarriage. It is often used for spontaneous sweating and excessive fetal movement due to spleen qi deficiency. *Cāng zhú* (Rhizoma Atractylodis) has a pungent flavor and dry nature. It is effective for transporting the spleen, and is often used for damp turbidity obstruction in the spleen of an excessive type. It is able to expel wind damp, relieve exterior syndromes via diaphoresis, and improve visual acuity. It is commonly used for *bi* due to wind damp; external invasion by wind cold complicated by damp; night blindness, and dim eyesight.

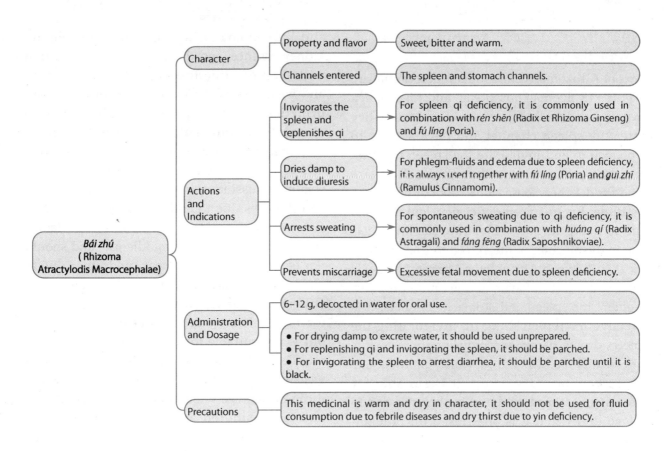

⑦ *Shān yào* (山药, Rhizoma Dioscoreae, Common
Yan Rhizome) ★ ★

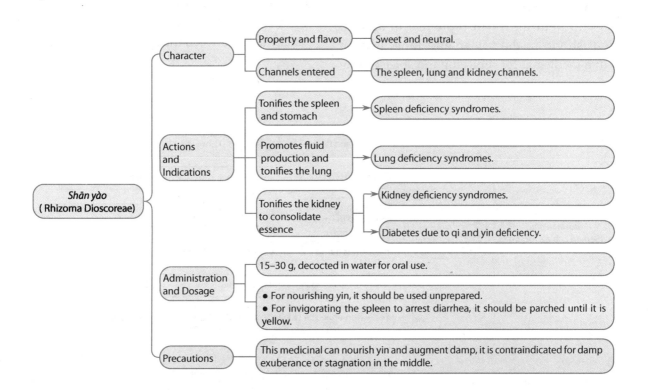

⑧ *Bái biǎn dòu* (白扁豆, Semen Lablab Album, White Hyacinth Bean) ★

Bái zhú (Rhizoma Atractylodis Macrocephalae), *shān yào* (Rhizoma Dioscoreae) and *bái biǎn dòu* (Semen Lablab Album) are sweet in flavor. They enter the spleen channel and have actions to replenish qi and invigorate the spleen to arrest diarrhea and reduce leukorrhagia. They are used for diarrhea, loose stools, poor appetite and lassitude due to spleen deficiency; leukorrhagia due to damp turbidity invading the lower *jiao* due to dysfunction of the spleen in transporting. *Bái zhú* (Rhizoma Atractylodis Macrocephalae) is bitter and sweet in flavor, and warm in property. It enters the spleen and stomach channels. It is effective for replenishing qi, invigorating the spleen, drying damp, and inducing diuresis. It is an essential medicinal to replenish qi, invigorate the spleen, and dry damp. It is suitable for loose stools caused by damp exuberance due to spleen deficiency. It is often used for phlegm-fluids and edema due to water retention caused by failure of the deficient spleen to transform water. Meanwhile, it can strengthen the right qi to arrest sweating and prevent miscarriage. It is commonly used for spontaneous sweating and excessive fetal movement due to spleen qi deficiency. *Shān yào* (Rhizoma Dioscoreae) is sweet and neutral. It can replenish qi as well as nourish yin in the spleen and lung. It is an effective medicinal for tonifying the spleen, lung and kidney channels. It can also consolidate kidney essence, and therefore is used for cough with dyspnea due to lung deficiency; aching and weakness of the waist and knees, frequent urination at night, spermatorrhea, premature ejaculation, and leukorrhagia with watery discharge due to kidney qi deficiency; emaciation, aching and weakness of the waist and knees and seminal emission due to kidney yin deficiency; and diabetes due to both qi and yin deficiency. *Bái zhú* (Rhizoma Atractylodis Macrocephalae) is suitable for damp in the middle *jiao*, and should not be used for internal heat syndromes due to yin deficiency. *Shān yào* (Rhizoma Dioscoreae) can nourish yin and augment damp, and can be used for internal heat syndromes due to yin deficiency, but is not suitable for damp exuberance in the middle. *Bái biǎn dòu* (Semen Lablab Album) has a weaker action in tonifying the spleen. However, it can harmonize the middle to transform damp, and is considered an effective medicinal to invigorate the spleen to transform damp. It can tonify the spleen without causing stagnation, and can remove damp without drying fluids. It is commonly used for loose stools, diarrhea and leukorrhagia due to damp exuberance from spleen deficiency. It is also used to treat vomiting, diarrhea, and distending pain induced by summer-heat damp impairing the middle, with disharmony between the spleen and stomach.

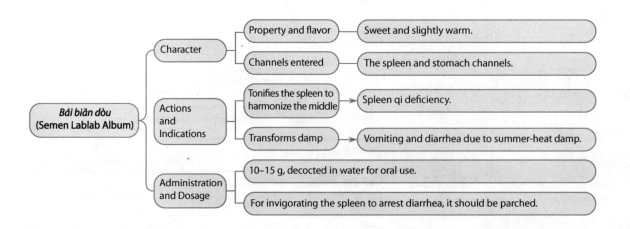

⑨ *Gān cǎo* (甘草, Radix et Rhizoma Glycyrrhizae, Licorice Root) ★★★

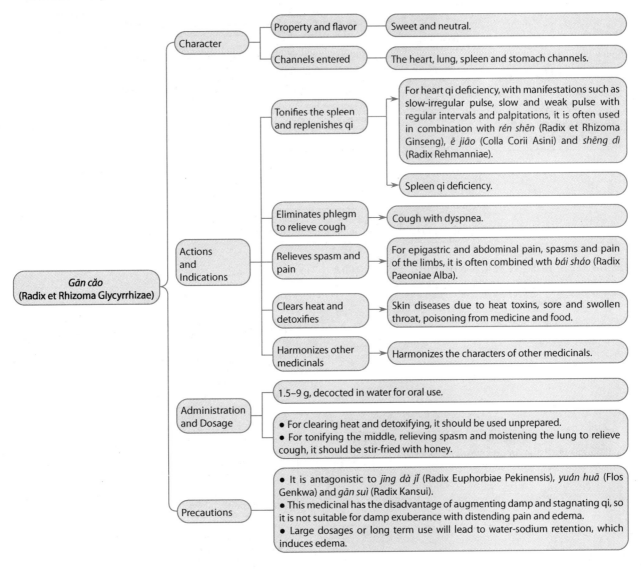

⑩ *Dà zǎo* (大枣, Fructus Jujubae, Chinese Date) ★★

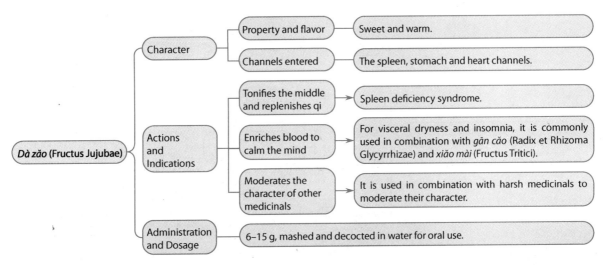

⑪ *Cì wǔ jiā* (刺五加, Radix et Rhizoma seu Caulis Acanthopanacis Senticosi, Manyprickle Acanthopanax)

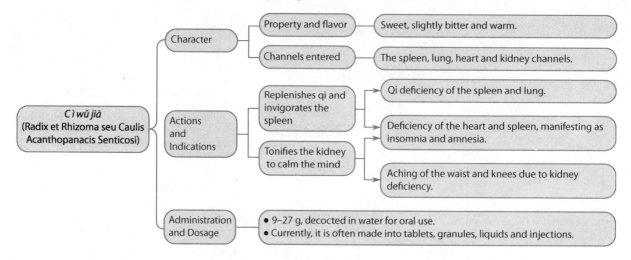

⑫ *Jiǎo gǔ lán* (绞股蓝, Rhizoma seu Herba Gynostemmatis Pentaphylli, Fiveleaf Gynostemma Herb or Root)

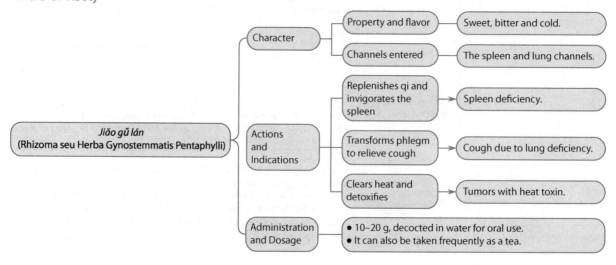

⑬ *Hóng jǐng tiān* (红景天, Radix et Rhizoma Rhodiolae Crenulatae, Gold Theragran)

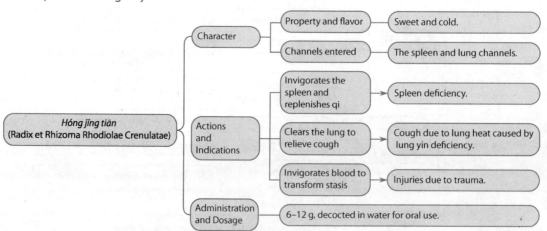

⑭ *Shā jí* (沙棘, Fructus Hippophae, Seabuckthorn Fruit)

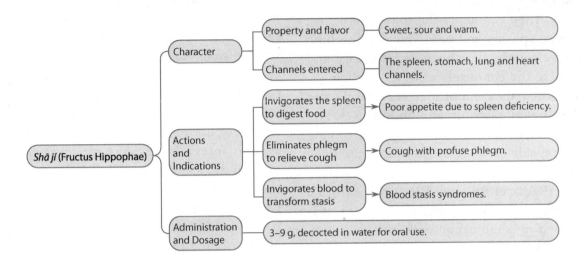

⑮ *Yí táng* (饴糖, Saccharum Granorum, Cerealose)

Dà zǎo (Fructus Jujubae) and *yí táng* (Saccharum Granorum) are sweet in flavor and warm in property. They enter the spleen and stomach channels to tonify the middle and replenish qi. They are used for lassitude, shortness of breath, and poor appetite caused by overstrain, internal injury, stomach and spleen deficiency, and deficiency of middle qi. They can strengthen the actions of tonifying the spleen and stomach when used with other common tonics. *Dà zǎo* (Fructus Jujubae) can nourish blood to calm the mind, and moderate the characters of other medicinals. It is used for a yellowish complexion due to blood deficiency, visceral dryness, and restlessness. It can reduce the side effects of harsh medicinals to protect the right qi. *Yí táng* (Saccharum Granorum) can relieve spasms and pain, and moisten the lung to relieve pain. It is used for spasms of the limbs, epigastric and abdominal pain due to middle deficiency, and dry cough with scanty phlegm due to lung deficiency.

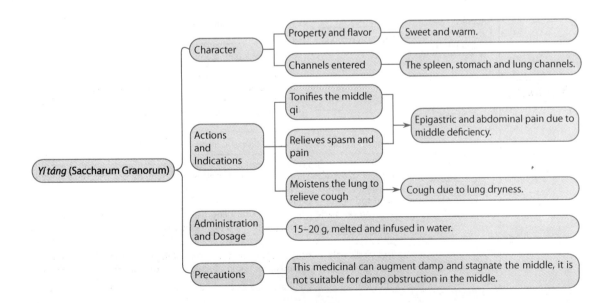

⑯ *Fēng mì* (蜂蜜, Mel, Honey) ★

Gān cǎo (Radix et Rhizoma Glycyrrhizae) and *fēng mì* (Mel) are sweet in flavor and neutral in property. They can tonify the spleen, replenish qi, relieve spasms and pain, moisten the lung to relieve cough, clear heat, and detoxify and harmonize the characters of other medicinals. Both medicinals are indicated for spasms and pain in the epigastrium and abdomen due to spleen qi deficiency; chronic cough due to lung deficiency; skin diseases; and for moderating the toxicity and harsh actions of other medicinals. *Gān cǎo* (Radix et Rhizoma Glycyrrhizae) has a better effect of relieving spasms and pain. It is often used in combination with *bái sháo* (Radix Paeoniae Alba) to treat spasms and pain in the epigastrium, abdomen and limbs due to various causes such as blood deficiency, blood stasis or cold congealing. It is effective for harmonizing the actions and characters of other medicinals. It is able to reduce the toxicity or harsh actions of other medicinals when used in a formula. These harsh medicinals include *fù zǐ* (Radix Aconiti Lateralis Praeparata) and *dà huáng* (Radix et Rhizoma Rhei). It can relieve spasms and pain, and therefore is used for abdominal pain induced by some medicinals such as *dà huáng* (Radix et Rhizoma Rhei). It can also ameliorate the unpleasant tastes of some medicinals with its sweet taste. In addition, *gān cǎo* (Radix et Rhizoma Glycyrrhizae) can replenish heart qi and eliminate phlegm to relieve cough. It is used for palpitations, slow-irregular pulse, slow and weak pulse with regular intervals due to heart qi deficiency; visceral dryness due to blood deficiency; cough and panting of a cold, heat, deficient or excess type if combined properly with other medicinals; it is also used for a sore and swollen throat, and poisoning from medicinals and food. *Fēng mì* (Mel) is moist in texture. It can moisten the intestines to promote defecation, and is used for constipation due to dry intestines. In addition, it is often used as an excipient in pills or extracts. Some Chinese medicinals are stir-fried with honey to strengthen their therapeutic effect of tonifying, and to harmonize their characteristics.

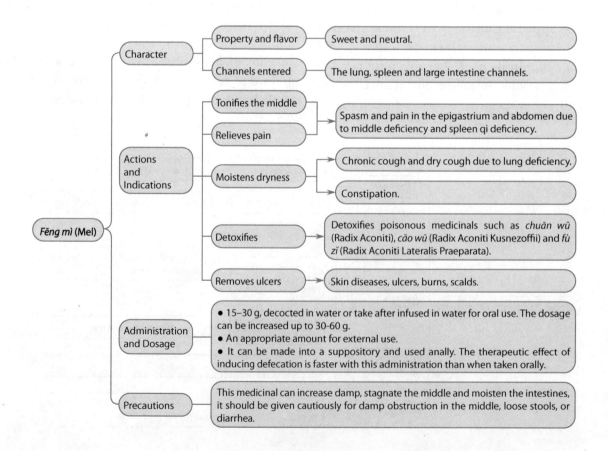

Section 2 Medicinals that Supplement Yang

Medicinals in this section are mostly sweet, pungent and salty in flavor, warm or hot in property, and enter the kidney channel. They have the actions of supplementing kidney yang so as to warm other internal organs and eliminate or improve symptoms caused by yang deficiency. They are indicated for aversion to cold, cold limbs, aching and weakness of the waist and knees, absence of libido, impotence, premature ejaculation, infertility, frequent urination, and enuresis due to kidney yang deficiency; cold pain in the epigastrium due to yang deficiency of the spleen and kidney; edema due to yang deficiency; deficiency of essence and blood due to deficiency of the liver and kidney, manifesting as dizziness, tinnitus, early graying of the hair, flaccidity of the extremities or the five kinds of delayed growth in infants, namely poor development, delayed closure of the fontanel in infants, delayed tooth eruption and delayed walking; deficient panting due to both lung and kidney deficiency, failure of the kidney to preserve qi; metrorrhagia, metrostaxis and leukorrhagia due to deficiency cold of kidney yang.

① *Lù róng* (鹿茸, Cornu Cervi Pantotrichum, Deer Velvet) ★ ★ ★

Addition: *Lù róng* (**Cornu Cervi Pantotrichum**), *lù jiǎo* (**鹿角, Cornu Cervi, Deer Antler**), *lù jiǎo jiāo* (**Colla Cornus Cervi**) and *lù jiǎo shuāng* (**Cornu Cervi Degelatinatum**) have the same origin. They come from the horn of the male *Cervus Nippon* Temminck or *C. elaphus* L., of the family Cervidae. They are salty in flavor and warm in property. They enter the kidney and liver channels. They can tonify the kidney in order to supplement, and are used for kidney deficiency manifesting as impotence, premature ejaculation, female sterility, frequent urination, dizziness, tinnitus, aching in the waist and knees, cold limbs, and low spirit. Their differences are as follows. *Lù róng* (Cornu Cervi Pantotrichum) is from the immature horn of the male *Cervus Nippon* Temminck or *C. elaphus* L., of the family

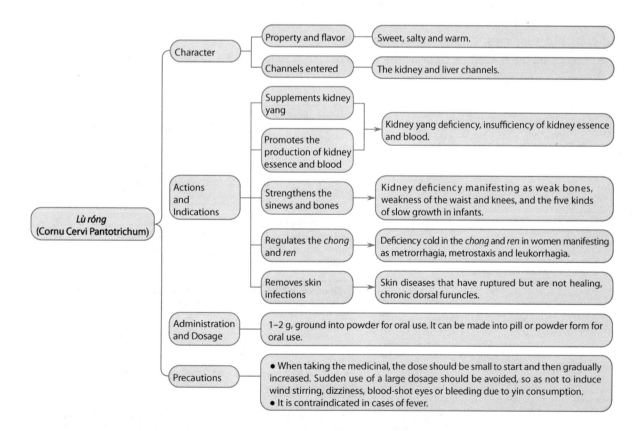

Cervidae. It is sweet in flavor, has a strong action in supplementing kidney yang, and in promoting production of kidney essence and blood. It is an essential medicinal to supplement kidney yang and promote production of kidney essence and blood, and can be used for various diseases caused by kidney yang deficiency, and kidney essence and blood deficiency. It can strengthen the bones and sinews, regulate the *chong* and *ren*, and remove skin infections. It is used for kidney yang deficiency, deficiency of kidney essence and blood, manifesting as flaccidity of the sinews and bones, weakness of the waist and knees, the five kinds of delayed growth in infants; deficiency cold in the *chong* and *ren* vessels in women, instability of the *dai* vessel manifesting as metrorrhagia, metrostaxis and leukorrhagia; skin diseases that have ruptured but have not healed, and chronic dorsal furuncles. *Lù jiǎo* (Cornu Cervi) is the ossific horn of a male deer. It has similar but weaker action than *lù róng* (Cornu Cervi Pantotrichum) in supplementing kidney yang, and strengthening the sinews and bones. It can be used instead of *lù róng* (Cornu Cervi Pantotrichum). It can invigorate the blood to remove stasis and reduce swellings, and is used for skin diseases, breast abscesses, pain due to blood stasis as well as pain in the lumbar vertebrae, sinews and bones. *Lù jiǎo jiāo* (Colla

Cornus Cervi) is the solid glue from a water extraction of deer horn. It is sweet and salty in flavor and warm in property. It is superior to *lù jiǎo* (Cornu Cervi), but is inferior to *lù róng* (Cornu Cervi Pantotrichum) in warming and nourishing the liver and kidney and promoting production of kidney essence and blood, and is effective for stopping bleeding. It is used for kidney yang deficiency, and kidney essence and blood deficiency, manifesting as emaciation; hematemesis, epistaxis, hematuria, metrorrhagia and metrostaxis of a deficiency cold type, and dorsal furuncles that are not healing. *Lù jiǎo shuāng* (Cornu Cervi Degelatinatum) is the residue after *lù jiǎo* (Cornu Cervi) is made into an extraction. It has a weaker action than *lù jiǎo* (Cornu Cervi) in supplementing kidney yang. However, it can consolidate kidney essence, stop bleeding, and promote wound healing. When used internally, it can treat metrorrhagia, metrostaxis and seminal emission. When used externally, it can treat bleeding due to trauma and skin diseases that have ruptured but that have not healed.

② *Zǐ hé chē* (紫河车, Placenta Hominis, Human Placenta) ★★

Lù róng (Cornu Cervi Pantotrichum) and *zǐ hé chē* (Placenta Hominis) can supplement kidney yang,

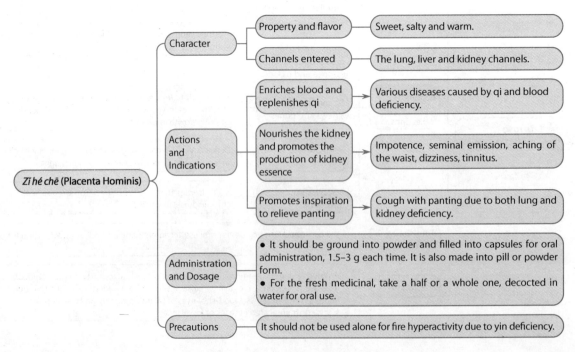

and promote the production of kidney essence and blood. They are effective medicinals for nourishing and strengthening the body. They are used for kidney yang deficiency, and deficiency of kidney essence and blood, manifesting as impotence, seminal emission, aching of the waist and legs, dizziness and tinnitus. *Lù róng* (Cornu Cervi Pantotrichum) has a strong action in supplementing kidney yang. It is used for severe cases of kidney yang deficiency and deficiency of kidney essence and blood. It can also strengthen the sinews and bones, regulate the *chong* and *ren* vessels, and remove skin infections. It is used for kidney yang deficiency, and deficiency of kidney essence and blood, manifesting as flaccidity of the sinews and bones, weakness of the waist and knees, the five kinds of delayed growth in infants; deficiency cold in the *chong* and *ren* vessels in women, instability of the *dai* vessel manifesting as metrorrhagia, metrostaxis and leukorrhagia; skin diseases after rupture that are not healing, and dorsal furuncles that are not healing. *Zǐ hé chē* (Placenta Hominis) has a strong action to nourish yin. It can improve the strength of both yin and yang, and is therefore used for various diseases caused by deficiency of kidney essence and blood. It can replenish qi and nourish blood, hence it is used for diseases caused by qi and blood deficiency, with manifestations such as delactation post-partum, a yellowish complexion, emaciation, lassitude; cough with dyspnea due to both lung and kidney deficiency.

③ *Yín yáng huò* (淫羊藿, Herba Epimedii, Epimedium Herb) ★ ★ ★

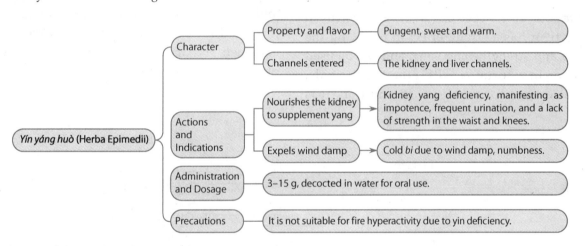

④ *Bā jǐ tiān* (巴戟天, Radix Morindae Officinalis, Morinda Root) ★ ★

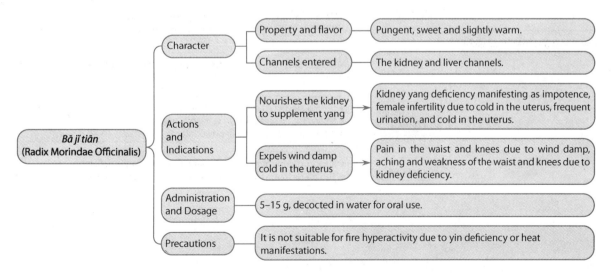

⑤ *Xiān máo* (仙茅, Rhizoma Curculiginis, Common Curculigo Rhizome)

Yín yáng huò (Herba Epimedii), *bā jǐ tiān* (Radix Morindae Officinalis) and *xiān máo* (Rhizoma Curculiginis) are pungent in flavor, and warm in property. They enter the kidney and liver channels. They have the actions of nourishing the kidney, supplementing kidney yang, strengthening the bones and sinews, and expelling wind damp. They are used for kidney yang deficiency, manifesting as impotence, female infertility, enuresis, frequent urination and flaccidity of the waist and knees; chronic cold *bi* due to wind damp with kidney deficiency, manifesting as aching of the waist and knees or flaccidity. These three medicinals are commonly used for mutual reinforcement. The differences are as follows: *Yín yáng huò* (Herba Epimedii) is pungent and sweet in flavor, and warm in property. It has a strong effect in tonifying the kidney and strengthening yang, and can be used alone or in a formula with other medicinals. It is also used for paralysis. In addition, it is commonly used for cough with dyspnea due to kidney yang deficiency and hypertension during menopause. *Bā jǐ tiān* (Radix Morindae Officinalis) is pungent and sweet in flavor, and slightly warm in property. It is inferior to *yín yáng huò* (Herba Epimedii) in tonifying the kidney and strengthening yang, however, it can promote the production of kidney essence and blood, and is therefore used for female infertility due to cold in the uterus, irregular menstruation and cold pain in the lower abdomen due to deficiency cold of the kidney and deficiency of kidney essence and blood. *Xiān máo* (Rhizoma Curculiginis) is pungent and hot, and toxic. It has a strong action in expelling wind damp, and is drier and hotter than *yín yáng huò* (Herba Epimedii) and *bā jǐ tiān* (Radix Morindae Officinalis). It will cause impairment to the yin if taken for a long time, and will cause dry lips and mouth. In addition, it is used for cold pain in the epigastrium and abdomen, and diarrhea caused by yang deficiency of the spleen and kidney.

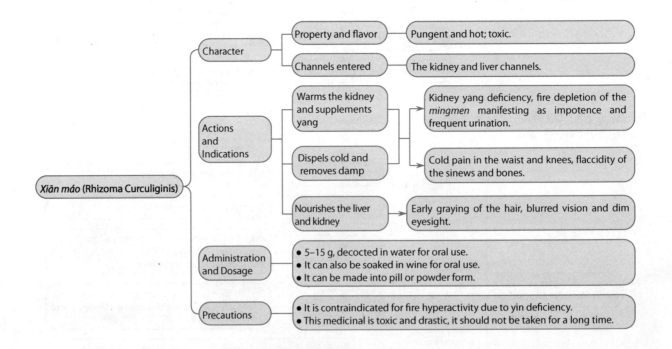

⑥ *Dù zhòng* (杜仲, Cortex Eucommiae, Eucommia Bark) ★★★

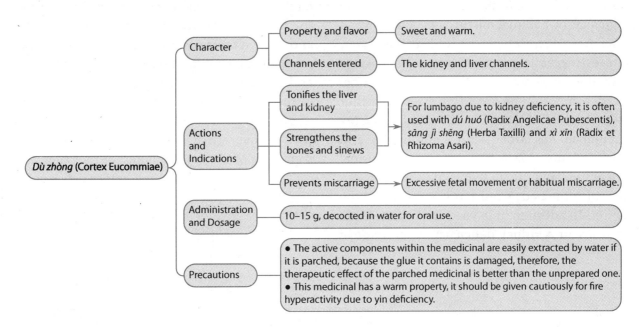

⑦ *Xù duàn* (续断, Radix Dipsaci, Himalayan Teasel Root) ★★★

Both *dù zhòng* (Cortex Eucommiae) and *xù duàn* (Radix Dipsaci) are sweet in flavor and warm in property. They enter the liver and kidney channels, and have the actions of tonifying the liver and kidney, strengthening the bones and sinews and preventing miscarriage. They are used for liver

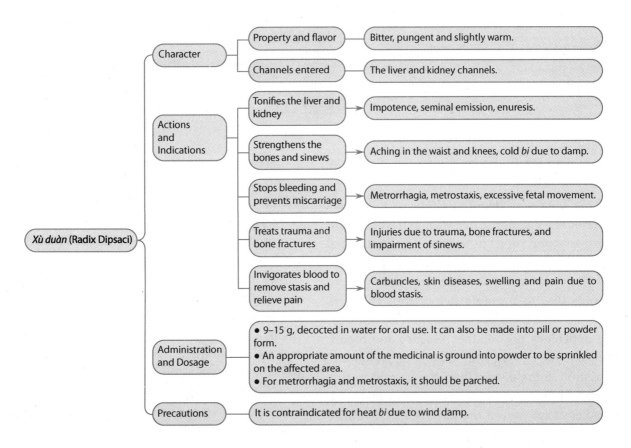

and kidney deficiency, manifesting as aching in the waist and knees, flaccidity of the lower limbs, excessive fetal movement, vaginal bleeding during pregnancy, or habitual miscarriage; kidney yang deficiency with deficiency cold in the lower, manifesting as impotence, seminal emission, spermatorrhea, enuresis and frequent urination. The two medicinals are often used together for mutual reinforcement. *Dù zhòng* (Cortex Eucommiae) has strong actions in tonifying and preventing miscarriage. It is an essential medicinal to treat lumbago due to kidney deficiency. It can strengthen the body's resistance and support the right qi. In addition, it is used for hypertension especially of a kidney deficiency type. *Xù duàn*

(Radix Dipsaci) has a bitter and pungent flavor. It is inferior to *dù zhòng* (Cortex Eucommiae) in tonifying and preventing miscarriage. It is effective for invigorating the blood, treating trauma and bone fractures, and therefore is commonly used for injuries due to trauma, bone fractures, and impairment of the sinews, and because of these actions, it is commonly in the field of traumatology. It is able to stop bleeding, and is used for metrorrhagia, metrostaxis and excessive menstruation due to instability of the *chong* and *ren* vessels caused by liver and kidney deficiency.

⑧ *Ròu cōng róng* (肉苁蓉, Herba Cistanches, Desertliving Cistanche) ★

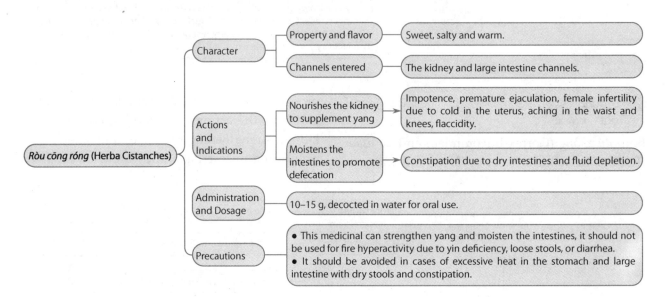

⑨ *Suǒ yáng* (锁阳, Herba Cynomorii, Songaria Cynomorium Herb)

Both *ròu cōng róng* (Herba Cistanches) and *suǒ yáng* (Herba Cynomorii) are sweet in flavor, warm in property, and moist in texture. They enter the kidney and large intestine channels to tonify the kidney in order to supplement yang and moisten the intestines to promote defecation. The two medicinals are used in combination for kidney yang deficiency with kidney essence and blood deficiency, manifesting with impotence, premature ejaculation, female infertility due to cold in the uterus, aching and flaccidity of the waist and knees; constipation in the elderly due to fluid

depletion with dry intestines. They are suitable for constipation due to dry intestines caused by kidney yang, kidney essence and blood deficiency. They are commonly used in pairs for mutual reinforcement. *Ròu cōng róng* (Herba Cistanches) has a moderate action, and is able to augment kidney essence and blood. It is considered an essential medicinal to supplement kidney yang and promote production of kidney essence and blood. *Suǒ yáng* (Herba Cynomorii) can moisten dryness and nourish the sinews. It is commonly used for flaccidity of the waist and knees, lack of strength of the bones and sinews and difficulty in walking due to deficiency of the liver and kidney.

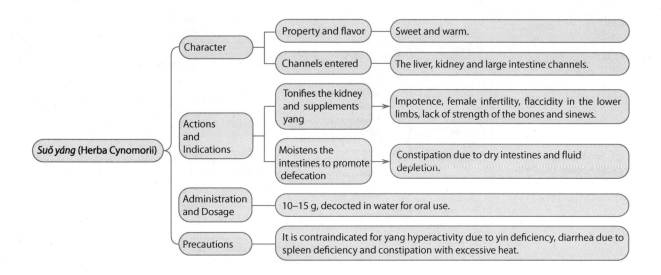

⑩ *Bǔ gǔ zhī* (补骨脂, Fructus Psoraleae, Psoralea Fruit) ★★

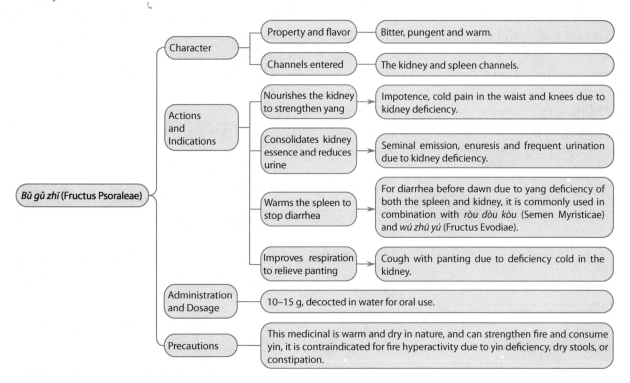

⑪ *Yì zhì rén* (益智仁, Fructus Alpiniae Oxyphyllae, Sharpleaf Glangal Fruit) ★

Both *bǔ gǔ zhī* (Fructus Psoraleae) and *yì zhì rén* (Fructus Alpiniae Oxyphyllae) are pungent in flavor, and warm or hot in property. They have the actions of tonifying the kidney to strengthen yang, consolidating kidney essence, reducing urine, and warming the spleen to stop diarrhea. They are used for kidney yang deficiency manifesting with seminal emissions, spermatorrhea, enuresis and frequent urination; constant diarrhea due to yang deficiency of the spleen and kidney. These two medicinals are commonly used together for mutual reinforcement. *Bǔ gǔ zhī* (Fructus Psoraleae) is pungent and bitter in flavor, warm and dry in property, and has a strong action in strengthening yang. It mainly tonifies the kidney

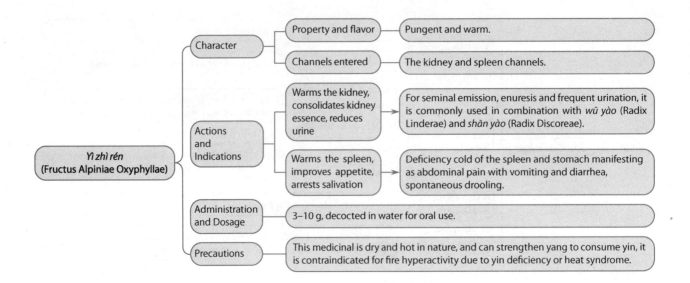

and strengthens yang, and is often used for kidney yang deficiency with fire depletion at the *mingmen*, manifesting with cold pain in the waist and knees and impotence. In addition, it is able to supplement kidney yang to improve respiration and relieve panting. It can be used for panting of a deficient type due to failure of the kidney to grasp the qi. *Yì zhì rén* (Fructus Alpiniae Oxyphyllae) is pungent in flavor and warm in property. It is inferior to *bǔ gǔ zhī* (Fructus

Psoraleae) in strengthening yang, and mainly acts on the spleen, and is effective for warming the spleen to promote appetite and arrest saliva. It is commonly used for deficiency cold of the spleen and stomach, manifesting as poor appetite, profuse saliva, infant's drooling, and cold pain in the abdomen.

⑫ *Tù sī zǐ* (菟丝子, Semen Cuscutae, Dodder Seed) ★ ★ ★

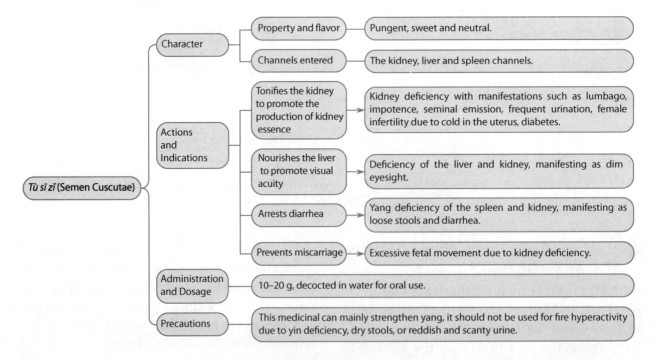

⑬ *Shā yuàn zǐ* (沙苑子, Semen Astragali Complanati, Flatstem Milkvetch Seed) ★

Both *tù sī zǐ* (Semen Cuscutae) and *shā yuàn zǐ* (Semen Astragali Complanati) are sweet

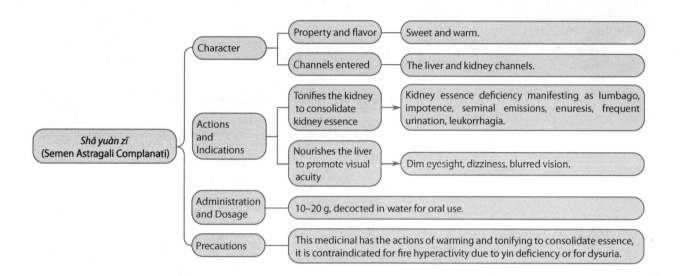

in flavor. They enter the liver and kidney channels, and have the actions of tonifying the kidney to supplement yang, consolidating kidney essence, reducing urine and nourishing the liver to promote visual acuity. Both of the medicinals are used for kidney deficiency, with symptoms such as lumbago, impotence, infertility, seminal emission, spermatorrhea, enuresis, frequent urination and leukorrhagia; both liver and kidney deficiency manifesting as dim eyesight and blurred vision. Clinically, the two medicinals are commonly used together for mutual reinforcement. *Tù sī zǐ* (Semen Cuscutae) is neutral in property, and is able to strengthen kidney yang and promote the production of kidney essence. It can tonify both yang and yin. It has actions of arresting diarrhea and preventing miscarriage. Therefore, it is used to treat loose stools and diarrhea due to both spleen and kidney deficiency; excessive fetal movement, vaginal bleeding during pregnancy due to liver and kidney deficiency; diabetes due to kidney deficiency. It is regarded as an effective medicinal to nourish the liver, kidney and spleen. *Shā yuàn zǐ* (Semen Astragali Complanati) is inferior to *tù sī zǐ* (Semen Cuscutae) in tonifying the liver and kidney. It is effective for consolidating kidney essence and reducing urine.

⑭ *Gé jiè* (蛤蚧, Gecko, Gecko) ★

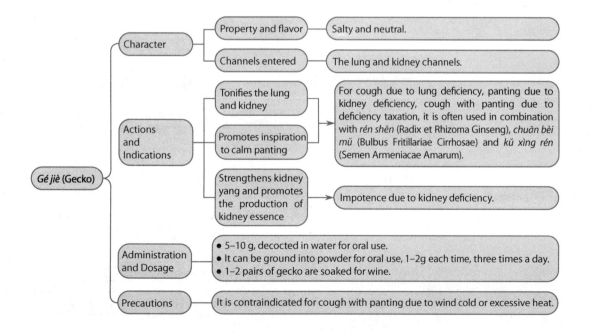

⑮ *Hé táo rén* (核桃仁, Semen Juglandis, English Walnut Seed)

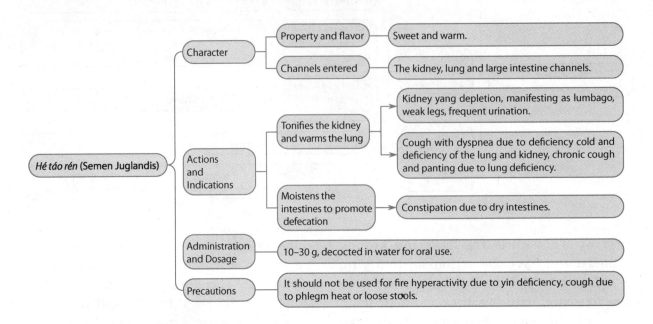

⑯ *Dōng chóng xià cǎo* (冬虫夏草, Cordyceps, Chinese Caterpillar Fungus) ★

Gé jiè (Gecko), *hé táo rén* (Semen Juglandis), *dōng chóng xià cǎo* (Cordyceps) and *zǐ hé chē* (Placenta Hominis) enter the lung and kidney channels. They can tonify the lung and kidney to relieve cough. They are often used for chronic cough and panting of a deficient type due to both lung and kidney deficiency failing to preserve qi. They are commonly used medicinals to treat cough and panting of a deficiency type. They are also used for kidney yang deficiency manifesting as impotence, seminal emission or aching in the waist and knees. *Gé jiè* (Gecko), is salty and neutral, and has a strong action in tonifying the lung and kidney, and promoting inspiration to calm panting. It is regarded as an essential medicinal to treat cough and panting of a deficient type. It can strengthen

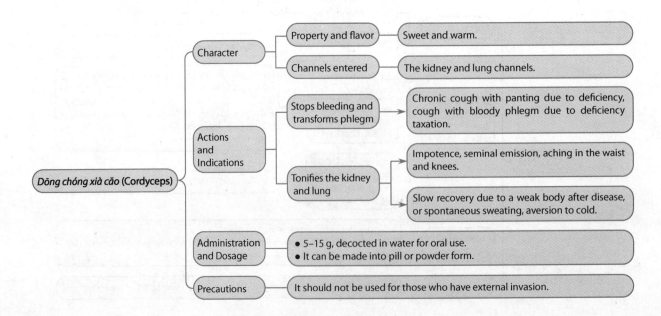

kidney yang as well as promote the production of kidney essence, and therefore is suitable for diseases caused by kidney yang, essence and blood deficiency. *Hé táo rén* (Semen Juglandis) is sweet in flavor, warm in property and moist in texture. It can moisten the intestines to promote defecation, and is used for constipation due to dry intestines resulting from fluid consumption. *Dōng chóng xià cǎo* (Cordyceps), sweet and neutral, is able to supplement kidney yang, nourish lung yin, stop bleeding, and transform phlegm. It is commonly used for cough with bloody phlegm due to deficiency taxation caused by lung yin deficiency. It is an effective medicinal for tonifying the lung and kidney. In addition, it is simmered with chicken, duck or pork to treat slow recovery after diseases due to a weak constitution, spontaneous sweating, and aversion to cold. *Zǐ hé chē* (Placenta Hominis) is sweet and salty in flavor, and warm in property. It can warm kidney yang as well as enrich kidney essence and blood. It is suitable for female infertility and impotence due to deficiency of kidney yang, essence and blood. In addition, it can replenish qi and nourish blood, and therefore is used for emaciation, lassitude, a yellowish complexion, and galactostasis postpartum due to qi and blood deficiency.

⑰ *Hú lú bā* (胡芦巴, Semen Trigonellae Callorhimi, Common Fenugreek Seed)

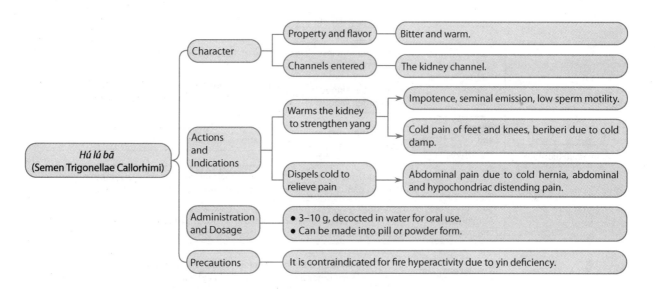

⑱ *Jiǔ cài zǐ* (韭菜子, Semen Allii Tuberosi, Tuber Onion Seed)

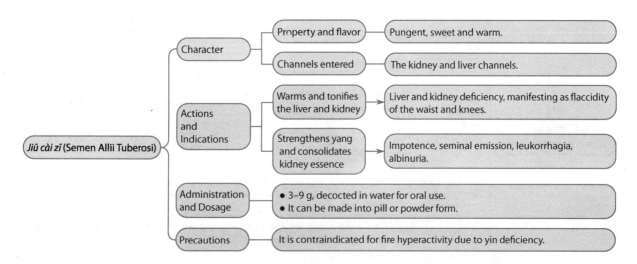

⑲ *Yáng qǐ shí* (阳起石, Actinolitum, Actinolite)

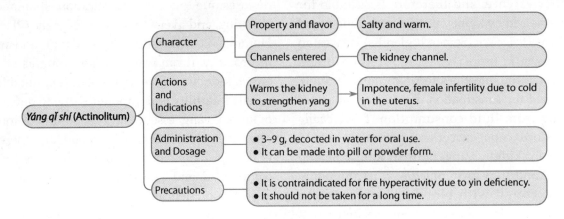

⑳ *Zǐ shí yīng* (紫石英, Fluoritum, Fluorite)

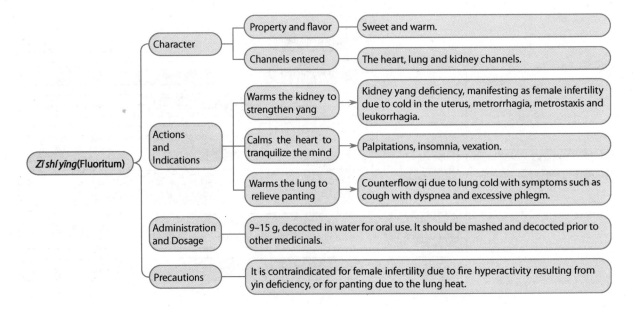

㉑ *Hǎi gǒu shèn* (海狗肾, Testes et Penis Callorhini, Ursine Seal's Testes and Penis)

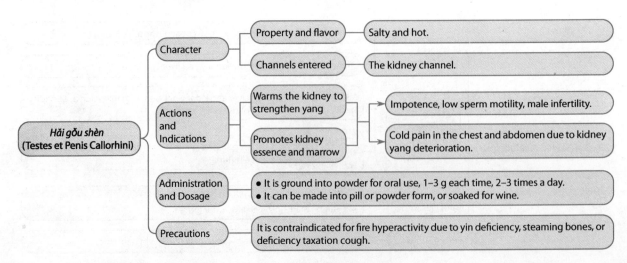

㉒ *Hǎi mǎ* (海马, Hippocampus, Sea-horse)

Hǎi gǒu shèn (Testes et Penis Callorhini) and *hǎi mǎ* (Hippocampus) are precious medicinals. They can tonify the kidney and strengthen yang, and are used for kidney yang deterioration manifesting as impotence, scanty sperm, female infertility due to cold in the uterus, aching and weakness in the waist and knees, and frequent urination. *Hǎi gǒu shèn* (Testes et Penis Callorhini) has a pure action in tonifying the kidney and promoting the production of kidney essence and marrow. *Huáng gǒu shèn* (黄狗肾, Testes et Penis Canis,

Dog's Testes and Penis) has a similar but inferior action to *hǎi gǒu shèn* (Testes et Penis Callorhini). It is more readily available and is less expensive, hence is it used instead of *hǎi gǒu shèn* (Testes et Penis Callorhini). *Hǎi mǎ* (Hippocampus) is able to invigorate blood to remove stasis and reduce swellings to relieve pain. It is used for abdominal masses due to blood stasis and injuries due to trauma. In addition, it is also used for panting due to kidney deficiency, dorsal furuncles, ulcers, and hemorrhage due to trauma.

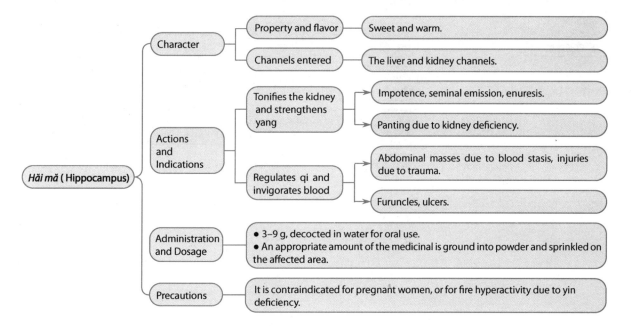

㉓ *Há ma yóu* (蛤蟆油, Oviductus Ranae, Chinese Woodfrog Oviduct)

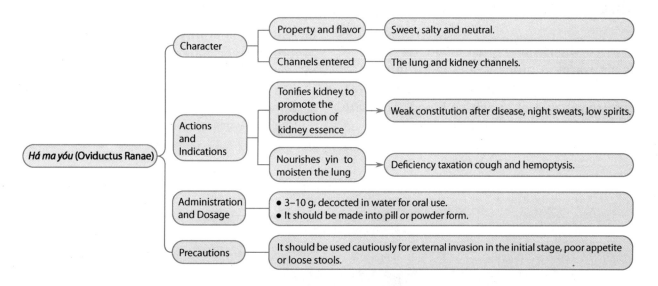

㉔ *Yáng hóng shān* (羊红膻, Radix Seu Herba Pimpinelae, Thellungianae Root or Herb)

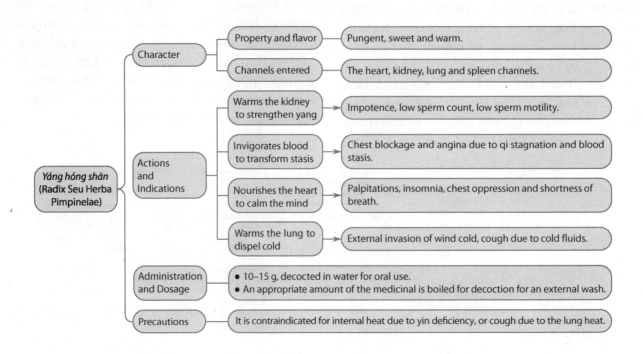

Yáng hóng shān
(Radix Seu Herba Pimpinelae)

- **Character**
  - **Property and flavor** — Pungent, sweet and warm.
  - **Channels entered** — The heart, kidney, lung and spleen channels.

- **Actions and Indications**
  - **Warms the kidney to strengthen yang** — Impotence, low sperm count, low sperm motility.
  - **Invigorates blood to transform stasis** — Chest blockage and angina due to qi stagnation and blood stasis.
  - **Nourishes the heart to calm the mind** — Palpitations, insomnia, chest oppression and shortness of breath.
  - **Warms the lung to dispel cold** — External invasion of wind cold, cough due to cold fluids.

- **Administration and Dosage**
  - 10–15 g, decocted in water for oral use.
  - An appropriate amount of the medicinal is boiled for decoction for an external wash.

- **Precautions** — It is contraindicated for internal heat due to yin deficiency, or cough due to the lung heat.

Section 3　Medicinals that Enrich Blood

Medicinals that enrich blood are sweet in flavor, warm in property and moist in texture. They enter the *xue* level of the heart and liver, and are capable of enriching blood. They are extensively used for various diseases caused by blood deficiency, manifesting with a pale or yellowish complexion, pale lips and nails, vertigo, tinnitus, palpitations, insomnia, amnesia, delayed menstruation, scanty light colored menstrual blood, or even amenorrhea, a light colored tongue, and a thready pulse.

① *Dāng guī* (当归, Radix Angelicae Sinensis, Chinese Angelica) ★ ★ ★

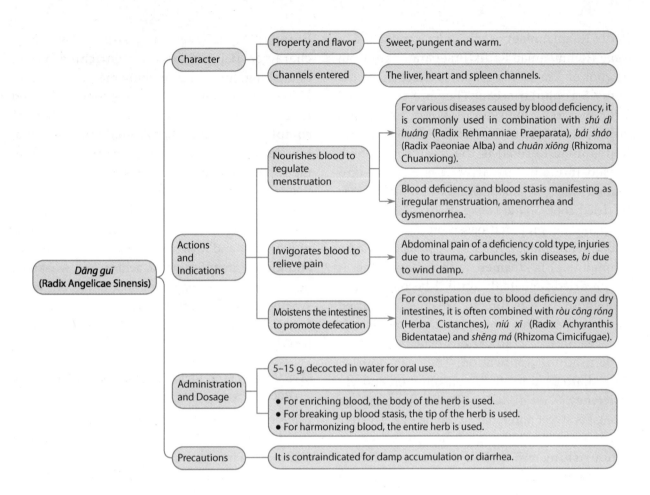

Dāng guī (Radix Angelicae Sinensis)

Character
- Property and flavor — Sweet, pungent and warm.
- Channels entered — The liver, heart and spleen channels.

Actions and Indications
- Nourishes blood to regulate menstruation
  - For various diseases caused by blood deficiency, it is commonly used in combination with *shú dì huáng* (Radix Rehmanniae Praeparata), *bái sháo* (Radix Paeoniae Alba) and *chuān xiōng* (Rhizoma Chuanxiong).
  - Blood deficiency and blood stasis manifesting as irregular menstruation, amenorrhea and dysmenorrhea.
- Invigorates blood to relieve pain
  - Abdominal pain of a deficiency cold type, injuries due to trauma, carbuncles, skin diseases, *bi* due to wind damp.
- Moistens the intestines to promote defecation
  - For constipation due to blood deficiency and dry intestines, it is often combined with *ròu cōng róng* (Herba Cistanches), *niú xī* (Radix Achyranthis Bidentatae) and *shēng má* (Rhizoma Cimicifugae).

Administration and Dosage
- 5–15 g, decocted in water for oral use.
- For enriching blood, the body of the herb is used.
- For breaking up blood stasis, the tip of the herb is used.
- For harmonizing blood, the entire herb is used.

Precautions
- It is contraindicated for damp accumulation or diarrhea.

---

②*Shú dì huáng* (熟地黄, Radix Rehmanniae Praeparata, Prepared Rehmannia Root) ★★★

Xiān dì huáng (鲜地黄, Radix Rehmanniae Recens, Fresh Rehmannia Root), *shēng dì huáng*

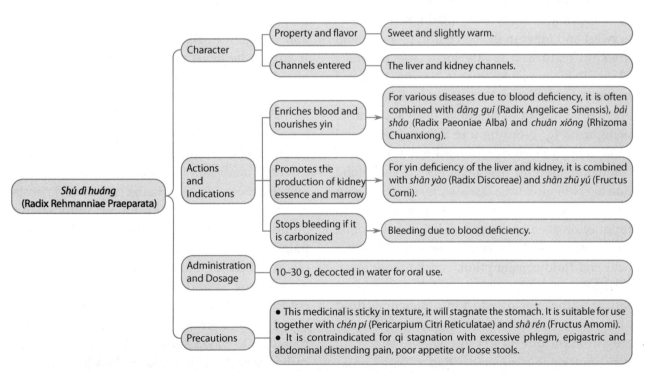

Shú dì huáng (Radix Rehmanniae Praeparata)

Character
- Property and flavor — Sweet and slightly warm.
- Channels entered — The liver and kidney channels.

Actions and Indications
- Enriches blood and nourishes yin
  - For various diseases due to blood deficiency, it is often combined with *dāng guī* (Radix Angelicae Sinensis), *bái sháo* (Radix Paeoniae Alba) and *chuān xiōng* (Rhizoma Chuanxiong).
- Promotes the production of kidney essence and marrow
  - For yin deficiency of the liver and kidney, it is combined with *shān yào* (Radix Discoreae) and *shān zhū yú* (Fructus Corni).
- Stops bleeding if it is carbonized
  - Bleeding due to blood deficiency.

Administration and Dosage
- 10–30 g, decocted in water for oral use.

Precautions
- This medicinal is sticky in texture, it will stagnate the stomach. It is suitable for use together with *chén pí* (Pericarpium Citri Reticulatae) and *shā rén* (Fructus Amomi).
- It is contraindicated for qi stagnation with excessive phlegm, epigastric and abdominal distending pain, poor appetite or loose stools.

(Radix Rehmanniae) or *gān dì huáng* and *shú dì huáng* (Rehmanniae Radix Praeparata) are from the root of *Rehmannia glutinosa* Libosch. of the family Scrophulariaceae. They are considered three different medicinals when processed with different methods. *Xiān dì huáng* (Radix Rehmanniae Recens) is the fresh root which is used immediately after it is dug up and cleaned. *Shēng dì huáng* (Radix Rehmanniae) is the dried root. *Shú dì huáng* (Radix Rehmanniae Praeparata) is prepared based on *shēng dì huáng* (Radix Rehmanniae). After *shēng dì huáng* (Radix Rehmanniae) is steamed with yellow wine, it is then dried repeatedly until it becomes black throughout, or it is directly steamed and dried until it is black and moist. The three medicinals are sweet in flavor. To various extents, they can all be used for tonification. They can nourish yin and are used for fluid consumption and yin deficiency. *Xiān dì huáng* (Radix Rehmanniae Recens) is sweet and bitter in flavor, and severely cold in property. Although it has a weak action in nourishing yin, it has a strong action in clearing heat, cooling blood and promoting fluid production. It is commonly used for various bleeding due to blood heat; fluid consumption due to febrile diseases manifesting as vexation and thirst; diabetes due to fluid consumption, and yin deficiency. *Shēng dì huáng* (Radix Rehmanniae) is sweet and bitter in flavor, cold in property and moist in texture. It is inferior to *xiān dì huáng* (Radix Rehmanniae Recens) in clearing heat and cooling blood, but is effective for nourishing yin and promoting fluid production. In addition to being used for bleeding due to blood heat, and fluid consumption due to febrile diseases, it is commonly used for heat invading the *ying* blood due to epidemic febrile diseases, manifesting with general fever, maculae, dry mouth, a crimson tongue, or even coma and delirium; epidemic febrile diseases in the later stage with lingering heat and fluid consumption, constant low fever, tidal fever, or stubborn diseases due to internal injury with fever due to yin deficiency; fluid and yin consumption due to febrile diseases, constipation due to dry intestines, and fluid consumption. *Shú dì huáng* (Radix Rehmanniae

Praeparata) is sweet and slightly warm in character. It is effective for enriching blood, nourishing yin, and promoting the production of kidney essence and marrow. It is commonly used for blood deficiency manifesting with a yellowish complexion, dizziness, palpitations, insomnia, low spirits, lassitude, irregular menstruation, metrorrhagia and metrostaxis; deficiency of the liver and kidney, and deficiency of kidney essence and blood, manifesting with vertigo, tinnitus, early graying of the hair, aching and weakness of the waist and knees; yin deficiency in the liver and kidney manifesting as aching and weakness of the waist and knees, seminal emission, night sweats, tinnitus, deafness, and diabetes. It is used for deficiency of yin, the kidney essence and blood.

③ *Bái sháo* (白芍, Radix Paeoniae Alba, White Peony Root) ★★★

Dāng guī (Radix Angelicae Sinensis) and *bái sháo* (Radix Paeoniae Alba) enter the liver and spleen channels. They can enrich blood and regulate menstruation, and are used for blood deficiency manifesting with a yellowish complexion, dizziness, palpitations, irregular menstruation, amenorrhea and dysmenorrhea. At the same time, they can relieve and are used, for pain. *Dāng guī* (Radix Angelicae Sinensis) is sweet and pungent in flavor, and warm in property. It enters the heart channel. It is able to enrich blood, invigorate blood, and dispel cold. It can be used for irregular menstruation, amenorrhea and dysmenorrhea due to blood deficiency, blood stasis or blood cold, especially of a cold stagnation and blood deficiency type. It is an essential medicinal to enrich blood and regulate menstruation. *Dāng guī* (Radix Angelicae Sinensis) is effective for enriching blood, invigorating blood and dispelling cold in order to relieve pain. Therefore, it is indicated for pain due to blood deficiency, blood stasis or deficiency cold, manifesting as abdominal pain of a deficiency cold type, pain and abdominal masses due to blood stasis, injuries due to trauma, swelling and pain due to blood stasis, *bi* due to wind damp, carbuncles, and skin diseases. In addition, it can

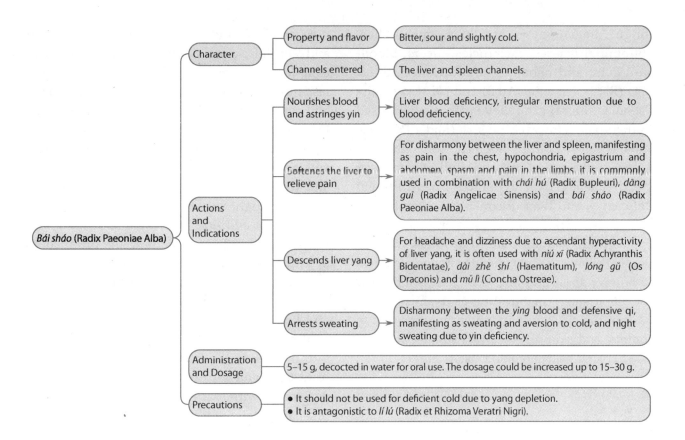

moisten the intestines to promote defecation. *Bái sháo* (Radix Paeoniae Alba) is bitter, sour and sweet in flavor, slightly cold in property. It is effective for nourishing blood and astringing yin. Therefore, it is suitable for blood deficiency and yin deficiency with heat manifestations. In addition, it can astringe liver yin, nourish blood, soften the liver, and relieve spasms and pain. It is indicated for liver yin deficiency, liver hyperactivity due to blood deficiency, liver qi constraint, and disharmony between the liver and spleen, manifesting as hypochondriac pain, and spasms and pain in the epigastrium, abdomen and limbs. In addition, *bái sháo* (Radix Paeoniae Alba) can suppress liver yang and astringe yin to arrest sweating. Therefore it is commonly used for ascendant hyperactivity of liver yang manifesting as headache, dizziness, vexation, and irritability; external invasion of wind cold leading to disharmony between the *ying* blood and *wei* qi, manifesting as sweating and aversion to cold; night sweats due to yin deficiency.

Bái sháo (Radix Paeoniae Alba) and *chì sháo* (Radix Paeoniae Rubra) are from the same plant. They are slightly cold in property. Physicians in ancient times believed that *bái sháo* (Radix Paeoniae Alba) was able to nourish and astringe, while *chì sháo* (Radix Paeoniae Rubra) was able to purge and disperse. *Bái sháo* (Radix Paeoniae Alba) is effective for nourishing blood to regulate menstruation, softening the liver to relieve pain, astringing yin to arrest sweating and suppressing liver yang. *Chì sháo* (Radix Paeoniae Rubra) is effective for clearing heat, cooling blood, invigorating blood to remove stasis, and clearing and purging liver fire. Clinically, *bái sháo* (Radix Paeoniae Alba) is indicated for various diseases caused by blood and yin deficiency and liver yang hyperactivity, manifesting as irregular menstruation, amenorrhea, dysmenorrhea, night sweats, spontaneous sweats, dizziness, tinnitus, vexation and irritability. *Chì sháo* (Radix Paeoniae Rubra) is indicated for various diseases caused by blood heat, blood stasis or liver fire, such as general fever with maculae, dry mouth, crimson tongue, hematemesis, epistaxis, amenorrhea, abdominal masses, carbuncles, ulcers, blood-shot eyes, and nebulae. In addition, both *bái sháo* (Radix Paeoniae Alba) and *chì sháo* (Radix Paeoniae Rubra) can relieve pain, and are used to treat pain. However, *bái sháo* (Radix Paeoniae Alba) is able to nourish blood and soften the liver to relieve spasm and pain. It is indicated for liver yin deficiency, liver hyperactivity with blood deficiency, and liver qi constraint, manifesting as hypochondriac pain, spasms and pain in the epigastrium, abdomen and four limbs. *Chì sháo* (Radix Paeoniae Rubra) is able to invigorate blood to remove stasis and relieve pain. It is indicated for blood stasis, manifesting as dysmenorrhea, pain in the chest and abdomen, injuries due to trauma, and skin diseases. It is suitable for pain due to blood heat and blood stasis.

④ *Ē jiāo* (阿胶, Colla Corii Asini, Donkey-hide Glue) ★ ★ ★

Both *shú dì huáng* (Radix Rehmanniae Praeparata) and *ē jiāo* (Colla Corii Asini) are essential medicinals to nourish blood. They can nourish blood and yin, and are used for blood and yin deficiency manifesting as a yellowish complexion, dizziness, palpitations, low spirits, lassitude, irregular menstruation, metrorrhagia and metrostaxis. *Shú dì huáng* (Radix Rehmanniae Praeparata) is sweet in flavor and slightly warm in property. It has actions of nourishing both liver and kidney yin, and is commonly used for aching and weakness in the waist and knees, seminal emission, night sweats, tinnitus, deafness, and diabetes. In addition, it is capable of tonifying the liver and kidney, promoting the production of kidney essence and blood, and therefore is used for dizziness, tinnitus, early graying of the hair, and aching and weakness in the waist and knees. *Ē jiāo* (Colla Corii Asini) is sweet, neutral and moist. It is effective for nourishing yin to moisten the lung, and is often used for lung heat and yin deficiency manifesting as dry cough with scanty phlegm, dry throat and phlegm containing blood; dry heat impairing the lung with symptoms such as dry cough without phlegm, dry nose and throat; yin consumption due to febrile diseases which leads to heart

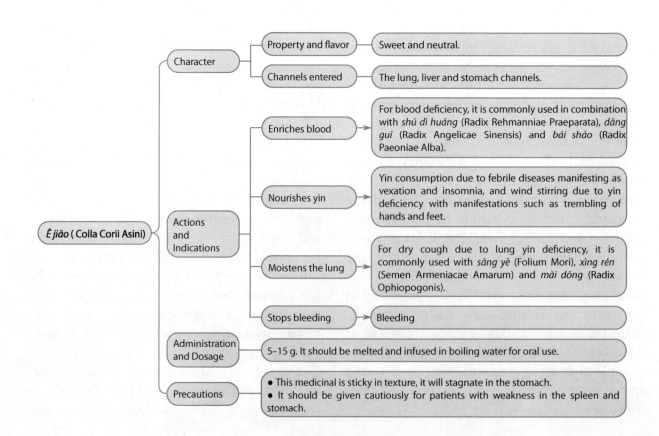

fire hyperactivity, manifesting as vexation and insomnia; depletion of yin with wind stirring due to epidemic febrile diseases in the later stage, manifesting as trembling of hands and feet. In addition, *ē jiāo* (Colla Corii Asini) is effective for stopping bleeding. It is used for hematemesis, epistaxis, hemoptysis, hemafecia, metrorrhagia, metrostaxis, and vaginal bleeding during pregnancy.

⑤ *Hé shǒu wū* (何首乌, Radix Polygoni Multiflori, Fleeceflower Root) ★ ★ ★

Both *shú dì huáng* (Radix Rehmanniae Praeparata) and *hé shǒu wū* (Radix Polygoni Multiflori) are sweet in flavor and slightly warm in property. They have the actions of tonifying the liver and kidney, promoting the production of kidney essence and blood. They are used for blood deficiency manifesting as a yellowish complexion, dizziness, palpitations, insomnia, irregular menstruation, metrorrhagia and metrostaxis; liver and kidney deficiency, and kidney essence and blood deficiency, manifesting with dizziness, tinnitus, early graying of the hair, and aching and weakness in the waist and knees. *Shú dì huáng* (Radix Rehmanniae Praeparata) has a strong action in tonifying. It is effective for nourishing

blood and yin, and promoting the production of kidney essence and blood. It is one of the main medicinals to nourish blood, tonify deficiency as well as nourish yin of the liver and kidney. It is also used for yin deficiency of the liver and kidney manifesting as aching and weakness in the waist and knees, seminal emission, night sweats, tinnitus, deafness and diabetes. It is often used in combination with *shān zhū yú* (Fructus Corni) and *shān yào* (Radix Discoreae). This medicinal is sticky in texture, therefore it will stagnate in the stomach. It can be used together with *chén pí* (Pericarpium Citri Reticulatae) and *shā rén* (Fructus Amomi). *Zhì hé shǒu wū* (Radix Polygoni Multiflori Praeparata) is inferior to *shú dì huáng* (Radix Rehmanniae Praeparata) in tonifying. However, it can astringe and consolidate the kidney, and is suitable for those who are too weak to be tonifyed. The unprepared medicinal has a weak action in tonifying but is able to prevent the recurrence of malaria, detoxify, and moisten the intestines to promote defecation. Therefore, it is often used for chronic malaria due to a weak constitution, qi and blood deficiency; carbuncles, scrofula; constipation due to old age, a weak body, and deficiency of kidney essence and blood.

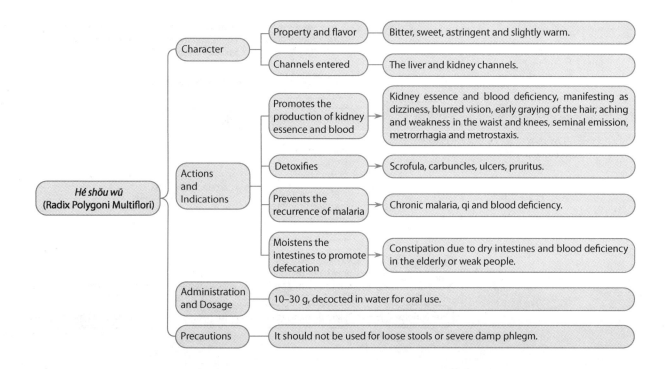

⑥ *Lóng yǎn ròu* (龙眼肉, Arillus Longan, Flesh of the Longan Fruit)

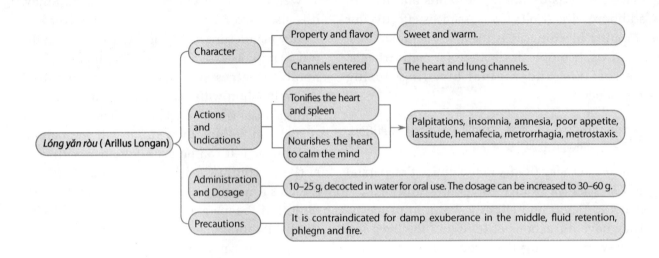

⑦ *Chǔ shí zǐ* (楮实子, Fructus Broussonetiae, Papermulberry Fruit)

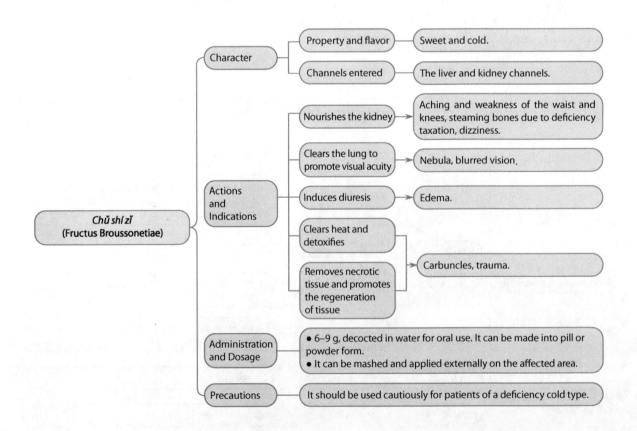

Section 4 Medicinals that Nourish Yin

Medicinals of this section are mostly sweet in flavor and cold in property. Some of the medicinals have a bitter flavor and can clear heat. Medicinals with the effect of nourishing yin in the lung and stomach mainly enter the lung and stomach channels. Medicinals with the effect of nourishing yin in the liver and kidney mainly enter the liver and kidney channels. A few medicinals enter the heart channel and can nourish heart yin. Medicinals in this section have the effect of nourishing yin, and can moisten dryness and clear heat. Nourishing yin includes nourishing lung yin, nourishing stomach (and spleen) yin, nourishing liver yin, nourishing kidney yin and nourishing heart yin. They are indicated for lung yin deficiency, stomach (spleen) yin deficiency, lung yin deficiency, and heart deficiency respectively. There are two major symptoms of yin deficiency syndromes: 1. Yin fluids failing to nourish the viscera and tissues, manifesting as dryness of the skin, throat, mouth, nose and eyes, or constipation due to dry intestines. 2. Internal heat due to yin deficiency, manifesting as tidal fever, night sweats, feverish sensation in five the centers, flushing of the cheeks, or yang hyperactivity due to yin deficiency manifesting as dizziness. There are special symptoms of yin deficiency in different internal organs: For lung deficiency, there are symptoms such as dry cough, scanty phlegm, hemoptysis and hoarseness. For stomach yin deficiency, there can be dry mouth and throat, insidious pain in the epigastrium, no desire to eat, discomfort in the epigastrium, dry vomiting, and hiccups. For spleen yin deficiency, which is mostly qi and yin deficiency in the spleen, there are manifestations such as poor appetite, abdominal distension after meals, constipation, dry lips with scanty fluids, dry vomiting, hiccups, a dry tongue and a scanty tongue coating. For liver yin deficiency, there can be dizziness, tinnitus, dry eyes, or numb limbs, spasms, and nail deformations due to malnutrition. For kidney yin deficiency, there are manifestations such as dizziness, tinnitus, deafness, loosening of the teeth, aching of the waist and knees, and seminal emission. For heart yin deficiency, there are manifestations such as palpitations, insomnia and frequent dreams.

① *Běi shā shēn* (北沙参, Radix Glehniae, Glehnia Root) ★ ★ ★

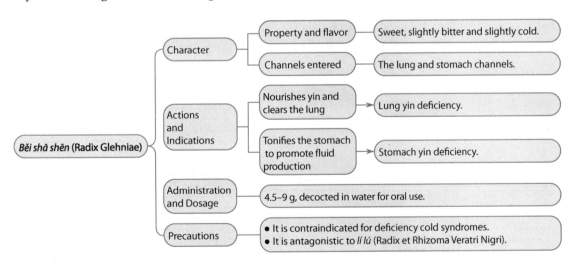

② *Nán shā shēn* (南沙参, Radix Adenophorae, Fourleaf Ladybell Root) ★ ★ ★

Běi shā shēn (Radix Glehniae) and *nán shā shēn* (Radix Adenophorae) are sweet in flavor, and slightly cold in property. They enter the lung and stomach channels. They have actions of nourishing yin, clearing the lung, tonifying the stomach, and promoting fluid production. They can be used for yin deficiency and lung dryness with heat, manifesting as dry cough, scanty phlegm, hemoptysis, dry throat and hoarseness; stomach yin deficiency with heat manifestations such as dry

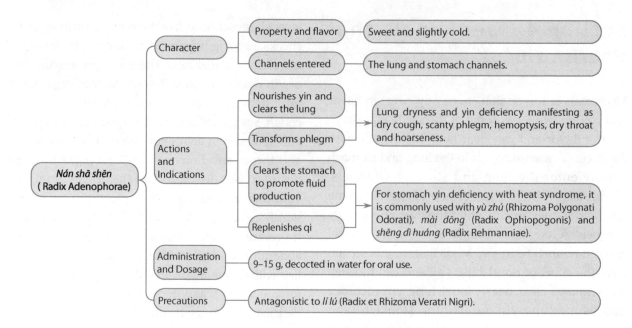

mouth, excessive drinking of water, poor appetite, dry stool, a scanty or peeled tongue coat, a red tongue with scanty fluids, stomachache, gastric distension, and dry vomiting. *Běi shā shēn* (Radix Glehniae) is from the root of *Glehnia littoralis* Fr. Schmidt *ex* Miq., of the family Umbelliferae. It has a stronger action in clearing and nourishing the lung and stomach, and is commonly used for the syndrome of yin deficiency in the lung and stomach with heat manifestations. *Nán shā shēn* (Radix Adenophorae) is the root of Adenophora tetraphylla (Thunb.) Fisch. or Adenophora stricta Miq., of the family Campanulaceae. It is inferior to *běi shā shēn* (Radix Glehniae) in clearing and nourishing the lung and stomach, however, it can replenish qi in the spleen and lung as well as transform phlegm. Therefore, it is suitable for qi and yin consumption in the lung, spleen and stomach, and sticky phlegm that is difficult to expectorate due to lung dryness.

③ *Bǎi hé* (百合, Bulbus Lilii, Lily Bulb) ★★

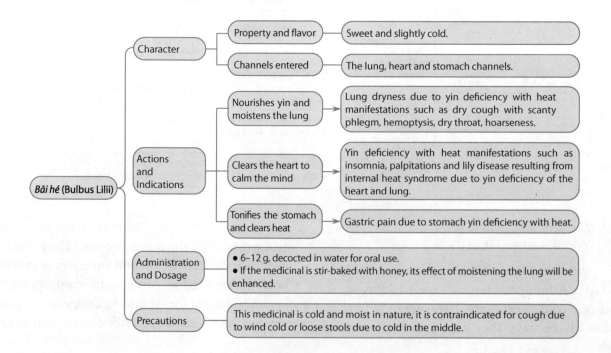

④ *Mài dōng* (麦冬, Radix Ophiopogonis, Dwarf Lilyturf Tuber) ★★★

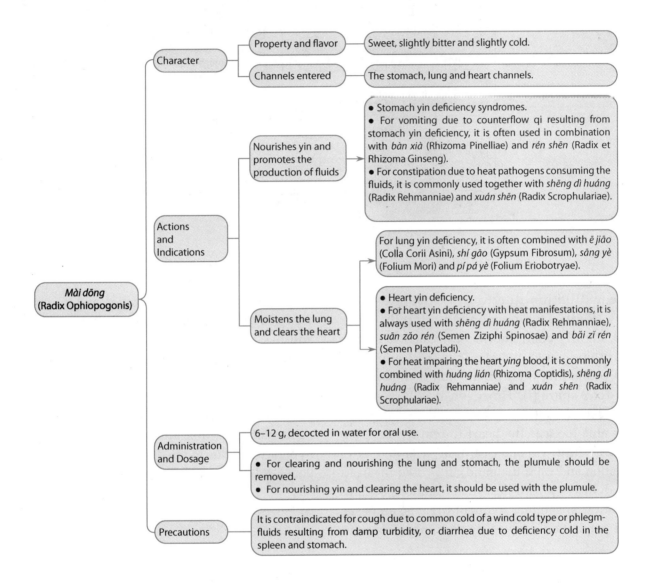

⑤ *Tiān dōng* (天冬, Radix Asparagi, Cochinchinese Asparagus Root) ★★

Mài dōng (Radix Ophiopogonis) and *tiān dōng* (Radix Asparagi) are from the root tuber of perennial herbs of the family Liliaceae. They are sweet and bitter in flavor, and cold in property. They enter the lung and stomach channels, and have actions of nourishing yin to moisten dryness, clearing the lung and promoting fluid production. The two medicinals can nourish lung yin, moisten lung dryness, clear lung heat,

nourish stomach yin, promote fluid production to relieve thirst, and increase fluids to promote defecation. They are used for yin deficiency and lung dryness with heat manifestations such as dry nose and throat, dry cough with scanty phlegm, hemoptysis, sore throat and hoarseness; heat impairing the stomach fluids or stomach, yin deficiency with heat manifestations such as a dry tongue, thirst, gastric pain, poor appetite, vomiting, hiccups, dry stool and diabetes; fluid consumption due to febrile diseases manifesting

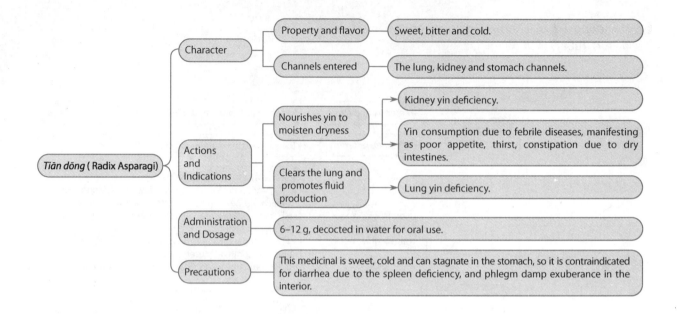

as constipation due to dry intestines. *Mài dōng* (Radix Ophiopogonis) is slightly bitter and slightly cold, and has a weaker action in nourishing yin to moisten dryness, clearing heat and promoting fluid production than *tiān dōng* (Radix Asparagi). However, it is less greasy than *tiān dōng* (Radix Asparagi). In addition, it is able to clear the heart to remove vexation (nourish heart yin and clear heart heat to remove vexation and calm the mind). It is used for heart yin deficiency with heat manifestations such as vexation, insomnia, frequent dreams, amnesia, and palpitations; as well as heat impairing heart *ying* blood manifesting as vexation and insomnia. *Tiān dōng* (Radix Asparagi) is bitter and cold, and has a stronger action in nourishing yin to moisten dryness, clearing fire and promoting fluid production. It can also nourish kidney yin and descend deficiency fire. It is used for kidney yin deficiency manifesting as dizziness, tinnitus, aching of the waist and knees as well as fire hyperactivity due to yin deficiency with steaming bones, tidal fever and seminal emissions.

⑥ *Shí hú* (石斛, Caulis Dendrobii, Dendrobium) ★★

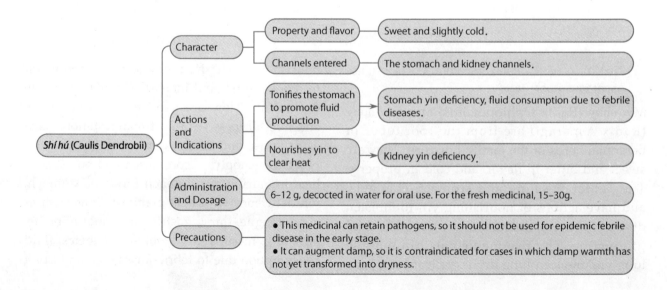

⑦ *Yù zhú* (玉竹, Rhizoma Polygonati Odorati, Fragrant Solomonseal Rhizome) ★★

Yù zhú (Rhizoma Polygonati Odorati) and *shí hú* (Caulis Dendrobii) are sweet in flavor and slightly cold in property. They enter the stomach channel and have the effect of tonifying the stomach and promoting fluid production to relieve thirst. They are used for fluid consumption due to febrile diseases, manifesting with low fever, vexation, thirst, dry mouth, dry throat, and a dry tongue with a blackish coating; stomach yin deficiency manifesting with thirst, dry throat, poor appetite, vomiting, hiccups, gastric upset, insidious pain or burning sensations in the stomach, and a bare tongue with a scanty coating. *Shí hú* (Caulis Dendrobii) enters the kidney channel, and can nourish kidney yin, brighten the eyes, strengthen the waist and knees, and descend deficiency fire.

They are both used for kidney yin deficiency manifesting as dim eyesight, flaccidity of the sinews and bones; fire hyperactivity due to yin deficiency manifesting as steaming bones with fever. *Yù zhú* (Rhizoma Polygonati Odorati) also enters the lung channel. It is effective for nourishing yin, moistening the lung, nourishing heart yin and clearing heart heat. It is used for yin deficiency and lung dryness with heat manifestations such as dry cough with scanty phlegm, hemoptysis and hoarseness; or heart yin impairment by heat manifesting as vexation, excessive sweating and palpitations. In addition, it can nourish yin without retaining pathogens, therefore is commonly used for cough due to wind warm pathogens in people with yin deficiency, or during warm winter days, with dry throat and phlegm retention.

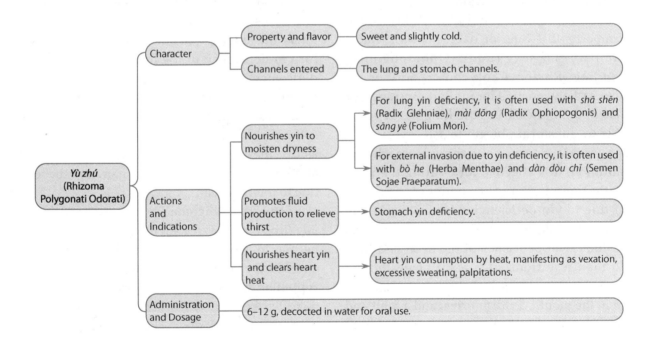

⑧ *Huáng jīng* (黄精, Rhizoma Polygonati, Solomonseal Rhizome) ★

Bǎi hé (Bulbus Lilii), *yù zhú* (Rhizoma Polygonati Odorati) and *huáng jīng* (Rhizoma Polygonati) are plants from the family Liliaceae. They have a sweet flavor and enter the lung and stomach channels to nourish yin, moisten the lung, and nourish stomach yin. They are used for yin deficiency and lung dryness with heat manifestations such as dry cough with scanty phlegm, hemoptysis, dry throat and hoarseness; yin consumption of the spleen and stomach, or stomach yin deficiency with heat manifestations such as dry mouth, poor appetite, insidious

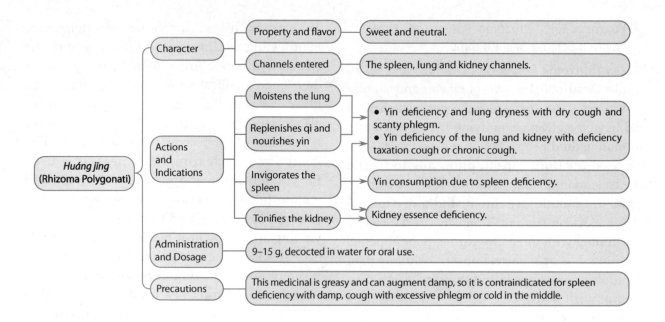

pain in the stomach, dry stools, a red tongue and a scanty coat. *Bǎi hé* (Bulbus Lilii) is cold in property. It is inferior to *běi shā shēn* (Radix Glehniae), *mài dōng* (Radix Ophiopogonis), *huáng jīng* (Rhizoma Polygonati) and *yù zhú* (Rhizoma Polygonati Odorati) in nourishing yin, moistening, and clearing the lung, however, it is able to transform phlegm to relieve cough. It has a weak action in nourishing stomach yin. In addition, it is effective for clearing the heart to calm the mind, and is commonly used for heat due to yin deficiency with insomnia and palpitations; and lily disease caused by internal heat due to yin deficiency of the heart and lung with manifestations such as brief periods of staring, inability to control the emotions, bitter taste in the mouth, reddish urine, and a faint and rapid pulse. *Yù zhú* (Rhizoma Polygonati Odorati) can nourish yin, moisten dryness and promote fluid production to relieve thirst. It is often used for diabetes due to fluid consumption from stomach heat. It can nourish yin without retaining pathogens, and is commonly used for cough due to wind warm pathogens in people with yin deficiency, or during warm winter days, with dry throat and phlegm retention. *Huáng jīng* (Rhizoma Polygonati) is sweet in flavor and neutral in property. It can nourish yin, moisten the lung,

replenish qi, invigorate the spleen and tonify kidney essence. It is an effective medicinal to tonify the lung, spleen and kidney. It is also used for yin deficiency in the lung and kidney with deficiency taxation cough or chronic cough; qi deficiency of the spleen and stomach manifesting as lassitude, poor appetite, and a deficient and soft pulse; kidney essence deficiency manifesting as dizziness, aching and weakness of the waist and knees, early graying of the hair; and diabetes due to internal heat.

Shān yào (Rhizoma Dioscoreae) and *huáng jīng* (Rhizoma Polygonati) are sweet in flavor and neutral in property. They enter the lung, spleen and kidney channels. They have the actions of replenishing qi and nourishing yin. Both are regarded as effective medicinals for tonifying the lung, spleen and kidney. They are used for cough due to lung deficiency; lumbago and weak feet due to kidney deficiency, and diabetes. *Shān yào* (Radix Discoreae) can mainly replenish qi and invigorate the spleen. It has an astringent nature, and therefore is suitable for spleen qi deficiency with loose stools, diarrhea, or leukorrhagia. It is capable of consolidating kidney essence, reducing urine and leukorrhagia, and is used for instability due to kidney deficiency manifesting as seminal emission, spermatorrhea, enuresis, frequent urination, and leukorrhagia. *Huáng jīng* (Rhizoma Polygonati) is more effective for nourishing yin, moistening the lung and tonifying the kidney than *shān yào* (Radix Discoreae). However, it is greasy and is contraindicated for cases with loose stools due to spleen deficiency. It is commonly used for dry cough due to yin deficiency; dry mouth, poor appetite, dry stools, and a red tongue without a coat caused by yin impairment of the spleen and stomach.

⑨ *Míng dǎng shēn* (明党参, Radix Changii, Medicinal Changium Root)

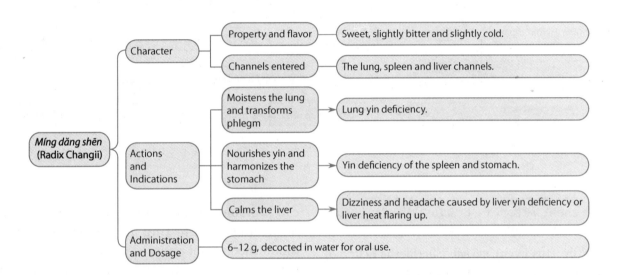

⑩ *Gǒu qǐ* (枸杞, Fructus Lycii, Barbary Wolfberry Fruit) ★★

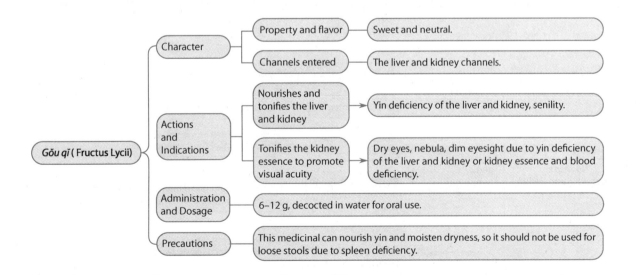

⑪ *Mò hàn lián* (墨旱莲, Herba Ecliptae, Yerbadetajo Herb) ★★★

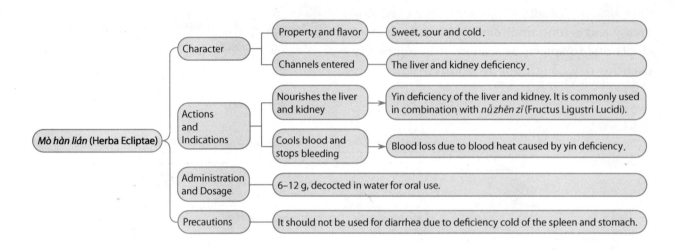

⑫ *Nǔ zhēn zǐ* (女贞子, Fructus Ligustri Lucidi, Glossy Privet Fruit) ★

Gǒu qǐ (Fructus Lycii), *mò hàn lián* (Herba Ecliptae) and *nǔ zhēn zǐ* (Fructus Ligustri Lucidi) are sweet in flavor. They enter the liver and kidney channels, and have the effect of nourishing the liver and kidney. They are used for yin deficiency of the liver and kidney manifesting as dizziness, tinnitus, early graying of the hair, aching and weakness in the waist and knees, seminal emissions, and diabetes. *Gǒu qǐ* (Fructus Lycii) and *nǔ zhēn zǐ* (Fructus Ligustri Lucidi) can promote visual acuity and are used for yin deficiency manifesting as dim eyesight and diminished visual acuity. *Gǒu qǐ* (Fructus Lycii) is neutral in property. It can promote the production of kidney essence and liver blood, and therefore is commonly used for dry eyes, nebulae and dim eyesight caused by yin deficiency of the liver and kidney, and deficiency of kidney essence and liver blood. It is able to nourish yin and moisten the lung, and is used for deficiency taxation cough due to yin deficiency. *Mò hàn lián* (Herba Ecliptae) has a cold property. It can cool blood

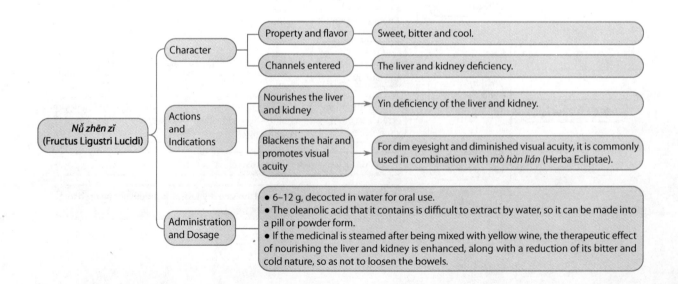

and stop bleeding, and is used for various types of bleeding due to blood heat with yin deficiency. *Nǚ zhēn zǐ* (Fructus Ligustri Lucidi) has a cool property. It can clear deficiency heat and is used for tidal fever and vexation due to internal heat with yin deficiency.

⑬ *Sāng shèn* (桑椹, Fructus Mori, Mulberry Root Bark)

Both *gǒu qǐ* (Fructus Lycii) and *sāng shèn* (Fructus Mori) are sweet in flavor. They enter the liver and kidney channels and have actions of tonifying the liver and kidney, promoting the production of kidney essence and liver blood. Both medicinals are used for liver and kidney deficiency, deficiency of kidney essence and liver blood, manifesting

as dizziness, tinnitus, deafness, early graying of the hair, insomnia, seminal emission, aching of the waist and knees, and diabetes. *Gǒu qǐ* (Fructus Lycii) is neutral in property. It is effective for improving visual acuity. It is therefore commonly used for dim eyesight and diminished visual acuity caused by liver and kidney deficiency. It is an essential medicinal to nourish the liver and kidney so as to promote visual acuity. It can nourish yin and moisten the lung. It is used for deficiency taxation cough due to yin deficiency. *Sāng shèn* (Fructus Mori) can promote fluid production and moisten the intestines. It is used for thirst due to fluid consumption and constipation due to yin and blood deficiency with dry intestines.

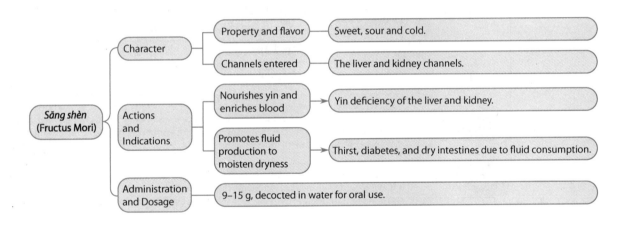

⑭ *Hēi zhī ma* (黑芝麻, Semen Sesami Nigrum, Black Sesame)

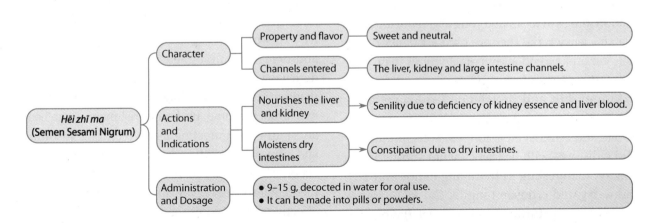

⑮ *Guī jiǎ* (龟甲, Carapax et Plastrum Testudinis, Tortoiseshell) ★★★

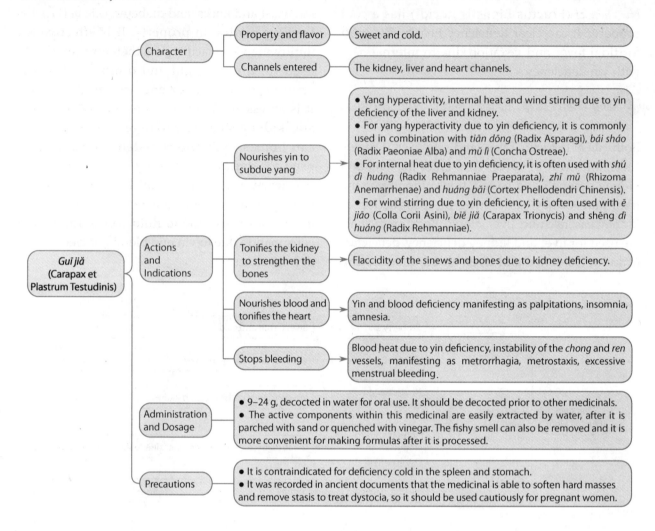

Character

- **Property and flavor** — Sweet and cold.
- **Channels entered** — The kidney, liver and heart channels.

Actions and Indications

- **Nourishes yin to subdue yang**
  - • Yang hyperactivity, internal heat and wind stirring due to yin deficiency of the liver and kidney.
  - • For yang hyperactivity due to yin deficiency, it is commonly used in combination with *tiān dōng* (Radix Asparagi), *bái sháo* (Radix Paeoniae Alba) and *mǔ lì* (Concha Ostreae).
  - • For internal heat due to yin deficiency, it is often used with *shú dì huáng* (Radix Rehmanniae Praeparata), *zhī mǔ* (Rhizoma Anemarrhenae) and *huáng bǎi* (Cortex Phellodendri Chinensis).
  - • For wind stirring due to yin deficiency, it is often used with *ē jiāo* (Colla Corii Asini), *biē jiǎ* (Carapax Trionycis) and *shēng dì huáng* (Radix Rehmanniae).
- **Tonifies the kidney to strengthen the bones** — Flaccidity of the sinews and bones due to kidney deficiency.
- **Nourishes blood and tonifies the heart** — Yin and blood deficiency manifesting as palpitations, insomnia, amnesia.
- **Stops bleeding** — Blood heat due to yin deficiency, instability of the *chong* and *ren* vessels, manifesting as metrorrhagia, metrostaxis, excessive menstrual bleeding.

Administration and Dosage

- • 9–24 g, decocted in water for oral use. It should be decocted prior to other medicinals.
- • The active components within this medicinal are easily extracted by water, after it is parched with sand or quenched with vinegar. The fishy smell can also be removed and it is more convenient for making formulas after it is processed.

Precautions

- • It is contraindicated for deficiency cold in the spleen and stomach.
- • It was recorded in ancient documents that the medicinal is able to soften hard masses and remove stasis to treat dystocia, so it should be used cautiously for pregnant women.

Guī jiǎ (Carapax et Plastrum Testudinis)

⑯ *Biē jiǎ* (鳖甲, Carapax Trionycis, Turtle Carapace) ★★★

Guī jiǎ (Carapax et Plastrum Testudinis) and *biē jiǎ* (Carapax Trionycis) are animal shells, and are salty in flavor and cold in property. They have the actions of nourishing yin to subdue yang and reducing fever of a deficiency type. They are used for deficiency of liver yin and ascendant hyperactivity of liver yang manifesting as headache and dizziness; deficiency of kidney yin and deficiency fire exuberance manifesting as steaming bones, tidal fever, night sweats and seminal emission; yin consumption by febrile diseases with deficiency wind stirring in the interior, manifesting as trembling hands and feet, and a dry, red crimson tongue. *Guī jiǎ* (Carapax et Plastrum Testudinis) has a sweet flavor, and enters the heart channel. It has a strong action in nourishing yin. It can also tonify the kidney to strengthen bones, stop bleeding, nourish blood and tonify the heart. It is often used for kidney deficiency with flaccidity of the waist and knees, weak sinews and bones, pidgeon chest in infants, frontal suture that has not closed, delayed eruption of teeth and delayed walking, etc.; blood heat due to yin deficiency, instability of the *chong* and *ren* vessels, manifesting as metrorrhagia, metrostaxis, excessive menstrual bleeding; under nourishment of the heart and kidney manifesting as palpitations, insomnia and amnesia. *Biē jiǎ* (Carapax Trionycis) has a strong action of clearing deficiency heat. It is an essential medicinal to treat fever due to yin deficiency. It is effective for softening hard masses and removing

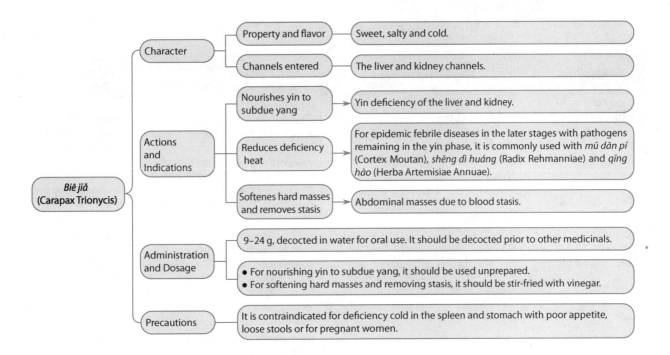

stasis, and is commonly used for abdominal masses due to blood stasis, chronic malaria, malarial nodules, splenohepatomegalia, and amenorrhea.

Actions of medicinals that tonify deficiency are summarized in the following tables (Tables 24-1~24-4):

Table 24-1: Summary of Actions of Medicinals that Replenish Qi:

Medicinal	Action in Common		Individual Character	
			Characteristic Actions	Other Actions
Rén shēn (Radix et Rhizoma Ginseng)	Sweet in flavor, warm or neutral in property, entering the spleen and lung channels. They can mainly replenish qi of the spleen and lung, and are indicated for lung qi deficiency and spleen qi deficiency	Replenishes qi of the spleen and lung, promotes fluid production to relieve thirst.	It has a strong effect of tonifyng. It is effective for greatly replenishing original qi. It is an essential medicinal to tonify deficiency and strengthen the body's resistance, and is regarded as the first choice to treat internal injury due to deficiency taxation. It can be used for deficiency of qi, blood and fluids.	Replenishes qi of the heart and kidney, calms and benefits the mind.
Dǎng shēn (Radix Codonopsis)			It has a similar but inferior action to *rén shēn* (Radix et Rhizoma Ginseng) in replenishing qi of the spleen and lung and promoting fluid production. It is an effective medicinal for tonifying the middle and replenishing qi. It can also nourish blood, and is always used instead of *rén shēn* (Radix et Rhizoma Ginseng) in common prescriptions that aim to replenish qi of the spleen and lung.	
Tài zǐ shēn (Radix Pseudostellariae)			It is inferior to *dǎng shēn* (Radix Codonopsis) in replenishing spleen and lung qi. It can also nourish yin and moisten the lung. It has the actions of both nourishing and clearing fire	
Xī yáng shēn (Radix Panacis Quinquefolii)			It has a slightly cool property. It is inferior to *rén shēn* (Radix et Rhizoma Ginseng) in replenishing qi. It is effective for nourishing yin, clearing heat and promoting fluid production. It is suitable for diseases caused by qi and yin deficiency with fire heat. It has the effect of both nourishing and clearing fire	

Table 24-1: Summary of Medicinals that Replenish Qi:

continued

Medicinal	Action in Common		Individual Character	
			Characteristic Actions	Other Actions
Huáng qí (Radix Astragali)	Sweet in flavor, warm or neutral in property, entering the spleen and lung channels. They can mainly replenish qi of the spleen and lung, and are indicated for lung qi deficiency and spleen qi deficiency.		It is inferior to *rén shēn* (Radix et Rhizoma Ginseng) in replenishing qi, which is similar to *dǎng shēn* (Radix Codonopsis). It is good at elevating yang to prevent the prolapse of internal organs, and is considered an essential medicinal to treat prolapse of internal organs due to qi deficiency.	Strengthens the defensive qi and consolidates the surface, induces diuresis to reduce edema, removes skin infections and promotes tissue regeneration
Bái zhú (Rhizoma Atractylodis Macrocephalae)		Replenishes qi and invigorates the spleen to arrest diarrhea and reduces leukorrhagia	It is effective for replenishing qi, invigorating the spleen, drying damp and inducing diuresis. It is an essential medicinal to replenish qi, invigorate the spleen and dry damp. It is suitable to treat diseases caused by damp exuberance due to spleen deficiency.	Consolidates the surface to arrest sweating, prevents miscarriage
Shān yào (Radix Discoreae)			It can tonify both qi and yin of the spleen and lung. It is suitable for diseases caused by both qi and yin deficiency of the spleen and lung. It is an effective medicinal with a neutral property for tonifying the spleen, lung and kidney.	Astringes the kidney essence to relieve enuresis and prevents seminal emission
Bái biǎn dòu (Semen Lablab Album)			It has a weak action in tonifying the spleen. It can harmonize the middle to transform damp. It is an effective medicinal for invigorating the spleen to transform damp. It is able to tonify the spleen without stagnating the stomach, and removes damp without drying fluids.	
Gān cǎo (Radix et Rhizoma Glycyrrhizae)		Invigorates the spleen, replenishes qi, relieves spasms and pain, moistens the lung to stop cough, clears heat, detoxifies, moderates the characters of other medicinals	It is effective for relieving spasms and pain and for moderating the characteristics of other medicinals.	Replenishes heart qi, removes phlegm to stop cough
Fēng mì (Mel)			Moistens intestines to promote defecation	
Dà zǎo (Fructus Jujubae)		Tonifies the middle and replenishes qi	Nourishes blood to calm the mind, moderates the characters of other medicinals	
Yí táng (Saccharum Granorum)			Relieves spasms and pain, moistens the lung to stop cough	
Cì wǔ jiā (Radix et Rhizoma seu Caulis Acanthopanacis Senticosi)		Replenishes qi and invigorates the spleen	Tonifies the kidney to calm the mind	
Jiǎo gǔ lán (Rhizoma seu Herba Gynostemmatis Pentaphylli)			Transforms phlegm to stop cough, clears heat, detoxifies	
Hóng jǐng tiān (Radix et Rhizoma Rhodiolae Crenulatae)			Clears the lung to stop cough, invigorates blood to transform stasis	
Shā jí (Fructus Hippophae)			Invigorates the spleen to digest food, transforms phlegm to stop cough, invigorates blood to remove stasis	

Table 24-2: Summary of Medicinals that Supplement Yang:

Medicinal	Action in Common	Individual Character		Other Actions
			Characteristic Actions	Other Actions
Lù róng (Cornu Cervi Pantotrichum)	Most of these are sweet, pungent and salty in flavor, warm or hot in property. They mainly enter the kidney channel, and have the effect of supplementing kidney yang. They are indicated for insufficiency of kidney yang.		It is effective for supplementing the kidney yang, promoting production of kidney essence and liver blood. It is an essential medicinal to supplement yang.	Strengthens the bones and sinews, regulates the chong and ren vessels, removes skin infections
Yín yáng huò (Herba Epimedii)		Tonifies the kidney to strengthen yang, strengthens the bones and sinews, expels wind damp	It has a strong action in tonifying the kidney and supplementing yang.	
Bā jǐ tiān (Radix Morindae Officinalis)			It has an inferior action in tonifying the kidney and supplementing yang, however, it is able to promote production of kidney essence and liver blood	
Xiān máo (Rhizoma Curculiginis)			It is toxic and has a strong action in expelling wind damp. It has a hot and dry nature, so it will cause impairment to yin if taken for a long time.	
Dù zhòng (Cortex Eucommiae)		Tonifies the liver and kidney, strengthens the bones and sinews, prevents miscarriage	It has a stronger action in tonifying and preventing miscarriage compared to xù duàn (Radix Dipsaci). It is an essential medicinal to treat lumbago due to kidney deficiency.	Reduces blood pressure
Xù duàn (Radix Dipsaci)			It has an inferior action in tonifying and preventing miscarriage. However, it is effective for activating blood, treating trauma and bone fractures. It is a commonly used medicinal in orthopedics and traumatology.	Stops bleeding
Ròu cōng róng (Herba Cistanches)		Tonifies the kidney to strengthen yang, moistens the intestines to promote defecation	It has a moderate action, which can promote production of kidney essence and liver blood. It is an effective medicinal for supplementing kidney yang, promoting the production of kidney essence and liver blood.	
Suǒ yáng (Herba Cynomorii)			It can moisten dryness to nourish the sinews. It is commonly used for flaccidity of the waist and knees, lack of strength in the sinews and bones and difficulty in walking due to deficiency of the liver and kidney.	
Bǔ gǔ zhī (Fructus Psoraleae)		Tonifies the kidney to strengthen yang, consolidates kidney essence and reduces urine, warms the spleen to arrest diarrhea	It has a strong action in strengthening yang. It is effective for tonifying the kidney to strengthen yang.	Improves inspiration to calm panting
Yì zhì rén (Fructus Alpiniae Oxyphyllae)			It has a stronger action than yì zhì rén (Fructus Alpiniae Oxyphyllae) in strengthening yang. It is effective for warming the spleen to improve the appetite and arrest salivation	
Tù sī zǐ (Semen Cuscutae)		Tonifies the kidney to strengthen yang, consolidates the kidney essence and reduces urine, nourishes the liver to promote visual acuity	It is neutral in property, and is able to supplement kidney essence and promote the production of kidney essence and liver blood. It can tonify both yin and yang. It can also arrest diarrhea and prevent miscarriage.	
Shā yuàn zǐ (Semen Astragali Complanati)			It is inferior to tù sī zǐ (Semen Cuscutae) in tonifying the liver and kidney. It is good at consolidating kidney essence, and reducing urine and leukorrhagia.	

Table 24-2: Summary of Medicinals that Supplement Yang:

continued

Medicinal	Action in Common		Individual Character	
			Characteristic Actions	**Other Actions**
Gé jiè (Gecko)	Most of these are sweet, pungent and salty in flavor, warm or hot in property. They mainly enter the kidney channel, and have the effect of supplementing kidney yang. They are indicated for insufficiency of kidney yang.	Tonifies the lung and kidney to relieve cough and panting	It has a strong action in tonifying the lung and kidney, and improving inspiration to calm panting. It is considered an essential medicinal to treat panting and cough of a deficiency type.	Promotes production of kidney essence and liver blood
Hé táo rén (Semen Juglandis)			Moistens the intestines to promote defecation	
Dōng chóng xià cǎo (Cordyceps)			It can tonify kidney and lung yin, stop bleeding, and transform phlegm.	
Zǐ hé chē (Placenta Hominis)			It can warm kidney yang, promote the production of kidney essence and liver blood, replenish qi and nourish blood	
Hú lú bā (Semen Trigonellae Callorhimi)		Tonifies the kidney to strengthen yang	It has a pure and strong action in tonifying the kidney to strengthen yang, and supplementing kidney essence and marrow.	
Hǎi mǎ (Hippocampus)			Invigorates blood to remove stasis, subdues swelling to relieve pain	
Hǎi gǒu shèn (Testis et Penis Callorhini)		Warms the kidney to strengthen yang	Dispels cold to relieve pain	
Yáng qǐ shí (Actinolitum)			It has a pure and strong action	
Jiǔ cài zǐ (Semen Allii Tuberosi)			It can tonify the liver, consolidate kidney essence, and reduce urine and leukorrhagia.	
Zǐ shí yīng (Fluoritum)			Calms the heart to tranquilize the mind, warms the lung to calm panting	
Yáng hóng shān (Radix Seu Herba Pimpinelae)			Invigorates blood to transform stasis, nourishes the heart to calm the mind, warms the lung to dispel cold	
Há ma yóu (Oviductus Ranae)			Tonifies kidney essence, nourishes yin and moistens the lung.	

Table 24-3: Summary of Medicinals that Nourish Blood:

Medicinal	Action in Common		Individual Character	
			Characteristic Actions	**Other Actions**
Dāng guī (Radix Angelicae Sinensis)	They mainly enter the *xue* level of the heart and liver, and have the effect of nourishing blood. They are indicated for blood deficiency syndromes.	Nourishes blood to regulate menstruation, relieves pain	It can nourish and invigorate blood, and dispel cold. It can be used for blood deficiency, blood stasis and blood cold manifesting as irregular menstruation, amenorrhea and dysmenorrhea. It is an essential medicinal to nourish blood and regulate menstruation. It can nourish blood, invigorate blood and dispel cold to relieve pain.	Moistens the intestines to promote defecation
Bái sháo (Radix Paeoniae Alba)			It is effective for nourishing blood and astringing yin. It is most suitable for blood deficiency and yin deficiency with heat manifestations. It is able to astringe liver yin, nourish blood and soften the liver to relieve spasms and pain.	Suppresses liver yang, astringes yin to arrest sweating

Table 24-3: Summary of Medicinals that Nourish Blood:

continued

Medicinal	Action in Common		Individual Character	
			Characteristic Actions	**Other Actions**
Shú dì huáng (Radix Rehmanniae Praeparata)	These mainly enter the *xue* level of the heart and liver, and have the effect of nourishing blood. They are indicated for blood deficiency syndromes.	Promotes kidney essence and liver blood	It has a strong action in tonifying. It is effective for nourishing blood and yin, promoting the production of kidney essence and liver blood, and supplementing marrow. It is an essential medicinal to nourish blood, tonify deficiency, and is the main medicinal to nourish yin of the liver and kidney. However, the medicinal is sticky and greasy, and will cause stagnation in the stomach.	
Hé shǒu wū (Radix Polygoni Multiflori)			It is inferior to *shú dì huáng* (Radix Rehmanniae Praeparata) in tonifying after being prepared. However, it is an astringent medicinal and can astringe to consolidate the kidney. It is most suitable for those who are too weak to be tonified, and is a good tonic medicinal. It has a weak action in tonifying when used unprepared, and can prevent the recurrence of malaria, detoxify, and moisten the intestines to promote defecation.	
Ē jiāo (Colla Corii Asini)		Nourishes blood	It has a strong action, and is an essential medicinal to nourish blood.	Nourishes yin to moisten the lung, stops bleeding
Lóng yǎn ròu (Arillus Longan)			Tonifies the heart and spleen, calms the mind	
Chǔ shí zǐ (Fructus Broussonetiae)			Nourishes the kidney, clears the liver, promotes visual acuity, induces diuresis	

Table 24-4: Summary of Medicinals that Nourish Yin:

Medicinal	Action in Common		Individual Character	
			Characteristic Actions	**Other Actions**
Běi shā shēn (Radix Glehniae)	These are sweet in flavor and cold in property, and enter the lung, stomach, liver and kidney channels. They mainly nourish yin and are indicated for deficiency syndromes of the lung, stomach, liver and kidney.	Nourishes yin to clear the lung, tonifies the stomach to promote fluids production	It has a stronger action in clearing and nourishing the lung and stomach, and is commonly used for yin deficiency of the lung and stomach with heat manifestations.	
Nán shā shēn (Radix Adenophorae)			Replenishes qi and transforms phlegm. It can tonify both qi and yin, and is suitable for both qi and yin consumption in the lung, spleen, and stomach, and sticky phlegm with difficult expectoration due to lung dryness.	
Bǎi hé (Bulbus Lilii)		Nourishes yin and moistens the lung, nourishes stomach yin	It has an inferior action in nourishing the stomach yin, moistening and clearing the lung. It can remove phlegm to stop cough.	Clears the heart to calm the mind
Yù zhú (Rhizoma Polygonati Odorati)			It is effective for nourishing yin, moistening dryness, and promoting fluids production to relieve thirst. It can nourish yin without retaining pathogens. It is commonly selected for external invasion due to yin deficiency.	Nourishes heart yin, clears heart heat
Huáng jīng (Rhizoma Polygonati)			It can nourish yin, moisten the lung, replenish qi, invigorate the spleen and tonify the kidney. It can tonify both qi and yin, and is an effective medicinal to tonify the lung, spleen and kidney.	

Table 24-4: Summary of Medicinals that Nourish Yin:

continued

Medicinal	Action in Common		Individual Character	
			Characteristic Actions	**Other Actions**
Mài dōng (Radix Ophiopogonis)	These are sweet in flavor and cold in property, and enter the lung, stomach, liver and kidney channels. They mainly nourish yin and are indicated for deficiency syndromes of the lung, stomach, liver and kidney.	Nourishes yin, moistens dryness, clears the lung and promotes fluids production	It has a weaker action in nourishing yin, moistening dryness, clearing heat and promoting fluid production compared with *tiān dōng* (Radix Asparagi). It also has a less greasy nature.	Clears the heart to remove vexation
Tiān dōng (Radix Asparagi)			It has a stronger action in nourishing yin, moistening dryness, clearing heat and promoting fluid production, but with a more greasy nature.	Nourishes kidney yin, descends deficiency fire
Shí hú (Caulis Dendrobii)			It is effective for nourishing stomach yin, promoting fluid production to relieve thirst, and clearing stomach heat.	Nourishes kidney yin, improves visual acuity, strengthens the waist and knees, descends deficient fire
Gǒu qǐ (Fructus Lycii)		Nourishes yin of the liver and kidney	Improves visual acuity	It can supplement kidney essence and liver blood and is effective for improving visual acuity.
Nǚ zhēn zǐ (Fructus Ligustri Lucidi)				Clears deficiency heat
Mò hàn lián (Herba Ecliptae)				Cools blood and stops bleeding
Guī jiǎ (Carapax et Plastrum Testudinis)		Nourishes yin to subdue yang, reduces deficiency fever	It has a stronger action in nourishing yin. It can also tonify the kidney to strengthen the bones, stop bleeding, nourish blood and tonify the heart.	
Biē jiǎ (Carapax Trionycis)			It has a strong action in nourishing yin. It is an essential medicinal to treat fever due to yin deficiency.	Softens hard masses to remove stasis
Sāng shèn (Fructus Mori)		Promotes production of kidney essence and liver blood, moistens the intestines to promote defecation	Promotes fluids production to moisten dryness	
Hēi zhī ma (Semen Sesami Nigrum)			It is nutritious and can promote the production of kidney essence and can nourish blood.	
Míng dǎng shēn (Radix Changii)			Moistens the lung to transform phlegm, nourishes yin to harmonize the stomach, calms the liver	

Tables for testing herbal knowledge of the actions and indications of medicinals that tonify deficiency are as follows (Tables 24-5~24-15, see p.427~434):

Table 24-5: Test your Herbal Knowledge of the Actions of Medicinals that Replenish Qi:

Actions ＼ Medicinal	Rén shēn	Xī yáng shēn	Dǎng shēn	Tài zǐ shēn	Huáng qí	Bái zhú	Shān yào	Bái biǎn dòu	Gān cǎo	Dà zǎo	Yí táng	Fēng mì
Replenishes lung qi												
Replenishes spleen qi												
Promotes fluid production												
Calms the mind												
Replenishes qi and nourishes yin												
Clears fire and promotes fluid production												
Greatly tonifies original qi												
Prevents miscarriage												
Replenishes qi to boost sinking yang												
Benefits defensive yang to consolidate the surface and arrests sweating												
Transforms damp												
Removes skin infections and promotes tissue regeneration												
Replenishes qi and invigorates the spleen												
Dries damp and promotes the flow of water												
Tonifies the spleen, lung and kidney												
Nourishes blood												
Preserves kidney essence and reduces leukorrhagia												
Invigorates the spleen												
Promotes the flow of water to reduce edema												
Clears summer-heat												
Tonifies the middle to relieve spasms and pain												
Replenishes qi and tonifies the middle												
Moistens the intestines to promote defecation												
Relieves spasms and pain												
Regulates the characteristics of other medicinals												
Nourishes blood to calm the mind												
Moderates the characteristics of other medicinals												
Clears heat and detoxifies												
Moistens the lung to stop cough												
Removes phlegm to stop cough												
Detoxifies												

Table 24-6: Test your Herbal Knowledge of the Actions of Medicinals that Supplement Yang (one):

Medicinal / Actions	Lù róng	Bā jǐ tiān	Yín yáng huò	Xiān máo	Bǔ gǔ zhī	Yì zhì rén	Hǎi gǒu shèn	Ròu cōng róng	Suǒ yáng	Gé jiè	Dōng chóng xià cǎo	Zǐ hé chē
Promotes the production of kidney essence and liver blood												
Tonifies kidney yang												
Strengthens the bones and sinews												
Regulates the *chong* and *ren* vessels												
Removes skin infections												
Tonifies the kidney to strengthen yang												
Expels wind damp												
Stops cough and calms panting												
Consolidates kidney essence and reduces urine												
Warms the spleen to arrest diarrhea												
Warms the kidney and supplements kidney essence												
Warms the spleen to arrest salivation												
Nourishes kidney essence and marrow												
Moistens the intestines to promote defecation												
Replenishs lung qi												
Expels cold damp												
Stops bleeding and transforms phlegm												
Improves inspiration to calm panting												
Replenishes qi and nourishes blood												

Table 24-7: Test your Herbal Knowledge of the Actions of Medicinals that Supplement Yang (two):

Medicinal / Actions	Hǎi mǎ	Tù sī zǐ	Shā yuàn zǐ	Dù zhòng	Xù duàn	Jiǔ cài zǐ	Yáng qǐ shí	Hú lú bā	Hé táo rén
Prevents miscarriage									
Invigorates the blood to remove stasis									
Reduces swelling to relieve pain									
Tonifies the kidney to consolidate kidney essence									
Treats trauma and bone fractures									
Arrests diarrhea									
Tonifies the kidney to supplement yang									
Tonifies the liver and kidney									
Strengthens the bones and sinews									
Stops bleeding									
Nourishes the liver to promote visual acuity									
Strengthens yang and consolidates kidney essence									
Warms the kidney to strengthen yang									

Table 24-7: Test your Herbal Knowledge of the Actions of Medicinals that Supplement Yang (two):

continued

Actions \ Medicinal	Hǎi mǎ	Tù sī zǐ	Shā yuàn zǐ	Dù zhòng	Xù duàn	Jiǔ cài zǐ	Yáng qǐ shí	Hú lú bā	Hé táo rén
Warms the kidney									
Dispels cold									
Relieves pain									
Warms the lung									
Moistens the intestines									

Table 24-8: Test your Herbal Knowledge of the Actions of Medicinals that Nourish Blood:

Actions \ Medicinal	Dāng guī	Shú dì huáng	Bái sháo	Hé shǒu wū	Ē jiāo	Lóng yǎn ròu
Nourishes blood to regulate menstruation						
Invigorates blood						
Regulates menstruation						
Consolidates the kidney and blackens hair						
Nourishes blood and yin						
Promotes production of kidney essence and marrow						
Enriches blood						
Calms the liver to relieve pain						
Astringes yin to arrest sweating						
Nourishes kidney essence and liver blood						
Relieves pain						
Tonifies the heart and spleen						
Moistens the intestines to promote defecation						
Stops bleeding						
Nourishes yin to moisten dryness						
Prevents the recurrence of malaria and detoxifies						
Nourishes blood to calm the mind						

Table 24-9: Test your Herbal Knowledge of the Actions of Medicinals that Nourish Yin:

Actions \ Medicinal	Běi shā shēn	Nán shā shēn	Bǎi hé	Mài dōng	Tiān dōng	Shí hú	Yù zhú	Huáng jīng	Gǒu qǐ	Mò hàn lián	Nǚ zhēn zǐ	Sāng shèn	Hēi zhī ma	Guī jiǎ	Biē jiǎ
Nourishes yin and clears the lung															
Tonifies the stomach and promotes fluid production															
Transforms phlegm															
Nourishes yin and clears heat															
Nourishes yin and moistens the lung															
Clears the heart to calm the mind															

Table 24-9: Test your Herbal Knowledge of the Actions of Medicinals that Nourish Yin:

continued

Actions \ Medicinal	Běi shā shēn	Nán shā shēn	Băi hé	Mài dōng	Tiān dōng	Shí hú	Yù zhú	Huáng jīng	Gŏu qĭ	Mò hàn lián	Nŭ zhēn zĭ	Sāng shèn	Hēi zhī ma	Guī jiă	Biē jiă
Nourishes yin and enriches blood															
Clears fire															
Promotes fluid production															
Replenishes qi															
Nourishes the kidney and moistens the lung															
Invigorates the spleen and replenishes qi															
Tonifies the liver and kidney															
Reduces deficiency fever															
Cools blood and stops bleeding															
Clears the heart to remove vexation															
Promotes fluid production															
Moistens the intestines to promote defecation															
Softens hard masses to remove stasis															
Nourishes yin to subdue yang															
Improves visual acuity															
Tonifies the kidney to strengthen the bones															
Stops bleeding															
Nourishes blood and tonifies the heart															
Nourishes kidney essence and liver blood															

Table 24-10: Test your Herbal Knowledge of the Indications of Medicinals that Replenish Qi:

Indications \ Medicinal	Rén shēn	Xī yáng shēn	Dăng shēn	Tài zĭ shēn	Huáng qí	Bái zhú	Shān yào	Bái biăn dòu	Gān căo	Dà zăo	Yí táng	Fēng mì
Deficiency taxation cough, bloody phlegm												
Lung qi deficiency												
Spleen qi deficiency												

Table 24-10: Test your Herbal Knowledge of the Indications of Medicinals that Replenish Qi:

continued

Medicinal / Indications	Rén shēn	Xī yáng shēn	Dǎng shēn	Tài zǐ shēn	Huáng qí	Bái zhú	Shān yào	Bái biǎn dòu	Gān cǎo	Dà zǎo	Yí táng	Fēng mì
Both qi and fluid deficiency												
Qi and blood deficiency												
Collapse syndrome due to qi deficiency												
Collapse of middle qi												
Spontaneous sweating due to a deficient exterior												
Internal organ dryness												
Skin diseases that have ruptured but are not healing												
Excessive fetal movement due to qi deficiency												
Qi deficiency of the lung and kidney												
Sore and swollen throat												
Diabetes												
Vomiting and diarrhea due to summer-heat damp												
Damp exuberance due to spleen deficiency												
Edema due to qi deficiency												
Spasms and pain of the epigastrium and abdomen												
Spasms and pain of the limbs												
Palpitations, slow-irregular pulse, or slow and weak pulse with regular intervals												
Cough with excessive phlegm												
Dry cough with scanty phlegm due to lung deficiency												
Internal heat due to yin deficiency												
Medicinal poisoning												
Food poisoning												
Yellowish complexion due to blood deficiency												
Spasms, epigastric and abdominal pain due to middle deficiency												
Skin diseases due to heat toxin												
Constipation due to dry intestines												
Poisoning by toxic medicinals such as chuān wū (Radix Aconiti), cǎo wū (Radix Aconiti Kusnezoffii) and fù zǐ (Radix Aconiti Lateralis Praeparata)												

Table 24-11: Test your Herbal Knowledge of the Indications of Medicinals that Supplement Yang (one):

Medicinal / Indications	Lù róng	Bā jǐ tiān	Yín yáng huò	Xiān máo	Bǔ gǔ zhī	Yì zhì rén	Gé jiè	Dōng chóng xià cǎo	Zǐ hé chē
Impotence, low sperm count due to kidney yang deficiency									
Metrorrhagia and metrostaxis due to deficiency cold in the *chong* and *ren* vessels									
Flaccidity of the sinews and bones due to deficiency of kidney essence and liver blood									
Headache and tinnitus									
Maldevelopment in infants									
Delayed closure of the fontanels, delayed teeth eruption, delayed walking									
Female infertility due to cold in the uterus									
Salivation in infants									
Skin diseases that have ruptured but are not healing									
Chronic dorsal furuncles									
Chronic *bi* due to wind damp with difficulty in walking									
Diarrhea due to yang deficiency of the spleen and kidney									
Frequent urination									
Diarrhea and salivation due to deficiency cold in the spleen and stomach									
Leukorrhea									
Cough with panting due to deficiency of the lung and kidney									
Aching in the lumbus and knees									
Deficiency panting due to the deficient kidney failing to preserve qi									
Seminal emission and spermatorrhea									
Constipation due to dry intestines									
Yellowish complexion and emaciation due to qi and blood deficiency									

Table 24-12: Test your Herbal Knowledge of the Indications of Medicinals that Supplement Yang (two):

Medicinal / Indications	Hé táo rén	Ròu cōng róng	Suǒ yáng	Tù sī zǐ	Shā yuàn zǐ	Dù zhòng	Xù duàn	Jiǔ cài zǐ	Hú lú bā
Impotence and low sperm count due to kidney yang deficiency									
Leukorrhagia									
Frequent urination, enuresis									

Table 24-12: Test your Herbal Knowledge of the Indications of Medicinals that Supplement Yang (two):

continued

Medicinal / Indications	Hé táo rén	Ròu cōng róng	Suǒ yáng	Tù sī zǐ	Shā yuàn zǐ	Dù zhòng	Xù duàn	Jiǔ cài zǐ	Hú lú bā
Flaccidity of the sinews and bones due to deficiency of kidney essence and liver blood									
Metrorrhagia, metrostaxis, excessive menstrual blood									
Dim eyesight due to deficiency of the liver and kidney									
Diarrhea due to yang deficiency of the spleen and kidney									
Excessive fetal movement due to deficiency of the liver and kidney									
Diabetes due to kidney deficiency									
Bi due to wind damp									
Female infertility due to cold in the uterus									
Constipation due to dry intestines									
Abdominal pain due to cold hernia									
Cold pain in the lower abdomen due to cold menstruation									
Beriberi due to cold damp									

Table 24-13: Test your Herbal Knowledge of the Indications of Medicinals that Enrich Blood:

Medicinal / Indications	Dāng guī	Shú dì huáng	Bái sháo	Hé shǒu wū	Ē jiāo	Lóng yǎn ròu
Yellowish complexion, dizziness and palpitations due to blood deficiency						
Irregular menstruation, metrorrhagia, metrostaxis						
Deficiency of liver yin						
Carbuncles, skin diseases						
Chronic malaria due to weak constitution						
Steaming bones and night sweats due to deficiency of kidney yin						
Seminal emission and diabetes due to deficiency of kidney yin						
Aching and weakness of the lumbus and knees due to deficiency of kidney essence and liver blood						
Pain						
Liver qi constraint						
Ascendant hyperactivity of liver yang						
Spontaneous sweating due to a deficient surface						
Constipation due to dry intestines and blood deficiency						
Various types of bleeding						
Dry cough due to yin deficiency						
Deficiency wind stirring due to yin consumption by febrile diseases						

Table 24-14: Test your Herbal Knowledge of the Indications of Medicinals that Nourish Yin (one):

Medicinal / Indications	Běi shā shēn	Nán shā shēn	Bǎi hé	Mài dōng	Tiān dōng	Shí hú	Yù zhú	Huáng jīng	Mài dōng	Gǒu qǐ
Lung deficiency and heat with dry cough and scanty phlegm										
Chronic and deficiency taxation cough										
Thirst and dry throat due to stomach yin deficiency, heat impairing stomach yin or fluid deficiency										
Yin consumption due to febrile diseases with low fever, vexation and thirst										
Dry throat and mouth due to deficiency of qi and fluids after diseases, or deficiency of the spleen and stomach										
Febrile diseases with remaining heat, vexation, palpitations, insomnia, frequent dreams										
Tidal fever, night sweats, seminal emissions										
Blurred vision due to yin deficiency of the liver and kidney										
Gastric insidious pain, gastric upset, dry vomiting										
Dark eyesight, flaccidity due to kidney deficiency										
Dizziness, aching and weakness of the lumbus and knees, early graying of the hair due to kidney deficiency and insufficiency of kidney essence										
Diabetes due to internal heat										

Table 24-15: Test your Herbal Knowledge of the Indications of Medicinals that Nourish Yin (two):

Medicinal / Indications	Mò hàn lián	Nǚ zhēn zǐ	Sāng shèn	Hēi zhī ma	Guī jiǎ	Biē jiǎ
Dizziness, early graying of the hair, lumbar aching and tinnitus due to yin deficiency of the liver and kidney						
Palpitations, insomnia and amnesia due to heart deficiency						
Fever and night sweats due to yin deficiency						
Yang hyperactivity due to yin deficiency						
Diabetes due to yin deficiency						
Constipation due to dry intestines						
Wind stirring and spasms of the limbs due to yin deficiency						
Flaccidity of the bones, delayed closure of the fontanel, delayed teeth eruption, delayed walking due to kidney deficiency						
Bleeding due to blood heat resulting from yin deficiency						
Abdominal masses due to blood stasis						
Malarial nodules						
Thirst due to fluid consumption						

Chapter 25
Astringent Medicinals

Concept

Medicinals whose principal effect is to induce astringency and arrest discharge are called astringent medicinals.

Characters and Actions

Medicinals in this chapter are mostly sour or astringent in flavor, and warm or neutral in property. They mainly enter the lung, spleen, kidney and large intestine channels. They have the actions of consolidating the exterior to stop excessive sweating, astringing the lung to stop cough, astringing the intestines to stop diarrhea, consolidating the kidney essence to reduce urination, stopping bleeding, and stopping leukorrhea.

Indications

Medicinals of this kind are mainly used for spontaneous sweating, night sweats, chronic cough, deficient panting, chronic diarrhea, chronic dysentery, seminal emission, spermatorrhea, enuresis, frequent urination, metrorrhagia, and leukorrhagia.

Combinations

The basic cause of qi collapse, indicated by bladder and bowel incontinence, spontaneous sweating and bleeding, spermatorrhea or leukorrhea, and cough, is right qi deficiency and weakness. Therefore, astringent medicinals are used to treat the branch. When using such medicinals, appropriate tonic medicinals should also be used so as to treat both the root and branch. For spontaneous sweating due to qi deficiency and night sweats due to yin deficiency, combine with medicinals for replenishing qi and nourishing yin. For chronic diarrhea and dysentery due to yang deficiency of the spleen and kidney, combine with medicinals with actions of warming and tonifying the spleen and kidney. For seminal emission, spermatorrhea, enuresis and frequent urination, combine with medicinals for tonifying the kidney. For instability of the *chong* and *ren* vessels with metrorrhagia and metrostaxis, combine with medicinals for tonifying the liver and kidney. For chronic cough and deficient panting due to impairment in the lung and kidney, combine with medicinals for tonifying the lung and kidney to improve inspiration. In a word, practitioners should search for basic causes of the disease and use medicinals in combination according to different syndromes. If this is done, then there will be good therapeutic effects.

Precautions

Astringent medicinals are astringent in flavor and can retain pathogens; therefore they should not be used for unresolved external pathogens, damp heat with diarrhea, dysentery, leukorrhagia, and bleeding as well as depressed heat retention. Some of the medicinals have the actions of clearing damp heat and resolving toxins, so alternative methods should be used for these conditions.

Classification

According to their different characters and clinical applications, astringent medicinals are divided into three categories: Medicinals that consolidate the exterior to stop sweating, medicinals that astringe the lung and large intestine, and medicinals that consolidate the kidney essence, reduce urination and stop leukorrhea.

Section 1   Medicinals that Consolidate the Exterior to Arrest Sweats

Medicinals in this section are often sweet in flavor and neutral in property. They mainly enter the lung and heart channels. They can regulate defensive qi and protect the interstices so as to consolidate the exterior to arrest sweating. They are commonly used for spontaneous sweating due to deficient qi failing to consolidate the exterior; and yin deficiency not checking yang, with yang heat forcing fluids to the exterior and causing night sweating.

① *Má huáng gēn* (麻黄根, Radix et Rhizoma Ephedrae, Ephedra Root) ★★

Má huáng (Herba Ephedrae) and *má huáng gēn* (Radix et Rhizoma Ephedrae) originate from *Ephedra sinica* stapf., E. *Intermedia* Schrenk et C.A. Mey., and E. *Equisetina* Bunge, of the family Ephedraceae. They have contrary actions because they come from different medicinal plant parts. *Má huáng* (Herba Ephedrae) is the stem. It is effective for releasing the exterior by inducing sweating. It is indicated for external invasion by wind cold, manifesting as aversion to cold, absence of sweating, fever, headache, and a floating and tense pulse. It can also diffuse the lung to calm panting and promote the flow of water to reduce edema. It is therefore used for cough and panting of a deficient type and edema accompanied by external invasion due to lung qi accumulation, which is caused by external pathogenic wind cold. *Má huáng gēn* (Radix et Rhizoma Ephedrae) is the root and rhizome. It is effective for consolidating the exterior to arrest sweating, and is indicated for spontaneous sweating due to qi deficiency, night sweating due to yin deficiency and deficient sweating postpartum. Of these two medicinals, one induces sweating and one stops sweating; their functions are not the same, and they should be differentiated for use.

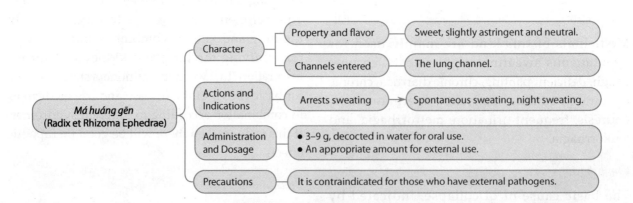

② *Fú xiǎo mài* (浮小麦, Fructus Tritici Levis, Blighted Wheat) ★★

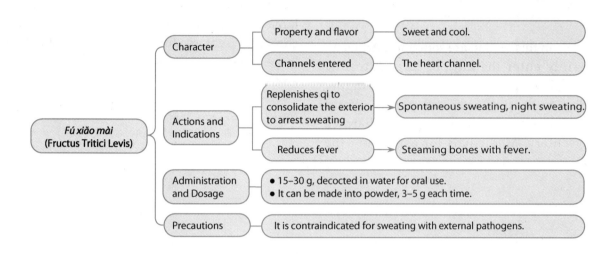

③ *Nuò dào gēn xū* (糯稻根须, Radix Oryzae Glutinosae, Glutinous Rice Rhizome and Root)

Má huáng gēn (Radix et Rhizoma Ephedrae), *fú xiǎo mài* (Fructus Tritici Levis) and *nuò dào gēn xū* (Radix Oryzae Glutinosae) can consolidate the exterior to arrest sweating. They are used for spontaneous sweating due to qi deficiency and night sweating due to yin deficiency. *Fú xiǎo mài* (Fructus Tritici Levis) and *nuò dào gēn xū* (Radix Oryzae Glutinosae) can also reduce deficiency fever, and are used for lingering deficiency fever, steaming bones and deficiency taxation fever. *Má huáng gēn* (Radix et Rhizoma Ephedrae) has a pure and strong action in arresting sweating, and is commonly used in clinic both internally or externally. *Fú xiǎo mài* (Fructus Tritici Levis) can replenish qi. *Nuò dào gēn xū* (Radix Oryzae Glutinosae) is able to tonify the stomach to promote fluid production, and is used for thirst due to yin deficiency after disease.

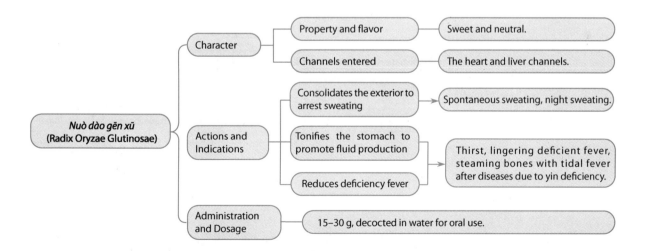

Section 2 Medicinals that Astringe the Lung and Large Intestine

Medicinals in this section are sour and astringent, and mainly enter the lung or large intestine channels. They have the actions of astringing the lung to stop cough and panting, and astringing the large intestine to arrest diarrhea and dysentery. Medicinals for astringing the lung are commonly used for cough and panting due to lung deficiency; panting of a deficiency type due to lung deficiency and kidney failing to preserve qi. Medicinals for astringing the large intestine are used for chronic diarrhea and chronic dysentery due to deficiency cold in the large intestine or deficiency cold in the spleen and kidney.

① *Wǔ wèi zǐ* (五味子, Fructus Schisandrae Chinensis, Chinese Magnoliavine Fruit) ★ ★ ★

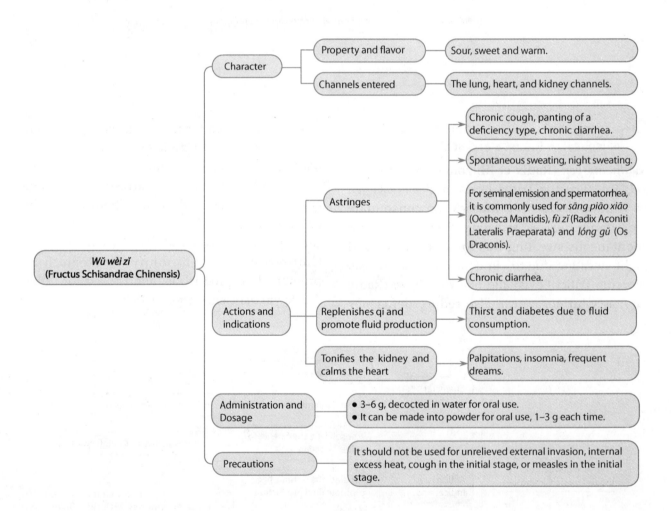

② *Wū méi* (乌梅, Fructus Mume, Smoked Plum)
　★ ★ ★

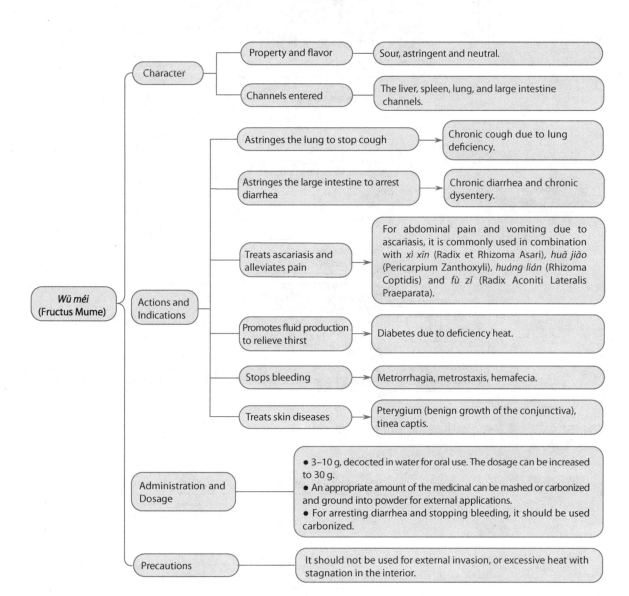

Character

- **Property and flavor** → Sour, astringent and neutral.
- **Channels entered** → The liver, spleen, lung, and large intestine channels.

Wū méi (Fructus Mume)

Actions and Indications

- **Astringes the lung to stop cough** → Chronic cough due to lung deficiency.
- **Astringes the large intestine to arrest diarrhea** → Chronic diarrhea and chronic dysentery.
- **Treats ascariasis and alleviates pain** → For abdominal pain and vomiting due to ascariasis, it is commonly used in combination with *xì xīn* (Radix et Rhizoma Asari), *huā jiāo* (Pericarpium Zanthoxyli), *huáng lián* (Rhizoma Coptidis) and *fù zǐ* (Radix Aconiti Lateralis Praeparata).
- **Promotes fluid production to relieve thirst** → Diabetes due to deficiency heat.
- **Stops bleeding** → Metrorrhagia, metrostaxis, hemafecia.
- **Treats skin diseases** → Pterygium (benign growth of the conjunctiva), tinea captis.

Administration and Dosage

- 3–10 g, decocted in water for oral use. The dosage can be increased to 30 g.
- An appropriate amount of the medicinal can be mashed or carbonized and ground into powder for external applications.
- For arresting diarrhea and stopping bleeding, it should be used carbonized.

Precautions → It should not be used for external invasion, or excessive heat with stagnation in the interior.

③ *Wǔ bèi zǐ* (五倍子, Galla Chinensis, Chinese Gall) ★

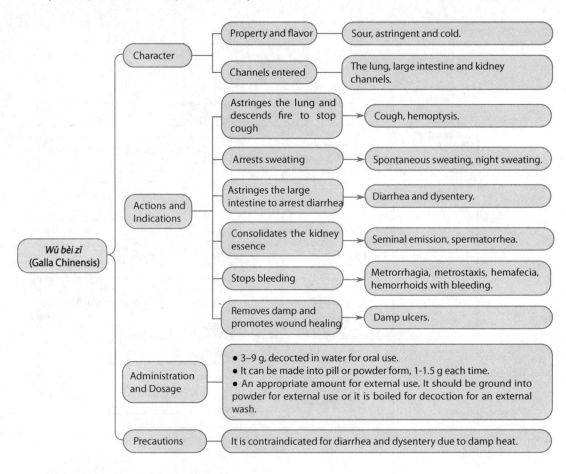

④ *Yīng sù qiào* (罂粟壳, Pericarpium Papaveris, Poppy Capsule)

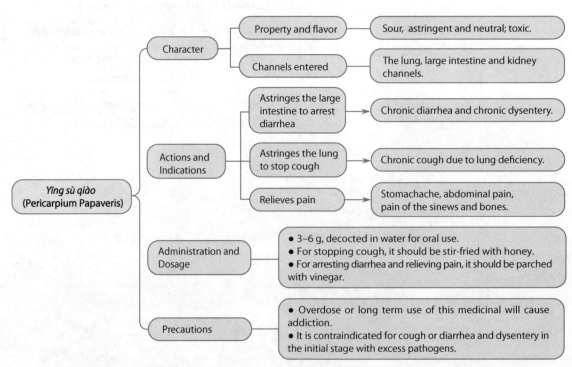

⑤ *Hē zǐ* (诃子, Fructus Chebulae, Medicine Terminalia Fruit) ★★

Wǔ wèi zǐ (Fructus Schisandrae Chinensis), *wǔ bèi zǐ* (Galla Chinensis), *wū méi* (Fructus Mume), *hē zǐ* (Fructus Chebulae) and *yīng sù qiào* (Pericarpium Papaveris) have the actions of astringing the lung to stop cough and astringing the large intestine to arrest diarrhea. They are used for chronic cough, chronic diarrhea and diarrhea due to lung deficiency. *Wǔ wèi zǐ* (Fructus Schisandrae Chinensis) and *wǔ bèi zǐ* (Galla Chinensis) can consolidate the kidney essence and arrest sweating. They are used for kidney deficiency failing to consolidate kidney essence with manifestations such as seminal emission, spontaneous sweating and night sweating. *Wǔ wèi zǐ* (Fructus Schisandrae Chinensis) is sour and sweet in flavor, warm in property and moist in texture. It has a strong action in astringing. It is able to astringe lung qi in the upper and nourish kidney yin in the lower. It is used for panting and cough due to both lung and kidney deficiency, and is regarded as an essential medicinal to treat chronic cough and deficiency panting. It can also replenish qi, promote fluid production, tonify the kidney and calm the heart. Therefore, it is used for thirst due to fluid consumption, diabetes due to yin deficiency; vexation, palpitations, insomnia and frequent dreams due to malnutrition of the heart or failure of the heart to communicate with the kidney. *Wǔ bèi zǐ* (Galla Chinensis) is sour and astringent in flavor and cold in property. It can descend fire and stop bleeding; remove damp and promote wound healing (when used externally). It can be used for cough with phlegm and hemoptysis due to lung heat; metrorrhagia, metrostaxis, hemorrhoids with bleeding; damp ulcers, and skin diseases. *Wū méi* (Fructus Mume) is sour and astringent in flavor, and neutral in property. It is able to relieve ascariasis and alleviate pain, and promote fluid production to relieve thirst and stop bleeding. It is used for abdominal pain and vomiting due to ascariasis; diabetes due to deficiency heat; metrorrhagia and metrostaxis. *Hē zǐ* (Fructus Chebulae) is bitter, sour and astringent in flavor, and neutral in property. It is capable of descending qi and relieving sore throat and loss of voice. It is commonly used for chronic cough and loss of voice due to lung deficiency; chronic cough and loss of voice due to phlegm heat stagnating in the lung. It is an essential medicinal to treat loss of voice. *Yīng sù qiào* (Pericarpium Papaveris) is sour and astringent in flavor, and neutral in property.

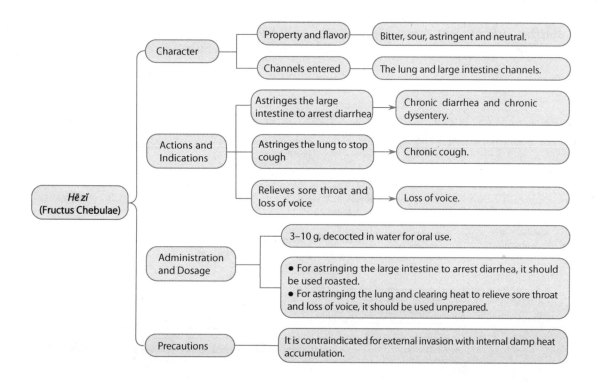

It is effective for relieving pain. It is commonly used for stomachache, abdominal pain and pain in the sinews and bones.

⑥ *Shí liú pí* (石榴皮, Pericarpium Granati, Pomegranate Rind)

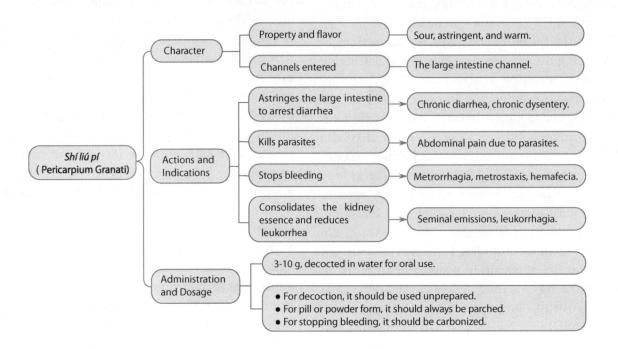

⑦ *Ròu dòu kòu* (肉豆蔻, Semen Myristicae, Nutmeg) ★★

Ròu dòu kòu (Semen Myristicae) and *hē zǐ* (Fructus Chebulae) can astringe the large intestine to arrest diarrhea. They are used for loose intestines with chronic diarrhea and chronic dysentery. *Ròu dòu kòu* (Semen Myristicae) is pungent and warm, and

is effective for warming the middle to promote qi flow. It is commonly used for distending pain in the epigastrium and abdomen, poor appetite and vomiting due to deficiency cold and qi stagnation in the middle *jiao*; and diarrhea before dawn due to yang deficiency in the spleen and kidney. *Hē zǐ* (Fructus Chebulae) is bitter, sour and astringent

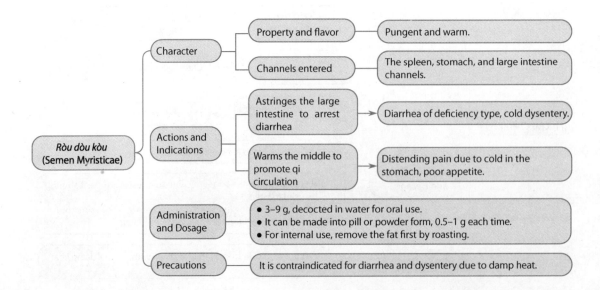

in flavor, and neutral in property. It is able to astringe the lung to stop cough, and descend qi to relieve sore throat and loss of voice. It is often used for chronic cough and loss of voice due to lung deficiency or phlegm heat accumulation in the lung.

Ròu dòu kòu (Semen Myristicae) and *bái dòu kòu* (Fructus Amomi Kravanh) are pungent in flavor and warm in property. They can warm the middle to promote qi flow. Both medicinals are used for deficiency cold and qi stagnation in the middle *jiao*, manifesting as epigastric and abdominal distending pain, poor appetite and vomiting. However, the two medicinals have different actions. *Ròu dòu kòu* (Semen Myristicae) is the ripe seed of the tree *Myristica fragrans* Houtt., of the family Myristicacene. It enters the large intestine channel and has a strong astringent action, and is effective for astringing the large intestine to arrest diarrhea. Therefore,

it is commonly used for chronic diarrhea due to deficiency cold of the spleen and stomach, and diarrhea before dawn due to yang deficiency of the spleen and kidney. *Bái dòu kòu* (Fructus Amomi Kravanh) is the ripe fruit of Amomum kravanh Pirreex Gagnep., or Amomum compactum Soland. Ex Maton., Zingiberaceae. It also enters the lung channel, and has a strong action in promoting qi flow. It is effective for transforming damp, and warming the stomach to relieve vomiting. It is commonly used for epigastric and abdominal distending pain, with no desire to eat due to damp obstruction in the middle *jiao* or qi stagnation in the spleen and stomach; damp warmth in the initial stage; and vomiting due to cold of the stomach.

⑧ *Chì shí zhī* (赤石脂, Halloysitum Rubrum, Halloysite) ★

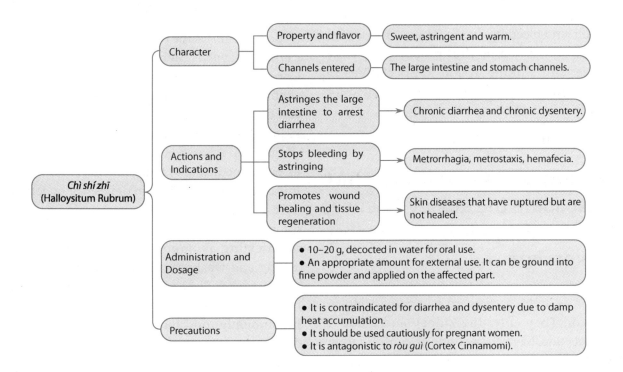

Chì shí zhī (Halloysitum Rubrum)

- **Character**
  - **Property and flavor** — Sweet, astringent and warm.
  - **Channels entered** — The large intestine and stomach channels.
- **Actions and Indications**
  - **Astringes the large intestine to arrest diarrhea** → Chronic diarrhea and chronic dysentery.
  - **Stops bleeding by astringing** → Metrorrhagia, metrostaxis, hemafecia.
  - **Promotes wound healing and tissue regeneration** → Skin diseases that have ruptured but are not healed.
- **Administration and Dosage**
  - 10–20 g, decocted in water for oral use.
  - An appropriate amount for external use. It can be ground into fine powder and applied on the affected part.
- **Precautions**
  - It is contraindicated for diarrhea and dysentery due to damp heat accumulation.
  - It should be used cautiously for pregnant women.
  - It is antagonistic to *ròu guì* (Cortex Cinnamomi).

⑨ *Yǔ yú liáng* (禹余粮, Limonitum, Limonite)

Chì shí zhī (Halloysitum Rubrum) and *yǔ yú liáng* (Limonitum) are sweet and astringent in flavor. They are able to astringe the large intestine to arrest diarrhea, stop bleeding and reduce

leukorrhea. They are used for instability of the lower *jiao* with slippery intestines, manifesting as chronic diarrhea, chronic dysentery, hemafecia, anal prolapse, metrorrhagia, metrostaxis and leukorrhagia. The two medicinals are often used

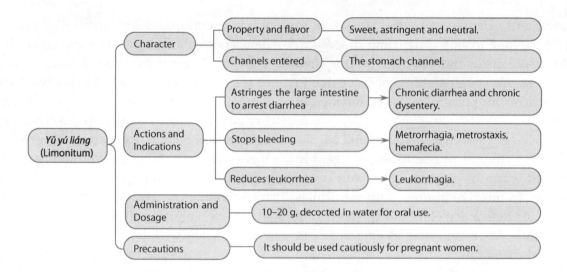

in combination for mutual reinforcement. *Chì shí zhī* (Halloysitum Rubrum) is warm in property. It can remove damp, promote wound healing and tissue regeneration when used externally. It is also used for skin diseases that have ruptured but are not healing, damp ulcers with watery effusion, and bleeding due to trauma. *Yǔ yú liáng* (Limonitum) has a neutral property, a heavy texture, and sinking action. It specializes in consolidating the lower *jiao*, and is indicated for qi collapse of the lower *jiao*.

Section 3 Medicinals that Consolidate the Kidney Essence, Reduce Urination and Arrest Leukorrhea

Medicinals in this section are sour and astringent in flavor. They enter the kidney and bladder channels and have the actions of consolidating kidney essence, reducing urination and arresting leukorrhea. Some of the medicinals are sweet in flavor and warm in property, and can nourish the kidney. Medicinals of this kind are indicated for instability of a deficient kidney manifesting as seminal emission, spermatorrhea, enuresis, frequent urination and leukorrhagia with watery discharge.

① *Shān zhū yú* (山茱萸, Fructus Corni, Asiatic Cornelian Cherry Fruit) ★ ★ ★

Shān zhū yú (Fructus Corni) and *wú zhū yú* (Fructus Evodiae) are warm in property and enter the liver channel. They have different origins and therefore have varied actions. *Shān zhū yú* (Fructus Corni) is the flesh of the deciduous arbor *Cornus officinalis* Sieb. Et Zucc., of the family Cornaceae. It is sour, and astringent in flavor, and slightly warm in property with a moist texture. It can tonify the kidney to promote production of kidney essence and warm the kidney to reinforce yang. It can nourish both yin and yang, and is an essential medicinal to tonify the liver and kidney. It is commonly used for yin deficiency in both the liver and kidney, manifesting as dizziness, aching lumbus and tinnitus; deficiency of kidney yang, manifesting as impotence, low sperm count, aching and weakness of the lumbus and knees, and dysuria. *Shān zhū yú* (Fructus Corni) can tonify the liver and kidney as well as astringe. It is commonly used for instability due to kidney deficiency, manifesting with seminal emission, spermatorrhea, enuresis, frequent urination; deficiency of the liver and kidney leading to instability of the *chong* and *ren* vessels, with manifestations such as metrorrhagia, metrostaxis, excessive menstrual bleeding, sweating, and collapse due to deficiency. *Wú zhū yú* (Fructus Evodiae) is from the nearly matured fruit of *Evodia rutaecarpa* (Juss) Benth, of the family

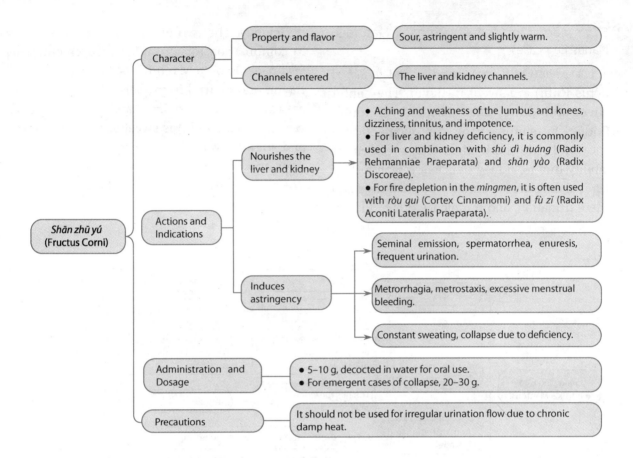

Rutaceae. It is pungent and bitter in flavor, and hot in property. It can both dispel cold in the liver and relieve liver qi constraint. It is able to dispel cold to relieve pain, and soothe the liver to descend qi. Therefore, it is commonly used for abdominal pain due to cold hernia; parietal headache, vomiting of saliva, cold pain in the epigastrium and abdomen caused by deficiency cold in the liver and stomach, leading to the adverse flow of turbid yin. It is considered an essential medicinal to treat various pains due to

cold stagnation in the liver channel. It can also dry damp, warm the middle to relieve vomiting, and strengthen yang to arrest diarrhea. It is often used for beriberi with swelling and pain due to cold damp, or upward rushing in the abdomen; vomiting due to cold in the stomach; vomiting and sour regurgitation due to liver constraint transforming into fire; and diarrhea before dawn due to yang deficiency of the spleen and kidney.

② *Fù pén zǐ* (覆盆子, Fructus Rubi, Raspberry) ★

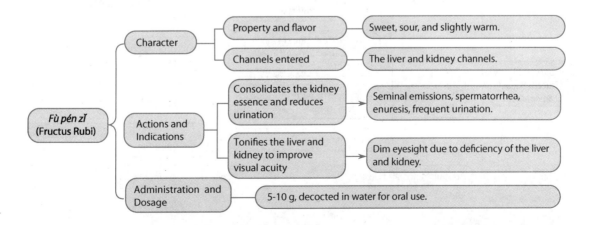

③ *Sāng piāo xiāo* (桑螵蛸, Ootheca Mantidis, Mantis Egg-case) ★★★

Sāng piāo xiāo (Ootheca Mantidis) and *fù pén zǐ* (Fructus Rubi) are sweet in flavor. They enter the liver and kidney channels, and can tonify the kidney to reinforce yang, consolidate kidney essence, and reduce urination. They are used for instability due to kidney deficiency, manifesting as seminal emission, spermatorrhea, enuresis and frequent urination; and impotence due to kidney deficiency. The two medicinals are often used in combination for mutual reinforcement. *Sāng piāo xiāo* (Ootheca Mantidis) is sweet and salty in flavor, and neutral in property. It is suitable for enuresis, frequent urination and leukorrhagia. *Fù pén zǐ* (Fructus Rubi) is sweet and sour in flavor, and slightly warm in property. It can tonify the liver and kidney, and is used for dim eyesight due to deficiency of the liver and kidney.

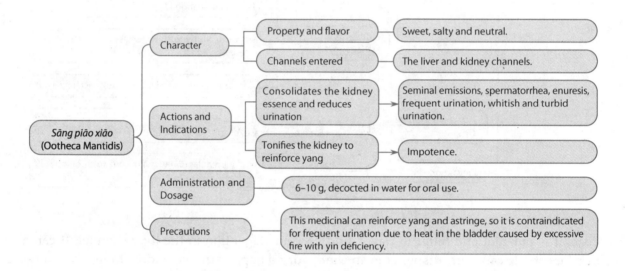

④ *Jīn yīng zǐ* (金樱子, Fructus Rosae Laevigatae, Cherokee Rose Fruit) ★

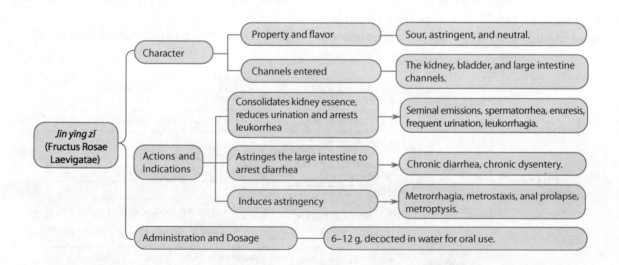

⑤ *Hǎi piāo xiāo* (海螵蛸, Endoconcha Sepiae, Cuttlebone)

Both *sāng piāo xiāo* (Ootheca Mantidis) and *hǎi piāo xiāo* (Endoconcha Sepiae) enter the liver and kidney, and have the actions of consolidating kidney essence, reducing urination and arresting leukorrhea. They are used for seminal emissions, spermatorrhea, enuresis, frequent urination and leukorrhagia. However, the two medicinals have different origins and therefore have varied actions. *Sāng piāo xiāo* (Ootheca Mantidis) is the egg case of *Tenodera sinensis* Saussure, *Statilia maculata* (Thunberg), or *Hierodula patellifera* (Serville), of the Mantis Branch. It is sweet and salty in flavor, and neutral in property. It is able to tonify the kidney so as to reinforce, and is used for various diseases caused by kidney yang

deficiency. It is suitable for enuresis and frequent urination, as well as impotence. *Hǎi piāo xiāo* (Endoconcha Sepiae) is the internal shell of the mollusk *sepiella maindroni* de Rochebrune., or *Sepia esculenta* Hoyle, of the family Sepidae. It is salty and astringent in flavor, and slightly warm in property. It has a strong action in inducing astringency. It is often used for seminal emissions and leukorrhagia. It can also stop bleeding, restrain the excessive secretion of gastric acid to relieve pain, remove damp and promote wound healing (when used externally). It is often used for metrorrhagia, metrostaxis, hematemesis, hemafecia, and bleeding due to trauma; vomiting of gastric acid with stomachache; damp ulcers, eczema, and ulcers that will not heal.

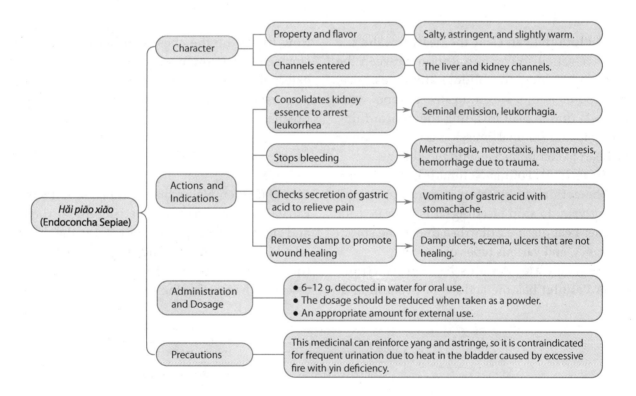

⑥ *Lián zǐ* (莲子, Semen Nelumbinis, Lotus Seed) ★★★

Addition: *Lián xū* (莲须, **Stamen Nelumbinis, Lotus Stamen**) has the effect of consolidating the kidney essence, and is indicated for seminal emission, spermatorrhea, leukorrhagia and frequent urination.

Lián fáng (莲房, **Receptaculum Nelumbinis, Lotus Receptacle**) can stop bleeding and transform stasis. It is indicated for metrorrhagia, metrostaxis, hemorrhoids with bleeding, postpartum abdominal pain due to blood stasis, and lochiostasis.

Lián zǐ xīn (莲子心, **Plumula Nelumbinis,**

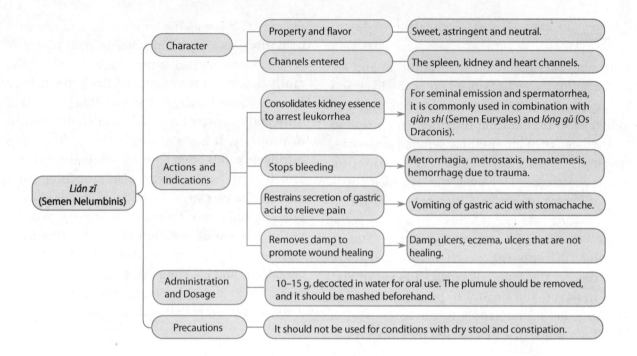

Lotus Plumule) can clear the heart to calm the mind, re-establish communication between the heart and kidney, consolidate kidney essence, and stop bleeding. It is indicated for coma and delirium due to heat invading the pericardium; insomnia and seminal emission due to failure of the heart to communicate with the kidney.

Hé yè (荷叶, **Folium Nelumbinis, Lotus Leaf)** has the actions of clearing summer-heat, and raising yang to stop bleeding. It is indicated for summer-heat diseases, diarrhea due to the spleen deficiency, and various types of bleeding.

Hé gěng (荷梗, **Petiolus Nelmbinis, Hindu Lotus Petiole)** has the actions of promoting qi flow to soothe the chest and harmonizing the stomach to prevent miscarriage. It is indicated for external invasion by summer-heat damp, chest oppression and discomfort, vomiting during pregnancy, and excessive fetal movement.

⑦ *Qiàn shí* (芡实, Semen Euryales, Gordon Euryale Seed) ★★

Lián zǐ (Semen Nelumbinis) and *qiàn shí* (Semen Euryales) are sweet and astringent in flavor, and neutral in property. They enter the spleen and kidney channels, and have the actions of tonifying the kidney to consolidate kidney essence, invigorating the spleen to arrest diarrhea,

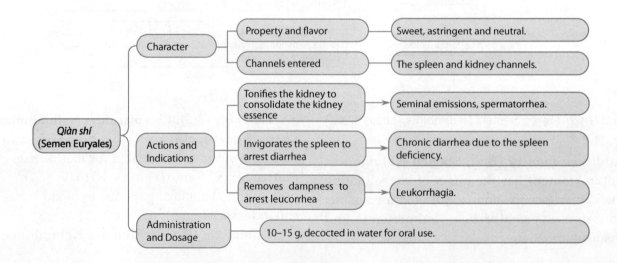

and stopping leukorrhea. For seminal emission, spermatorrhea, enuresis and frequent urination due to kidney deficiency, they are always used in combination with *lóng gǔ* (Os Draconis) and *mǔ lì* (Concha Ostreae). They can also be used in combination for chronic diarrhea, poor appetite and leukorrhagia due to spleen deficiency, or constant leukorrhagia due to both spleen and kidney deficiency. *Lián zǐ* (Semen Nelumbinis) mainly tonifies the spleen and has a stronger action than *qiàn shí* (Semen Euryales), which is known as "*the fruit for tonifying the spleen*". Meanwhile, it also enters the heart channel, and can nourish the heart to calm the mind, and reestablish communication between the heart and the kidney. It is used for deficiency vexation, palpitations, and insomnia due to failure of the heart to communicate with the kidney. *Qiàn shí* (Semen Euryales) mainly tonifies the kidney. It is inferior to *lián zǐ* (Semen Nelumbinis) in tonifying. However, it can remove damp. It is able to astringe without drying fluids, stagnating the stomach or retaining damp. Therefore it is commonly used for chronic diarrhea and leukorrhagia due to damp exuberance with spleen deficiency. It can also be used for leukorrhagia due

to damp heat when combined with medicinals for clearing heat and drying damp or medicinals for draining damp.

⑧ *Cì wei pí* (刺猬皮, Corium Erinacei, Hedgehog Skin)

Jīn yīng zǐ (Fructus Rosae Laevigatae) and *cì wei pí* (Corium Erinacei) can consolidate kidney essence and reduce urination. They specialize in consolidating the lower *jiao* without tonifying. They are used for seminal emission, spermatorrhea, enuresis and frequent urination. *Jīn yīng zǐ* (Fructus Rosae Laevigatae) is sour and astringent in flavor, and neutral in property. It has a stronger action of astringing compared with *cì wei pí* (Corium Erinacei). It can also arrest leukorrhea and astringe the large intestine to stop diarrhea. It is used for metrorrhagia, metrostaxis, leukorrhagia, chronic diarrhea and chronic dysentery. *Cì wei pí* (Corium Erinacei) is bitter and neutral with a descending action. It can stop bleeding by astringing and transform stasis to relieve pain. Therefore, it is used for hemafecia, hemorrhoids with bleeding, as well as stomachache and vomiting due to qi stagnation and blood stasis.

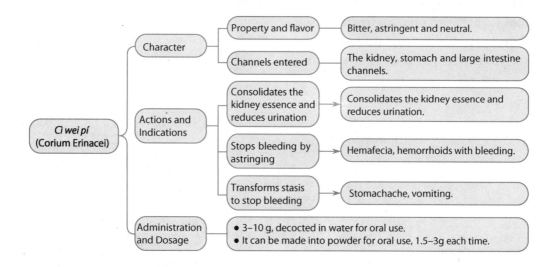

⑨ *Chūn pí* (椿皮, Cortex Ailanthi, Ailanthus Bark or Root Bark)

Both *chūn pí* (Cortex Ailanthi) and *shí liú pí* (Pericarpium Granati) have the actions of astringing the large intestine to arrest diarrhea, stopping

bleeding, arresting leukorrhea and killing parasites. They are used for chronic diarrhea, chronic dysentery, hemafecia, metrorrhagia, metrostaxis, leukorrhagia and abdominal pain due to ascariasis. In addition, they can kill parasites to relieve itching

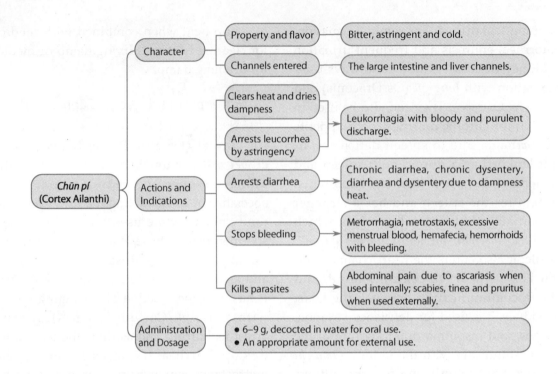

and are used for scabies, tinea and pruritus when used externally. *Chūn pí* (Cortex Ailanthi) is bitter and astringent in flavor, and cold in property. It is effective for clearing heat and drying damp. It is often used for diarrhea and dysentery due to damp heat, leukorrhea with a yellowish, thick discharge; metrorrhagia, metrostaxis and excessive menstrual bleeding due to blood heat. *Shí liú pí* (Pericarpium Granati) is sour and astringent in flavor, warm in property. It is effective for astringing the large intestine to arrest diarrhea, and is often used for chronic diarrhea and dysentery. In addition, it can consolidate kidney essence by astringing and is used for seminal emission and spermatorrhea.

⑩ *Jī guān huā* (鸡冠花, Flos Celosiae Cristatae, Cockcomb Flower)

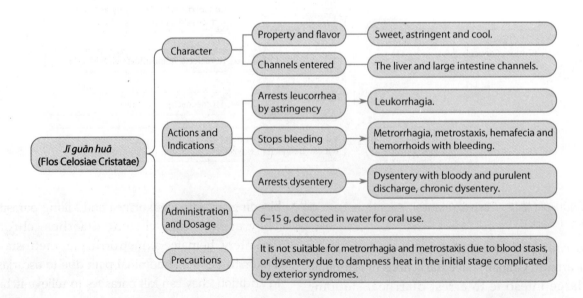

Actions of astringent medicinals are summarized in the following table (Table 25-1):

Table 25-1: Summary of Astringent Medicinals:

Medicinal	Action in Common		Individual Character	
			Characteristic Actions	Other Actions
Má huáng gēn (Radix et Rhizoma Ephedrae)	These are usually sour and astringent in flavor, warm or neutral in property. They mainly enter the lung, spleen, kidney and large intestine channels. They have the effect of astringing and are used to arrest discharge.	Consolidates the exterior to arrest sweating, indicated for spontaneous sweating and night sweating	It has a pure and strong action, which can arrest sweating when used internally and externally.	
Fú xiǎo mài (Fructus Tritici Levis)		Reduces deficient fever	Replenishes qi	
Nuò dào gēn xū (Radix Oryzae Glutinosae)			Benefits the stomach to promote fluid production	
Wǔ wèi zǐ (Fructus Schisandrae Chinensis)		These are medicinals with the actions of astringing the lung and large intestine. They can astringe the lung to stop cough, astringe the large intestine to arrest diarrhea and dysentery.	These astringe the lung to stop cough, astringe the large intestine to arrest diarrhea	Consolidates kidney essence, arrests sweating. It has a strong action in astringing, and is an essential medicinal to treat chronic cough and deficiency panting.	Replenishes qi and promotes fluid production, tonifies the kidney and calms the heart.
Wǔ bèi zǐ (Galla Chinensis)				Consolidates kidney essence, arrests sweating, descends qi, stops bleeding by astringing. Removes damp and promotes wound healing when used externally.	
Wū méi (Fructus Mume)				Relieves ascariasis to stop pain, promotes fluid production to relieve thirst, arrests metrorrhagia and stops bleeding	
Hē zǐ (Fructus Chebulae)				Descends qi to relieve sore throat and loss of voice, is an essential medicinal to treat loss of voice	
Yīng sù qiào (Pericarpium Papaveris)				Toxic, is effective for relieving pain	
Shí liú pí (Pericarpium Granati)			Astringes the large intestine to arrest diarrhea	Kills parasites, stops bleeding by astringing	
Ròu dòu kòu (Pericarpium Granati)				It is effective for warming the middle to promote the flow of qi.	
Chì shí zhī (Halloysitum Rubrum)			Astringes the large intestine to arrest diarrhea, stops bleeding by astringency, arrests leukorrhea	Removes damp, promotes wound healing and tissue regeneration	
Yǔ yú liáng (Limonitum)				It has a heavy texture, and specializes in consolidating and astringing the lower *jiao*.	

Table 25-1: Summary of Astringent Medicinals:

continued

Medicinal	Action in Common			Individual Character	
				Characteristic Actions	Other Actions
Shān zhū yú (Fructus Corni)	These are usually sour and astringent in flavor, warm or neutral in property. They mainly enter the lung, spleen, kidney and large intestine channels. They have the effect of astringing and are used to arrest discharge	These are medicinals for consolidating kidney essence, reducing urination and arresting leukorrhea. They are indicated for seminal emission, spermatorrhea, enuresis, frequent urination and leukorrhagia with watery discharge caused by instability and kidney deficiency		It can tonify the liver and kidney as well as astringe. It has a warm property and moderate tonic action. It is an essential medicinal to nourish yin and yang, consolidate kidney essence to arrest discharge.	
Sāng piāo xiāo (Ootheca Mantidis)			Tonifies the kidney to reinforce yang, consolidates kidney essence and reduces urination	It is suitable to treat enuresis, frequent urination and leukorrhagia.	
Fù pén zǐ (Fructus Rubi)				Tonifies the liver and kidney to improve visual acuity	
Hǎi piāo xiāo (Endoconcha Sepiae)			Consolidates kidney essence and arrests leukorrhea	It has a strong astringing action, but cannot tonify.	Stops bleeding by astringing, checks excessive secretion of gastric acid to relieve pain, relieves damp and promotes wound healing
Jīn yīng zǐ (Fructus Rosae Laevigatae)				It has a strong astringing action	Reduces urination, arrests leukorrhea, astringes the large intestine to arrest diarrhea
Lián zǐ (Semen Nelumbinis)			Tonifies the kidney to consolidate kidney essence, invigorates the spleen to arrest diarrhea, arrests leukorrhea	It can mainly tonify the spleen, and has a stronger tonifying action than *qiàn shí* (Semen Euryales).	Nourishes the heart to calm the mind, promotes communication between the heart and kidney
Qiàn shí (Semen Euryales)				It can mainly tonify the kidney. Although it has a milder tonifying action than *Lián zǐ* (Semen Nelumbinis), it can remove damp and astringe without drying fluids, stagnating the stomach or retaining damp. It is commonly used for chronic diarrhea and leukorrhagia due to spleen deficiency with damp exuberance.	
Chūn pí (Cortex Ailanthi)			Arrests leukorrhea by astringing, stops bleeding, arrests diarrhea and dysentery	It is effective for clearing heat and drying damp. It is often used for diarrhea, dysentery and leukorrhagia with purulent and bloody discharge due to damp heat.	
Jī guān huā (Flos Celosiae Cristatae)				It is commonly used for leukorrhagia.	
Cì wei pí (Semen Euryales)				Consolidates kidney essence, reduces urination, stops bleeding by astringing, transforms stasis to relieve pain	

Tables for testing your herbal knowledge
of astringent medicinals are as follows (Tables
25-2~25-5):

Table 25-2: Test your Herbal Knowledge of the Actions of Astringent Medicinals (one):

Actions \ Medicinal	Wǔ wèi zǐ	Wū méi	Wǔ bèi zǐ	Yīng sù qiào	Hē zǐ	Shí liú pí	Ròu dòu kòu	Chì shí zhī	Yǔ yú liáng
Astringes the lung and nourishes the kidney									
Arrests sweating									
Promotes fluid production to relieve thirst									
Calms the mind to tranquilize the mind									
Astringes the lung to stop cough									
Astringes the large intestine to arrest diarrhea									
Relieves ascariasis to relieve pain									
Astringes kidney essence to arrest diarrhea									
Descends fire									
Consolidates kidney essence to arrest discharge									
Stops bleeding by astringing									
Relieves pain									
Relieves sore throat and loss of voice									
Kills parasites									
Warms the middle to promote qi flow									
Stops bleeding									
Promotes wound healing and tissue regeneration									
Arrests leukorrhea									

Table 25-3: Test your Herbal Knowledge of the Actions of Astringent Medicinals (two):

Actions \ Medicinal	Shān zhū yú	Fù pén zǐ	Sāng piāo xiāo	Hǎi piāo xiāo	Jīn yīng zǐ	Lián zǐ	Qiàn shí	Má huáng gēn	Fú xiǎo mài	Nuò dào gēn xū
Removes damp and promotes wound healing										
Astringes										
Tonifies the kidney										
Invigorates the spleen to arrest diarrhea										
Tonifies the kidney to reinforce yang										
Consolidates kidney essence and arrests leukorrhea										
Stops bleeding by astringing										
Restrains excessive gastric acid to relieve pain										
Tonifies the liver and kidney										
Astringes the large intestine to arrest diarrhea										

Table 25-3: Test your Herbal Knowledge of the Actions of Astringent Medicinals (two):

continued

Actions \ Medicinal	Shān zhū yú	Fù pén zǐ	Sāng piāo xiāo	Hǎi piāo xiāo	Jīn yīng zǐ	Lián zǐ	Qiàn shí	Má huáng gēn	Fú xiǎo mài	Nuò dào gēn xū
Tonifies the kidney to consolidate kidney essence										
Reduces deficiency fever										
Arrests leukorrhea										
Nourishes the heart										
Consolidates kidney essence and reduces urination										
Removes damp to arrest leukorrhea										
Arrests sweating										
Replenishes qi										
Removes heat										
Tonifies the spleen to arrest diarrhea										

Table 25-4: Test your Herbal Knowledge of the Indications of Astringent Medicinals (one):

Indications \ Medicinal	Wǔ wèi zǐ	Wǔ méi	Wǔ bèi zǐ	Yīng sù qiào	Hē zǐ	Shí liú pí	Ròu dòu kòu	Chì shí zhī	Yǔ yú liáng
Metrorrhagia, metrostaxis									
Cough and panting due to liver and kidney deficiency									
Thirst due to fluid consumption									
Diabetes due to internal heat									
Spontaneous sweating, night sweating									
Seminal emissions, spermatorrhea									
Anal prolapse									
Palpitations, insomnia, frequent dreams									
Abdominal pain and vomiting due to ascariasis									
Chronic cough due to lung deficiency									
Hemafecia, hemorrhoids with bleeding									
Ulcers, furuncles									
Loss of voice									
Stomachache, abdominal pain, pain of the sinews and bones									
Ascariasis, enterobiasis, taeniasis									
Distending pain, poor appetite and vomiting due to stomach cold									
Skin diseases that have ruptured but are not healing									
Damp ulcers with watery effusion									
Chronic diarrhea									
Leukorrhagia									

Table 25-5: Test your Herbal Knowledge of the Indications of Astringent Medicinals (two):

Medicinal / Indications	Shān zhū yú	Fù pén zǐ	Sāng piāo xiāo	Hǎi piāo xiāo	Jīn yīng zǐ	Lián zǐ	Qiàn shí	Má huáng gēn	Fú xiǎo mài	Nuò dào gēn xū
Dizziness due to liver and kidney deficiency										
Collapse with excessive sweating										
Impotence due to kidney yang deficiency										
Seminal emission, enuresis										
Metrorrhagia, metrostaxis										
Lumbar aches, tinnitus										
Chronic diarrhea, chronic dysentery										
Dim eyesight due to liver and kidney insufficiency										
Leukorrhagia										
Steaming bones with fever										
Hemorrhage due to trauma										
Vomiting of gastric acid with stomachache										
Damp ulcers, eczema										
Ulcers that are not healing										
Diabetes due to internal heat										
Poor appetite due to spleen deficiency										
Vexation, palpitations and insomnia due to failure of the heart to communicate with the kidney										
Spontaneous sweating, night sweating										
Hematemesis, hemafecia										

Chapter 26
Emetics

Concept

Medicinals whose principle effect is to treat diseases caused by poisonous materials, food, or phlegm retention in the stomach or above the chest and diaphragm are called emetics.

Character and Actions

Medicinals of this chapter are usually sour, bitter and pungent in flavor and enter the stomach channel. They act to cause vomiting of poisonous materials, foods, and phlegm-fluids.

Indications

Medicinals in this chapter are indicated for the accidental ingestion of poisons which are then retained in the stomach prior to digestion; gastric distending pain due to food retention; phlegm-fluids obstruction in the chest and diaphragm or throat that cause dyspnea; phlegm-turbidity invading upwards that cloud the clear orifices and lead to epilepsy and madness.

Precautions

Emetics have drastic actions and are toxic; therefore they can impair the stomach and the right qi, so they are used only for cases that have both a pattern of excess and excess manifestations. To ensure their safe use and efficiency, when using emetics doctors should start with a small dosage, and then gradually increase the dosage. Large dosages are prohibited. At the same time, emetics should be discontinued as long as the condition is improving. Successive or long-term use of these medicinals should be avoided so as not to cause side effects such as poisoning or excessive vomiting. If the therapeutic effect is not as strong as desired, the patient can drink hot water or tickle their throat with a feather to induce vomiting. If there is constant vomiting after taking the medicinals, they should be discontinued immediately. Active measures should be taken in cases of emergency. After vomiting, the patient should rest, and the immediate intake of food should be avoided. After the stomach function has recovered, liquid food or easily digestible food should be given to nourish the stomach qi. Eating greasy and spicy food is prohibited. Emetics are prohibited for the elderly, the weak, infants, during pregnancy, for women postpartum, for patients with blood loss, dizziness, palpitations, deficiency taxation cough, and panting. As the emetics have violent actions and will always cause suffering to patients after they ingest them, they are rarely used in modern clinical practice.

① *Cháng shān* (常山, Radix Dichroae, Dichroa Root) ★★

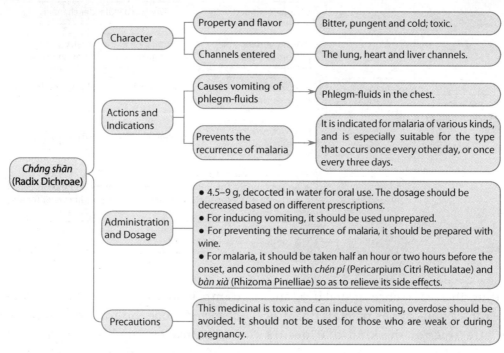

② *Guā dì* (瓜蒂, Pedicellus Melo, Muskmelon Fruit Pedicel) ★★

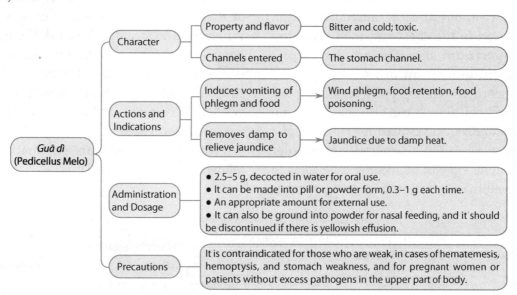

③ *Dǎn fán* (胆矾, Chalcanthitum, Chalcanthite) ★★

Cháng shān (Radix Dichroae), *guā dì* (Pedicellus Melo) and *dǎn fán* (Chalcanthitum) are toxic. They have the actions of inducing the vomiting of poisonous food, retained food, phlegm or saliva. They are used for the accidental ingestion of poisonous substances which are then retained in the stomach prior to digestion; gastric distending pain due to food retention; phlegm-fluids obstruction in the chest and diaphragm or throat that cause dyspnea; phlegm-turbidity invading upwards that cloud the clear orifice and lead to epilepsy and madness. *Cháng shān* (Radix Dichroae) is effective for inducing the vomiting of phlegm and saliva, and is indicated for phlegm-fluids in the chest. It is also effective

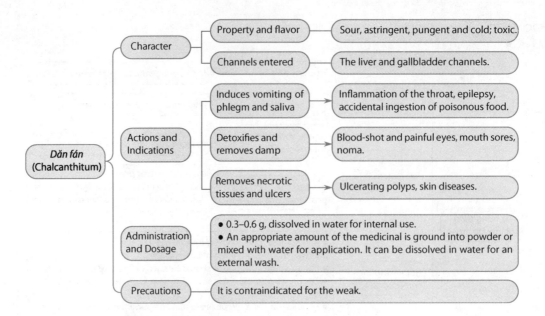

	Character	Property and flavor	Sour, astringent, pungent and cold; toxic.
		Channels entered	The liver and gallbladder channels.
Dǎn fán (Chalcanthitum)	Actions and Indications	Induces vomiting of phlegm and saliva	Inflammation of the throat, epilepsy, accidental ingestion of poisonous food.
		Detoxifies and removes damp	Blood-shot and painful eyes, mouth sores, noma.
		Removes necrotic tissues and ulcers	Ulcerating polyps, skin diseases.
	Administration and Dosage	• 0.3–0.6 g, dissolved in water for internal use. • An appropriate amount of the medicinal is ground into powder or mixed with water for application. It can be dissolved in water for an external wash.	
	Precautions	It is contraindicated for the weak.	

for preventing the recurrence of malaria, and is suitable for various types of malaria; it is especially effective for the kind that occurs once every other day, three times a day. *Guā dì* (Pedicellus Melo) is effective for inducing the vomiting of hot phlegm, and retained food. It is indicated for various diseases caused by phlegm heat retention in the chest and food retention in the epigastrium, manifesting as epilepsy, madness, inflammation of the throat with panting, gastric distending pain, vexation, poor appetite, and belching. It can also remove damp to relieve jaundice, and is used for jaundice of a damp heat type. It can be ground into powder and used alone via a nasal feeding tube so as to release a yellowish effusion in order to remove damp heat to treat jaundice. It can also be decocted alone, or ground into powder for oral use for treating jaundice. *Dǎn fán* (Chalcanthitum) is effective for inducing vomiting of phlegm and saliva, and is indicated for wind phlegm obstruction, inflammation of the throat, epilepsy or the accidental ingestion of poisonous food. When used externally, it can detoxify, remove damp, remove necrotic tissues and ulcers, and is used for blood-shot and painful eyes, mouth sores, ulcerative gingivitis, as well as failure of swellings to rupture, and abnormal growth of the conjuntiva with pain.

Actions of emetics are summarized in the following table (Table 26-1):

Table 26-1: Summary of Emetics:

Medicinal	Action in Common	Individual Character	
		Characteristic Actions	Other Actions
Cháng shān (Radix Dichroae)	Toxic, induces the vomiting of poisonous substances, retained food, phlegm or saliva	It is effective for inducing the vomiting of phlegm and saliva, and is indicated for phlegm-fluids accumulation.	Prevents the recurrence of malaria
Guā dì (Pedicellus Melo)		It is effective for inducing the vomiting of hot phlegm, or retained food, and is indicated for various diseases caused by phlegm heat accumulated in the chest, food retention in the stomach.	Removes damp to relieve jaundice
Dǎn fán (Chalcanthitum)		It is effective for inducing the vomiting of wind phlegm and poisonous substances, and is indicated for wind phlegm accumulation, inflammation of the throat, epilepsy, or accidental ingestion of poisonous food.	Detoxifies, removes damp, removes necrotic tissues when used externally

Tables to test your herbal knowledge of actions and indications of emetics are as follows (Tables 26-2 and 26-3):

Table 26-2: Test your Herbal Knowledge of Actions of Emetics:

Medicinal / Actions	Cháng shān	Guā dì	Dǎn fán
Induces the vomiting of phlegm and saliva			
Prevents the recurrence of malaria			
Induces the vomiting of phlegm and food			
Removes damp to relieve jaundice			
Detoxifies, removes damp			
Removes necrotic tissues			

Table 26-3: Test your Herbal Knowledge of Indications of Emetics:

Medicinal / Indications	Cháng shān	Guā dì	Dǎn fán
Phlegm-fluids in the chest			
Inflammation of the throat			
Phlegm heat accumulated in the chest			
Necrotic tissues			
Jaundice of a damp heat type			
Epilepsy and convulsions due to wind phlegm			
Malaria			
Blood shot and painful eyes			
Mouth sores, noma			
Swellings without ulceration			
Food retention in the stomach			

Chapter 27
Medicinals that Attack Toxins, Kill Parasites and Stop Itching

Concept

Medicinals whose principle effect is to attack toxins to treat sores, kill parasites and stop itching are called medicinals that attack toxins, kill parasites and stop itching.

Indications

Medicinals of this kind are usually used in the departments of external medicine, dermatology and otorhinolaryngology. They treat such things as ulcers, carbuncles, furuncles, scabies, tinea, eczema, otopyorrhea (chronic otitis media with eardrum perforation and purulent discharge), syphilis, insect and snake bites, and cancerous masses.

Precautions

Medicinals of this kind are mostly used both externally and internally. The application method varies according to the different disease present.

The medicinals can be ground into a fine powder and then sprinkled on the affected area, decocted for an external wash, ground for a hot application, used for a bath or rinsing the mouth, ground and mixed with oil or water for applications, made into an ointment for smearing, or made into patent medicine twists or suppositories. When such medicinals are used internally, they should be made into a pill or powder form to allow them to melt and be absorbed gradually. Medicinals in this chapter have a range of toxicities, and they are used based on the theory of *"removing toxic material by using toxic medicinals"*. Whether they are used externally or internally, doctors should tightly control the dosage. Overdose or long-term use should be avoided so as not to induce side effects. During the process of preparing the prescriptions, it is important to abide by processing and preparation standards, in order to reduce toxicity and ensure medication safety.

① *Xióng huáng* (雄黄, Realgar, Realgar) ★ ★ ★

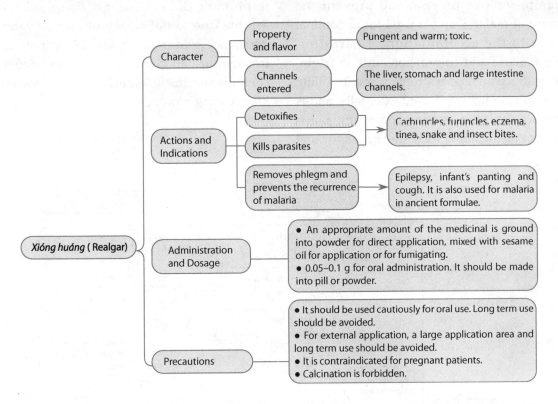

② *Liú huáng* (硫黄, Sulphur, Sulphur) ★ ★ ★

Both *xióng huáng* (Realgar) and *liú huáng* (Sulpur) are toxic medicinals with the actions of attacking toxins and killing parasites, and when applied externally are commonly used for scabies, tinea and chronic ulcers. *Xióng huáng* (Realgar) has a strong action in detoxifying to treat ulcers, and is indicated for carbuncles, furuncles and poisonous

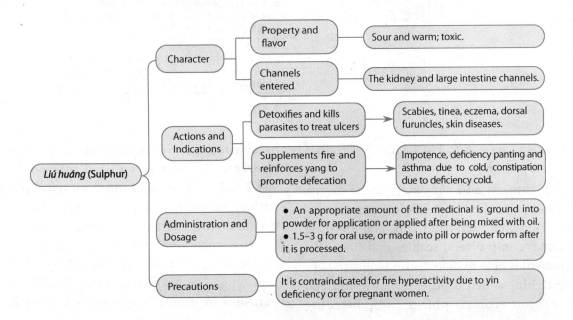

snake bites. In addition, it is able to kill parasites, dry damp, remove phlegm and prevent the recurrence of malaria, and is used for abdominal pain due to the accumulation of parasites, asthma, malaria and convulsions due to fright. *Liú huáng* (Sulphur) has a strong action in killing parasites to stop itching if used externally, and is used for scabies, tinea, eczema and pruritus. It is an essential medicinal to treat scabies. As for oral use, it can supplement fire and reinforce yang to promote defecation. It is also used for cold asthma due to deficiency of kidney yang, and deficiency cold in the lower *jiao*; impotence and frequent urination due to kidney deficiency; and constipation in the elderly due to deficiency of kidney yang with deficiency cold.

③ *Bái fán* (白矾, Alumen, Alum) ★★

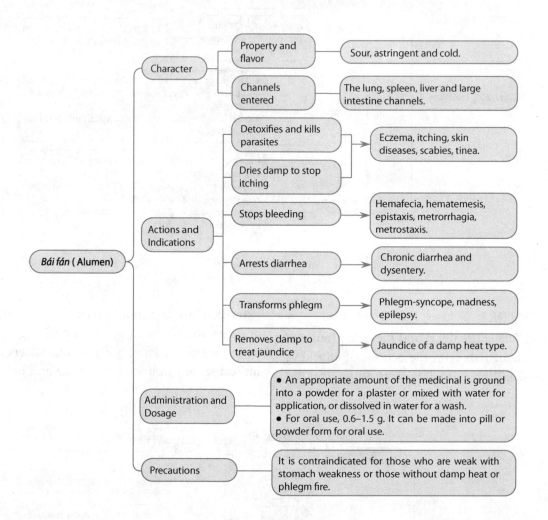

④ *Shé chuáng zǐ* (蛇床子, Fructus Cnidii, Common Cnidium Fruit) ★★

Bái fán (Alumen) and *shé chuáng zǐ* (Fructus Cnidii) are not toxic. They can kill parasites to stop itching when used externally, and are used for eczema, damp ulcers, scabies and tinea. *Bái fán* (Alumen) is able to detoxify and kill parasites to stop itching when used externally, and can clear heat to transform phlegm, stop bleeding by astringing, and astringe the large intestine to arrest diarrhea when used internally. It is also used for diseases caused by wind phlegm, such as syncope, epilepsy, madness, hemafecia, metrorrhagia, metrostaxis, hemorrhage due to trauma, chronic diarrhea and dysentery, anal prolapse, metroptosis, and jaundice of a damp heat type. *Shé chuáng zǐ* (Fructus Cnidii) can kill parasites to stop itching when used externally,

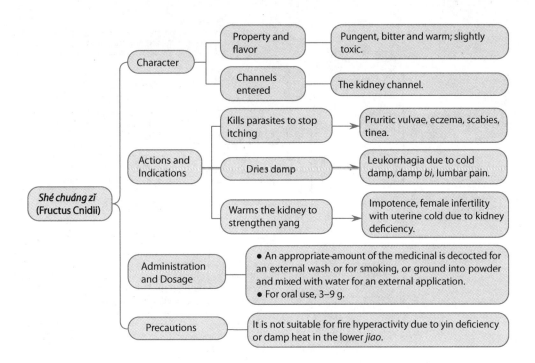

and warm the kidney to strengthen yang, dispel cold and expel wind damp when used internally. It is also used for kidney yang deficiency manifesting as impotence, female infertility, leukorrhagia of a cold damp kind, damp *bi*, and aching of the low back.

⑤ *Chán sū* (蟾酥, Venenum Bufonis, Toad Venom) ★★

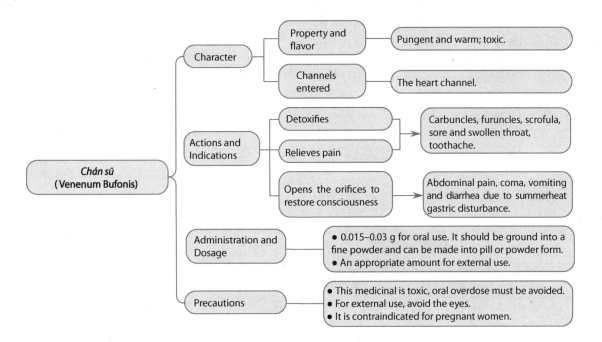

⑥ *Zhāng nǎo* (樟脑, Camphora, Camphor) ★

Chán sū (Venenum Bufonis) and *zhāng nǎo* (Camphora) are pungent in flavor, and warm or hot in property. They have migrating actions and can open the orifices to restore consciousness and repel foulness. Both medicinals are used for abdominal pain, vomiting, diarrhea or even coma due to summer-heat damp or improper diet. *Chán*

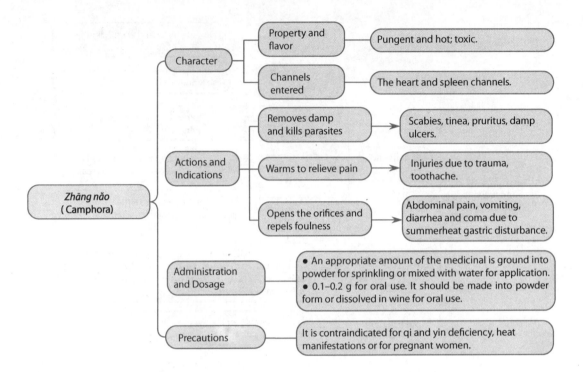

sū (Venenum Bufonis) has effective actions for attacking toxins and reducing swellings to relieve pain. It is also used for malignant skin tumors, ulcers, carbuncles, furuncles, scrofula, scarlet fever, sores due to wind, acute tonsillitis, sore and swollen throat, and toothache. In addition, in recent years it has been used for various types of carcinomas, such as liver cancer, intestinal cancer, leukemia and skin cancer; and it is efficient when used both externally and internally. *Zhāng nǎo* (Camphora) is able to remove damp, kill parasites and warm to relieve pain when used externally. Therefore it is used for scabies, tinea, pruritus, ulcerations, toothache, and injuries due to trauma.

⑦ *Mù biē zǐ* (木鳖子, Semen Momordicae, Cochinchina Momordica Seed) ★

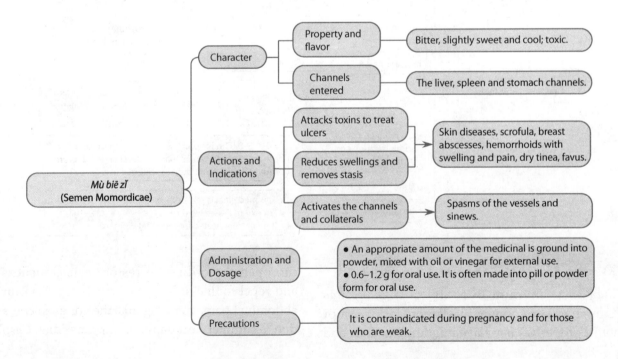

⑧ *Tǔ jīng pí* (土荆皮, Cortex Pseudolaricis, Golden Larch Bark) ★★

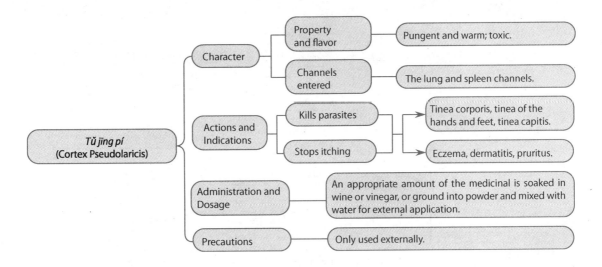

⑨ *Fēng fáng* (蜂房, Nidus Vespae, Honeycomb) ★★

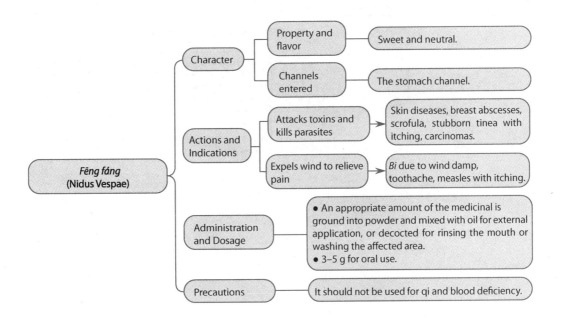

⑩ *Dà suàn* (大蒜, Bulbus Allii, Garlic Bulb) ★★

Fēng fáng (Nidus Vespae) and *dà suàn* (Bulbus Allii) have the actions of detoxifying and killing parasites. They are used for carbuncles, furuncles, scabies and tinea. *Fēng fáng* (Nidus Vespae) can also dispel wind to relieve pain and stop itching, and is used for *bi* due to wind damp, insidious rashes, pruritus and toothache. In addition, it is used for malignant tumors. *Dà suàn* (Bulbus Allii) can detoxify, kill parasites, reduce swellings, and arrest dysentery. It is used for diarrhea, dysentery, tuberculosis, pertussis, ancylostomiasis and enterobiasis.

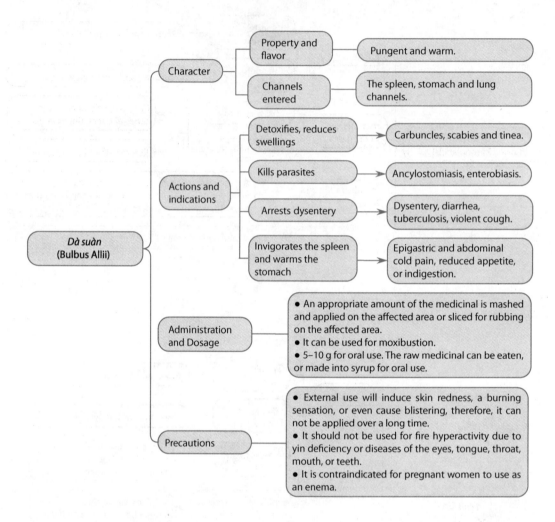

Character
- Property and flavor → Pungent and warm.
- Channels entered → The spleen, stomach and lung channels.

Dà suàn (Bulbus Allii)

Actions and indications
- Detoxifies, reduces swellings → Carbuncles, scabies and tinea.
- Kills parasites → Ancylostomiasis, enterobiasis.
- Arrests dysentery → Dysentery, diarrhea, tuberculosis, violent cough.
- Invigorates the spleen and warms the stomach → Epigastric and abdominal cold pain, reduced appetite, or indigestion.

Administration and Dosage
- An appropriate amount of the medicinal is mashed and applied on the affected area or sliced for rubbing on the affected area.
- It can be used for moxibustion.
- 5–10 g for oral use. The raw medicinal can be eaten, or made into syrup for oral use.

Precautions
- External use will induce skin redness, a burning sensation, or even cause blistering, therefore, it can not be applied over a long time.
- It should not be used for fire hyperactivity due to yin deficiency or diseases of the eyes, tongue, throat, mouth, or teeth.
- It is contraindicated for pregnant women to use as an enema.

Actions of medicinals that attack toxins, kill parasites and stop itching are summarized in the following table (Table 27-1):

Table 27-1: Summary of Medicinals that Attack Toxins, Kill Parasites and Stop Itching:

Medicinal	Action in Common		Individual Character	
			Characteristic Actions	Other Actions
Xióng huáng (Realgar)	Most of these are toxic. They can attack toxins, kill parasites and stop itching. They are indicated for skin diseases and facial diseases.	Detoxifies, kills parasites	It has a strong action in detoxifying to treat ulcers.	Kills parasites, dries damp, removes phlegm, prevents the recurrence of malaria
Liú huáng (Sulphur)			It has a strong action in killing parasites and stopping itching when used externally. It is often used for scabies, tinea, eczema and pruritus, and is regarded as an essential medicinal to treat scabies.	Supplements fire, strengthens yang to promote defecation when used internally.
Bái fán (Alumen)		Non-toxic, kills parasites and stops itching when used externally	Clears heat to transform phlegm, stops bleeding by astringing, astringes the large intestine to arrest diarrhea when used internally	
Shé chuáng zǐ (Fructus Cnidii)			Warms the kidney to strengthen yang, dispels cold, dispels wind, dries damp when used internally	
Chán sū (Venenum Bufonis)		Opens the orifices to restore consciousness, repels foulness	Attacks toxins, subsides swelling to relieve pain	
Zhāng nǎo (Camphora)			Removes damp, kills parasites, warms to relieve pain when used externally	
Fēng fáng (Nidus Vespae)		Attacks toxins, kill parasites	Dispels wind to relieve pain, stops itching	
Dà suàn (Bulbus Allii)			Reduces swellings, arrests dysentery	
Mù biē zǐ (Semen Momordicae)			Attacks toxins to treat ulcers, reduces swellings and removes stasis	
Tǔ jīng pí (Cortex Pseudolaricis)			Specializes in killing parasites to stop itching, indicated for tinea of various kinds	

Tables to test your herbal knowledge of the actions and indications of medicinals that attack toxins, kill parasites and stop itching are as follows (Tables 27-2 and 27-3):

Table 27-2: Test your Herbal Knowledge of the Actions of the Medicinals that Attack Toxins, Kill Parasites and Stop Itching:

Actions / Medicinal	Xióng huáng	Liú huáng	Bái fán	Shé chuáng zǐ	Tǔ jīng pí	Fēng fáng	Dà suàn
Detoxifies							
Dispels wind to relieve pain							
Detoxifies, kills parasites, stops itching							
Supplements fire, reinforces yang to promote defecation							
Transforms phlegm							
Warms the kidney to strengthen yang							
Arrests diarrhea							
Kills parasites to stop itching							
Stops bleeding							
Attacks toxins, kills parasites							
Dispels wind, dries damp							
Kills parasites							
Reduces swellings							
Arrests dysentery							

Table 27-3: Test your Herbal Knowledge of the Indications of the Medicinals that Attack Toxins, Kill Parasites and Stop Itching:

Indications / Medicinal	Xióng huáng	Liú huáng	Bái fán	Shé chuáng zǐ	Tǔ jīng pí	Fēng fáng	Dà suàn
Chronic diarrhea and dysentery							
Eczema, scabies, tinea							
Snake and insect bites							
Abdominal pain due to the accumulation of parasites							
Asthma of a cold type due to kidney yang deficiency							
Bi due to wind damp							
Constipation due to deficiency cold							
Carbuncles, furuncles							
Hemafecia, metrorrhagia, metrostaxis, bleeding due to trauma							
Epilepsy, convulsions and madness due to wind phlegm							
Female infertility due to cold of the uterus							
Diarrhea, dysentery							
Measles, syphilis							
Tinea of various kinds							
Scrofula							
Impotence							
Insidious rashes with itching							
Toothache due to wind fire							
Pruritic vulvae							
Tuberculosis, pertussis							
Hook worms, pinworms							

Chapter 28
Medicinals that Draw out Toxins, Expel Pus and Rejuvenate Flesh

Concept

Medicinals used externally for removing toxins and necrotic tissue, and promoting tissue regeneration and wound healing are referred to as medicinals that draw out toxins, expel pus and rejuvenate flesh.

Indications

Medicinals of this kind are indicated for carbuncles, furuncles and skin diseases that have ruptured but have difficult pus discharge, or with necrotic tissue, difficulty in tissue regeneration, carcinomas, and syphilis. Some of the medicinals are also commonly used for eczema, pruritus, mouth sores, inflammation of the throat, blood-shot eyes and nebulae.

Precautions

The application method of such medicinals varies according to different pathological conditions and usages. They are ground into powder for sprinkling, mixed with oil for applications, made into medicinal twists, made into ointments, or applied to the eyes, throat, nose or ears. Most of the medicinals are minerals, heavy metals, or are processed. Most of them are harshly toxic or strongly irritable, so their dosage and administration should be strictly controlled. They should not be used in overdose or for a long period of time externally. Some of the medicinals are not suitable to be applied on the face, head or mucus membranes, so as not to induce side effects and ensure safety. The ones that contain arsenic, mercury and lead have severe side effects, and therefore should be noted.

① *Shēng yào* (升药, Hydrargyrum Oxydatum Crudum, Mercuric Oxide) ★★★

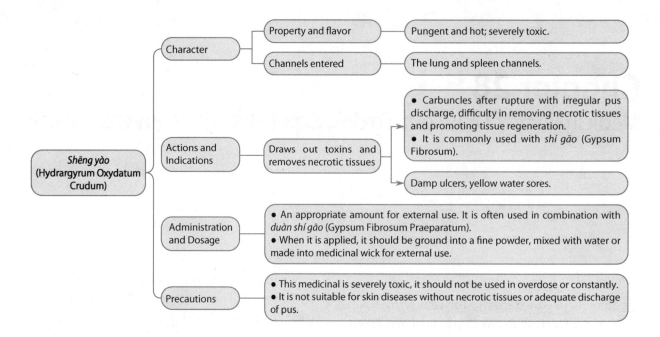

② *Qīng fěn* (轻粉, Calomelas, Calomel)

Shēng yào (Hydrargyrum Oxydatum Crudum) and *qīng fěn* (Calomelas) are medicinals that contain mercury. However, they have different actions. *Shēng yào* (Hydrargyrum Oxydatum Crudum) is pungent and hot with a severe toxicity. It is effective for drawing out toxins, removing necrotic tissues, and expelling pus. It is indicated for carbuncles after rupture but with restricted pus discharge; difficulty in removing necrotic tissues, and promoting tissue regeneration. It is a commonly used medicinal in

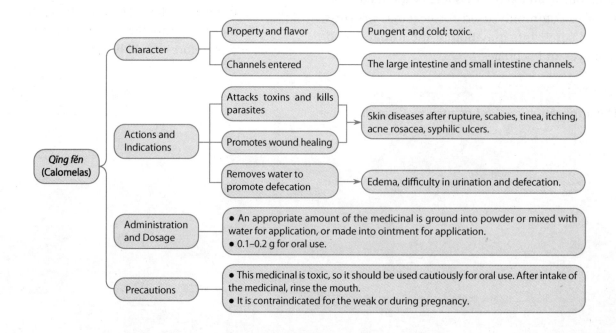

traumatology and is often used with *duàn shí gāo* (Gypsum Fibrosum Praeparatum) in a powdered form. *Qīng fěn* (Calomelas) is pungent and cold with a severe toxicity. It has a strong action in attacking toxins, killing parasites and promoting wound healing when used externally, and is used for scabies, tinea, syphilis and skin diseases after rupture. It is used internally to promote urination and defecation, to remove water to reduce edema, and is used for edema and constipation of an excess type.

③ *Pí shí* (砒石, Arsenicum, Arsenolite) ★

Both *pí shí* (Arsenicum) and *xióng huáng* (Realgar) contain arsenic. They are pungent in flavor, warm or hot in property, and toxic. *Pí shí* (Arsenicum) is pungent, severely hot and severely toxic. It can remove necrotic tissue externally; remove phlegm to calm panting internally. It is indicated for tinea, ulcers, scrofula, noma, hemorrhoids, ulcerations with necrotic tissues; and asthma due to cold phlegm. *Xióng huáng* (Realgar) is pungent, warm and toxic. It is able to detoxify, kill parasites, dry damp, remove phlegm and prevent the recurrence of malaria. It is indicated for carbuncles, furuncles, eczema, scabies, tinea, snake or insect bites; abdominal pain due to the accumulation of parasites; a pruritic anus due to enterobiasis; asthma, malaria, and epilepsy due to fright.

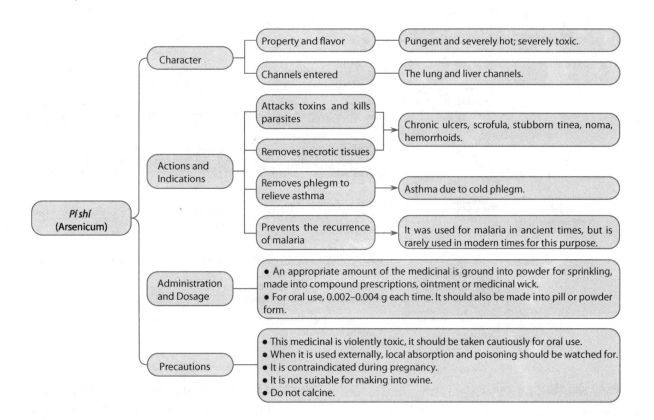

④ *Qiān dān* (铅丹, Minium, Lead Oxide) ★

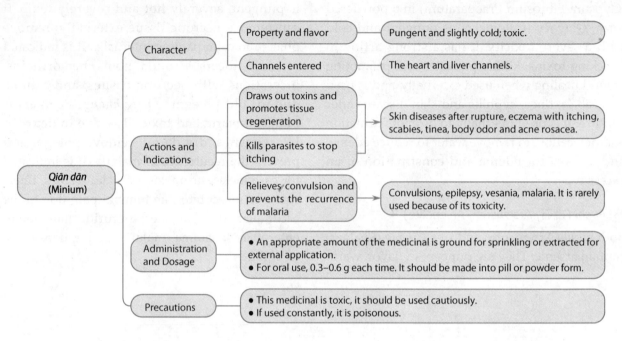

⑤ *Lú gān shí* (炉甘石, Calamina, Smithsonite) ★★

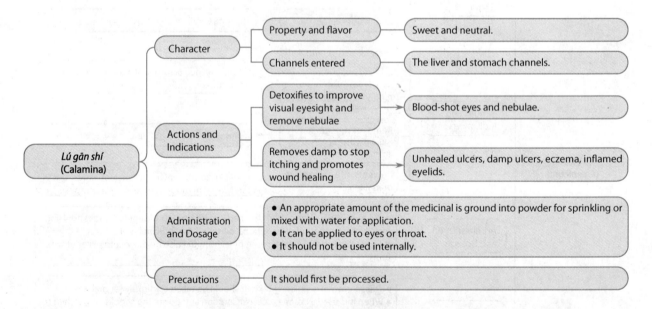

⑥ *Péng shā* (硼砂, Borax, Borax) ★★

Lú gān shí (Calamina) and *péng shā* (Borax) can detoxify and remove necrotic tissues. They are only slightly irritating and are therefore commonly used in ophthalmology. They are used for blood-shot eyes and nebulae. *Lú gān shí* (Calamina) is neutral in property and has a small action in detoxifying. It is exclusively for external use. It is

effective for detoxifying, improving visual acuity, removing nebulae, removing damp, promoting tissue regeneration, and healing wounds. It is indicated for blood-shot eyes, nebulae, ocular disease with wind syndrome; non-healing ulcers, damp ulcers, eczema and pruritus. It is a commonly used medicinal in ophthalmology and traumatology. *Péng shā* (Borax) is cool in property.

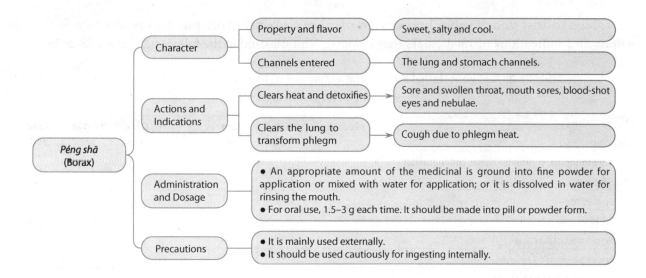

It is effective for clearing heat and detoxifying when used externally, and is indicated for sore and swollen throat, mouth sores, blood-shot eyes and nebulae. It is also a commonly used medicinal in ophthalmology and traumatology. It is able to clear the lung to transform phlegm when used internally, and is used for yellow and sticky phlegm and incomplete expectoration due to phlegm heat accumulation.

Actions of medicinals that draw out toxins, expel pus and rejuvenate flesh are summarized in the following table (Table 28-1):

Table 28-1: Summary of Medicinals that Draw out Toxins, Expel Pus and Rejuvenate Flesh:

Medicinal	Action in Common		Individual Character	
			External Use	**Internal Use**
Shēng yào (Hydrargyrum Oxydatum Crudum)	Most of these are toxic. They have the actions of drawing out toxins, removing necrotic tissues, promoting wound healing and tissue regeneration. They are indicated for skin diseases after rupture but with irregular discharge, or unhealed ulcers, carcinomas, syphilis, etc.	Medicinals containing mercury	It has a strong toxicity, it is effective for drawing out toxins, removing necrotic tissues, expelling pus discharge, and is regarded as a essential medicinal in traumatology. It is used exclusively for external application	
Qīng fěn (Calomelas)			It is very toxic, and has a strong action in attacking toxins, killing parasites and promoting wound healing.	Promotes urination and defecation, removes water to reduce edema
Lú gān shí (Calamina)		Detoxifies and preserves from decay and is slightly irritating, commonly used medicinals in ophthalmology	It has a moderate and mild action in detoxifying. It is exclusively provided for external use. It is effective for detoxifying, improving visual acuity, removing nebulae, removing damp to promote tissue regeneration and wound healing	
Péng shā (Borax)			It is effective for clearing heat and detoxifying. It is a commonly used medicinal in laryngology and ophthalmology.	Clears the lung to transform phlegm
Pí shí (Arsenicum)			With a great toxicity, it can attack toxins, kill parasites and remove necrotic tissue when used externally.	Removes phlegm to relieve asthma, prevents the recurrence of malaria
Qiān dān (Minium)			It is able to draw out toxins, promote tissue regeneration, kill parasites and stop itching	

Tables to test your herbal knowledge of actions and indications of medicinals that draw out toxins, expel pus and rejuvenate flesh are summarized in the following (Tables 28-2~28-3):

Table 28-2: Test your Herbal Knowledge of Actions of Medicinals that Draw out Toxins, Expel Pus and Rejuvenate Flesh:

Actions \ Medicinal	Shēng yào	Qīng fěn	Pí shí	Qiān dān	Lú gān shí	Péng shā
Draws out toxins, promotes tissue regeneration						
Attacks toxins						
Kills parasites						
Clears heat and detoxifies						
Removes necrotic tissues						
Removes phlegm to relieve asthma						
Kills parasites to stop itching						
Detoxifies, improves visual acuity and removes nebulae						
Removes damp, promotes tissue regeneration and wound healing						
Promotes wound healing						
Clears the lung to transform phlegm						

Table 28-3: Test your Herbal Knowledge of Indications of Medicinals that Draw out Toxins, Expel Pus and Rejuvenate Flesh:

Indications \ Medicinal	Shēng yào	Qīng fěn	Pí shí	Qiān dān	Lú gān shí	Péng shā
Carbuncles that have ruptured but have irregular pus discharge						
Scabies and tinea						
Syphilis						
Chronic ulcers						
Scrofula						
Noma						
Hemorrhoids						
Ulcers with necrotic tissues						
Asthma due to cold phlegm						
Damp ulcers						
Blood-shot eyes, nebulae, ocular diseases with wind syndrome						
Sore and swollen throat						
Mouth sores						
Cough with thick phlegm due to phlegm heat accumulation in the lung						

Index by Disease Names and Symptoms

A

abdominal cold pain 18
abdominal distending pain and fullness 145
abdominal distension 108, 151
abdominal distension after meals 411
abdominal distension due to malnutrition 146
abdominal edema 196
abdominal fullness 229
abdominal hard masses 126, 228, 301, 302, 303
abdominal masses 116, 122, 145, 153, 283, 286, 288, 289, 291, 326, 327, 347, 357, 403, 408, 421
abdominal masses and fullness 160
abdominal pain 54, 92, 94, 99, 107, 113, 116, 122, 126, 127, 145, 151, 162, 193, 201, 205, 216, 218, 220, 222, 233, 234, 235, 258, 271, 287, 299, 321, 327, 372, 374, 390, 406, 441, 442, 445, 449, 462, 463
abdominal pain due to ascariasis 260
abdominal pain due to the accumulation of parasites 151, 471
abdominal pain during menstrual bleeding 276, 277
abdominal pain post-partum 126, 230
abnormal growth of the conjuntiva 458
abnormal growths 113
abnormal or difficult childbirth 372, 374
abscesses of the internal organs 107
absence of libido 391
absence of sweating 436
accumulation of parasites 151, 462
aching and flaccidity of the waist and knees 396
aching and weakness of the lumbus and knees 444
aching and weakness of the waist and knees 386, 391, 406, 416
aching in the shoulders and back 158
aching joints all over the body 159
aching joints and bones 168, 169
aching joints of the shoulders and limbs 54
aching lumbus 444
aching of the waist and legs 393
aching of the waist and knees 293, 294, 394, 411, 414, 419
acid regurgitation 93
acute and chronic convulsions 366
acute convulsions in infants 364, 366
adverse flow of qi and fire 286
agitation 80, 146
alternate chills and fever 68, 92, 267
amenorrhea 54, 108, 122, 126, 145, 153, 199, 202, 204, 206, 218, 271, 283, 286, 287, 288, 289, 291, 292, 293, 299, 300, 301, 303, 327, 334, 346, 372, 374, 404, 406, 407, 408, 421
amnesia 193, 347, 350, 351, 357, 375, 380, 382, 383, 404, 414, 420
anal prolapse 68, 229, 443
anal, uterine and stomach prolapse 384
ancylostomiasis 254, 260, 465
anger 146
angina 232, 271, 333, 374
angina due to chest blockage 287
aphasia 168
aphonia 110
ascariasis 254, 257, 260, 441, 449
ascites 146, 332
asthma 26, 36, 230, 231, 291, 333, 366, 462, 471
aversion to cold 53, 54, 55, 56, 60, 63, 64, 66, 69, 70, 184, 193, 199, 213, 217, 218, 391, 401, 407, 436

B

belching 226, 228, 235, 245, 249, 317, 331, 358, 359, 458
beriberi 148, 163, 164, 168, 174, 199, 219, 258, 324, 445
bi 109, 204, 271, 284, 287, 288, 298, 303, 314, 334, 351, 365, 366, 384, 394, 406, 463, 465
bi in the joints 283
bi of a wind cold type 158
bitter taste 68, 93, 219, 233, 234, 267
bitter taste in the mouth 93, 416

bleeding 81, 104, 265, 276, 286, 321, 435, 441, 447, 448, 449, 462

bleeding due to trauma 104, 119, 262, 296, 299, 347, 392, 447

blood heat 321

blood in the stools 87, 94

blood loss 384

blood stasis 109, 153, 170, 206, 228, 232, 296, 299, 303, 372, 374, 392, 403, 406, 421

blood-shot and painful eyes 122, 458

blood-shot eyes 18, 63, 93, 144, 145, 146, 205, 265, 293, 323, 472, 473

blood-shot, swollen and painful eyes 94, 103, 128, 198, 355, 356, 359, 362, 363, 366, 374

bloody and purulent discharge 94, 299

bloody and purulent stools 113

bloody discharge 265

bloody phlegm 83, 101

blurred vision 66, 88, 185, 293, 346, 355, 356, 399

body aches 53

body lice 330

boils 103

bone fractures 296, 297, 299, 302, 351, 396

breast abscesses 87, 94, 103, 116, 227, 228, 269, 319, 321, 351, 392

breast distending pain 116, 226, 235, 359

breast distending pain before menstruation 237

breast distending pain or masses 228

breast swellings with pain 375

brief lactation 238

burns 81, 124, 145, 265, 273, 374

C

cancerous masses 460

carbuncles 20, 103, 104, 123, 153, 171, 264, 268, 273, 287, 292, 293, 303, 314, 315, 351, 362, 372, 375, 406, 408, 409, 460, 461, 464, 465, 469, 471

carbuncles after rupture 470

carbuncles on the surface of the body 107

carcinoma 97

cardiac and abdominal pain 327, 334

cardiac cold pain 217

cardiac pain 216, 233, 235, 238, 321

cardiac spasm 160

cardiogenic edema 196

cerebral artery spasm 333

cestodiasis 254, 260

chest and abdominal pain 249, 284, 288, 301

chest and epigastric fullness and distress 55

chest and epigastric masses and distress 89

chest and hypochondriac distending pain 233, 234, 359

chest and hypochondriac pain 229, 284, 288

chest blockage 216, 217, 229, 230, 233, 235, 238, 271

chest distension 187

chest distress 65, 69, 235

chest distress and pain 226

chest oppression 92, 193, 199, 227, 267, 321, 328, 379, 382

chest oppression and discomfort 323, 448

chest pain 83, 101, 107, 193, 227, 323

chills 216

cholelithiasis 286

chronic and acute convulsions in infants 362

chronic convulsions 354

chronic otitis media 460

chronic stubborn bi 366

chyluria 127, 197, 204, 206

cirrhosis 36

clenched fists 372, 374

cold bi 372, 374

cold body 374

cold excess congealed in the chest 153

cold feeling in the back 216

cold hernia 218, 220, 445

cold in the uterus 217, 220, 277, 394,

396, 403

cold limbs 213, 217, 221, 391

cold low back 26

cold pain 221

cold pain in the abdomen 218, 398

cold pain in the chest and abdomen 374

cold pain in the epigastrium 213, 391

cold pain in the epigastrium and abdomen 276, 394, 445

cold pain in the loins and knees 213

cold pain in the lower abdomen 220, 394

cold pain in the waist and knees 215, 217, 398

cold phlegm 471

cold uterus 213

coldness of the limbs 18

collapse 444

coma 80, 85, 93, 119, 121, 124, 128, 144, 145, 286, 289, 311, 321, 354, 362, 364, 371, 372, 373, 374, 375, 406, 448, 463

common cold 60, 68, 119, 258

conjunctival congestion 63, 65, 66, 85, 87, 88

constant diarrhea 397

constant vomiting 54

constipation 65, 81, 87, 92, 121, 145, 146, 151, 204, 205, 206, 226, 229, 230, 258, 260, 291, 321, 323, 327, 328, 351, 401, 406, 409, 411, 414, 462

constipation in the elderly 146, 396

convulsion of the four limbs 57

convulsions 25, 93, 101, 124, 146, 318, 346, 351, 357, 359, 361, 362, 364, 366, 371

convulsions due to fright 462

convulsions in infants 161, 321, 372, 374

convulsions of the limbs 357

coronary artery disease 36, 333, 374

cough 25, 26, 36, 54, 55, 60, 63, 65, 66, 70, 81, 83, 101, 107, 108, 110, 126, 127, 150, 151, 185, 193, 194, 202, 206, 213, 216, 221, 226, 227,

230, 235, 249, 260, 266, 267, 268,
291, 299, 311, 312, 314, 316, 317,
318, 319, 321, 322, 323, 326, 327,
328, 330, 331, 332, 333, 351, 379,
380, 381, 384, 386, 390, 393, 394,
416, 435, 438, 441, 443
cough from over-strain 319
cough with bloody phlegm 401
counterflow of lung qi 327
counterflow qi into the abdomen
219
craniofacial infections 121
cutaneous pruritus 170
cyanotic complexion 371, 374

D

damp heat 286
damp sores 92, 119, 127
damp turbidity obstruction 384
damp ulcers 169, 185, 190, 199, 201,
233, 267, 299, 346, 356, 357, 441,
444, 447, 462, 472
damp-warmth 190
dark maculae 291
dark purplish ecchymoses 119
deafness 93, 298, 346, 359, 375, 406,
408, 409, 411, 419
decline of *mingmen* fire 216
decreased urine production 384
defecation of an excess type 332
deficiency cold 276, 406
deficiency distension in the
epigastrium and abdomen 378
deficiency of essence and blood 391
deficiency panting 346, 359
deficiency taxation cough 327, 328,
418
deficiency taxation fever 437
deficient asthma 218
deficient panting 391
deformity of joints 366
delactation 303
delayed closure of the fontanel in
infants 391
delayed eruption of teeth 420
delayed menstruation 404
delayed walking 391, 420

delactation 393
delirium 80, 85, 93, 119, 121, 124,
128, 144, 145, 289, 362, 366, 371,
406, 448
dementia 375
depression 85, 226
devitalization 53
diabetes 69, 81, 93, 121, 380, 383, 386,
399, 406, 408, 409, 413, 416, 418,
419, 441
diaphragm fluid retention 317
diarrhea 26, 54, 57, 68, 69, 79, 89, 92,
94, 96, 99, 104, 108, 109, 127, 162,
184, 186, 187, 190, 191, 193, 198,
199, 213, 216, 221, 222, 226, 228,
229, 230, 233, 238, 258, 267, 273,
276, 277, 298, 382, 384, 386, 394,
399, 416, 435, 438, 441, 442, 443,
448, 449, 450, 462, 463, 465
diarrhea before dawn 219, 442, 443
diarrhea or dysentery with
abdominal pain 249
difficult pus discharge 469
difficult to expectorate 318
difficulty in defecation and urination
151, 153
difficulty in removing necrotic
tissues 470
difficulty in tissue regeneration 469
difficulty in walking 396
difficulty lying down in bed 328, 332
dim eyesight 355, 356, 384, 399, 415,
418, 419, 446
diminished spirit 213
diminished visual acuity 418, 419
diphtheria 121
discharge 60, 61
discomfort in the epigastrium 411
distended abdomen due to
malnutrition 108, 127
distending hypochondriac pain 68
distending pain 229, 249
distending pain and fullness in the
epigastrium and abdomen 238
distending pain in the chest,
hypochodrium, epigastrium and
abdomen 235, 237

distending pain in the epigastrium
and abdomen 442
distending pain of the breasts 238
distension and fullness 148, 258
distension and oppression in the
chest and diaphragm 314
distension in the head 265
distention 375
distress 374, 375
diuresis 99
dizziness 26, 66, 68, 87, 88, 94, 146,
170, 193, 265, 267, 346, 355, 356,
357, 358, 359, 362, 375, 382, 383,
384, 391, 393, 406, 407, 408, 409,
411, 414, 416, 418, 419, 444
dizziness, tinnitus 391
dorsal furuncles 317, 392, 393, 403
dropsy 115
drowsiness 375
dry and painful eyes 185
dry cough 83, 321, 389, 408, 411, 413,
415, 417
dry cough with sticky phlegm 319
dry cough without phlegm 408
dry eyes 411, 418
dry intestines 81, 291, 396, 401, 406,
411, 414
dry lips 92
dry lips and mouth 318, 394
dry lips with scanty fluids 411
dry mouth 121, 122, 126, 406, 407,
411, 415, 417
dry mouth and throat 411
dry nose and throat 408, 413
dry stools 145, 205, 268, 416, 417
dry throat 125, 267, 351, 408, 415
dry throat and hoarseness 411
dry vomiting 411, 412
dryness of the skin, throat, mouth,
nose and eyes 411
dysentery 79, 89, 92, 94, 96, 97, 99,
104, 108, 109, 113, 119, 127, 151,
162, 184, 199, 213, 221, 229, 230,
238, 258, 265, 267, 273, 299, 435,
438, 442, 443, 449, 450, 462, 465
dysentery with blood 273
dysentery with inability to eat 375

dysfunction of the limbs 119

dysmenorrhea 54, 69, 108, 122, 126, 204, 218, 220, 234, 235, 249, 271, 283, 284, 286, 287, 288, 289, 291, 292, 293, 299, 301, 303, 327, 334, 346, 406, 407, 408

dysphagia 119

dyspnea 36, 81, 110, 126, 127, 150, 151, 185, 196, 202, 213, 216, 221, 226, 230, 249, 291, 314, 317, 318, 321, 322, 326, 327, 328, 379, 380, 381, 383, 384, 386, 393, 394, 456, 457

dysuria 54, 70, 104, 115, 145, 168, 174, 190, 191, 193, 196, 198, 201, 213, 216, 218, 268, 274, 293, 294, 326, 332, 347, 366, 444

dysuria during pregnancy 96

dysuria post partum 293

E

ear pain with pustular discharge 128

earaches with pus discharge 374

eardrum perforation 460

early graying of the hair 268, 391, 406, 408, 409, 416, 418, 419

ecchymoses 119, 121, 122, 126

eczema 81, 92, 93, 95, 119, 124, 160, 163, 168, 169, 170, 185, 199, 201, 206, 222, 265, 267, 447, 460, 462, 469, 471, 472

edema 54, 55, 70, 85, 104, 115, 148, 150, 151, 153, 164, 168, 174, 184, 190, 191, 193, 196, 198, 199, 216, 217, 258, 267, 268, 292, 293, 294, 324, 326, 331, 334, 384, 386, 391

edema of a yang excess type 146

edema of the face and limbs 196

emaciation 108, 127, 258, 378, 386, 392, 393, 401

enlarged abdomen 127, 258

enlargement of the spleen and liver 326

enterobiasis 254, 258, 260, 330, 465, 471

enuresis 174, 213, 216, 217, 235, 249, 298, 334, 346, 357, 391, 394, 396, 397, 399, 416, 435, 444, 446, 447, 449

epidemic febrile diseases 406

epigastric and abdominal pain 288

epigastric and abdominal cold pain 217

epigastric and abdominal distending pain 186, 187, 226, 228, 230, 233, 234, 235, 301, 443

epigastric and abdominal distending pain and fullness 229

epigastric and abdominal distension and fullness 89, 182, 183, 184, 228, 245

epigastric and abdominal fullness 375

epigastric and abdominal fullness and masses 375

epigastric and abdominal pain 233, 235, 287, 389

epigastric and abdominal stagnation 314

epigastric cold pain 220, 222

epigastric fullness 182, 184

epigastric pain 160

epilepsy 101, 124, 146, 222, 286, 311, 314, 315, 317, 318, 321, 346, 351, 357, 359, 361, 362, 364, 366, 371, 375, 456, 457, 458, 462, 471

epilepsy due to fright 104

epistaxis 57, 66, 85, 92, 93, 101, 110, 119, 121, 122, 124, 125, 126, 127, 144, 145, 205, 258, 262, 263, 264, 265, 267, 268, 270, 273, 286, 294, 332, 359, 392, 408, 409

erysipelas 65, 97, 101, 103

excessive appetite 93

excessive drinking of water 412

excessive fetal movement 174, 267, 268, 276, 277, 384, 386, 396, 399, 448

excessive menstrual bleeding 268, 420, 444, 450

excessive menstrual blood 94, 174, 274

excessive menstruation 396

excessive saliva 184

excessive sputum 268

excessive sweating 415, 435

excessive tearing 63, 65, 87, 88, 359,

362, 364

excessive uterine bleeding 92, 94, 174

expectoration of foul and fishy sputum 323

expectoration of purulent and bloody discharge 321

expectoration of purulent sputum 327

expectoration of thick phlegm 317

expectoration of yellow and sticky sputum 330

expectoration of yellow and thick sputum 326, 332

external contraction of wind cold 158

external invasion 384, 448

external invasion due to deficiency 382

F

facial distortion 161, 168, 311, 314, 315, 366

failure of swellings to rupture 458

fainting 315, 317

fasciolopsis 260

fatigue 182

favus 234

febrile diseases 289, 291, 321, 408

feelings of fullness and discomfort in the chest and hypochondria 68

female infertility 276, 277, 394, 396, 403, 463

female sterility 391

fetal death 372, 374

fetal movement 54, 92

fever 53, 54, 55, 56, 60, 64, 65, 66, 68, 69, 70, 79, 80, 81, 85, 89, 92, 93, 97, 99, 101, 113, 121, 122, 124, 125, 127, 128, 145, 168, 184, 193, 218, 267, 362, 364, 366, 371, 372, 406, 415, 436, 437

fever after noon 328

fever receding without sweat 122, 124, 125

fever that worsens at night 119

feverish sensation in five the centers

411

feverish sensation in the palms and soles 124

fish bones caught in the throat 160

flaccidity 173, 182, 185, 394

flaccidity of the extremities 391

flaccidity of the lower limbs 293, 294, 396

flaccidity of the sinews and bones 392, 393, 415

flaccidity of the waist and knees 394, 396, 420

fluid consumption 401, 406, 441

fluid depletion 396

fluid retention 150

fluid retention in the chest and hypochondria 332

flushing 18, 92, 218, 355, 371, 372

flushing of the cheeks 411

flushing swollen face 101

food retention 113, 227, 228, 230, 456, 457

forehead pain 60

forgetfulness 194

foul and turbid discharge 185

frequent dreams 346, 347, 350, 351, 354, 357, 375, 382, 411, 414, 441

frequent urination 174, 213, 216, 217, 235, 249, 298, 334, 346, 357, 391, 394, 396, 397, 399, 403, 416, 435, 444, 446, 447, 449, 462

frequent urination at night 386

fright 344

frontal suture 420

fullness 374

fullness and distension of the chest 68

furuncles 103, 104, 273, 362, 372, 392, 460, 461, 464, 465, 469, 471

furuncles on the back of the body 218

G

galactostasis 359

galactostasis postpartum 401

gallstones 206

gastric cold pain 55

gastric dilation 229

gastric distending pain 456, 457, 458

gastric distension 412

gastric fullness 56

gastric pain 160, 356, 413

gastric upset 415

general aching 158

general body aches 60

general coldness 371

general fever 121, 126, 322, 407

general itching 201

general pain 351

general pruritus 163

German measles 163

goiter 87, 311, 318, 319, 324, 325, 357

H

habitual miscarriage 396

habitual constipation 146

hangovers 196

hard breast masses 227

head lice 330

headache 26, 53, 54, 55, 56, 57, 60, 61, 63, 64, 65, 66, 68, 81, 87, 88, 93, 99, 101, 144, 146, 158, 159, 160, 170, 184, 193, 199, 219, 265, 284, 288, 293, 294, 314, 315, 322, 323, 328, 355, 359, 362, 364, 366, 372, 374, 407, 436

heat 121

heat attacking the pericardium 362

heat *bi* 289

heat diarrhea 69

heaviness 328

heaviness of the body 193, 199

heavy body 56, 57, 69

heavy or chronic uterine bleeding 57

hemafecia 57, 92, 96, 113, 119, 121, 262, 383, 409, 443, 447, 449, 462

hematemesis 57, 66, 92, 93, 101, 110, 119, 121, 122, 124, 125, 126, 127, 144, 145, 205, 258, 262, 263, 264, 265, 267, 268, 270, 272, 273, 276, 277, 286, 294, 359, 392, 408, 409, 447

hematuria 113, 119, 121, 125, 127, 197, 201, 202, 206, 258, 262, 263, 264, 267, 268, 271, 273, 326, 392

hemiparalysis 169, 271, 283, 311, 314, 366, 384

hemiplegia 161, 168

hemoptysis 66, 144, 145, 262, 264, 265, 267, 268, 270, 272, 273, 332, 409, 411, 413, 415, 441

hemorrhage 26, 258

hemorrhage due to trauma 403, 462

hemorrhage in the middle jiao 216

hemorrhoids 87, 89, 94, 127, 265, 330, 362, 441, 447, 449, 471

hemorrhoids with bleeding 96

hepatic abscesses 108

hernia 226, 228

hernia pain 233, 235

hernia with bearing-down distending pain 249

hernia with pain 234, 235

hiccups 26, 83, 219, 221, 240, 331, 358, 359, 411, 413, 415

high blood pressure 94

high fever 18, 63, 144, 289

hoarseness 323, 366, 411, 413, 415

hookworms 260

hot phlegm 314

hot stranguria 96, 99

hyperlipidemia 333

hypertension 170, 265, 330, 332, 333

hypochondriac distending pain 54, 65, 89, 93, 128, 226, 228, 235

hypochondriac pain 93, 219, 227, 233, 288, 317, 407, 408

I

impairment of the sinews 162, 297, 299, 302, 396

impotence 213, 215, 217, 220, 382, 383, 391, 393, 394, 396, 398, 399, 400, 403, 444, 446, 447, 462, 463

inability to control the emotions 416

inability to eat 54

incomplete expectoration 65, 473

incomplete expectoration of scanty and sticky sputum 321

incomplete expectoration of thick discharge 321

indigestion 245, 249

indistinct maculae 289

indistinct skin rashes 293

indolence of speech 380, 381, 383, 384

infant night-crying 65

infant's carbuncles 362

infant's drooling 398

infections on the body surface 60, 65

infertility 391, 399

inflammation of the throat 101, 153, 171, 317, 351, 458, 469

inflammation of the throat with panting 458

inflexible joints 160, 168, 171, 365

ingestion of poisonous food 458

restricted pus discharge 470

injuries 126, 206

injuries due to trauma 122, 145, 160, 164, 170, 171, 204, 237, 268, 269, 271, 283, 286, 287, 289, 291, 292, 293, 296, 297, 299, 301, 302, 327, 334, 347, 372, 396, 403, 406, 408, 464

insect or snake bites 97

insidious pain in the epigastrium 411

insidious pain or burning sensations in the stomach 415

insidious rashes 465

insomnia 26, 69, 88, 93, 99, 119, 124, 128, 193, 218, 269, 289, 290, 321, 344, 346, 347, 350, 351, 354, 356, 357, 359, 375, 380, 382, 383, 404, 406, 409, 411, 414, 419, 420, 441, 448, 449

internal injury 273, 406

internal stirring of liver wind 354

intestinal abscesses 103, 107, 116, 122, 126, 193, 194, 205, 287, 321, 327

intestinal cancer 464

intestinal distomiasis 254

irregular defecation 245, 249

irregular menstrual flow 292

irregular menstruation 54, 65, 69, 202, 226, 235, 237, 276, 277, 283, 286, 288, 289, 291, 292, 293, 327, 394, 406, 407, 408, 409

irritability 26, 69, 346, 355, 356, 357,

358, 359, 362, 364, 407

itching 196, 206, 222, 260, 346, 351, 356, 357, 359, 449, 462, 465

itchy throat 66

J

jaundice 85, 89, 92, 95, 104, 110, 115, 127, 145, 168, 190, 203, 204, 205, 233, 234, 267, 268, 286, 334, 462

jin kou li (dysentery with inability to eat) 375

joint and general body pain 60

joint pain 57

joint, shoulder and back pain in the upper part of body 60

K

kidney deficiency 399, 403

kidney yang deficiency 216, 394

L

lack of lactation 116

lack of strength of the bones and sinews 396

lack of sweating 55, 60

lassitude 183, 184, 193, 228, 273, 377, 378, 379, 380, 381, 383, 384, 386, 389, 393, 401, 406, 408, 416

leprosy 61, 161

leukemia 464

leukorrhagia 60, 94, 96, 127, 174, 184, 185, 190, 193, 194, 205, 206, 267, 298, 334, 346, 357, 384, 386, 391, 392, 393, 399, 416, 417, 435, 443, 444, 446, 447, 449, 463

leukorrhagia 92

leukorrhea 276, 277, 334, 435, 450

lingering heat 406

lingering low fever 125

lithiasis 206

liver heat 293

liver wind stirring in the interior 354

lochia 145

lochiostasis 292, 293, 447

lockjaw 362, 372, 374

loose intestines 442

loose stools 26, 182, 217, 228, 233,

234, 378, 381, 383, 384, 386, 399

loosening of the teeth 411

loss of appetite 249

loss of hair 268

loss of voice 323, 441, 443

low fever 415

low sperm count 444

low spirits 183, 217, 273, 377, 379, 380, 382, 391, 406, 408

low voice 379, 380, 381, 383, 384

lower abdominal pain 218

lumbago 399, 416

lung and kidney deficiency 393

lung deficiency 416, 441

lung dryness 260

lung heat 266, 267, 268, 299

M

maculae 69, 97, 101, 258, 362, 364, 406, 407

madness 119, 456, 457, 458, 462

malaria 69, 113, 228, 258, 273, 409, 421, 458, 462, 471

malarial nodules 421

malignant skin tumors 464

malignant tumors 465

malnutrition 411

malnutrition induced distended abdomen 249, 257, 258, 260

mammary abscesses 303

masses 228, 375

masses in the breast 227

measles 63, 64, 68, 70, 124, 160, 169, 359

measles with itching 366

menopause 394

menstrual spotting 92, 94

mental disorders 357

mental disturbance 351

metroptosis 462

metrorrhagia 113, 121, 122, 258, 262, 263, 264, 265, 267, 268, 270, 273, 274, 276, 277, 288, 346, 357, 359, 383, 391, 392, 393, 396, 406, 408, 409, 420, 435, 441, 443, 444, 447, 449, 450, 462

metrostaxis 113, 121, 122, 258, 262,

263, 264, 265, 267, 268, 270, 273, 274, 276, 277, 288, 346, 357, 359, 383, 391, 392, 393, 396, 406, 408, 409, 420, 435, 441, 443, 444, 447, 449, 450, 462

migraines 314, 315, 366

mouth sores 85, 93, 101, 128, 145, 146, 199, 294, 299, 346, 362, 372, 374, 458, 469, 473

multiple abscesses 311, 312

mumps 97, 101, 258

N

nail deformations 411

nasal obstruction 54, 60, 61

nausea 55, 56, 92, 182, 183, 184, 226, 227, 228, 235, 237, 245, 249, 314

nebula 65, 87, 88, 94, 122, 355, 356, 359, 363, 408, 418, 469, 472, 473

necrotic tissue 469, 471

nephritic edema 36

nephritis 293

night blindness 185, 355, 384

night fever 121, 122

night sweating 81, 126, 127, 193, 357

night sweats 36, 93, 121, 122, 124, 127, 346, 347, 351, 406, 407, 408, 409, 411, 420, 435

night-blindness 356

no appetite 187, 228, 245, 267, 328

no desire to eat 411

no sweating 36

nocturnal fever 124, 125

noma 471

non-healing ulcers 356, 472

numb limbs 169, 283, 411

numbness 54, 160, 161, 170, 171, 312, 317, 365, 384

numbness in the limbs and trunk 311

O

obstinate sores 153

obstinate tinea 150, 153

ocular disease 472

opisthotonus 57, 361

oppression in the chest and

diaphragm 317, 328

oral bitterness 355

orbital pain 60

orchidoptosis 220

otopyorrhea 460

P

pain 57, 145, 160, 170, 171, 226, 228, 296, 299, 327, 334, 351, 374, 375, 392, 445, 458

pain and abdominal masses 406

pain due to cancer 160

pain due to hernia 227

pain due to stasis 284

pain in the chest and abdomen 271

pain in the body and joints 317

pain in the chest, hypochondria and abdomen 271

pain in the chest, hypochondrium, epigastrium and abdomen 235, 286

pain in the epigastrium and abdomen 390

pain in the epigastrium, abdomen and four limbs 408

pain in the lumbar vertebrae, sinews and bones 392

pain in the sinews and bones 442

pain of the four limbs 57

pain upon palpation 321

pain with blood stasis 164

painful sensations in the limbs and joints 289

pale complexion 18

pale lips and nails 404

pale or yellowish complexion 384, 404

palpitations 54, 193, 194, 213, 218, 269, 289, 344, 346, 347, 350, 351, 356, 357, 359, 375, 377, 379, 382, 383, 384, 390, 404, 406, 408, 409, 414, 415, 420, 441, 449

panting 311, 312, 317, 327, 331, 332, 333, 359, 382, 390, 398, 403, 435, 438

paralysis 300, 303, 394

paralysis and flaccidity of feet and knees 293

parasite accumulation 222

parasites 201, 234

parietal headache 445

pertussis 465

phlegm 55, 213, 227, 311, 315, 316, 317, 354, 375, 389, 408, 441

phlegm fire disturbing the heart 344

phlegm heat 109, 366

phlegm heat accumulation 473

phlegm heat obstruction 374

phlegm heat stagnating in the lung 441

phlegm nodes 94

phlegm nodules 53

phlegm obstruction 153, 218, 286, 321

phlegm-fluids 184, 190, 191, 384, 386

phlegm-fluids accumulation 317

phlegm-fluids in the chest 457

phlegm-fluids obstruction in the chest and diaphragm or throat 456, 457

phlegm-turbidity 456, 457

phlegm-turbidity accumulation 371

photophobia 87, 88, 362, 364

pidgeon chest in infants 420

plum pit qi 230, 237

poisoning 390

poisoning from seafood 54

poisonous snake bites 160, 205, 206, 233, 314, 315, 461

poisonous substances 457

polydypsia 121

poor appetite 55, 56, 68, 108, 182, 183, 184, 186, 193, 222, 228, 233, 234, 235, 237, 378, 380, 381, 383, 384, 386, 389, 398, 411, 412, 413, 415, 416, 417, 442, 443, 449, 458

poor appetite and digestion 235

poor development 391

poor digestion 228

post-operative pain 160

postpartum abdominal pain 54, 145, 204, 271, 283, 284, 286, 288, 289, 291, 292, 293, 299, 302, 303, 327, 346, 447

premature ejaculation 386, 391, 396

prickly heat 199

profuse and thin sputum 216

profuse menstrual blood 276, 277, 288

profuse menstruation 122

profuse phlegm 317, 321, 322, 328, 351

profuse saliva 398

profuse secretion of gastric acid 357

profuse sputum 222, 227, 235, 249

profuse white phlegm 312

prolapse 26, 357, 462

prolapse of the internal organs 230, 378, 384

promoting tissue regeneration 470

pruritic anus 471

pruritic vulvae 94, 201, 222

pruritus 61, 63, 64, 71, 93, 95, 161, 450, 462, 464, 465, 469, 472

puffiness 293, 378

puffiness of the limbs 213

pulmonary abscesses 83, 107, 108, 193, 194, 267, 319, 328, 351

pulmonary and intestinal abscesses 291

purplish black ecchymoses 123, 124

purplish dark measles 124

purplish menstrual blood with clots 288

purpura 262, 267

purulent and bloody expectoration 108

purulent and bloody stools 99, 127

purulent and foul expectoration 107

purulent discharge 460

purulent expectoration 83, 193, 267

putrid breath 184

Q

qi stagnation 228, 230, 374

R

rashes 25, 123, 124

red swelling pain in the joints 96

red swellings 289

red, swollen, painful, and inflexible joints 97

reddish scanty urine 83

reddish urine 89, 92, 93, 116, 199, 203, 416

renal prolapse 68

restlessness 69, 93, 119, 121, 194, 269, 344, 346, 351, 354, 356, 357, 359, 375, 389

retching 219

retention of the lochia 372, 374

retention of urine 366

rhagades 273

roundworm 95, 260

runny nose 60, 61

rupture 374

S

salivation 182

scabies 61, 95, 146, 153, 161, 170, 260, 268, 330, 450, 460, 461, 462, 464, 465, 471

scalds 81, 119, 124, 145, 204, 206, 265, 268, 273, 374

scalds, burns 97

scanty and reddish urine 85, 89, 199, 201

scanty light colored menstrual blood 404

scanty phlegm 83, 334, 408, 411, 413, 415

scanty sperm 403

scanty sweating 69

scanty urine 85

scarlet fever 464

schistosomiasis 254, 260

scrofula 87, 94, 99, 104, 108, 116, 121, 150, 196, 303, 311, 315, 318, 319, 324, 325, 357, 366, 409, 464, 471

scrotal swelling and pain 93

seminal emission 93, 121, 122, 124, 193, 215, 217, 346, 347, 357, 386, 392, 393, 396, 397, 399, 400, 406, 408, 409, 411, 414, 416, 418, 419, 420, 435, 441, 444, 446, 447, 448, 449, 450

sepsis 128

septicemia 93

severe and chronic abdominal

masses 300

severe blood loss 382

severe pain in the vertex 60

severe thirst 68

shortness of breath 60, 70, 377, 379, 380, 381, 382, 383, 384, 389

shortness of breath worsening with activity 379

shortness of breath worsening with movement 378

skin cancer 464

skin diseases 287, 299, 347, 374, 392, 393, 441, 469, 471

skin diseases that have ruptured but have not healed 346

skin rashes 101, 126, 346, 351, 357

sleeping curled up in a ball 217

slight aversion to cold 99

sluggish digestion 193

snake bites 103, 104, 115, 153

snake or insect bites 471

sore and swollen throat 63, 323, 346, 372, 374, 390, 464, 473

sore mouth 69

sore throat 87, 92, 101, 323, 413

sores 25, 96, 103, 104, 153, 168, 273

sores due to wind 464

sores without pus 119

sour regurgitation 128, 182, 219, 226, 235, 245, 249, 445

spasm of muscles 57

spasm of the limbs 61

spasm of the sinews 57

spasms 160, 162, 351, 361, 362, 364, 366, 371, 372, 390, 408, 411

spasms and pain in the epigastrium, abdomen and limbs 407

spasms of sinews and vessels 168, 366

spasms of the hands and feet 364

spasms of the limbs 361, 389

spasms of the sinews and muscles 169, 170, 171

spermatorrhea 213, 215, 217, 249, 346, 357, 386, 396, 397, 399, 416, 435, 444, 446, 447, 449, 450

spitting of saliva 219

splenohepatomegalia 357, 421

spontaneous sweating 36, 346, 357, 383, 384, 386, 401, 435, 437, 441

spotting 174

stabbing and fixed pain in the chest, abdomen and head 283

stabbing pain in the chest and abdomen 299

stabbing pain in the heart and abdomen 346

stabbing pain in the lower abdomen 288

stagnation 328

stagnation and oppression in the chest and diaphragm 321

stagnation in the epigastrium 317

stagnation of the breast collaterals 116

staring 351, 416

stasis 292, 299, 300, 301

stasis of milk in the mammary glands 199

steaming bone fevers 93

steaming bones 121, 124, 125, 126, 127, 193, 414, 415, 420, 437

steaming bones with fever 122

steaming bones with tidal fever 168

stiff neck 361

stomach cold 314

stomach heat 266, 267, 268

stomach prolapse 68, 229

stomachache 170, 232, 326, 357, 412, 442, 447, 449

stranguria 83, 85, 89, 104, 108, 113, 115, 119, 127, 190, 193, 194, 196, 197, 198, 199, 201, 202, 204, 206, 249, 264, 266, 267, 271, 293, 294, 303, 326, 347

stroke 161, 168, 169, 271, 283, 303, 314, 317, 318, 321, 362, 366, 371, 374, 384

stubborn diseases 406

stubborn phlegm 321

stubborn tinea 160

subcutaneous diseases 346

subcutaneous edema 332

summer heat 374

superficial nodules 99, 104, 121, 150, 303, 312, 314, 315, 325, 357, 366

suppurating infections 79, 85, 97, 99, 101, 110, 113, 115, 116, 118, 145, 150, 152, 170, 204, 206, 233, 238, 269, 289

suppurative infection 20

susceptibility to falls 361

sweating 26, 80, 213, 217, 218, 407, 444

sweating due to deficiency 379

sweet and greasy tastes 184

swelling 103, 104, 145, 170, 171, 206, 273, 296, 299, 324, 327, 334, 351, 374, 375, 384, 445

swelling and pain 108, 287, 301, 321, 406

swelling and pain due to stasis 302

swelling and pain in ears and eyes 93

swelling and redness of the head 121

swelling of the ears with pustular discharge 89

swelling pain 54, 116, 122, 163, 228, 237, 258, 265, 271, 292, 303, 351

swelling pain due to stasis 283

swelling pain in the feet and knees 185

swelling pain of the gums 60, 81

swelling pain or bleeding 330

swelling pains 268, 271

swollen and painful eyes 145, 146, 293, 355, 364

swollen and painful feet 219

swollen and painful gums 110, 294, 362

swollen and painful gums and throat 205

swollen and sore gums 145

swollen and sore throat 69, 101, 104, 108, 109, 110, 116, 119, 121, 124, 146, 206, 362, 366

swollen and sore throat and gums 144

swollen feet 168

swollen head 101

syncope 54, 318, 371, 374, 462

syphilis 460, 469, 471

T

tapeworms 258, 260

tendon spasms 162

tenesmus 92, 99, 113, 127, 151, 229, 230, 238, 258

testicular swelling and pain 227

testicular swelling pain 234, 249, 324

tetanus 161, 168, 314, 315, 366

tetanus with spasms 361

the five kinds of delayed growth in infants 392, 393

the retention of urine 323, 347

thick sputum 318

thin discharge 276, 277

thirst 18, 63, 64, 68, 69, 79, 80, 81, 83, 85, 92, 101, 121, 125, 199, 266, 267, 268, 351, 380, 381, 383, 406, 413, 415, 437, 441

thoracic accumulation 314, 317

throat swelling and pain 97

tidal fever 124, 126, 127, 193, 406, 411, 414, 419, 420

tinea 61, 95, 146, 153, 161, 170, 196, 260, 268, 317, 330, 450, 460, 461, 462, 464, 465, 471

tinea capitis 150, 234

tinea of the vulvae 124

tinea tonsure 150

tinnitus 298, 346, 355, 359, 375, 391, 393, 404, 406, 407, 408, 409, 411, 414, 418, 419, 444

tonsillitis 464

toothache 60, 69, 87, 160, 170, 298, 464, 465

trauma 85, 288

trembling 361

trembling hands and feet 420

trembling with fear 346

trichomonas vaginalis 254, 260, 330

tuberculosis 465

tuberculous pleurisy 36

tumors 116

twilight blindness 356

tympanites 153

U

ulcerated skin 265
ulcerated skin with yellow exudation 96
ulcerated sores 81
ulcerations 464, 471
ulcerative gingivitis 299, 458
ulcers 116, 168, 171, 196, 206, 260, 268, 273, 283, 292, 293, 303, 319, 351, 403, 408, 447, 460, 461, 464, 471
ulcers in the lower limbs 119
unconsciousness 372, 374
underdevelopment of children 173
urine retention 384
urolithiasis 197, 201, 206, 249, 326
urticaria 61, 63, 64, 71
uterine cold 276
uterine prolapse 68, 229

V

vaginal bleeding 92
vaginal bleeding during pregnancy 174, 267, 268, 276, 277, 396, 399, 409
vaginal discharge 26
vague pain in the epigastrium and abdomen 53
vertigo 54, 294, 312, 314, 315, 361, 362, 364, 404, 406
vexation 79, 80, 81, 83, 85, 88, 92, 93, 99, 119, 121, 124, 125, 127, 128, 146, 196, 199, 266, 267, 268, 289, 321, 346, 347, 351, 356, 357, 358, 359, 362, 364, 371, 380, 406, 407, 409, 414, 415, 419, 449, 458
vicarious menstruation 286
violent pain in the chest and abdomen 372, 374
visceral dryness 389, 390
vitiligo 359
vomiting 26, 54, 55, 68, 83, 85, 89, 92, 93, 127, 128, 162, 182, 183, 184, 186, 187, 213, 219, 220, 221, 222, 226, 227, 228, 231, 233, 235, 237, 240, 245, 249, 266, 267, 268, 271, 277, 314, 317, 321, 331, 358, 359, 382, 386, 413, 415, 441, 442, 443, 445, 449, 463
vomiting and diarrhea 56
vomiting during pregnancy 448
vomiting of gastric acid 326, 447
vomiting of phlegm and saliva 314
vomiting of saliva 445
vomiting of water 232

W

waist pain 240
watery discharge 386, 444
watery effusion 299, 444
weak constitution 409
weak feet 416
weak sinews and bones 420
weakness of the waist and knees 392, 393
wet sores 95
wheezing 213
wheezing phlegm 362
white and turbid discharge 334
whitish and thin expectoration 213
whitish or yellowish complexion 377
wind cold *bi* 53
wind damp 271, 287, 289, 303, 406
wind damp type pruritus 60
wind edema 332
wind heat 258
wind phlegm 314
wind phlegm obstruction 458
wind retention in the *shaoyin* channel 159
wind syndrome 472
withered hair 127
wounds 108

Y

yang deficiency 391
yang deficiency of the spleen and kidney 397
yellow and sticky phlegm 473
yellow and thick expectoration 318
yellow eyes and skin 203
yellow leukorrhea 89
yellowish complexion 258, 273, 378, 382, 389, 393, 401, 406, 408, 409
yellowish, thick discharge 450
yin abscesses 53
yin deficiency 407, 417, 437, 441

Index by Chinese Medicinals — Pin Yin Names

A

Ā wèi 251
ǎi dì chá 333
ài yè 30, 275, 276, 277

B

bā dòu 35, 36, 152
bā jǐ tiān 393, 394
bā jiǎo 219
bā jiǎo huí xiāng 219
bái biǎn dòu 386
Bǎi bù 329
bái dòu kòu 186, 443
Bái fán 462
Bái fù zǐ 314
Bái guǒ 332, 333
Bǎi hé 412, 415
bái huā shé shé cǎo 115
bái jí 35, 272
bài jiàng cǎo 107
Bái jiè zǐ 315, 316
bái liǎn 35, 118
bái máo gēn 266, 267
Bái qián 317, 321
bái sháo 27, 33, 35, 390, 406, 407
Bái tóu wēng 112, 113
bái wēi 125
bái xiān pí 95
bái zhǐ 58, 59
bái zhú 33, 384, 386
bǎi zǐ rén 348, 350
bàn biān lián 115

bǎn lán gēn 100, 101
Bān máo 302
bàn xià 35, 312, 314, 321
bàn xià qū 314
bào mù shén 194
Běi dòu gēn 109
bèi mǔ 318
běi shā shēn 411, 416
Bì bá 222
Bì chéng qié 222
Bì xiè 203
Biǎn xù 200, 201
biē jiǎ 420
bīng láng 256, 257
bīng piàn 373
bò he 12, 23, 26, 28, 63, 64
bǔ gǔ zhī 397

C

cán shā 162
cāng ěr zǐ 60, 61
cāng zhú 12, 184, 384
cǎo dòu kòu 187
cǎo guǒ 187
cǎo jué míng 355
cǎo wū 30, 35, 36, 160, 214
cè bǎi yè 266, 267
chái hú 26, 33, 67, 68
Chán sū 463
chán tuì 64
cháng shān 29, 457
chē qián zǐ 198
chén pí 12, 28, 227

chén xiāng 231
Chéng liǔ 62
chì fú líng 193
chì sháo 35, 122, 407
chì shí zhī 36, 443
chì zhú 384
chóng lóu 104
chòu wú tóng 169
Chǔ shí zǐ 410
chuān bèi mǔ 12, 35, 36, 318
Chuān liàn zǐ 232, 233
Chuān mù tōng 199
chuān niú xī 293
chuān shān jiǎ 303
Chuān shān lóng 172
chuān wū 12, 30, 35, 36, 160, 214
Chuān xīn lián 99
chuān xiōng 11, 12, 13, 284, 287, 289
chuí pén cǎo 205
chūn pí 94, 449
cì jí lí 359
cí shí 20, 345, 346, 358
cì wei pí 449
Cì wǔ jiā 388
cōng bái 41, 61, 237

D

dà dòu huáng juǎn 69
Dà fù pí 238
dà huáng 12, 26, 144, 204, 268, 390
dà huí xiāng 219
Dà jì 263
Dà qīng yè 100, 101

dà suàn 465

dà xuè téng 107

dà zǎo 22, 41, 387, 389

dài zhě shí 26, 358, 359

dàn dòu chǐ 69

dǎn fán 457

Dǎn nán xīng 313

dān shēn 35, 289

dàn zhú yè 84

dāng guī 12, 23, 34, 404, 406

dǎng shēn 12, 18, 22, 28, 381, 384

dāo dòu 239, 240

dào yá 247, 248

Dēng xīn cǎo 203

Dì ěr cǎo 205

dì fū zǐ 201

dì gǔ pí 125, 127

dì huáng 12

Dì jǐn cǎo 114

Dì lóng 365, 366

dì yú 264, 265

Dīng gōng téng 165

dīng xiāng 35, 219, 220

dōng chóng xià cǎo 400

Dōng guā pí 194, 196

Dōng kuí zǐ 202

dú huó 158, 159

dú jiǎo lián 30

dù zhòng 395

Duàn lóng gǔ 357

duàn shí gāo 471

E

É bù shí cǎo 62

ē jiāo 12, 408

é zhú 300, 301

ér chá 299

F

fǎ bàn xià 314

Fān bái cǎo 115

fān hóng huā 291

fān xiè yè 146

fáng fēng 57, 168

fáng jǐ 167, 168

fěi zǐ 259

Fēng fáng 465

fēng mì 390

Fēng xiāng zhī 288

Fó shǒu 235

fú líng 12, 191, 193

Fú líng pí 191

fù pén zǐ 445, 446

fú píng 70

Fú shén 192

fú xiǎo mài 437

fù zǐ 12, 18, 23, 30, 34, 35, 214, 215, 216, 382, 390

G

gān cǎo 18, 30, 35, 36, 387, 390

gān dì huáng 406

gān jiāng 18, 28, 33, 215, 216, 220

Gān sōng 239

gān suì 30, 35, 36, 149, 150

gǎo běn 59

Gǎo lì shēn 380

gāo liáng jiāng 220

gé gēn 20, 23, 68

Gé jiè 28, 399, 400

Gé shān xiāo 250

gōng dīng xiāng 220

gǒu jǐ 173, 297

gǒu qǐ 12, 417, 418, 419

gōu téng 27, 363, 364

gǔ huí xiāng 219

Gǔ jīng cǎo 87

gǔ suì bǔ 297

gǔ yá 247, 248

guā dì 457

guā lóu 30, 35, 319, 321

guā lóu pí 319

guā lóu rén 319

guā lóu shuāng 319

Guān bái fù 314

Guān mù tōng 199

guàn zhòng 102, 257

Guī jiǎ 420

guì zhī 19, 23, 33, 53

H

Há ma yóu 403

hǎi fēng téng 164, 170

hǎi fú shí 325

Hǎi gé qiào 325

Hǎi gǒu shèn 402, 403

hǎi jīn shā 201

hǎi mǎ 403

hǎi piāo xiāo 447

Hǎi tóng pí 170

hǎi zǎo 35, 323, 324

Hàn fáng jǐ 168

Hán shuǐ shí 82

hè cǎo yá 257, 259

Hé gěng 448

hé huān pí 350

hè shī 258, 259

hé shǒu wū 409

hé táo rén 400

hé yè 41, 448

hē zǐ 441, 442

Hēi zhī ma 419

Hóng dà jǐ 149

hóng huā 290, 291

Hóng jǐng tiān 388

hóng shēn 380

hòu pò 184, 230

hú huáng lián 127

hú jiāo 221

hú lu 195, 196

Hú lú bā 401

hǔ pò 346

Hú Suī 62

Hú tuí zǐ yè 335

hǔ zhàng 204, 205

Huā jiāo 221

Huà jú hóng 227

huā ruǐ shí 270

huà shān shēn 30, 334

huá shí 198

huái huā 265

Huái jiǎo 265

huái niú xī 293

huáng bǎi 22, 92

Huáng gǒu shèn 403

huáng jīng 36, 415, 416

huáng lián 11, 12, 22, 26, 33, 91, 321

huáng qí 12, 22, 23, 26, 34, 383, 384

huáng qín 28, 33, 90, 267

Huáng yào zǐ 324

huí xiāng 219

huǒ má rén 147
Huò xiāng 183

J

Jì cài 197
Jī gǔ cǎo 206
Jī guān huā 450
Jì mù 275
jī nèi jīn 248, 249
Jī shǐ téng 250
Jī xuè téng 294
jiāng bàn xià 314
jiāng cán 366
jiāng huáng 285
jiàng xiāng 270
Jiǎo gǔ lán 388
jié gěng 27, 28, 322, 323
Jǐn dēng lóng 110
Jīn guǒ lǎn 111
jīn qián bái huā shé 162
jīn qián cǎo 204, 205
jīn qiáo mài 107
Jīn yín huā 97, 99
Jīn yīng zǐ 446, 449
jīng dà jǐ 35, 36, 149, 150
jīng jiè 56, 57
jǐng tiān sān qī 268
Jiǔ cài zǐ 401
Jiǔ xiāng chóng 239
Jú hé 227
jú huā 12, 26, 66
Jú luò 227
Jú yè 227
jú yè sān qī 268
jué míng zǐ 87, 355

K

Kǔ dòu zǐ 96
kǔ liàn pí 255, 257
Kǔ shēn 95
kǔ xìng rén 327, 328
kuǎn dōng huā 329
kūn bù 324
Kūn míng shān hǎi táng 165

L

lái fú zǐ 248

láng dú 35
Lǎo guàn cǎo 171
Léi gōng téng 171
léi wán 257
Lí lú 35
lì zhī hé 233
Lián fáng 447
lián qiào 98, 99
Lián xū 447
Lián zǐ 447, 448
Lián zǐ xīn 447
Líng xiāo huā 295
Líng yáng jiǎo 361, 362, 364
Líng zhī 348
liú huáng 35, 461
liú jì nú 299
Lóng chǐ 346
lóng dǎn cǎo 93
lóng gǔ 345, 346, 356
Lóng yǎn ròu 410
Lóu gū 197
lòu lú 105, 116
Lǜ dòu 119
Lú gān shí 472
lú gēn 41, 82, 83, 266
lú huì 146
lù jiǎo 391
lù jiǎo jiāo 391
Lù lù tōng 166
Lù róng 391, 392
Lù xián cǎo 175
lǜ è méi 236, 237
Luó bù má 360
Luó hàn guǒ 334
luò shí téng 170

M

mǎ bó 109
mǎ chǐ xiàn 112, 113
Mǎ dōu líng 330
má huáng 22, 26, 27, 28, 36, 52, 53, 55, 70, 436
má huáng gēn 436, 437
mǎ qián zǐ 30, 296
Mǎ wěi lián 97
mài dōng 382, 413, 416
mài yá 247, 248

Màn jīng zǐ 67
Mǎn shān hóng 335
máng xiāo 26, 145, 146
Māo zhuǎ cǎo 317
Méi gui huā 236, 237
méng chóng 301
Méng shí 326
Mì méng huā 88
mì tuó sēng 35
Míng dǎng shēn 417
mò hàn lián 418
mò yào 287
Mù biē zǐ 464
mǔ dān pí 121, 122, 125
mǔ dīng xiāng 220
mù fáng jǐ 168
Mù guā 162
Mù hú dié 111
mǔ lì 356
Mù xiāng 230, 233, 234
Mù zéi 71

N

Nán guā zǐ 256, 259
nán shā shēn 411
niú bàng zǐ 64
niú huáng 362, 372
niú xī 12, 293
nǚ zhēn zǐ 418
nuò dào gēn xū 437

O

ǒu jié 274

P

pàng dà hǎi 323
páo jiāng 216, 276
pèi lán 183
péng shā 472
pí pá yè 330
pí shí 471
pī shuāng 31, 35
Pí xiāo 146
pò xiāo 35
Pú gōng yīng 102, 103
pú huáng 270

Q

Qí shé 161
qiàn cǎo 269, 270
Qiān dān 472
qián hú 321
qiān jīn zǐ 152
Qiān lǐ guāng 117
Qiān nián jiàn 174
qiān niú zǐ 35, 36, 151
qiàn shí 448
qiāng huó 28, 58, 59, 158
Qín jiāo 167
Qín pí 94
qīng bàn xià 314
qīng dài 101
qīng fěn 470
qīng fēng téng 164
Qīng guǒ 110
Qīng hāo 124, 125
qīng mù xiāng 233
qīng pí 227
Qīng xiāng zǐ 88
Qú mài 200, 201
quán guā lóu 319
quán shēn 104
quán xiē 365, 366

R

Rěn dōng téng 97
rén shēn 12, 13, 30, 35, 36, 379, 380,
    381, 383
ròu cōng róng 23, 396
Ròu dòu kòu 442, 443
ròu guì 18, 26, 33, 36, 216
Rǔ xiāng 286, 287

S

Sān kē zhēn 96
sān léng 36, 301
sān qī 12, 13, 268, 270
sāng bái pí 331
sāng jì shēng 173
sāng piāo xiāo 446, 447
sāng shèn 419
sāng yè 65, 66
Sāng zhī 168, 170

Shā jí 389
shā rén 12, 186
shā shēn 35
shā yuàn zǐ 398
shān cí gū 116
shān dòu gēn 109
shān yào 12, 18, 385, 386, 416
Shān zhā 246, 248
Shān zhū yú 444
shāng lù 30, 151
shé chuáng zǐ 462
Shè gān 108, 109
Shè xiāng 372, 373
Shēn jīn cǎo 163
shén qū 246, 248
shēng dì huáng 119, 120, 405
shēng jiāng 41, 54, 216
shēng jiāng pí 54, 216
shēng jiāng zhī 54, 216
shēng má 23, 26, 68
Shēng shài shēn 380
Shēng tiě luò 360
Shēng yào 470
shí chāng pú 373, 375
shì dì 240
shí gāo 18, 23, 26, 80, 81
shí hú 414, 415
shí jué míng 26, 355, 356
Shǐ jūn zǐ 255, 257
shí liú pí 449
Shí nán yè 176
shí wéi 201
shǒu wū téng 349, 350
shú dì huáng 34, 405, 406, 408, 409
shuǐ niú jiǎo 123
shuǐ yín 31, 35
shuǐ zhì 301
Sī guā luò 172
sì jì qīng 118
Sōng jié 163
Sōng zǐ rén 148
sū hé xiāng 373
sū mù 297, 299
sū yè 23, 28
sū zǐ 27
Suān zǎo rén 347, 350
suō luó zǐ 237

suǒ yáng 22, 396

T

tài zǐ shēn 381
tán xiāng 231
Táng shēn 380
táo rén 291, 327
tiān dōng 413
tiān huā fěn 30, 35, 83
tiān má 30, 364
tiān nán xīng 313, 314
tián qī 13
Tiān xiān téng 238
Tián xìng rén 327
tiān zhú huáng 321
tíng lì zǐ 331
tōng cǎo 199
Tǔ biē chóng 296, 301
tǔ dà huáng 268
Tǔ fú líng 106
Tǔ jīng pí 465
tù sī zǐ 398

W

wǎ léng zǐ 325
wáng bù liú xíng 294, 303
wèi jiāng 216
Wěi líng cài 114
wēi líng xiān 159
wǔ bèi zǐ 440, 441
wú gōng 41, 366
Wǔ jiā pí 173
wǔ líng zhī 36, 287
wū méi 22, 28, 439, 441
wū shāo shé 161
wǔ wèi zǐ 12, 33, 382, 438, 441
wū yào 232, 234
wú yí 259
wú zhū yú 218, 444

X

xī jiǎo 36, 124
xī xiān cǎo 169
xì xīn 12, 35, 59
xī yáng shēn 380
xià kū cǎo 86, 93
Xià tiān wú 288

Xiān ài yè 276

Xiān dì huáng 405

xiān hè cǎo 272

xiān máo 394

xiāng fù 234

xiāng jiā pí 195, 196

xiāng rú 55

xiāng yuán 235

xiǎo huí xiāng 218, 219

xiǎo jì 263

xiè bái 237, 321

Xié cǎo 349

xīn yí 23, 61

xìng rén 22

xióng dǎn 117, 362

xióng huáng 31, 461, 471

xú cháng qīng 159

xù duàn 395

xuán fù huā 316, 359

xuán míng fěn 146

xuán shēn 35, 120

Xuè jié 298, 299

Xuě lián huā 175

Xuě shàng yī zhī hāo 166

xuè yú tàn 274

Xún gǔ fēng 163

Y

yā dǎn zǐ 113

yá xiāo 36

yā zhí cǎo 85

yán hú suǒ 285, 287

Yáng hóng shān 404

yáng jīn huā 333

Yáng qǐ shí 402

yáng tí 267, 268

yě jú huā 103

Yě shān shēn 380

Yì mǔ cǎo 292

yí táng 389

yì yǐ rén 192, 193

yì zhì rén 397

yín chái hú 126, 127

Yīn chén 204, 205

Yín xìng yè 332

Yín yáng huò 393, 394

yīng sù qiào 440, 441

yǔ bái fù 314

yù jīn 35, 285

yù lǐ rén 147

yù mǐ xū 194, 196

Yú xīng cǎo 106, 107

yǔ yú liáng 443

yù zhú 415

yuán huā 35, 36, 150

yuǎn zhì 27, 350, 375

Yuè jì huā 295

Z

zào jiá 316

zào jiǎo cì 20

zào xīn tǔ 277

zé lán 292

zé qī 196

zé xiè 28, 193

zhāng nǎo 463

zhè bèi mǔ 12, 35, 36, 318

Zhēn zhū 363

Zhēn zhū cǎo 207

zhēn zhū mǔ 356

zhǐ jù zǐ 195, 196

zhī mǔ 18, 30, 81

zhǐ qiào 229

zhǐ shí 33, 229, 230

zhī zǐ 18, 85

zhú lì 54, 320, 321

Zhú lì bàn xià 314

zhū líng 192, 193

zhù má gēn 267

zhú rú 320, 321

zhū shā 27, 344, 346

Zhú yè 84

zhú yè juǎn xīn 85

Zǐ bèi chǐ 357

zǐ cǎo 123

zǐ hé chē 392, 400

zǐ huā dì dīng 103

Zǐ rán tóng 297, 299

Zǐ shí yīng 402

zǐ sū 328

Zǐ sū gěng 54, 328

Zǐ sū yè 54, 328

zǐ sū zǐ 328

zǐ wǎn 329

zǐ zhū 273, 274

Zōng lǘ tàn 273, 274

Index by Chinese Medicinals – Pharmaceutical Names

A

Actinolitum 402
Agkistrodon 161
Aloe 146
Alumen 462
Arillus Longan 410
Arisaema cum Bile 313
Arsenicum 31, 35, 471
Aspongopus 239

B

Bombyx Batryticatus 366
Borax 472
Borneolum Syntheticum 373
Bulbus Allii 465
Bulbus Allii Fistulosi 41, 61, 237
Bulbus Allii Macrostemi 237, 321
Bulbus Fritillariae Cirrhosae 12, 35, 36, 318
Bulbus Fritillariae Thunbergii 12, 35, 36, 318
Bulbus Lilii 412, 415
Bungarus Parvus 162

C

Cacumen Platycladi 266, 267
Cacumen Tamaricis 62
Calamina 472
calcined Os Draconis 357
Calculus Bovis 362, 372
Calomelas 470

Calyx Kaki 240
Calyx seu Fructus Physalis 110
Camphora 463
Carapax et Plastrum Testudinis 420
Carapax Trionycis 420
Catechu 299
Caulis Aristolochiae Manshuriensis 199
Caulis Bambusae in Taenia 320, 321
Caulis Clematidis Armandii 199
Caulis Dendrobii 414, 415
Caulis Erycibes 165
Caulis Lonicerae Japonicae 97
Caulis Perillae 328
Caulis Perillae 54
Caulis Piperis Kadsurae 164, 170
Caulis Polygoni Multiflori 349, 350
Caulis Sargentodoxae 107
Caulis Sinomenii 164
Caulis Spatholobi 294
Caulis Trachelospermi 170
Chalcanthitum 457
Chlorite-schist 326
Cinnabaris 27, 344, 346
Colla Corii Asini 12, 408
Colla Cornus Cervi 391
Concha Arcae 325
Concha Cypraeae Violacae 357
Concha Haliotidis 26, 355, 356
Concha Margaritiferae Usta 356
Concha Meretricis seu Cyclinae 325
Concha Ostreae 356

Concretio Silicea Bambusae 321
Cordyceps 400
Corium Erinacei 449
Cornu Bubali 123
Cornu Cervi 391
Cornu Cervi Pantotrichum 391, 392
Cornu Rhinocerotis 36, 124
Cornu Saigae Tataricae 361, 362, 364
Cortex Acanthopanacis 173
Cortex Ailanthi 94, 449
Cortex Albiziae 350
Cortex Cinnamomi 18, 26, 33, 36, 216
Cortex Dictamni 95
Cortex Erythrinae 170
Cortex Eucommiae 395
Cortex Fraxini 94
Cortex Lycii 125, 127
Cortex Magnoliae Officinalis 184, 230
Cortex Meliae 255, 257
Cortex Mori 331
Cortex Moutan 121, 122, 125
Cortex Periplocae 195, 196
Cortex Phellodendri Chinensis 22, 92
Cortex Pseudolaricis 465
Cortex Zingiberis Officinalis 216
Crinis Carbonisatus 274
Cutis Poriae 191

D

defatted Semen Trichosanthis 319

Dens Draconis 346

E

Endoconcha Sepiae 447

Endothelium Corneum Gigeriae Galli 248, 249

Eupolyphaga seu Steleophaga 296, 301

Exocarpium Benincasae 194, 196

Exocarpium Citri Grandis 227

F

Faeces Bombycis 162

Faeces Trogopterori 36, 287

Flos Buddlejae 88

Flos Campsis 295

Flos Carthami 290, 291

Flos Caryophylli 35, 219, 220

Flos Celosiae Cristatae 450

Flos Chrysanthemi 12, 26, 66

Flos Chrysanthemi Indici 103

Flos Daturae 333

Flos Eriocauli 87

Flos Farfarae 329

Flos Genkwa 35, 36, 150

Flos Inulae 316, 359

Flos Lonicerae Japonicae 97, 99

Flos Loropetali Chinensis 275

Flos Magnoliae 23, 61

Flos Mume 236, 237

Flos Rosae Chinensis 295

Flos Rosae Rugosae 236, 237

Flos Sophorae 265

Fluoritum 402

Folium Apocyni Veneti 360

Folium Artemisiae Argyi 30, 275, 276, 277

Folium Callicarpae Formosanae 273, 274

Folium Citri Reticulatae 227

Folium Clerodendri 169

Folium Eriobotryae 330

Folium Ginkgo 332

Folium Illics Purpureae 118

Folium Isatidis 100, 101

Folium Mori 65, 66

Folium Nelumbinis 41, 448

Folium Perillae 23, 28, 54

Folium Perillae 328

Folium Photiniae 176

Folium Phyllostachydis Henonis 84

Folium Pyrrosiae 201

Folium Rhododendri Daurici 335

Folium Sennae 146

fresh Folium Artemisiae Argyi 276

Fructus Alpiniae Oxyphyllae 397

Fructus Amomi 12, 186

Fructus Amomi Kravanh 186, 443

Fructus Anisi Stellati 219

Fructus Arctii 64

Fructus Aristolochiae 330

Fructus Aurantii 229

Fructus Aurantii Immaturus 33, 229, 230

Fructus Broussonetiae 410

Fructus Bruceae 113

Fructus Canarii 110

Fructus Cannabis 147

Fructus Carpesii 258, 259

Fructus Caryophylli 220

Fructus Chaenomelis 162

Fructus Chebulae 441, 442

Fructus Citri 235

Fructus Citri Sarcodactylis 235

Fructus Cnidii 462

Fructus Corni 444

Fructus Crataegi 246, 248

Fructus Evodiae 218, 444

Fructus Foeniculi 218, 219

Fructus Forsythiae 98, 99

Fructus Gardeniae 18, 85

Fructus Gleditsiae 316

Fructus Hippophae 389

Fructus Hordei Germinatus 247, 248

Fructus Jujubae 22, 41, 387, 389

Fructus Kochiae 201

Fructus Lagenariae 195, 196

Fructus Ligustri Lucidi 418

Fructus Liquidambaris 166

Fructus Litseae 222

Fructus Lycii 12, 417, 418, 419

Fructus Malvae 202

Fructus Momordicae 334

Fructus Mori 419

Fructus Mume 22, 28, 439, 441

Fructus Oryzae Germinatus 247, 248

Fructus Perillae 27

Fructus Perillae 328

Fructus Piperis 221

Fructus Piperis Longi 222

Fructus Psoraleae 397

Fructus Quisqualis 255, 257

Fructus Retinervus Luffae 172

Fructus Rosae Laevigatae 446, 449

Fructus Rubi 445, 446

Fructus Schisandrae Chinensis 12, 33, 382, 438, 441

Fructus Setariae Germinatus 247, 248

Fructus Sophorae 265

Fructus Toosendan 232, 233

Fructus Tribuli 359

Fructus Trichosanthis 30, 35, 319, 321

Fructus Tritici Levis 437

Fructus Tsaoko 187

Fructus Ulmi Macrocarpae Praeparata 259

Fructus Viticis 67

Fructus Xanthii 60, 61

Frusta Ferri 360

G

Galla Chinensis 440, 441

Ganoderma 348

Gecko 28, 399, 400

Glauberitum 82

Gryllotalpa 197

Gypsum Fibrosum 18, 23, 26, 80, 81

Gypsum Fibrosum Praeparatum 471

H

Haematitum 26, 358, 359

Halloysitum Rubrum 36, 443

Herba Abri 206

Herba Agastachis 183

Herba Agrimoniae 272

Herba Andrographis 99

Herba Ardisiae Japonicae 333

Herba Aristolochiae 238

Herba Aristolochiae Mollissimae

163

Herba Artemisiae Annuae 124, 125

Herba Artemisiae Anomalae 299

Herba Artemisiae Scopariae 204, 205

Herba Capsellae 197

Herba Centipedae 62

Herba Cirsii 263

Herba Cistanches 23, 396

Herba Commelinae 85

Herba Coriandri Sativi 62

Herba Cynomorii 22, 396

Herba Dianthi 200, 201

Herba Ecliptae 418

Herba Ephedrae 22, 26, 27, 28, 36,
    52, 53, 55, 70, 436

Herba Epimedii 393, 394

Herba Equiseti Hiemalis 71

Herba Erodii 171

Herba et Gemma Agrimoniae 257,
    260

Herba Eupatorii 183

Herba Euphorbiae Humifusae 114

Herba Euphoribiae Helioscopiae 196

Herba Hedyotis Diffusae 115

Herba Houttuyniae 106, 107

Herba Hyperici Japonici 205

Herba Leonuri 292

Herba Lobeliae Chinensis 115

Herba Lophatheri 84

Herba Lycopi 292

Herba Lycopodii 163

Herba Lysimachiae 204, 205

Herba Menthae 12, 23, 26, 28, 63, 64

Herba Moslae 55

Herba Paederiae 250

Herba Patriniae 107

Herba Phyllanthi Urinariae 207

Herba Plantaginis 199

Herba Polygoni Avicularis 200, 201

Herba Portulacae 112, 113

Herba Potentillae Chinensis 114

Herba Potentillae Discoloris 115

Herba Pyrolae 175

Herba Saussureae Lanicepsis 175

Herba Schizonepetae 56, 57

Herba Sedi 205

Herba Sedi Aizoon 268

Herba Senecionis Scandentis 117

Herba seu Radix Cirsii Japonici 263

Herba Siegesbeckiae 169

Herba Spirodelae 70

Herba Taraxaci 102, 103

Herba Taxilli 173

Herba Violae 103

Hippocampus 403

Hirudo 301

Hydrargyrum 31, 35

Hydrargyrum Oxydatum Crudum
    470

I

Indigo Naturalis 101

K

Korean Ginseng 380

L

Lasiosphaera seu Calvatia 109

Lignum Aquilariae Resinatum 231

Lignum Dalbergiae Odoriferae 270

Lignum Pini Nodi 163

Lignum Santali Albi 231

Lignum Sappan 297, 299

Limonitum 443

Lithargyrum 35

M

Magnetitum 20, 345, 346, 358

Margarita 363

Massa Medicata Fermentata 246, 248

Medulla Junci 203

Medulla Tetrapanacis 199

Mel 390

Minium 472

Mirabilitum 35, 36, 146

Moschus 372, 373

Mylabris 302

Myrrha 287

N

Natrii Sulfas 26, 145, 146

Natrii Sulfas Exsiccatus 146

Nidus Vespae 465

Nodus Nelumbinis Rhizomatis 274

O

Olibanum 286, 287

Omphalia 257

Ootheca Mantidis 446, 447

Ophicalcitum 270

Os Draconis 345, 346, 356

Oviductus Ranae 403

P

Pedicellus Melo 457

Pericarpium Arecae 238

Pericarpium Citri Reticulatae 12, 28,
    227

Pericarpium Citri Reticulatae Viride
    227

Pericarpium Granati 449

Pericarpium Papaveris 440, 441

Pericarpium Trichosanthis 319

Pericarpium Zanthoxyli 221

Periostracum Cicadae 64

Petiolus Nelmbinis 448

Petiolus Trachycarpi 273, 274

Pheretima 365, 366

Placenta Hominis 392, 400

Plumula Nelumbinis 447

Pollen Typhae 270

Polyporus 192, 193

Poria 12, 191, 193

Poria Rubra 193

Pseudobulbus Cremastrae seu Pleiones
    116

Pumex 325

Pyritum 297, 299

R

Radix Achyranthis Bidentatae 12,
    293

Radix Aconiti 12, 30, 35, 36, 160, 214

Radix Aconiti Brachypodi 166

Radix Aconiti Coreani 314

Radix Aconiti Kusnezoffii 30, 35, 36,
    160, 214

Radix Aconiti Lateralis Praeparata
    12, 18, 23, 30, 34, 35, 214, 215, 216,
    382, 390

Radix Adenophorae 411

Radix Ampelopsis 35, 118

Radix Angelicae Dahuricae 58, 59

Radix Angelicae Pubescentis 158, 159

Radix Angelicae Sinensis 12, 23, 34, 404, 406

Radix Aristolochiae 233

Radix Arnebiae 123

Radix Asparagi 413

Radix Astragali 12, 22, 23, 26, 34, 383, 384

Radix Aucklandiae 230, 233, 234

Radix Berberidis 96

Radix Boehmeriae 267

Radix Bupleuri 26, 33, 67, 68

Radix Changii 417

Radix Cocculi Trilobi 168

Radix Codonopsis 12, 18, 22, 28, 381, 384

Radix Curcumae 35, 285

Radix Cyathulae 293

Radix Cynanchi Wilfordii 250

Radix Dichroae 29, 457

Radix Dipsaci 395

Radix et Rhizoma Asari 12, 35, 59

Radix et Rhizoma Asteris 329

Radix et Rhizoma Clematidis 159

Radix et Rhizoma Cynanchi Atrati 125

Radix et Rhizoma Cynanchi Paniculati 159

Radix et Rhizoma Ephedrae 436, 437

Radix et Rhizoma Gentianae 93

Radix et Rhizoma Ginseng 12, 13, 30, 35, 36, 379, 380, 381, 383

Radix et Rhizoma Ginseng Indici 380

Radix et Rhizoma Ginseng Rubra 380

Radix et Rhizoma Glycyrrhizae 18, 30, 35, 36, 387, 390

Radix et Rhizoma Nardostachyos 239

Radix et Rhizoma Notoginseng 12, 13, 268, 270

Radix et Rhizoma Rhei 12, 26, 144, 204, 268, 390

Radix et Rhizoma Rhodiolae Crenulatae 388

Radix et Rhizoma Rubiae 269, 270

Radix et Rhizoma Salviae Miltiorrhizae 35, 289

Radix et Rhizoma seu Caulis Acanthopanacis Senticosi 388

Radix et Rhizoma Sophorae Tonkinensis 109

Radix et Rhizoma Thalictri Baicalensis 97

Radix et Rhizoma Veratri Nigri 35

Radix Euphorbiae Fischerianae 35

Radix Euphorbiae Pekinensis 35, 36, 149, 150

Radix Gentianae Macrophyllae 167

Radix Glehniae 35, 411, 416

Radix Gynura 268

Radix Isatidis 100, 101

Radix Kansui 30, 35, 36, 149, 150

Radix Knoxiae 149

Radix Linderae 232, 234

Radix Morindae Officinalis 393, 394

Radix Ophiopogonis 382, 413, 416

Radix Oryzae Glutinosae 437

Radix Paeoniae Alba 27, 33, 35, 390, 406, 407

Radix Paeoniae Rubra 35, 122, 407

Radix Panacis Quinquefolii 380

Radix Peucedani 321

Radix Physochlainae 30, 334

Radix Phytolaccae 30, 151

Radix Platycodonis 27, 28, 322, 323

Radix Polygalae 27, 350, 375

Radix Polygoni Multiflori 409

Radix Pseudostellariae 381

Radix Puerariae Lobatae 20, 23, 68

Radix Pulsatillae 112, 113

Radix Ranunculi Ternati 317

Radix Rehmanniae 12, 119, 120, 405, 406

Radix Rehmanniae Praeparata 34, 405, 406, 408, 409

Radix Rehmanniae Recens 405

Radix Rhapontici 105, 116

Radix Rumicis Japonici 267, 268

Radix Sanguisorbae 264, 265

Radix Saposhnikoviae 57, 168

Radix Scrophulariae 35, 120

Radix Scutellariae 28, 33, 90, 267

Radix Seu Herba Pimpinelae 404

Radix Sophorae Flavescentis 95

Radix Stellariae 126, 127

Radix Stemonae 329

Radix Stephaniae Tetrandrae 167, 168

Radix Stephaniae Tetrandrae 168

Radix Tinosporae 111

Radix Trichosanthis 30, 35, 83

Radix Tripterygii Wilfordii 171

Radix Tripterygium Hypoglaucum 165

Ramulus Cinnamomi 19, 23, 33, 53

Ramulus Mori 168, 170

Ramulus Uncariae Cum Uncis 27, 363, 364

Realgar 31, 461, 471

Receptaculum Nelumbinis 447

Resina Ferulae 251

Resina Liquidambaris 288

Rhizoma Acori Tatarinowii 373, 375

Rhizoma Alismatis 28, 193

Rhizoma Alpiniae Officinarum 220

Rhizoma Anemarrhenae 18, 30, 81

Rhizoma Arisaematis 313, 314

Rhizoma Atractylodis 12, 184, 384

Rhizoma Atractylodis Macrocephalae 33, 384, 385, 386

Rhizoma Belamcandae 108, 109

Rhizoma Bistortae 104

Rhizoma Bletillae 35, 272

Rhizoma Chuanxiong 11, 12, 13, 284, 287, 289

Rhizoma Cibotii 173, 297

Rhizoma Cimicifugae 23, 26, 68

Rhizoma Coptidis 11, 12, 22, 26, 33, 91, 321

Rhizoma Corydalis 285, 287

Rhizoma Curculiginis 394

Rhizoma Curcumae 300, 301

Rhizoma Curcumae Longae 285

Rhizoma Cyperi 234

Rhizoma Cyrtomii 102, 257

Rhizoma Dioscoreae 12, 18, 385, 386, 416

Rhizoma Dioscoreae Bulbiferae 324

Rhizoma Dioscoreae Hypoglaucae 203

Rhizoma Dioscoreae Nipponicae 172

Rhizoma Drynariae 297

Rhizoma et Radix Cynanchi Stauntonii 317, 321

Rhizoma et Radix Notopterygii 28, 58, 59, 158

Rhizoma et Radix Valerianae Pseudoofficinalis 349

Rhizoma Fagopyri Dibotryis 107

Rhizoma Gastrodiae 30, 364

Rhizoma Homalomenae 174

Rhizoma Imperatae 266, 267

Rhizoma Ligustici 59

Rhizoma Menispermi 109

Rhizoma Paridis 104

Rhizoma Phragmitis 41, 82, 83, 266

Rhizoma Picrorhizae 127

Rhizoma Pinelliae 35, 312, 314, 321

Rhizoma Pinelliae Fermentatum 314

Rhizoma Polygonati 36, 415, 416

Rhizoma Polygonati Odorati 415

Rhizoma Polygoni Cuspidati 204, 205

Rhizoma seu Herba Gynostemmatis Pentaphylli 388

Rhizoma Smilacis Glabrae 106

Rhizoma Sparganii 36, 301

Rhizoma Typhonii 30, 314

Rhizoma Zingiberis 18, 28, 33, 215, 216, 220

Rhizoma Zingiberis Praeparatum 276

Rhizoma Zingiberis Recens 41, 54, 216

roasted Rhizoma Zingiberis 216

S

Saccharum Granorum 389

Sanguis Draconis 298, 299

Sargassum 35, 323, 324

Sclerotium Poriae Pararadicis 192, 194

Scolopendra 41, 366

Scorpio 365, 366

Semen Aesculi 237

Semen Allii Tuberosi 401

Semen Alpiniae Katsumadai 187

Semen Arecae 256, 257

Semen Armeniacae Amarum 22, 327, 328

Semen Armeniacae Dulce 327

Semen Astragali Complanati 398

Semen Canavaliae 239, 240

Semen Cassiae 355

Semen Cassiae 87, 355

Semen Celosiae 88

Semen Citri Reticulatae 227

Semen Coicis 192, 193

Semen Crotonis 35, 36, 152

Semen Cucurbitae 256, 259

Semen Cuscutae 398

Semen Euphorbiae 152

Semen Euryales 448

Semen Ginkgo 332, 333

Semen Hoveniae 195, 196

Semen Juglandis 400

Semen Lablab Album 386

Semen Lepidii 331

Semen Litchi 233

Semen Momordicae 464

Semen Myristicae 442, 443

Semen Nelumbinis 447, 448

Semen Oroxyli 111

Semen Persicae 291, 327

Semen Pharbitidis 35, 36, 151

Semen Phaseoli Radiati 119

Semen Pini Koraiensis 148

Semen Platycladi 348, 350

Semen Pruni 147

Semen Raphani 248

Semen Sesami Nigrum 419

Semen Sinapis 315, 316

Semen Sojae Germinatus 69

Semen Sojae Praeparatum 69

Semen Sterculiae Lychnophorae 323

Semen Strychni 30, 296

Semen Torreyae 259

Semen Trichosanthis 319

Semen Trigonellae 401

Semen Vaccariae 294, 303

Semen Ziziphi Spinosae 347, 350

Sophora Alopecuroides 96

Spica Prunellae 86, 93

Spina Gleditsiae 20

Spora Lygodii 201

Squama Manitis 303

Stamen Nelumbinis 447

Stigma Croci 291

Stigma Maydis 194, 196

Styrax 373

Succinum 346

Succus Bambusae 54, 320, 321

Succus Rhizomatis Zingiberis 54, 216

Sugared Ginseng 380

Sulphur 35, 461

Sun-dried Ginseng 380

T

Tabanus 301

Talcum 198

Terra Flava Usta 277

Testes et Penis Callorhini 402, 403

Testes et Penis Canis 403

Thallus Laminariae 324

Thorny Elaeagnus Leaf 335

U

Ursi Fel 117, 362

V

Vascular Aurantii 227

Venenum Bufonis 463

Z

Zaocys 161

图书在版编目（CIP）数据

中药学图表解（英文）/ 钟赣生主编．—北京：人民
卫生出版社，2009. 2
（中医基础学科图表解丛书）
ISBN 978-7-117-10640-5

Ⅰ．中…　Ⅱ．钟…　Ⅲ．中药学—中医学院—教学参
考资料—英文　Ⅳ．R28

中国版本图书馆 CIP 数据核字（2008）第 144847 号

中药学图表解（英文）

主　　编：钟赣生
出版发行：人民卫生出版社（中继线 +8610-6761-6688）
地　　址：中国北京市丰台区方庄芳群园三区 3 号楼
邮　　编：100078
网　　址：http://www.pmph.com
E - mail：pmph @ pmph.com
发　　行：pmphsales @ pmph.com
购书热线：+8610-6769-1034（电话及传真）
开　　本：889×1194　1/16
版　　次：2009 年 2 月第 1 版　2009 年 2 月第 1 版第 1 次印刷
标准书号：ISBN 978-7-117-10640-5/R・10641

版权所有，侵权必究，打击盗版举报电话：**+8610-8761-3394**
（凡属印装质量问题请与本社销售部联系退换）